DHHS: Department of Health and Human Services

DIA: Department of Industrial Accidents

DME: durable medical equipment

DMERC: durable medical equipment regional carrier/contractor

DN: discrepancy notice

DNFB: discharged—not final billed (balance)

DNS: did not show

DOB: date of birth

DOI: date of injury; Department of Insurance

DOS: date of service

DRGs: diagnosis-related groups

DSM-IV-TR: *Diagnostic and Statistical Manual of Mental Disorders, Fourth Edition, Text Revision*

DX: diagnosis

E & M codes, E/M codes: evaluation and management codes

ECF: extended care facility

ECP: electronic claims processor

ED: emergency department

EDI: electronic data interchange

EHR: electronic health record

EIN: employer identification number

ELOS: estimated length of stay

EMC: electronic media claims

EMG: emergency

EMR: electronic medical record

EMS: emergency medical services

EOB: explanation of benefits

EOC: episode of care; evidence of coverage; explanation of coverage

EOM: end of month

EOY: end of year

EPF: expanded problem focused

EPO: exclusive provider organization

EPSDT: Early and Periodic Screening, Diagnosis, and Treatment (program)

ERA: electronic remittance advice

ERISA: Employee Retirement Income Security Act

ERM: electronic records management

ESRD: end-stage renal disease

EVC: eligibility verification confirmation

Ex: examination

F & A: findings and award

FA: fiscal agent

FCA: False Claims Act

FCRA: Fair Credit Reporting Act

FCS: Facility Coding Specialist

FECA: Federal Employees' Compensation Act

FEHBP: Federal E_____ _____ _____ ts Pr_

FE_

FE_

FFS:

FH:

FI: fis_

FICA: _____al Insurance Contributions Act

FL: form locator

FMC: foundation for medical care

FMLA: Family and Medical Leave Act of 1993

FP: family practitioner

FY: fiscal year

GAF: geographic adjustment factor

GP: general practitioner

GPCI: Geographic Practice Cost Indices

GSP: global surgery policy

H & P: history and physical

HBA: health benefits advisor

HCF: health care finder

HCPCS: Healthcare Common Procedure Coding System

HEDIS: Health Plan Employer Data and Information Set

HFSA: health care flexible spending account

HHC: home health care

HICN: health insurance claim number

HIM: health information management

HIPAA: Health Insurance Portability and Accountability Act of 1996

HL7: Health Level Seven

HMO: health maintenance organization

HPI: history of present illness

HPSA: health professional shortage area

HSA: health service agreement; health systems agency; health savings account

ICD-9-CM: *International Classification of Diseases, Ninth Revision, Clinical Modification*

ICD-10-CM: *International Classification of Diseases, Tenth Revision, Clinical Modification*

ICD-10-PCS: *International Classification of Diseases, Tenth Revision, Procedural Coding System*

ICU: intensive care unit

ID card: identification card

IME: independent medical evaluation; independent medical evaluator; independent medical examiner

IP: inpatient

IPA: independent (or individual) practice association

IPPE: initial preventive physical examination

continued on inside back cover

FORDNEY'S
MEDICAL INSURANCE
DICTIONARY
for Billers and Coders

BAKER COLLEGE OF
CLINTON TWP. LIBRARY

MARILYN TAKAHASHI FORDNEY, CMA-AC (AAMA)
Formerly Instructor of Medical Insurance, Medical
Terminology, Medical Machine Transcription,
and Medical Office Procedures
Ventura College
Ventura, California

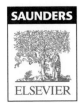

SAUNDERS

ELSEVIER

SAUNDERS
ELSEVIER

11830 Westline Industrial Drive
St. Louis, Missouri 63146

FORDNEY'S MEDICAL INSURANCE DICTIONARY   ISBN: 978-1-4377-0026-8
FOR BILLERS AND CODERS
Copyright © 2010 by Saunders, an imprint of Elsevier Inc.

Notice

Neither the Publisher nor the Author assumes any responsibility for any loss or
injury and/or damage to persons or property arising out of or related to any use of
the material contained in this book. It is the responsibility of the treating practitioner,
relying on independent expertise and knowledge of the patient, to determine the best
treatment and method of application for the patient.

The Publisher

Library of Congress Cataloging-in-Publication Data

Fordney, Marilyn Takahashi.
  Fordney's medical insurance dictionary for billers and coders / Marilyn Takahashi
Fordney.
    p.; cm.
  ISBN 978-1-4377-0026-8 (pbk.: alk. paper)
1. Health insurance claims–Dictionaries. 2. Medical fees–Dictionaries. I. Title.
II. Title: Medical insurance dictionary for billers and coders.
  [DNLM: 1. Insurance, Health, Reimbursement–United States–Dictionary–
English. 2. Forms and Records Control–United States–Dictionary–English.
3. Insurance Claim Reporting–United States–Dictionary–English.
W 13 F712f 2010]
  HG9386.F67 2010
  368.38'2003–dc22   2009004374

Executive Editor: Susan Cole
Associate Developmental Editor: Melissa Gladback
Editorial Assistant: Elizabeth Fergus
Publishing Services Manager: Patricia Tannian
Senior Project Manager: Kristine Feeherty
Design Direction: Kimberly Denando

Printed in the United States of America

Last digit is the print number: 9 8 7 6 5 4 3 2 1

Working together to grow
libraries in developing countries

www.elsevier.com | www.bookaid.org | www.sabre.org

ELSEVIER   BOOK AID International   Sabre Foundation

With love, respect, and gratitude, I dedicate this first edition to my husband, Sándor Havasi, a linguist who enjoys words and has an intellectual curiosity for names from many cultures.

In 1975 when I began writing *Insurance Handbook for the Medical Office*, I looked for a dictionary that contained health insurance words, phrases, acronyms, and abbreviations. Over 30 years later, I still cannot find one that meets my needs. I also discovered that when I researched a word, I had to go to various websites to obtain the information. There is not a single location that has everything.

Throughout the years as I wrote and updated my textbooks to new editions, I accumulated numerous words and in many instances developed the definitions from scratch. As the fields of health insurance, billing, and procedural and diagnostic coding have evolved, they have become more complex and the changes continue to come more rapidly than in prior decades. I also noticed that whenever I attended workshops and seminars on these subjects, the speakers would use abbreviations as a convenience. Many attendees would look puzzled and raise a hand to ask for the expanded definition of the abbreviation; some would be too shy to ask. In this dictionary, I have tried to include the terms most likely to confront those involved with medical insurance, billing, and coding issues.

An additional problem is that a U.S. president is elected every four years and the political party in power makes changes to policies, procedures, and terminology. For example, many words in federal programs are changed or updated to newer titles. This is somewhat confusing and problematic when you read an article and think you have come across a new term but in actuality it is a new name for an already existing health insurance word. The multiple large corporate takeovers have also made it difficult to keep track of the names of various professional organizations. This pocket dictionary addresses these problems by indicating if a word or professional organization was formerly known by another name.

One of the major difficulties in health insurance is trying to understand the technical jargon. I have attempted to break this down in layman's terms so the definitions are concise and can be easily understood, but in a few instances some explanations are longer than the technical version.

This comprehensive pocket reference book is a compilation of terms that provides a key source of information for instructors, novice students, and long-time practitioners in the field of medical insurance, billing, and coding. It is also useful for consumers because many tend not to read their insurance policies and those who do read them do not know the meaning of various terms, clauses, and phrases. This reference is also helpful to business owners who need a good reference to assist them when making an insurance purchase decision. Insurance agents may find the dictionary a necessity when marketing and servicing health insurance products or answering questions from clients.

In this reference book, you will find words related to private care, managed care, federal health insurance programs, HIPAA compliance and security, diagnostic and procedural coding, credit and collection, ethics and legality, Internet jargon, informal expressions, electronic claims processing, professional organizations and associations, and federal legislative acts. This reference will assist you with spelling of abbreviations and words. Where needed, figures, tables, and boxes are included to visually clarify the definition of words and phrases.

Experts who perform medical insurance billing and coding reviewed all entries. This extensive review process resulted in the refinement of more than 7,500 definitions that reflect current knowledge and practice. The user will find valuable tips related to billing and coding for some of the definitions.

All abbreviations are cross referenced so you can locate their meaning as well as their translation. A list of abbreviations commonly used in health care appears on the inside front and back covers of this book.

Marilyn Takahashi Fordney

ACKNOWLEDGMENTS

I am thankful to many individuals on the staff at Elsevier for guidance and support in getting this project to its fruition. I express particular appreciation to Susan Cole, executive editor; Melissa Gladback and Elizabeth Fergus, associate developmental editors; and Kristine Feeherty, project manager, for coordination of this project. I gratefully acknowledge the work of Kimberly Denando, Art and Design, for the design of this first edition.

I wish to express gratitude to the principal reviewers who provided additional information about some of the entries and inserted corrections and comments. I take pride in listing my principal reviewers for this first edition:

Yaladie Cosme Rodriguez, CPC, AAPC
HCIM Instructor
New Horizons Learning Center
Las Marias, Puerto Rico

Tiffany Sorenson, RMA
Instructor
Certified Careers Institute
Salt Lake City, Utah

Cynthia Stahl, CPC, CCS-P, CPC-H
Lead Instructor, Medical Billing and Coding
MedTech College
Indianapolis, Indiana

Alphabetical Order

All entries (words, phrases, abbreviations, and acronyms) are in alphabetical order, are bold faced, and have cross-references where needed. Abbreviations and acronyms are cross-referenced to locate the full definition.

Abbreviations

Most abbreviations are shown preferably without punctuation and appear either capitalized or in lower case depending on what is most commonly seen in the literature. They may have numerous meanings in addition to what is stated in this dictionary because most clinical meanings are not shown.

Cross-References

Where an entry is fully defined by another term, a reference instead of a definition is provided— for example: **AAPC** See *American Academy of Professional Coders (AAPC)*. By following cross-references, you can quickly locate entries that may be closely associated with the word you look up, so always take the time to go to the cross-referenced word or words.

Italics

Italic type is used to highlight cross-references, for titles of publications, and for words or phrases that have a special meaning.

Parentheses

Parentheses are used to show when an acronym or an abbreviation is commonly used.

Meaning

The most common meaning has been provided for most words. Frequently, the same word will have several similar but slightly different meanings. If a word has more than one commonly accepted meaning, a number precedes the additional definitions.

Spelling

This dictionary assists with spelling and optional spelling of words.

Organization and Associations

Those that retain an active role in the field of medical insurance billing and coding are included in the dictionary, along with a brief statement of their purpose. They are also listed by abbreviations and acronyms. Appendix 2 contains a quick reference to various professional associations for billers and coders.

Figures, Tables, and Boxes

Figures, tables, and boxes are shown to help the reader gain understanding, to visually clarify the definition of words and phrases, and to help relate abstract concepts to the real world of insurance and billing. Appendix 1 contains a compilation of anatomical illustrations, surgical words, fracture terminology, and body planes for quick reference.

CONTENTS

Preface, *p. vi*

Alphabetical Listing of Terms, *pp. 1-327*

Appendix 1: **Anatomical Illustrations for Coders,** *p. 328*
Appendix 2: **Professional Associations,** *p. 351*

Credits, *p. 354*

A

A "Tier" See *Tier, A.*

A1 HCPCS Level II modifier that may be used with CPT or HCPCS Level II codes indicating dressing for one wound. Use of this modifier affects Medicare payment.

A2 HCPCS Level II modifier that may be used with CPT or HCPCS Level II codes indicating dressing for two wounds. Use of this modifier affects Medicare payment.

A3 HCPCS Level II modifier that may be used with CPT or HCPCS Level II codes indicating dressing for three wounds. Use of this modifier affects Medicare payment.

A4 HCPCS Level II modifier that may be used with CPT or HCPCS Level II codes indicating dressing for four wounds. Use of this modifier affects Medicare payment.

A5 HCPCS Level II modifier that may be used with CPT or HCPCS Level II codes indicating dressing for five wounds. Use of this modifier affects Medicare payment.

A6 HCPCS Level II modifier that may be used with CPT or HCPCS Level II codes indicating dressing for six wounds. Use of this modifier affects Medicare payment.

A7 HCPCS Level II modifier that may be used with CPT or HCPCS Level II codes indicating dressing for seven wounds. Use of this modifier affects Medicare payment.

A8 HCPCS Level II modifier that may be used with CPT or HCPCS Level II codes indicating dressing for eight wounds. Use of this modifier affects Medicare payment.

A9 HCPCS Level II modifier that may be used with CPT or HCPCS Level II codes indicating dressing for nine or more wounds. Use of this modifier affects Medicare payment.

AA HCPCS Level II modifier that may be used with CPT or HCPCS Level II codes indicating anesthesia performed by anesthetist. Use of this modifier affects Medicare payment.

AAA See *Area Agency on Aging (AAA).*

AAAASF See *American Association for Accreditation of Ambulatory Surgery Facilities, Inc. (AAAASF).*

AAAHC See *Accreditation Association for Ambulatory Healthcare (AAAHC).*

AAFP See *American Academy of Family Physicians (AAFP).*

AAHomecare See *American Association for Homecare (AAHomecare).*

AAHP See *American Association of Health Plans (AAHP).*

AAMA See *American Association of Medical Assistants (AAMA).*

AAOS See *American Academy of Orthopaedic Surgeons (AAOS).*

AAPA See *American Academy of Physician Assistants (AAPA).*

AAPC See *American Academy of Professional Coders (AAPC).*

AAPCC See *adjusted average per capita cost (AAPCC).*

AAPPO See *American Association of Preferred Provider Organizations (AAPPO).*

AARP See *American Association of Retired People (AARP).*

AB See *Aid to the Blind (AB).*

abandonment 1. To intentionally relinquish rights or claim to property with no intention of possession in the future. 2. To discontinue medical care by a provider without proper notice after accepting a patient.

ABC codes See *alternative billing codes (ABCs).*

ABCs See *alternative billing codes (ABCs).*

ABD See *adverse benefit determination (ABD).*

aberrancy Medical services that differ from what is considered usual or normal when compared with the national average.

A/B jurisdictions Fifteen regions in the United States assigned to Medicare Administrative Contractors (MACs) for receiving and processing insurance claims for Medicare Parts A and B. See Figure A-1.

ABMT See *autologous bone marrow transplant (ABMT).*

ABN See *Advance Beneficiary Notice (ABN).*

ABN-G See *Advance Beneficiary Notice (ABN).*

ABN-L See *Advance Beneficiary Notice (ABN).*

absolute assignment Permanent transfer of ownership of a life insurance policy from one individual to another. See also *assignment.*

absolute bankruptcy See *straight petition in bankruptcy.*

abstract 1. To select information from a patient's medical record looking at hard copy or via electronic equipment for statistical purposes or for submission of an insurance claim for reimbursement. 2. Report prepared by the patient's attending physician at the conclusion of a patient's hospital stay that summarizes the diagnosis, treatment, and results and outlines any further treatment after discharge. This is known as a *discharge summary.* 3. See *case summary card.*

abstractor Individual who selects and extracts information from a patient's medical record electronically from computer files or manually from paper files. Coded diagnoses may be used to track morbidity and

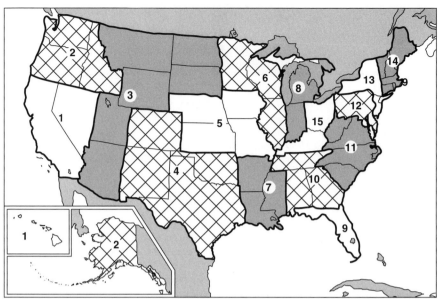

Figure A-1 Medicare Parts A/B Jurisdictions of Medicare Administrative Contractors (MACs). *Jurisdiction 1:* American Samoa, California, Guam, Hawaii, Nevada, and Northern Mariana Islands. *Jurisdiction 2:* Alaska, Idaho, Oregon, and Washington. *Jurisdiction 3:* Arizona, Montana, North Dakota, South Dakota, Utah, and Wyoming. *Jurisdiction 4:* Colorado, New Mexico, Oklahoma, and Texas. *Jurisdiction 5:* Iowa, Kansas, Missouri, and Nebraska. *Jurisdiction 6:* Illinois, Minnesota, and Wisconsin. *Jurisdiction 7:* Arkansas, Louisiana, and Mississippi. *Jurisdiction 8:* Indiana and Michigan. *Jurisdiction 9:* Florida, Puerto Rico, and U.S. Virgin Islands. *Jurisdiction 10:* Alabama, Georgia, and Tennessee. *Jurisdiction 11:* North Carolina, South Carolina, Virginia, and West Virginia. *Jurisdiction 12:* Delaware, District of Columbia, Maryland, New Jersey, and Pennsylvania. *Jurisdiction 13:* Connecticut and New York. *Jurisdiction 14:* Maine, Massachusetts, New Hampshire, Rhode Island, and Vermont. *Jurisdiction 15:* Kentucky and Ohio.

mortality, infectious disease, and index disease information for the purpose of quality of care and utilization review in a facility. Another purpose is that extracted data may be used for submission of insurance claims.

abuse Under the Medicare program, incidents or practices, not usually considered fraudulent, that are inconsistent with accepted sound medical business or fiscal practices (e.g., billing for noncovered services, excessive charges, improper billing practices, billing Medicare beneficiaries at a higher rate than other patients, submitting bills to Medicare instead of to third-party payers that are primary, billing for medically unnecessary services, violating the Medicare participation agreements, coding at a higher level of service than was actually provided, overusing medical services).

abuse, personal When another person intentionally causes another individual mental or physical harm or pain.

AC See *affiliated contractor (AC)*.

ACAAI See *American College of Allergy, Asthma and Immunology (ACAAI)*.

Academy of Managed Care Pharmacy (AMCP) National professional society dedicated to the concept and practice of pharmaceutical care in managed health care environments. AMCP's mission is to promote the development and application of pharmaceutical care in order to ensure appropriate health care outcomes for all individuals. Its sole purpose is to represent the views and interest of managed care pharmacy.

accelerated benefits Life insurance policy rider that allows the insured, under certain circumstances, to receive the proceeds of a life insurance policy before he or she dies, such as terminal or catastrophic illness, need for long-term care, or confinement to a nursing home. Also called *living benefits*.

accelerated payment Temporary partial advanced monies to medical providers because of delays in payments of insurance claims.

acceptability Individual's or group's overall assessment of medical care available to him or her. The individual appraises such things as the cost, quality, results, and convenience of medical care, as well as provider attitudes in determining the acceptability of health services provided. See also *access* and *availability*.

acceptance Insured's decision to enter into an insurance contract at the terms offered by the insurance company.

accepting assignment 1. Under Medicare Part B, an agreement in which a Medicare participating physician agrees to accept 80% of the approved charge from the fiscal intermediary and 20% of the approved charge from the patient, after the patient's deductible has been met. 2. Transfer of the legal interest in an insurance policy to another individual, usually when property is sold; or in life insurance only valid with consent of the insurance company. 3. Transfer of an individual's right to collect an amount payable under an insurance contract.

access Refers to an individual's ability to obtain needed medical care such as location of facilities, transportation, hours of operation, cost of care, availability of medical services, and acceptability of services to the patient.

access fee Per member per month (PMPM) amount of money paid by a health insurer to a network to use that network's providers.

accessibility of services Ability to obtain medical care and services when a patient is in need of them.

accessory dwelling unit (ADU) Separate housing arrangement within single-family home. The ADU is a complete living unit and includes a private kitchen and bath.

accident An unexpected, unforeseen happening causing injury traceable to a definite time and place.

accident and health insurance Insurance for accidental injury or accidental death that includes benefits payable in case of disease.

accident insurance Health insurance that insures an individual if he or she suffers a loss due to accidental bodily injury. Insurance benefits can replace part of earned income lost through disability caused by the accidental injury. Accident insurance also may pay for medical expenses and indemnity for death or loss of limbs or sight from an accident.

accident perils Insurance grouping used by health insurance underwriters to assess the type and degree of danger represented by a specific occupation such as exposure to fire, use of dangerous machinery, handling of heavy objects, and the risk of falling.

accidental bodily injury Unintended, unexpected, and unforeseeable cause of a physical injury sustained as the result of an accident.

accidental death and dismemberment (AD&D) Insurance policy provision that protects the insured if he or she suffers loss of sight or loss of limb(s) or death by accident. This is a supplementary benefit rider or endorsement that provides for an amount of money in addition to the basic death benefit of a life insurance policy. Some AD&D riders pay one half of the benefit amount if the insured loses one limb or the sight in one eye.

accidental death and dismemberment (ADD) coverage Insurance plan benefit in the event of loss of life, limb, or eyesight from an accident that is a supplementary benefit to a group term life insurance plan.

accidental death benefit (ADB) rider Supplementary benefit provision that gives an amount of money (lump sum) in addition to the basic death benefit of a life insurance policy and is payable only if the insured dies from an accident. This is often referred to as "double indemnity" when the additional amount is equal to the face amount of the policy.

accidental means provision Rider in a life insurance policy stating that an accidental death benefit is payable if the insured's death was the result, directly and independently of all other causes, of bodily injury caused solely by external, violent, and accidental means. The "means" that caused the mishap must be accidental to claim benefits under the policy.

accidental result provision Rider in a life insurance policy stating that an accidental death benefit is payable if the insured's death was the result, directly and independently of all other causes, of accidental bodily injury.

accommodation Type of hospital room (e.g., private, semiprivate, ward, intensive care unit).

accommodation revenue code Three-digit code used by facilities to identify a specific accommodation or ancillary charge on a hospital or skilled nursing facility bill to a third-party payer. Also see *revenue code*.

account Formal record of all transactions made on an individual's financial record, listing debits, credits, and balance; may be computerized, or in a medical practice using a manual bookkeeping system, this term is referred to as a *ledger, ledger card, financial accounting record*, or *patient account ledger*.

account balance carried forward See *beginning balance*.

account number See *group number*.

accountable health plan (AHP) Component of managed competition that functions as both provider and insurer (payer) of health care services. AHPs compete with other AHPs to provide the most cost-effective benefits package and the best quality of care. AHPs have preventive programs and emphasize wellness. Providers either own, work for, or contract with these health plans. Also known as *accountable health partnership (AHP), integrated delivery system (IDS), integrated health system (IHS), integrated health delivery system (IHDS), community accountable healthcare network (CAHN), integrated service networks (ISN), health purchasing alliance (HPA), community care network (CCN)*, and *organized delivery systems*.

accounting See *bookkeeping*.

accounts receivable (AR) 1. Total amount of money owed by patients to a business for professional services rendered by a provider or medical group. 2. Money owed to a hospital facility from patients, insurance companies, managed care plans, and government programs.

accounts receivable (AR) journal See *day sheet.*

accounts receivable (A/R) transaction Miscellaneous Medi-Cal accounting transactions as a result of cost settlements, state audits, or refund checks received by the fiscal intermediary.

accreditation 1. Seal of approval; evaluative process whereby a program of study or an institution is recognized by an external body as meeting certain predetermined standards. Accreditation may either be permanent or may be given for a specified period of time. 2. Related to hospitals, it means that a facility meets certain standards of quality. These standards are set by private, nationally recognized groups that check on the quality of care (staff and equipment) at health care facilities usually every 3 years. Accreditation can be awarded by two organizations: The Joint Commission (formerly known as *Joint Commission of Accreditation of Health Care Organization [JCAHO]*) and the American Osteopathic Association (AOA). State or federal governments can recognize accreditation in lieu of, or as the basis for, licensure or other mandatory approvals. Also see *certification.*

Accreditation Association for Ambulatory Health Care (AAAHC) The Accreditation Association for Ambulatory Health Care, also known as the *Accreditation Association* or *AAAHC*, was formed in 1979 to assist ambulatory health care organizations improve the quality of care provided to patients. AAAHC is the leader in ambulatory health care accreditation and accredits more than 2500 organizations in a wide variety of ambulatory health care settings including ambulatory and office-based surgery centers, managed care organizations, and Indian and student health centers. With a single focus on the ambulatory care community, the Accreditation Association offers organizations a cost-effective, flexible, and collaborative approach to accreditation. The Accreditation Association's mission is to maintain its position as the preeminent leader in developing standards to advance and promote patient safety, quality, value, and measurement of performance for ambulatory health care through peer-based accreditation processes, education, and research.

accreditation cycle for M+C deeming Duration of the Centers for Medicare and Medicaid Services' (CMS) recognition of the validity of an accrediting organization's determination that a Medicare+Choice organization (M+CO) is "fully accredited."

accreditation for deeming Some states use the findings of private accreditation organizations, in part or in whole, to supplement or substitute for state oversight of some quality-related standards. This is referred to as "deemed compliance" with a standard.

accreditation for participation State requirement that managed care plans must be accredited to participate in the Medicaid managed care program.

accredited To have a seal of approval. Being accredited means that a facility or health care organization has met certain quality standards. These standards are set by private, nationally recognized groups that check on the quality of care at health care facilities and organizations. Organizations that accredit Medicare Managed Care Plans include the National Committee for Quality Assurance, The Joint Commission, and the American Accreditation HealthCare Commission/Utilization Review Accreditation Commission (URAC).

accredited hospital A facility that meets certain standards of quality. These standards are set by private, nationally recognized groups that check on the quality of care (staff and equipment) at health care facilities usually every 3 years. Accreditation can be awarded by two organizations: The Joint Commission and the American Osteopathic Association (AOA). The Joint Commission has six levels—the lowest is not accredited and the highest is accredited with commendation. AOA has several levels, the lowest level being denial of accreditation and the highest being accreditation with resurvey within 3 years. State or federal governments can recognize accreditation in lieu of, or as the basis for, licensure or other mandatory approvals.

accredited record technician (ART) See *Registered Health Information Technician (RHIT).*

Accredited Standards Committee X12 (ASC X12) Organization accredited by the American National Standards Institute (ANSI) for the development, maintenance, and publication of electronic data exchange national standards. Also called *X12.*

accrete 1. Medicare term that means the addition of new enrollees to a health plan. 2. In managed care plans, this is an enrollment term. 3. In accounting, this term means accrue.

accrual Funds set aside for a benefit plan's expenses by estimating data of the claims system and the plan's prior history.

accrual accounting Accounting method that requires business organizations to report income in the period earned and to deduct expenses in the period incurred.

accrue 1. When a right is vested in a person, that right is said to accrue (to go) to the benefit of that person. 2. To report a transaction in the time period to which its effect relates.

accrued benefit Amount of benefit in a pension plan that has accumulated on behalf of an individual plan participant at any particular time.

accrued income Earnings on a stated sum of money that continues to increase until the money is paid out.

accumulated cost of insurance One factor used when calculating life insurance reserves. The formula is the accumulated cost of insurance equals the net single premium paid at the end of the term of coverage by the surviving insureds to give death benefits on the insureds who died during the term.

accumulated dividends Accrued funds payable to policy owners but left with life insurance company to build up and earn interest.

accumulated funding deficiency Amount by which a qualified pension plan fails to meet the minimum funding legal standards. A plan with an accumulated funding deficiency is subject to a penalty tax and enforcement provisions. Also called *funding deficiency*.

accumulated value Amount of money invested plus the interest earned.

accumulation 1. Percentage added to insurance benefits given as a reward or incentive to the insured because of continuous renewal of the policy. This may be added as a provision in some health insurance policies. 2. Total number of services used by a patient under an insurance plan that limits costs or office visits.

accumulation at interest Option under which a life insurance policy dividends are retained on deposit with the insurer to accrue interest. Also called *accumulation option*.

accumulation option See *accumulation at interest*.

accumulation period 1. Time during which premiums are payable on a deferred annuity contract. 2. Precise time period during which the insured must incur eligible medical expenses that satisfy a required deductible. This applies to major medical or comprehensive medical plans.

accumulation units Ownership shares in a variable annuity's separate account fund. An individual pays premiums for a variable annuity and these premiums are credited to the purchaser's account (accumulation units). After the accumulation period ends, these units are used to buy annuity units. See also *annuity units*.

accuracy Pertaining to medical data in hospital or medical office settings, the degree to which the information is correct, precise, and free of errors.

ACER See *annual contractor evaluation report (ACER)*.

ACF See *alternative care facility (ACF)*.

ACG See *ambulatory care group (ACG)*.

ACGs See *adjusted clinical groups (ACGs)*.

ACH See *automated clearinghouse (ACH)*.

ACLS See *Advanced Cardiac Life Support (ACLS) certification*.

ACMCS See *American College of Medical Coding Specialists (ACMCS)*.

acquired In a medical sense, clinically indicates a condition produced by outside influences and not genetically.

acquired immune deficiency syndrome (AIDS) Fatal disease caused by a virus (human immunodeficiency virus [HIV]) that damages the body's immune system. It deprives the body of its own natural defenses to fight illness and infection. Also see *human immunodeficiency virus (HIV)*.

acquisition cost 1. Total cost to the company of setting up a new business such as commissions to agents and brokers, supervision costs, sales promotion expenses, and cost of secretarial work. 2. In health insurance, the cost of selling, underwriting, and issuing a new insurance policy (administrative costs, brokers' commissions, advertising, and medical fees). Also called *policy acquisition costs*.

ACR See *adjusted community rating (ACR)*.

ACS See *Advanced Coding Specialist (ACS)*.

ACS contract See *administrative services only (ASO) agreement*.

act 1. Generally refers to the Social Security Act, and titles referred to are titles of that Act. 2. Term for legislation that passed through Congress and was signed by the President or passed over his veto. Also called *law* or *statute*.

act of God Accident or event that results from natural causes without human intervention and could not be prevented by foresight such as flood, lightning, earthquake, tornado, or storm.

active 1. In business, producing profit or interest (active funds). 2. In insurance, may refer to a group or individual member or subscriber's status that is currently in effect.

active duty family members (ADFM) Spouse and dependents of an active member of the United States government military services (e.g., Army, Navy, Air Force, Marines, Coast Guard). This phrase is used more frequently in the TRICARE health care program.

active duty service member (ADSM) Active member of the United States government military services (e.g., Army, Navy, Air Force, Marines, Coast Guard).

actively-at-work provision Rider in a group insurance contract that states if an employee is absent from work due to illness, injury, or other specific reasons, on the date the employee's coverage is due to begin, then insurance will not begin until the date the employee returns to work. For a dependent, a plan may require that, if in the hospital on the effective date, that date is deferred until the dependent's release from hospital.

activities of daily living (ADLs) 1. Physical nonoccupational activities used to determine eligibility for long-term care such as bathing, continence, dressing, eating, mobility, transferring in and out of bed or a chair, using the toilet, and walking. ADLs are used to measure how dependent a person may be on requiring assistance in performing any or all of these activities. Compare with *instrumental activities of daily living (IADLs)*. 2. In workers' compensation cases, these activities may include self-care, communication, physical activity, sensory function, hand functions, travel, sexual function, sleep, and social and recreational activities.

actual acquisition cost Prescription drug program phrase that means the actual cost of a drug to the pharmacy or to the managed care plan that contracts with the pharmacist.

actual cash value Insurance provision in which the policy owner receives a dollar amount that is equal to the replacement value of damaged property minus the depreciation.

actual charge 1. Fee the physician charges for service or supplier bills for a supply item at the time the insurance claim is submitted to the insurance company or government payer. 2. In the Medicare program, the fee is often more than the amount Medicare approves. See *approved charge* and *assignment.*

actuarial Statistical calculations used to establish a managed care plan's rates and premiums based on future projections of utilization and cost for a specific member or subscriber population.

actuarial assumptions 1. Characteristics used in calculating the risks and costs of a plan (i.e., age, sex, and occupation of enrollees; location; utilization rates; and service costs) to calculate premium rates and reserves. 2. In relation to pension plans, these assumptions affect the amount of the yearly contribution to adequately fund a defined benefit pension plan (DBPP).

actuarial balance Difference between the summarized income rate and the summarized cost rate over a given valuation period.

actuarial cost method Method of calculating the annual amount a plan sponsor must contribute to fund a specific set of defined benefit pension plan (DBPP) benefits for a group of participants.

actuarial deficit Negative actuarial balance.

actuarial department Section in a life and health insurance company that oversees the company and is operated on a mathematically sound basis. This department calculates premium and dividend rates, establishes a company's reserve liabilities, and figures nonforfeiture, surrender, and loan values. Its research predicts mortality and morbidity rates, and this helps sets the guidelines for selecting risks and establishes the profits of the company's products.

actuarial rates One-half the expected monthly cost of the supplemental medical insurance (SMI) program for each aged enrollee (for the aged actuarial rate) and one-half the expected monthly cost for each disabled enrollee (for the disabled actuarial rate) for the duration the rate is in effect.

actuarial soundness 1. Measure of the adequacy of hospital insurance and supplementary medical insurance (SMI) financing as determined by the difference between trust fund assets and liabilities for specified periods. 2. A pension fund is considered to be actuarially sound when the amount of money in the fund and the current level of contributions to the fund are sufficient to meet the liabilities that have accrued and are accruing on a current basis.

actuarial status Measure of the adequacy of the financing as determined by the difference between assets and liabilities at the end of the periods for which financing was established.

actuarial valuation Dollar value of a pension plan's assets and liabilities as determined by the actuary. The value is based on statistical probability. It is used to establish if the assets are adequate to fund the plan's liabilities. If not, the plan sponsor must increase its contributions to make up the deficiency. If the assets are more than necessary, the plan sponsor can reduce contributions. Also called *plan valuation.*

actuary Technical expert of life insurance who can apply the theory of probability to calculate policy reserves and mortality, morbidity, dividends, premium, and lapse rates. An actuary prepares statistical studies and reports.

acuity 1. Clearness or sharpness of perception such as visual acuity. 2. Measure of a patient's severity of illness to establish nurse staffing requirements.

acupressure Chinese massage that uses deep pressure over meridian points to relieve pain.

acupuncture Ancient Chinese practice of insertion of long, fine needles into specific exterior body locations (meridians) to relieve pain, to induce surgical anesthesia, and for therapeutical purposes.

acupuncturist Individual who practices acupuncture.

acute Refers to a medical condition that runs a short but relatively severe course. To report for billing purposes, documentation must establish medical necessity of services rendered.

acute care Medical services that are generally provided for a short period of time to treat a certain illness or condition. This type of care can include short-term hospital stays, doctor's visits, surgery, and x-rays.

acute care facility Facility that gives continuous professional medical care to patients during an acute condition, injury, or sudden onset of illness or disease.

acute care services Immediate medical services for the examination, diagnosis, care, and treatment of a patient because of severe episodes of illness. Usually, acute care is given in a hospital by specialized personnel and use of sophisticated technical equipment. It may be intensive care, critical care, or emergency care.

acute illness Sickness that is usually of short-term duration and that often comes on quickly.

Acute Long Term Hospital Association (ALTHA) Organization formed to protect patient access to quality long-term hospital care; formerly known as *Long Term Acute Care Hospital Association of America (LTACHA).* Long Term Acute Care Hospitals (LTACHs) are hospitals that provide patients with acute care for extended inpatient stays (defined by federal statute as an average of 25 days or more). ALTHA works to protect the rights of medically complex patients and the hospitals that treat them by educating federal and state regulators, members of Congress, and health care industry colleagues. ALTHA also works to increase quality of care by sharing and improving best practices among its hospital members.

AD 1. HCPCS Level II modifier that may be used with CPT or HCPCS Level II codes indicating physician supervision for more than four concurrent anesthesia procedures. Use of this modifier affects Medicare payment. 2. Abbreviation for administrative director. See *administrative director (AD)*.

AD&D See *accidental death and dismemberment (AD&D)*.

ADA See *American Dental Association (ADA); Americans with Disabilities Act (ADA)*.

ADB See *accidental death benefit (ADB) rider*.

ADD See *accidental death and dismemberment (ADD) coverage*.

add-on code Procedural code in the CPT book that is preceded with a plus (+) symbol indicating the code may be reported in addition to the parent or primary procedure code number (see Box A-1). Add-on codes are never reported for stand-alone services but are reported secondarily in addition to the primary procedure.

add-on code symbol (+) Symbol used in the procedure code book titled *Current Procedural Terminology (CPT)* to indicate the code may be reported in addition to the primary procedure code number.

addition Individual who becomes insured after the effective date of a group insurance policy.

additional benefits Health care services not covered by Medicare and reductions in premiums or cost sharing for Medicare-covered services. Additional benefits are specified by the Medicare Advantage (MA) Organization and are offered to Medicare beneficiaries at no additional premium. Those benefits must be at least equal in value to the adjusted excess amount calculated in the adjusted or average community rate (ACR). An excess amount is created when the average payment rate exceeds the adjusted community rate (as reduced by the actuarial value of coinsurance, copayments, and deductibles under Parts A and B of Medicare). The excess amount is then adjusted for any contributions to a stabilization fund. The remainder is the adjusted excess, which is used to pay for services not covered by Medicare and/or is used to reduce charges otherwise allowed for Medicare-covered services. Additional benefits can be subject to cost sharing by plan enrollees. Additional benefits can also be different for each MA plan offered to Medicare beneficiaries.

Box A-1 ADD-ON CODE		
Parent code	11000	Biopsy of skin … single lesion each separate/additional lesion (list separately in addition to code for primary procedure)
Add-on code	+11101	

additional diagnosis See *secondary diagnosis* and *other diagnoses*.

additional documentation request (ADR) Form issued by a Medicare administrative contractor (MAC) to a provider asking for more information in a patient's medical record so that coverage, coding, and payment determination can be made concerning a claim.

additional insurance option See *additional term insurance option* and *fifth dividend option*.

additional term insurance option Option in a life insurance policy in which current dividends are used as a net single premium to purchase 1-year term insurance to maintain level protection for a period up to the insured's retirement age. This is often used with a split-dollar plan. Also called *additional insurance option* or *fifth dividend option*.

additions, deletions, revisions (ADR) Commonly used acronym in relation to a hospital charge description master (CDM); also called *charge master*.

addressable Under HIPAA rules, implementation specification under the security rule related to encrypted electronic mail that contains the patient's protected health information. The provider must implement the specification as stated in the rule, implement protections equivalent to the rule, or clearly document why the implementation specification does not apply.

ADEA See *Age Discrimination in Employment Act of 1967 (ADEA)*.

adequate care See *due care*.

adequate rates Charges that generate insurance premiums that are enough to cover incurred claims, operational costs, risk charges, and contingency reserve funds.

ADFM Abbreviation in the TRICARE program that means active duty family members.

ADGs See *aggregated diagnosis groups (ADGs)*.

adhesion Band of scar tissue of two adjacent structures that are usually separate from each other. This condition may occur as the result of surgery, infection, or injury.

adjudicate Processing of an insurance claim by an insurance company through a series of edits for determination of coverage (benefits) and issue of payment to the provider or patient.

adjudication Process of the final determination of the issues involving settlement of an insurance claim as payable, partially payable, or denied; also known as *claim settlement*.

adjunct codes CPT codes that are referred to in the Medicine Section as Special Services, Procedures and Reports and fall under the category of Miscellaneous Services. They are important to consider when billing because these codes provide the reporting physician with a means of identifying special services and reports that are provided in addition to the basic services provided such as handling of laboratory specimens, telephone calls, seeing patients after hours, office emergency services, supplies and materials, special reports, travel, and educational services rendered to patients.

adjustable life insurance policy Life insurance contract that allows the policy owner to change the policy's plan by changing the amount of the coverage or premium. The insurance company calculates the plan of insurance based on the chosen death benefit and premium. An adjustable life insurance policy can use a plan that ranges from a term insurance policy of short duration to a limited-payment whole life insurance policy.

adjusted average per capita cost (AAPCC) Estimated average cost of Medicare benefits in a given region for an individual. It is based on criteria such as age, sex, institutional status, Medicaid, disability, and end-stage renal disease (ESRD) status. Centers for Medicare and Medicaid Services (CMS) uses AAPCC as a basis for making monthly payments to managed care plans.

adjusted clinical groups (ACGs) System developed by Johns Hopkins University that is a comprehensive family of measurement tools designed to help explain and predict how health care resources are delivered and consumed. ACGs are based on building blocks called aggregated diagnosis groups (ADGs). See *aggregated diagnosis groups (ADGs)*.

adjusted community rate (ACR) Annual calculation of premium (payment rates) that health plans would have received for their Medicare enrollees to provide Medicare-covered benefits if paid their private market premiums. This is done to adjust subsequent year supplemental benefits or premiums to return any excess Medicare revenue above the ACR to enrollees. Also called *average community rate (ACR)*. See *adjusted average per capita cost (AAPCC)*.

adjusted community rating (ACR) Used by managed care plans to determine group rates for each group's expected use of medical services during an upcoming contract period. Also known as *factored rating* or *community rating by class (CRC)*.

adjusted drug benefit list Schedule showing names of a small amount of drugs often prescribed to long-term patients that can be modified from time to time by the managed care or insurance plan. Also called a *drug maintenance list*.

adjusted gross charges 1. Accounts receivable amount showing the write-off portion from the total gross charges of amounts that by law or provider contract cannot be collected. 2. Medicare approved amount is the adjusted gross charge.

adjusted historical payment basis (AHPB) Average payment for the service in a locality under the current system. AHPB is based on the average prevailing charge Medicare paid all physicians in a particular geographic area for a specific service. "Adjusted" means reduced by a percent to ensure that the fee schedule phase-in is budget neutral. Medicare carriers used ADPBs to figure blended payment rates during the transition period before implementation of the RBRVS system of payment.

adjusted payment rate (APR) Amount of money that the Centers for Medicare and Medicaid Services will pay Medicare risk health maintenance organizations (HMOs) to cover a Medicare beneficiary. The rate is taken from the adjusted average per capita cost (AAPCC) based on health risk factors for the beneficiaries.

adjuster 1. Employed representative of the insurance company who is responsible for handling insurance claims as they are received from patients and medical practices and who determines the dollar amount of a claim or debt. 2. In industrial cases, a representative of the insurer who investigates, evaluates, and negotiates the patient's insurance claim and acts for the company in the settlement of claims. Adjusters may be employees of the insurance company or an individual operating independently and hired by a company to adjust a particular loss. Also called *claims administrator, claims examiner, claims processor, claim representative,* or *health insurance adjuster.*

adjustment 1. Posting an entry to a patient's financial account to indicate a change to the balance due such as additional payment, partial payment, courtesy adjustment, write off, discount. 2. Change made to correct an error in billing, processing of a claim, or as a result of a retroactive rate change (e.g., late charges for a previously submitted bill). These situations may be found by either claims personnel or by the provider. Possible errors that would allow adjustments to be processed include overpayment, underpayment, or payments to the wrong provider.

adjustment codes Special codes used by insurance carriers to explain the reason an insurance claim or a medical service was paid differently than the billed amount.

adjustment reasons Reference list of coded explanations of changes made to a paid insurance claim. The codes detail and clarify all services reported and eliminate having to generate a separate letter of explanation.

adjustments to payment rates Changes or modifications to the base payment rates to allow for differences in providers' situations that affect their costs of giving medical services. These adjustments are to accommodate differences in local prices for products and services, delivery of specialized types of care, or atypical characteristics of beneficiaries.

adjuvant technique Additional technique(s) that may be required at the time a bypass graft is created to improve patency of the lower extremity autogenous or synthetic bypass graft or fistula. Use of CPT codes 35685 and 35686 are add-on codes and should be reported with a code for the primary procedure performed.

ADLs See *activities of daily living (ADLs)*.

administration Policies, procedures, and management of functions related to the operation of an insurance plan by the insurance company after it becomes effective. In some situations, the insurance claims processing and payment may be administered by a separate entity.

administrative agent See *insurance carrier*.

administrative allowance Fee paid to an agent or administrator for overseeing and managing an insured's policy that would normally be handled by the insurance company.

administrative code sets 1. Code sets that characterize a general business situation, rather than a medical condition or service. 2. Under the Health Insurance Portability and Accountability Act (HIPAA), a phrase that refers to nonclinical or nonmedical code sets. Compare with medical code sets.

administrative costs General phrase that refers to Medicare operating expenses (salaries, facilities, equipment, rent, utilities) and the federal share of the states' expenditures for administration of the Medicaid program

administrative data Information that is collected, processed, and stored in automated information systems. Administrative data include enrollment or eligibility information, claims information, and managed care encounters. The claims and encounters may be for hospital and other facility services, professional services, prescription drug services, laboratory services, and so on.

administrative director (AD) In workers' compensation insurance, the head of the Division of Workers' Compensation.

administrative expenses Operating costs incurred by the Department of Health and Human Services (HHS) and the Department of the Treasury in administering the supplemental medical insurance (SMI) program and the provisions of the Internal Revenue Code relating to the collection of contributions. Such administrative expenses, which are paid from the SMI trust fund, include expenditures for contractors to determine costs of, and make payments to, providers, as well as salaries and expenses of Centers for Medicare and Medicaid Services (CMS).

administrative guidelines Health insurance plan document that gives detailed explanations of the plan's benefits, how to file insurance claims, payment of claims, deductibles, prescription drug plan, coordination of benefits, administrative rules, and so on.

administrative law judge (ALJ) Hearings officer who presides at a Level 4 hearing between providers of services, or beneficiaries, and Medicare contractors. Such situations occur when there is an appeal of a denied Medicare insurance claim, as well as appeals from proposed Office of the Inspector General (OIG) exclusions.

administrative loading See *administrative expenses*.

administrative manual Reference book of instructions given to the insurance policyholder by the insurance company that explains the duties of the plan administrator.

administrative medical assistant Person who, under the direction of a physician, performs various routine front office tasks in a hospital, clinic, or other health facility. These duties may consist of scheduling patients for appointments, answering the telephone, interviewing and registering the patient, filing documents, billing, completing insurance claims, bookkeeping, and so on. Also see *clinical medical assistant*.

administrative services only (ASO) agreement Contract between a self-funded insurance plan and an insurance company or third-party administrator (TPA) whereby the insurance company provides administrative services only and assumes no risk. Usually, this is an employer's group health insurance program and it retains financial responsibility for payment of the insurance claims. Services include actuarial activities, benefit plan design, claim processing, data recovery and analysis, employee benefits communication, financial advice, medical care conversions, preparation of data for federal reports, and stop-loss coverage. Also known as *ACS contract*.

administrative services organization (ASO) Association that provides only administrative services for a self-funded insurance company or entity such as billing, practice management, and marketing.

administrative simplification (AS) Title II, Subtitle F, of HIPAA, which gives Health and Human Services (HHS) the authority to mandate the use of standards for the electronic exchange of health care data; to specify what medical and administrative code sets should be used within those standards; to require the use of national identification systems for health care patients, providers, payers (or plans), and employers (or sponsors); and to specify the types of measures required to protect the security and privacy of personally identifiable health care information. This is also the name of Title II, Subtitle F, Part C of HIPAA.

Administrative Simplification Compliance Act Statute that was signed into law on December 27, 2001, as Public Law 107-105. It provides a 1-year extension to Health Insurance Portability and Accountability Act (HIPAA)–covered entities to meet electronic and code set transaction requirements. It allows the Secretary of the Department of Health and Human Services (HHS) to exclude providers from Medicare if they are not compliant with the HIPAA electronic and code set transaction requirements and to prohibit Medicare payment of paper claims received after October 16, 2003, except under certain situations.

administrative subpoenas Subpoenas issued in the course of administrative proceedings or investigations seeking the disclosure of medical records or other patient health information such as hearings before disciplinary boards to revoke professional licenses, proceedings before state agencies to determine the propriety of facility license citations, and disputes before administrative law judges about proper Medicare or Medicaid reimbursement.

administrator 1. Individual appointed by a court to manage and settle a deceased person's estate. 2. Third-party entity or individual responsible for the management of a group insurance program. Responsibilities include accounting, certificate issuance, and insurance claim reimbursement. 3. In a 401(k) defined-contribution pension plan, a company that processes employees' contributions, mails statements, ensures compliance with federal tax law, and handles other bureaucratic chores. 4. In the Medicare and Medicaid programs, the title of the director of the Centers for Medicare and Medicaid Services (CMS).

admission Registration of a patient either as an inpatient or outpatient for receiving medical services in a health care facility. The patient is given a register number. An admission can be either a direct admission, a direct admission from the emergency department, or transfer-in from another medical facility. See also *inpatient admission, outpatient admission,* and *newborn admission.*

admission and disposition report Daily hospital report that shows patients gained and lost in census, changes in status, and numerical strengths of transient patients and boarders.

admission certification Method of assuring that only those patients who need hospital care are admitted. Certification can be granted before admission (pre-admission) or shortly after (concurrent). Length of stay for the patient's diagnosed problem is usually assigned on admission under a certification program.

admission date The month, day, and year the patient is admitted to the hospital as an inpatient or as an outpatient for services or tests. Admission date is inserted in Field 12 of the Uniform Bill (UB-04) inpatient hospital billing claim form. The electronic version requires an eight-character date listing year, month, and day: 20XX0328. For an admission notice for hospice care for a Medicare patient, enter the effective date of election of hospice benefits.

admission-discharge-transfer system Computer software program used by hospitals to keep track of patients from the time of admission to time of discharge or transfer to another facility.

admission process Registration of a patient either as an inpatient or outpatient for receiving medical services in a health care facility. Admissions staff give the patient a registration number and obtain demographic, insurance, and medical information, which is entered into the computer system.

admission review Review a patient's medical case for appropriateness and necessity of admissions.

admission wire Blue Cross and Blue Shield phrase; a formal notice sent by a host plan to the home plan that one of their members has been admitted into a plan hospital in the host plan's area and a request for membership information. See also *approval wire.*

admissions per 1000 (APT) Method used to compare the number of hospital admissions for defined populations for a specific period of time, usually 1 year. APT is commonly used by managed care plans to evaluate utilization management performance. Admissions per 1000 formula: number of hospital admissions for a population divided ($\div$) by the number of persons in that population, and the result multiplied ($\times$) by 1000.

admitted company Insurance company that is licensed by the state and authorized to conduct business within that state.

admitted reinsurer Reinsurer licensed to accept reinsurance in a given region in the United States. Also called an *authorized reinsurer.*

admitting diagnosis Initial identification of the condition for which the patient is admitted to the hospital as an inpatient.

admitting diagnosis code Three- to five-digit numeric diagnostic code number that indicates the patient's diagnosis at the time of inpatient hospital admission.

admitting physician Patient's provider of medical services who arranges for the patient's admission to a hospital or facility.

adoptee Individual who has been adopted.

adoption 1. To take into one's own family by legal process and raise as one's own child. 2. To take up and use an idea or practice as one's own.

adoptive parent One who becomes the legal parent of a child who was not born to him or her, such as a stepparent or relative.

ADPL-BASS See *average daily patient load—bassinet (ADPL-BASS).*

ADPL-IP See *average daily patient load—inpatient (ADPL-IP).*

ADPL-TOT See *average daily patient load—total (ADPL-TOT).*

ADR See *alternative dispute resolution (ADR), average daily revenue (ADR), additional documentation request (ADR),* and *additions, deletions, revisions (ADR).*

ADS See *alternative delivery system (ADS).*

ADSM See *active duty service member (ADSM).*

ADU See *accessory dwelling unit (ADU).*

adult care home Type of licensed adult board and care residence that offers housing and personal care services for 3 to 16 residents. Services may include meals, supervision, and transportation. The home may be a single family house. Such a residence is licensed as an *adult family home* or *adult group home.* Also called *board and care home* or *group home.*

adult day care Daytime community-based program for functionally impaired adults that provides a variety of health, social, and related support services in a protective setting.

adult foster care (AFC) Residential assistance for individuals older than the age of 18 who no longer can live alone and care for themselves and do not need daily nursing supervision. AFC is provided on a 24-hour basis in a state licensed homelike facility with 5 to 10 residents. AFC homes are categorized as assisted living centers and give general supervision and personal care services. They assist with self-administration of medications and assist with supervision of self-treatment of a physical disorder. Also called *domiciliary care*. See also *assisted living center (ALC)* and *activities of daily living (ADL)*.

adult living care facility Used when billing medical services rendered at a residential care facility that houses Medicare beneficiaries who cannot live alone but who do not need around-the-clock skilled medical services. The facility services do not include a professional medical component.

adult primary policy Insurance policy that shows the name of the patient (insured or subscriber) as the policyholder.

adult secondary policy Insurance policy that shows the name of the patient as a dependent on a second insurance policy.

Advance Beneficiary Notice (ABN) Agreement given to the patient to read and sign before rendering a service if the participating physician thinks that it may be denied for payment because of medical necessity or limitation of liability by Medicare. The patient agrees to pay for the service. ABNs only apply if the patient is in the original Medicare program. They do not apply if the patient is in a Medicare managed care plan or private fee-for-service plan. May be referred to as an ABN-G (i.e., ABNs used by providers, physicians, practitioners, and suppliers). An ABN is also known as a *waiver of liability agreement, responsibility statement*, or *notice of noncoverage*. ABN-L refers to ABNs used when only laboratory services are being delivered. HHABN is an ABN used for home health services.

advance check Check sent to the provider before filing of an insurance claim for medical services or billing statement for an insurance examination.

advance coverage decision Determination that the patient's private fee-for-service plan makes on whether or not it will pay for a particular medical service.

advance directive As specified in the Patient Self-Determination Act, this is a legal document prepared by an individual that gives directions about his or her wishes in the event he or she becomes incapacitated and not able to make decisions. It designates a person to make medical decisions. An advance directive includes such documents as do-not-resuscitate (DNR) order, durable power of attorney, right to die document, and living will. Also called *health care advance directive* or *living will*.

advance funding Process in which an employer who is sponsoring a pension plan deposits money in a fund during the participants' working years to guarantee payment of pension benefits to the plan's participants when they retire.

advanced billing concept (ABC) codes See *alternative billing codes (ABCs)*.

Advanced Cardiac Life Support (ACLS) certification Certification of those professionals who take care of seriously injured or ill patients.

Advanced Coding Specialist (ACS) Certification offered by the Board of Advanced Medical Coding (BAMC) to physician and facility coders who successfully complete the qualifying examination. See *Board of Advanced Medical Coding (BAMC)*.

advanced registered nurse practitioner (ARNP) Registered nurse who has advanced education and clinical training in a health care specialty area.

advanced underwriting department Insurance company home office division that is responsible for giving technical and sales help to insurance agents about estate planning and business insurance. Also known as *estate planning department*.

adverse benefit determination (ABD) Denied or incorrectly paid health benefit under HMO, PPO, or POS managed care plans that follow federal regulations mandated under the Employee Retirement Income Security Act (ERISA).

adverse effect Unfavorable, detrimental, or pathologic reaction to a drug that occurs when appropriate doses are given to humans for prophylaxis (prevention of disease), diagnosis, or therapy.

adverse selection Method or process used in a managed care contract where there is a risk of enrolling members who are sicker than assumed and may use expensive medical services more often.

advisor In a 401(k) defined-contribution pension plan, a firm that helps the employer choose a provider, select the investment options, and make any other decisions about the plan.

Advisory Council on Social Security Prior to the enactment of the Social Security Independence and Program Improvements Act of 1994 (Public Law 103-296) on August 15, 1994, the Social Security Act required the appointment of an Advisory Council every 4 years to study and review the financial status of the Old Age, Survivors, and Disability Insurance (OASDI) and Medicare programs. Its report on the financial status of the OASDI program was submitted on January 6, 1997. Under the provisions of the Public Law, this was the last Advisory Council to be appointed.

advocate Individual who gives the patient support or protects his or her rights.

AE HCPCS Level II modifier that may be used with CPT or HCPCS Level II codes indicating service performed by a registered dietitian. Use of this modifier affects Medicare payment.

AEP See *annual election period (AEP)* and *appropriateness evaluation protocol (AEP)*.

aesthetic surgery See *cosmetic surgery*.

AEVS See *automated eligibility verification system (AEVS)*.

AF HCPCS Level II modifier that may be used with CPT or HCPCS Level II codes indicating service performed by a specialty physician. Use of this modifier affects Medicare payment.

AFC See *adult foster care (AFC)*.

AFDC See *Temporary Assistance to Needy Families (TANF)* (formerly *Aid to Families with Dependent Children*).

AFEHCT See *Association for Electronic Health Care Transactions (AFEHCT)*.

affiliate Corporation in which a majority of the stock is owned by any or all of the stockholders, directors, or officers of another corporation. These individuals also own a majority of the stock in that other corporation.

affiliated contractor (AC) Medicare carrier, fiscal intermediary (FI), or other contractor such as a durable medical equipment regional carrier (DMERC) that shares some or all of the provider service carrier's (PSC's) jurisdiction in which the affiliated contractor performs non-PSC Medicare functions such as claims processing or education.

affiliated entities Under the privacy rule, allows several entities to be treated as a single covered entity. Only one consent is necessary, which binds all of the affiliated entities.

affiliated health care provider See *participating provider (par)* or *participating physician*.

affiliated hospital See *hospital affiliation*.

affiliation period Length of time managed care plan members must wait before receiving benefits. It is an alternative to preexisting condition exclusions seen in insurance plans. Under the Health Insurance Portability and Accountability Act (HIPAA), an affiliation period may not last longer than 2 months or, if a late enrollee, 3 months. It begins on the member's date of enrollment. If a member changes coverage more than 3 months after the enrollment date, the new plan cannot impose an affiliation period.

aforesaid As previously stated.

AFS See *alternative financing system (AFS)*.

AG HCPCS Level II modifier that may be used with CPT or HCPCS Level II codes indicating services performed by a primary physician. Use of this modifier affects Medicare payment.

against medical advice (AMA) Discharge status of a patient who leaves the hospital before being released by a physician.

age analysis Procedure of systematically arranging the accounts receivable, by age, from the date of service.

age break Phrase used in insurance rating purposes that relates to the grouping of age categories (e.g., females age 18-25).

age change Date halfway between natural birth dates when the age of an individual changes to the next higher age. It is referred to when an individual is purchasing life insurance; the insurance age being the nearer birthday. When purchasing an annuity, the annuity age considered is the last previous birthday.

Age Discrimination in Employment Act of 1967 (ADEA) Federal legislation that protects employees age 40 and older and requires employers to offer employees 65 years or older the same employment and health insurance benefits as offered to younger employees. ADEA prohibits an individual from being fired based on age and prevents employers from forcing employees to retire at age 65. ADEA also prohibits employers from stopping contributions or accrual of benefits to pension plans after workers reach age 65.

age distribution System of establishing insurance rates for eligible or insured employees under a group life plan by their insurance year of birth, attained age, or actual year of birth.

age limits Minimum or maximum ages in which an insurance company or managed care plan will not accept applications or renew policies.

age of majority Age at which an individual has the legal capability of being responsible for his or her actions (e.g., enter into a contract or vote in a national election). In most states the age of majority is 21 years, but in some it is 18 because of enactment in 1972 of the 26th Amendment of the U.S. Constitution, which allowed 18-year-olds to vote in federal elections. Also known as *legal majority* or *emancipated minor*.

age restriction In a health care plan when there is a limitation of benefits when the patient reaches a certain age.

age/sex factor Measurement in actuarial underwriting that uses age and sex risk of medical costs of a population relative to another population.

age/sex rates (ASRs) In a managed care contract, a structure of capitation payments based on members' ages and genders. ASRs are used to calculate premiums for the purpose of group billing. Also called *table rates*.

age/sex rating See *age/sex rates (ASRs)*.

aged Under Social Security, an individual 65 years and older whose income and resources are within supplemental security income (SSI) limitations.

aged enrollee Individual age 65 or older who is enrolled in the supplemental medical insurance (SMI) program.

agency See *insurance company*.

agency agreement Contract between a principal and an agent that explains the scope of the insurance agent's authority. See *agent*.

agency company Insurance company that markets products via independent or self-employed agents.

Agency for Healthcare Research and Quality (AHRQ) Formerly Agency for Health Care Policy and Research (AHCPR), which is part of the U.S. Department of Health and Human Services. It is the lead agency charged with supporting research designed to improve the quality of health care, reduce its cost, and broaden access to essential services. AHRQ's broad programs of research bring practical, science-based information to medical practitioners and to consumers and other health care purchasers. AHRQ's mission is to improve the quality, safety, efficiency, and effectiveness of health care for all Americans.

agency system Method in which insurance companies use commissioned agents to sell and deliver individual insurance policies. It is the most common system and has branch office distribution and general agency distribution systems. Also called *ordinary agency system.*

agent 1. Individual who is authorized by another person, the principal, to act on the principal's behalf for contracts with third parties. 2. Insurance company representative licensed by the state that sells insurance policies and services the policyholder for the insurer. There are independent agents and exclusive agents. Life insurance agents may also be called *life underwriters.* Also called *insurance agent, insurance broker,* or *field underwriter.*

agent of record Insurance individual (agent or broker) recognized by the insurer as the one to whom the commission is to be paid.

agent's statement Section of the insurance application form where the insurance agent reports data that he or she knows or suspects about the potential insured that is not stated by the applicant.

aggravation In workers' compensation, change in a preexisting condition that causes a temporary or permanent increase in disability or creates a need for additional or different medical treatment. An aggravation may be caused by either a new injury or by work activity involving a physical, chemical, or biological factor.

aggregate amount In a managed care contract, the maximum amount (limit) for which a member is insured for any single event.

aggregate indemnity Maximum amount for which an insured may collect for any disability, period of disability, or covered medical service under an insurance policy.

aggregate stop loss Agreement in a managed care plan to relieve the amount of liability for insurance claims that are in excess of the amount anticipated for the contract year. Also see *stop loss.*

aggregate stop loss insurance Insurance coverage that becomes effective when an employer who has self-insurance has its total group medical insurance claims reach a specific threshold chosen by the employer. This threshold is a percentage of its yearly predicted group health claim costs.

aggregated diagnosis groups (ADGs) Under a system developed by Johns Hopkins University called *adjusted clinical groups (ACGs)*, ACGs are a comprehensive family of measurement tools designed to help explain and predict how health care resources are delivered and consumed. ACGs are based on building blocks called *aggregated diagnosis groups (ADGs).* ADGs are a grouping of diagnosis codes that are similar in terms of severity and likelihood of persistence of the health condition over time. There are two categories of ADGs, ambulatory diagnostic groups–major diagnostic category (ADG-MDC) and ambulatory diagnostic groups–hospital dominant (ADG-HosDom).

aging accounts receivable (A/R) report Document used to determine outstanding balances from each patient's account showing status of 30, 60, 90, or 120 days from the date of insurance claim submission. It can be generated by using the date an insurance claim was filed to assess the age of the claim in days. Sometimes referred to as an *aging report.*

aging report 1. Document that reports the status of insurance claims to the provider of the medical services and identifies individual transactions that need to be followed up (e.g., appeal or resubmit a corrected a claim). 2. See *aging accounts receivable (A/R) report.*

AGPA See *American Medical Group Association (AMGA).*

agreed medical evaluator (AME) Physician who is certified by the Industrial Medical Council (IMC) and conducts medicolegal evaluations of injured workers in workers' compensation cases for insurance companies or workers' compensation appeals board. AMEs are agreed on by the employer and a referee (represents the employee) or appeals board at the expense of one of the parties to resolve disputed medical issues. The AME is referred by the parties in a workers' compensation proceeding. The report of an AME is considered the evidence of both parties. The AME renders an unbiased opinion about the degree of disability of an injured worker. May be referred to as *independent medical evaluator (IME)* or *qualified medical evaluator (QME).*

agreement Legal document signed by two or more individuals that contains specific mutual understandings.

AH HCPCS Level II modifier that may be used with CPT or HCPCS Level II codes indicating services performed by a clinical psychologist. Use of this modifier affects Medicare payment.

AHA See *American Hospital Association (AHA).*

AHBP See *adjusted historical payment basis (AHBP).*

AHCA See *American Health Care Association (AHCA).*

AHCPR See *Agency for Healthcare Research and Quality (AHRQ),* formerly Agency for Health Care Policy and Research (AHCPR).

AHIMA See *American Health Information Management Association (AHIMA)*.

AHIP See *America's Health Insurance Plans (AHIP)*.

AHP See *allied health professional (AHP)* and *accountable health plan (AHP)*.

AHRQ See *Agency for Healthcare Research and Quality (AHRQ)*, formerly Agency for Health Care Policy and Research (AHCPR).

AIC See *amount-in-controversy (AIC) requirements*.

Aid to Families with Dependent Children (AFDC) See *Temporary Assistance to Needy Families (TANF)*.

Aid to the Blind (AB) A group that is entitled to benefits under the Medi-Cal program.

Aid to the (permanently) Disabled (ATD) A group that is entitled to benefits under the Medi-Cal program.

AIDS See *acquired immune deficiency syndrome (AIDS)*.

AIHD See *Association for Integrity of Healthcare Documentation (AIHD)*.

airplane insurance Insurance that is purchased by commercial airlines and consists of property insurance on airplanes and liability insurance for passengers and persons not passengers. It is for negligent acts or omissions by the airline that may result in bodily injuries or property damages.

AJ HCPCS Level II modifier that may be used with CPT or HCPCS Level II codes indicating services performed by a clinical social worker. Use of this modifier affects Medicare payment.

AK HCPCS Level II modifier that may be used with CPT or HCPCS Level II codes indicating services provided by a nonparticipating physician. Use of this modifier affects Medicare payment.

AKS Abbreviation that may be defined as *anti-kickback statute*. See *Stark I Regulations* and *Stark II Regulations*.

albumin One of a class of simple proteins in the blood. The level of albumin may reflect the amount of protein intake in food.

ALC See *assisted living center (ALC)*.

aleatory That which depends on an uncertain event.

aleatory contract Agreement in which one of the parties may recover a larger value than the value lost, which is dependent on the occurrence of a future contingency.

ALF Abbreviation that means assisted living facility. See *assisted living center (ALC)*.

algorithm Rule or procedure containing conditional logic for solving a problem or accomplishing a task. Guideline algorithms concern rules for evaluating patient care against published guidelines. Criteria algorithms concern rules for evaluating criteria compliance. Algorithms may be expressions in written form, graphic outlines, diagrams, and flow charts that describe each step in the work or thought process.

alien Individual not a citizen or national of the United States but belonging to another country or people; a foreigner. May be referred to as an *immigrant* when a person from another country comes to settle.

alien carrier See *alien insurer*.

alien company See *alien insurer*.

alien insurer Insurance company residing and incorporated under the laws of a foreign country (e.g., Canada, England). Also called *alien carrier* or *alien company*.

alignment of incentives Phrase used in a managed care contract to describe the financial arrangements between physicians and hospital facilities that let both parties share in the risks and rewards of controlling costs and increasing income.

ALJ See *administrative law judge (ALJ)*.

all-clause deductible Insurance policy provision in which the deductible is met by a collection of eligible expenses incurred for any variety of covered claims within a given time period.

all-inclusive rate In a managed care contract, a flat fee charged daily by a facility (per diem rate) or for a total hospital stay. For submitting a Uniform Bill (UB-04) claim, revenue codes are 0100 (all-inclusive room and board plus ancillary) and 0101 (all-inclusive room and board). This is commonly billed by state psychiatric hospitals.

all-lines exclusive agency system See *multiple-line agency (MLA) system*.

all patient diagnosis-related group (APDRG or AP-DRG) Diagnosis-related group (DRG) system that is an enhancement of the original DRGs. It includes groupings for pediatric and maternity cases and services for HIV-related conditions and other special cases.

all-payer health care system State system that helps in determining equal uniform prices on medical and hospital services across all providers and all public and private payers, for instance, a common fee schedule. Also referred to as *all-payer system*.

all-payer system See *all-payer health care system*.

alleged father See *presumptive father*.

alliance 1. Health insurance purchasing entity (public or private) that enrolls subscribers or members within a given region, collects premiums, enforces rules that manage health plans, and purchases subscribers' or members' insurance from participating health plans. 2. Organization or group of employers that pools resources to buy health care goods and services. Also known as a *purchasing group*. See *consumer health alliances*. 3. Formal, mutual arrangement of companies, providers, or institutions, established to further common goals.

allied health professional (AHP) Health care provider who is not licensed as a doctor of medicine or osteopathy (e.g., nurse practitioner, physician assistant, chiropractor, medical assistant).

allied lines Type of property insurance that may be purchased with a fire insurance policy.

allocated benefits Insurance policy provision in a group contract in which specific hospital and medical benefits such as x-rays, dressings, and drugs will be paid as shown in a schedule with a maximum amount payable for all such services.

allocation Assignment of overhead costs such as financial, operational, and personnel salaries to different departments in a hospital facility, managed care plan, or insurance company depending on usage of physical space, staffing size, and other fair and reasonable considerations. Also called *allocation of overhead*.

allocation of overhead See *allocation*.

allocation of risk Method used by insurers in which uninsurable small employers are equitably assigned among insurance companies.

allopathy Medical therapy in which a disease or abnormal condition is treated by creating an environment that is opposite to or incompatible with the disease or condition that the patient suffers. An example would be the use of antibiotic drugs given to patients to fight a disease caused by bacteria to which the drugs are antagonistic. Allopathic physicians are Doctors of Medicine (MDs).

allowable charge 1. In the Medicare program, the fee schedule amount for a medical service that is published annually by the Centers for Medicare and Medicaid Services (CMS). This fee is based on relative value units (RVUs) taking into consideration the physician's work RVU, the practice expense RVU, and the malpractice insurance RVU. To bring the fees in line for the region where the physician practices and to adjust for regional overhead and malpractice costs, each of the RVUs is adjusted for each Medicare local carrier by geographic practice cost indices (GPCIs), pronounced "gypsies." Sometimes this is called the *approved charge*. 2. Amount on which TRICARE figures the patient's cost-share for covered care. This is based on 75% to 80% of the allowable charge.

allowable expense Insurance policy provision under coordination of benefits that defines any medically necessary, reasonable, or customary item of expense and is a benefit of one or more of the insurance plans under which an individual is insured.

allowed amount Maximum dollar value the insurance company assigns to each procedure or service on which payment is based. Typically, a percent (e.g., 80%) of the allowed amount is paid by the insurance carrier. Also called *approved charge* or *approved amount*. See also *maximum allowable* and *maximum allowable charge (MAC)*.

allowed charge Individual charge determined by an insurance carrier for a covered supplemental medical insurance (SMI) medical service or supply.

allowed condition In workers' compensation cases, a condition recognized as a direct result of an industrial injury or occupational illness.

ALOS See *arithmetic mean length of stay (AMLOS)*.

alphabetical index In the *International Classification of Diseases, Ninth Revision, Clinical Modification (ICD-9-CM)* code book, an alpha list of diagnoses located in Volume 2. This assists in trying to choose an accurate diagnostic code for a medical case.

alphabetical index to External Causes of Injury and Poisoning In the *International Classification of Diseases, Ninth Revision, Clinical Modification (ICD-9-CM)* code book, an alpha list of causes and places of injuries and poisoning, located at the back of Volume 2. This assists in trying to choose an accurate diagnostic code for an injury or poisoning case.

altering patient records Unethical and illegal practice of changing or adding an amendment to a patient's medical records either to obtain more reimbursement or due to a pending audit or legal review of records.

alternate beneficiary Individual entitled to the proceeds of a life insurance policy if no primary beneficiary is living when the insured dies. Also called *contingent beneficiary, secondary beneficiary*, or *successor beneficiary*.

alternate delivery system (ADS) 1. Any health care delivery system other than traditional fee-for-service (e.g., health maintenance organization [HMO], preferred provider organization [PPO], individual practice association [IPA]). 2. Provision of health services in settings that are more cost effective than an inpatient, acute-care hospital such as skilled and intermediate nursing facilities, hospice program, and in-home services.

alternate financing mechanism See *alternative funding mechanism*.

alternate treatment plan Strategy for treatment of a patient other than in a hospital.

alternate valuation date For tax purposes, the value of a decedent's estate is made as of the date of death. However, the estate executor may elect to value all estate assets 6 months from the date of death, the alternate valuation date.

alternative billing codes (ABCs) System of coding for integrative health care that consists of five-character alphabetic symbols with appended two-character practitioner modifiers that represent the practitioner type. These codes represent more than 4000 integrative health care products and services (Box A-2). ABC codes include the following specialty areas: acupuncturist, body work, chiropractic, conventional nursing, indigenous medicine, mental health care, minority health care, oriental medicine, physical medicine, spiritual and prayer-based healing, Ayurvedic medicine, botanical medicine, clinical nutrition, holistic dentists and physicians, homeopathy, massage therapy, midwifery, naturopathic medicine, osteopathic medicine, and somatic educational. ABCs were used to bill for these services as a pilot study maintained by Alternative Link, Inc. As of October 16, 2006, Alternative Link discontinued its pilot study. Covered entities under

The following description illustrates the coding hierarchy of ABC code with modifier:

CEBAM-1G High-risk pregnancy identification, Antepartum, Midwifery, Practice specialties

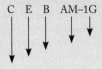

C   E   B   AM–1G

HIPAA may not use the codes in HIPAA transactions but may use the codes for non-HIPAA transactions. Also called *advanced billing concept (ABC) codes*. See also *integrative health care* and *alternative medicine*. Website: www.alternativelink.com

alternative care 1. Nontraditional medical care given by providers such as acupuncturists. 2. Medical care received instead of inpatient hospitalization (e.g., outpatient surgery, home health care, skilled nursing facility care).

alternative care facility (ACF) Assisted living facility for elderly who do not need nursing care. ACFs have private and semiprivate rooms for residents and are usually near shopping and entertainment resources.

alternative delivery system (ADS) Phrase that indicates any other health care system other than the traditional fee-for-service or indemnity insurance.

alternative dispute resolution (ADR) Method or procedure used to settle insurance claims other than through a lawsuit. See also *arbitration*.

alternative financing system (AFS) Another system for financing medical services that is different from a fee-for-service method (e.g., capitation).

alternative funding mechanism Method designed to provide the account with a more favorable cash flow (e.g., self-funding and deferred premiums).

alternative medicine Nontraditional medical care given by providers such as acupuncture, aroma therapy, chiropractic, diet, exercise, faith healing, homeopathy, Indian Ayurvedic medicine, massage, meditation, mind/body therapies, nutritional and herbal medicine, stress management, and therapeutic touch. A number of health insurance companies and managed care organizations have begun to provide insurance coverage for a few of these alternative therapies. Alternative billing codes (ABCs) are used to bill for these services. Also see *integrative health care* and *alternative billing codes (ABCs)*. Website: www.alternativelink.com

alternative work assignment In workers' compensation case, the placement of an injured worker in another job with the same employer as a temporary or permanent accommodation to the workers' disability.

ALTHA See *Acute Long Term Hospital Association (ALTHA)*.

Alzheimer's disease Progressive, irreversible disease characterized by degeneration of the brain cells and severe loss of memory, causing the individual to become dysfunctional and dependent on others for basic living needs.

AM HCPCS Level II modifier that may be used with CPT or HCPCS Level II codes indicating services performed by a physician associated with a team. Use of this modifier affects Medicare payment.

AMA See *American Medical Association (AMA); against medical advice (AMA)*.

ambulance (air or water) Air or water vehicle specifically designed, equipped, and staffed for life-saving assistance and transportation of the sick or injured.

ambulance fee schedule In the Medicare program, a fee schedule for the payment of ambulance services that became effective April 1, 2002. This involves a 5-year transition during which payment is based on a blended amount—part fee schedule and part provider or supplier's reasonable cost.

ambulance (land) Land vehicle specifically designed, equipped, and staffed for life-saving assistance and transportation of the sick or injured.

ambulatory 1. A patient capable of moving without assistance. Also see *activities of daily living (ADLs)*. 2. Descriptive term used when services are provided to a patient in a physician's office, clinic, or hospital outpatient department.

ambulatory care All types of health services that are provided on an outpatient basis, in contrast to services provided in the home or to persons who are inpatients. Although many inpatients may be ambulatory, the term *ambulatory care* usually implies that the patient must travel to a location to receive services that do not require an overnight stay. Many services that once required hospitalization are now considered ambulatory care. Sometimes called *outpatient care*.

ambulatory care clinic See *ambulatory care facility*.

ambulatory care evaluation Confidential utilization review and medical audit process in which physicians review an ambulatory care facility to assure the quality of medical care, services, and procedures. This peer review process may be done by the local medical society or other organization approved by the medical society in a specific locale.

ambulatory care facility Outpatient hospital or free-standing medical or dental treatment facility that provides medical care on an outpatient basis, without an overnight stay. It offers diagnostic, therapeutic, and rehabilitative services; preventive care; emergency medicine; and minor surgery to individuals. See *emergency center*. Also called *ambulatory surgery center, clinic, day surgery, free-standing surgical center, outpatient facility, primary care center,* or *urgent care center*.

ambulatory care group (ACG) See *ambulatory patient groups (APGs)*.

ambulatory care sensitive conditions (ACSC) Medical conditions for which physicians broadly concur that a substantial proportion of these cases should not advance to the point where hospitalization is necessary if the patients are treated in a timely fashion with adequate primary care and managed properly on an outpatient basis.

ambulatory diagnostic groups (ADG) See *aggregated diagnosis groups (ADGs)*.

ambulatory patient Individual who is receiving medical services and is able to walk or ambulate in a wheelchair.

ambulatory patient care groups See *ambulatory payment classification (APC) system*.

ambulatory patient groups (APGs) Classification system by case types used until 2000 as a payment method developed for the Centers for Medicare and Medicaid Services (CMS). It was replaced with ambulatory surgery categories (ASCs) and later replaced by the ambulatory payment classification (APC) system.

ambulatory payment classes See *ambulatory payment classification (APC) system*.

ambulatory payment classification (APC) system 1. Method developed by the Centers for Medicare and Medicaid Services (CMS) for outpatient hospital reimbursement based on procedures that have similar clinical characteristics and similar costs rather than on diagnoses. 2. Medicare's outpatient prospective payment system (OPPS) for hospital outpatient services that became effective August 1, 2000. Depending on the services given, hospital facilities may be paid for more than one APC for an encounter. APC information is updated and released twice a year in the *Federal Register*. Also called *ambulatory payment classes, ambulatory patient classifications (APCs)*, and *ambulatory patient care groups*.

ambulatory payment classifications (APCs) See *ambulatory payment classification (APC) system*.

ambulatory surgery Operative procedure performed on a patient as an outpatient in which he or she is admitted, treated, and released on the same day from the facility. Also referred to as *outpatient surgery*.

ambulatory surgery categories (ASCs) ASCs were adopted to replace ambulatory patient groups (APGs) for outpatient or 1-day surgery cases that were derived from the surgery section of the CPT. Later, this was replaced by the ambulatory payment classification (APC) system.

ambulatory surgery center (ASC) Licensed free-standing facility, other than a physician's office, at which outpatient medical services are provided on an ambulatory basis (e.g., diagnosis, treatment, same-day surgery, rehabilitation). ASCs are hospital based (or sponsored) or independently owned (or sponsored). Surgery of an uncomplicated nature that traditionally was done on an inpatient basis but can be performed with equal efficiency without hospital admission is now being done in an ASC. To receive payment for

Medicare patients, the facility must have an agreement with the Centers for Medicare and Medicaid Services (CMS) and meet specific requirements. ASCs are paid according to nine different payment groups based only on their cost similarities. Also called *surgicenter* or *ambulatory surgical center*.

ambulatory surgery program Facility's schedule for the performance of elective surgical procedures on patients admitted and discharged on the same day the procedure is performed.

ambulatory surgical center (ASC) See *ambulatory surgery center (ASC)* and *free-standing surgical center*.

ambulatory utilization review (AUR) Evaluation and analysis of the medical necessity, appropriateness, and efficiency of medical services given in an ambulatory facility. Utilization review is typically performed by a utilization review committee.

ambulatory visit See *outpatient visit*.

ambulatory visit groups (AVGs) AVGs were replaced by ambulatory patient groups (APGs) as an outpatient classification system by Health Systems International (HSI). Then ambulatory surgery categories (ASCs) were adopted, replacing APGs for outpatient or 1-day surgery cases that were derived from the surgery section of the CPT. Later this was replaced by the ambulatory payment classification (APC) system.

ambulatory weighted unit See *relative weighted product (RWP)*.

AMCP See *Academy of Managed Care Pharmacy (AMCP)*.

AMCRA See *American Association of Health Plans (AAHP)*.

AME See *agreed medical evaluator (AME)* and *average monthly earnings (AME)*.

amendment 1. Additional entry inserted into a patient's existing chart or progress note to correct data or to add more information. 2. Legal document or a clause added to a contract in which the terms of the contract are increased, limited, or decreased. Also called *endorsement* or *rider*.

amendments and corrections Under HIPAA's final privacy rule, an amendment to a patient's medical record indicates that the data are in dispute while retaining the original information, while a correction to a medical record alters or replaces the original record.

America's Health Insurance Plans (AHIP) National organization that was formed as a result of a merger of the Health Insurance Association of America (HIAA), Group Health Association of America (GHAA), American Managed Care and Review Association (AMCRA), and American Association of Health Plans (AAHP). Their member companies offer insurance coverage for medical expenses, long-term care, disability income, dental, supplemental, stop-loss, and reinsurance to consumers, employers, and public purchasers. Its purpose is to represent the interests of their members on legislative and regulatory issues at the federal and state levels, and with the media, consumers, and employers. They provide information and services such as newsletters, publications, a magazine, and on-line services. They also conduct education, research, and quality assurance programs and engage in a host of other activities to assist their members. AHIP participates in the maintenance of some code sets including the HCPCS Level II codes.

American Academy of Family Physicians (AAFP) AAFP and its members are committed to care that is equitable for all people; centered on the whole person within the context of family and community; based on science, technology, and best available evidence; supported by lifelong professional learning; and grounded in respect and compassion for the individual. AAFP's vision is to transform health care to achieve optimal health for everyone. The mission of the AAFP is to improve the health of patients, families, and communities by serving the needs of members with professionalism and creativity.

American Academy of Orthopaedic Surgeons (AAOS) Nonprofit organization for orthopaedic surgeons and allied health professionals.

American Academy of Physician Assistants (AAPA) National organization that represents physician assistants (PAs) in all specialties and all employment settings. Its membership also includes PA students and supporters of the profession. Its mission is to promote quality, cost-effective, accessible health care and the professional and personal development of PAs.

American Academy of Professional Coders (AAPC) National organization composed of medical coders and billers. It offers examinations for becoming a Certified Professional Coder (CPC), Certified Professional Coder-Apprentice (CPC-A), Certified Professional Coder-Hospital (CPC-H), and Certified Professional Coder-Payer (CPC-P).

American Association for Accreditation of Ambulatory Surgery Facilities, Inc. (AAAASF) National organization established in 1980 to develop an accreditation program to standardize and improve the quality of medical and surgical care in ambulatory surgery facilities while assuring the public of high standards for patient care and safety in an accredited facility. Its mission is to develop and implement standards of excellence to ensure the highest quality of patient care through an accreditation program that serves both the medical community and the public interest by establishing a means for measuring medical competence and providing an external source for evaluating patient safety in the ambulatory surgery setting. AAAASF accreditation has been approved by some State Departments of Health in lieu of State Licensure. Many private insurance carriers recognize accreditation by AAAASF for reimbursement of covered procedures.

For insurance carriers that require Medicare certification, AAAASF has a separate program to evaluate and approve facilities for certification by Medicare, using the same peer inspection process that is used for regular accreditation.

American Association for Homecare (AAHomecare) Organization for the home care industry that includes intravenous therapy, medical services and manufacturers, and health providers. AAHomecare was created through the merger of the Health Industry Distributors Association's Home Care Division (HIDA Home Care), the Home Health Services and Staffing Association (HHSSA), and the National Association for Medical Equipment Services (NAMES).

American Association for Medical Transcription (AAMT) See *Association for Integrity of Healthcare Documentation (AIHD)*.

American Association of Health Plans (AAHP) In 2003 the Health Insurance Association of America (HIAA), Group Health Association of America (GHAA), and the American Managed Care and Review Association (AMCRA) merged with American Association of Health Plans (AAHP) and created what is now known as *America's Health Insurance Plans (AHIP)*. See *America's Health Insurance Plans (AHIP)*.

American Association of Medical Assistants (AAMA) National organization composed of medical assistants, medical assisting students, and medical assisting educators with state and local chapters. It (1) promotes education for clinical and administrative medical assistants, (2) establishes educational requirements for national certification and continuing education requirements for recertification, and (3) is recognized by the American Medical Association.

American Association of Preferred Provider Organizations (AAPPO) National association of network-based preferred provider organizations (PPOs) and affiliate organizations established in 1983 that puts control in the hands of the physician and patient, therefore empowering both results in the best care. PPOs provide easy access to quality care from the right doctor, providing the right care at the right time. AAPPO promotes and supports the PPO industry, consumers enrolled in PPOs, and the collaborative effort of the industry to reduce health care costs. Member organizations include PPOs, provider organizations, network-based health plans, affiliate organizations, and specialty networks including chiropractic, dental, laboratory, mental health, ophthalmic, pharmacy, physical therapy, and workers' compensation.

American Association of Retired People (AARP) A nonprofit organization protecting the rights and needs of retired individuals.

American College of Allergy, Asthma and Immunology (ACAAI) Professional association of allergists and immunologists. Established in 1942, the ACAAI is dedicated to improving the quality of patient care in allergy and immunology through research, advocacy, and professional and public education. The ACAAI's goals are to (1) improve the quality of patient care in allergy, asthma, and immunology; (2) maintain and advance the diagnostic and therapeutic skills of members and foster their appropriate application; (3) sponsor and conduct educational and scientific programs and publications; (4) develop and disseminate educational information for members, patients, health plan purchasers and administrators, and other physicians and health professionals.

American College of Medical Coding Specialists (ACMCS) Nonprofit professional coders organization that offers certification as a Physician Coding Specialist (PCS), Facility Coding Specialist (FCS), and Coding Specialist for Payors (CSP).

American College of Surgeons (ACS) Nonprofit scientific and educational association of surgeons that was founded in 1913 to improve the care of the surgical patient by setting high standards for surgical education and practice. Examples of activities conducted by ACS include educational programs such as the Clinical Congress and standard-setting programs in cancer and trauma care.

American College of Surgeons Professional Association (ACSPA) Affiliated nonprofit corporation founded by the American College of Surgeons (ACS) Board of Regents in 2002 to develop new products and services to benefit surgeons and their patients. An initial and major component of ACSPA's efforts is the formation of a political action committee (PAC) that will work to improve the legislative and regulatory climate in which surgeons practice.

American Dental Association (ADA) Professional organization for dentists that has guidelines for completion and submission of a dental claim form. The ADA maintains the Current Dental Terminology (CDT) medical code set. The ADA and the Dental Content Committee (DeCC), which it hosts, have formal consultative roles under the Health Insurance Portability and Accountability Act (HIPAA).

American Group Practice Association (AGPA) See *American Medical Group Association (AMGA).*

American Health Care Association (AHCA) Nonprofit federation of affiliated state health organizations, together representing more than 10,000 nonprofit and for-profit assisted living, nursing facility, developmentally disabled, and subacute care providers that care for more than 1.5 million elderly and disabled individuals nationally. AHCA represents the long-term care community to the nation at large—to government, business leaders, and the general public. It also serves as a force for change within the long-term care field, providing information, education, and

administrative tools that enhance quality at every level. At its Washington, D.C., headquarters, the association maintains legislative, regulatory, and public affairs, as well as member services staffs that work both internally and externally to assist the interests of government and the general public, as well as member providers.

American Health Information Management Association (AHIMA) National professional organization for promoting the art and science of medical record management and improving the quality of comprehensive health information for the welfare of the public. AHIMA offers educational services and professional certifications for coding and sponsors some compliance educational seminars.

American Hospital Association (AHA) Organization formed in 1913 to advance the health of individuals and communities through leading, representing, and serving health care provider organizations that are accountable to the community and committed to health improvement. AHA maintains the central office on ICD-9-CM, answers coding questions, and publishes the *Coding Clinic for ICD-9-CM.* AHA hosts the National Uniform Billing Committee (NUBC), which has a formal consultative role under HIPAA.

American Institute of Certified Public Accountants (AICPA) National voluntary association of certified public accountants.

American Managed Care Review Association (AMCRA) See *American Association of Health Plans (AAHP).*

American Medical Association (AMA) National professional society of physicians formed in 1847 that develops and promotes medical practice, research, and education on behalf of patients and physicians. The AMA publishes the *Physician's Current Procedural Terminology (CPT)* code book and maintains the coding system. AMA is the secretariat of the National Uniform Claim Committee (NUCC), which has a formal consultative role under HIPAA.

American Medical Group Association (AMGA) Organization founded in 1950 that represents medical groups including some of the nation's largest, most prestigious integrated health care delivery systems. AMGA advocates for the multispecialty medical group model of health care delivery and for the patients served by medical groups through innovation and information sharing, benchmarking, leadership development, and continuous striving to improve patient care. Headquartered in Alexandria, Virginia, AMGA is the strategic partner for medical groups providing a comprehensive package of benefits including political advocacy, educational and networking programs and publications, benchmarking data services, and financial and operations assistance. It was formerly known as *American Association of Medical Clinics (AAMC)* and became American Group Practice Association

(AGPA). Then in mid-1996 it merged with Unified Medical Group Association (UMGA) to form the American Medical Group Association (AMGA).

American Medical Informatics Association (AMIA) Professional organization that promotes the development and use of medical informatics for patient care, teaching, research, and health care administration.

American National Standards (ANS) National standards developed and approved by organizations accredited by the American National Standards Institute (ANSI).

American National Standards Institute (ANSI) Nonprofit accredited organization founded in 1979 that approves all national standards. It formed the Accredited Standards Committee X12 (ASC X12), which is responsible for establishing electronic communication standards for banking, insurance, and health care. It handles health care–related standards including claims and remittance mandated by the Health Insurance Portability and Accountability Act of 1996. ANSI accredits other standards-setting committees and oversees their compliance with an open rule-making process that they follow to qualify for ANSI accreditation.

American Nursing Association (ANA) Professional organization representing registered nurses (RNs) through 54 constituent member associations. ANA advances the nursing profession by fostering high standards of nursing practice, promoting the economic and general welfare of nurses in the workplace, projecting a positive and realistic view of nursing, and by lobbying the Congress and regulatory agencies on health care issues affecting nurses and the public.

American Osteopathic Association (AOA) Member association founded in 1897 that represents osteopathic physicians (DOs). AOA serves as the primary certifying body for DOs and is the accrediting agency for all osteopathic medical colleges and health care facilities. AOA's mission is to advance the philosophy and practice of osteopathic medicine by promoting excellence in education, research, and the delivery of quality, cost-effective health care within a distinct, unified profession. AOA stands firmly behind osteopathic physicians' ethical and professional responsibilities to patients and the medical profession.

American Psychiatric Association (APA) International professional organization of psychiatrists and related medical specialists that renders services for people with mental disease, mental retardation, and substance-related disorders.

American Psychological Association (APA) Professional organization for advancement of psychology as a science and profession and promotes health, education, and human welfare.

American Society for Testing and Materials (ASTM) National standards group that formed the ASTM Committee E31 on Health Care Informatics.

It published general guidelines for development of standards for health care identifiers.

American Society of Anesthesiologists (ASA) National association of anesthesiologists that maintains and publishes guidelines for coding anesthesia services.

American Standard Code for Information Interchange (ASCII) Common computer coding system used for data communications that uses 128 numbers for a set of letters and characters, leaving 128 numbers as extras in an eight-bit byte. Programmers use the extra characters to create graphic characters, applicable to specific computers. The abbreviation is commonly pronounced "AS-key."

Americans with Disabilities Act (ADA) Federal law that provides disabled employees equal treatment regarding the "terms, conditions, and privileges" of employment including the right to a harassment-free work environment.

AMIA See *American Medical Informatics Association (AMIA).*

AMLOS See *arithmetic mean length of stay (AMLOS).*

amortization Process of the gradual retirement of an outstanding debt by making periodic payments over a stated period of time.

amount billed Fee charged for the medical services rendered to a patient by a provider and submitted or transmitted by the provider on an insurance claim form. When the provider is billing, this total charge is inserted in Block 28 of the CMS-1500 insurance claim form. When the hospital is billing, this total charge is inserted in Field 47 of the UB-04 insurance claim form.

amount, duration, and scope Medicaid parameters defining a state's benefits. Because each state has different Medicaid plans, these benefits will vary from state to state.

amount-in-controversy (AIC) requirements In the Medicare program, the dollar amount of a medical service that has been denied and then appealed by the provider and patient to the insurance carrier for redetermination.

AMPS See *automated Medicaid payment system (AMPS).*

ANA See *American Nursing Association (ANA).*

anatomic modifiers In Healthcare Common Procedure Coding System (HCPCS) Level II coding, two alphanumeric characters placed after the usual five-digit CPT procedure code number. These modifiers are used to identify specific anatomical parts of the body when the CPT procedure code does not include that information. HCPCS modifiers are accepted by insurance carriers nationally and are updated annually by the Centers for Medicare and Medicaid Services (CMS).

anchor group Large medical group composed of multispecialists with multidisciplines that under managed care contracts handle the bulk of treatments and referrals of member patients and carry most of the clinical risk. Also called *key groups* or *core groups.*

ancillary Supplemental health care service required as part of giving other care such as anesthesia, laboratory, pharmacy, and radiology; other than routine hospital services (room, board, medical and nursing services).

ancillary charge Fee for an ancillary service that is sometimes billed as an additional service such as anesthesia, laboratory, pharmacy, or radiology charge and which may exceed the managed care plan's maximum allowable.

ancillary medical provider Medical professional with a limited license to practice medicine and therapy who may bill for these services. See also *nurse practitioner (NP), physician extender (PE),* and *physician assistant (PA).*

ancillary medical services 1. Supportive professional services other than room, board, and routine hospital services that are incidental to the hospital stay and provided by the facility such as ambulance, anesthesia, blood administration, drugs, laboratory tests, pharmacy, operating room, x-rays, medical, surgical, and central supplies; physical, occupational, and speech therapy; and inhalation therapies. Also called *inpatient ancillary services.* 2. In a medical office setting, ancillary medical services may consist of diagnostic tests such as x-rays or laboratory tests.

ancillary services See *ancillary medical services.*

and Word that is one of the conventions used in the diagnostic code book titled *International Classification of Diseases, Tenth Revision, Clinical Modification (ICD-10-CM).* When the term "and" is used in a narrative statement, it represents and/or. This convention does not appear in the former ICD-9-CM code books.

anemia Condition occurring when the blood is deficient in red blood cells and/or hemoglobin, which decreases the oxygen-carrying capacity of the blood.

anesthesia Partial or complete absence of normal sensation in the body. Anesthesia induced for medical purposes may be topical, local, regional, or general and should always be given by a doctor or a specially trained nurse.

anesthesia formula Payment formula is performed by taking the base anesthesia procedure units and adding them to the time reported, as well as units for physical status modifiers, qualifying circumstances, and any other allowed units or charges. This sum is multiplied by a conversion factor.

anesthesia minutes of service See *anesthesia time.*

anesthesia section Division of the *Current Procedural Terminology (CPT)* code book that contains information about anesthesia services.

anesthesia time Surgical time period during a procedure in which an anesthesiologist and anesthetist, or both, participate. The elapsed time is documented and begins when the anesthesiologist prepares the patient for the operation and ends when the patient is taken to the hospital recovery room. Also called *anesthesia minutes of service.*

anesthesiologist Doctor of Medicine (MD) who specializes in anesthesiology, the medical specialty concerned with the pharmacological, physiological, and clinical aspects of anesthesia and related fields.

anesthesiology Study of the administration of anesthesia drugs or gas to produce nerve blocks or loss of sensation in a patient.

anesthetist Individual who administers anesthesia drugs or gas to a patient before or during an operative procedure.

anniversary See *anniversary date.*

anniversary date 1. Start of a benefit year for an insured subscriber group; date on which a policy was issued. 2. Date an employee begins a new year of employment. Also called *anniversary* or *policy anniversary.*

announcement material Brochures, bulletins, memos, and advertisements used to solicit, enroll, and explain an insurance program.

annual completion factor Computation adjustment of 12 months of incurred and paid insurance claims to 12 months of expected incurred insurance claims. See *incurred claims* and *expected incurred claims.*

annual contractor evaluation report (ACER) Under the Medicare program, this is a yearly assessment report of a provider who contracts to render medical services to Medicare beneficiaries.

annual cost of living increase Social Security benefits and supplemental security income payments increased each year to keep pace with increases in the cost of living (inflation).

annual deductible See *deductible.*

annual election period (AEP) For Medicare beneficiaries, this is a time of year, during the month of November, in which all Medicare+Choice health plans are open and accepting new members. Enrollment begins the following January. See *election period.*

annual maximum Highest dollar amount that an insurance company will pay on all claims experienced in 1 year for an insured as stated in the insurance contract.

annual statement End-of-year report of an insurance company to the state insurance department that shows assets, liabilities, receipts, disbursements, and other financial data.

annually renewable term (ART) insurance See *yearly renewable term (YRT) insurance.*

annuitant 1. Individual who receives annuity payments. 2. Person whose lifetime is used as a measurement for establishing the length of time benefits are payable under a life annuity.

annuity 1. Contract that provides an income for a period of time such as a specific number of years or for life. 2. Right to give or receive a series of payments of an amount of money. Originally this was done on an annual basis, but currently payments may be made periodically during a year or over a certain period of time. Some types of annuities are *deferred annuity,* *immediate annuity, single premium annuity, variable annuity, whole life annuity,* and *life annuity.*

annuity certain Contract that provides an income for a specific number of years, regardless of life or death.

annuity consideration Payment, or one of the regular periodic payments, an annuitant makes for an annuity.

annuity period Time between each benefit payment in an annuity contract.

annuity units Ownership shares in a variable annuity's separate account fund after the accumulation period ends. Annuity units are purchased with accumulation units and are used to establish benefit payment amounts. See also *accumulation units.*

ANS See *American National Standards (ANS).*

ANSI See *American National Standards Institute (ANSI).*

ANSI 835 See *electronic remittance advice (ERA).*

antepartum Pregnancy time period between conception and the onset of labor.

anterior (A) Located in the front or toward the belly surface of the body.

anteroposterior (AP) Located front to back.

anteroposterior and lateral (AP and L) Phrase used in describing two x-ray projections or views (front to back and side) in the radiological examination.

Anti-Kickback Act of 1986 See *Stark I Regulations* and *Stark II Regulations.*

antimarkup rule Medicare regulation that limits the amount that can be billed by a physician or group practice for the technical component of diagnostic tests (excluding clinical diagnostic tests performed by clinical laboratories) that are performed by an outside supplier.

antirebate law Statute in most states that it is illegal practice by an insurance agent to discount or return any portion of his or her commission to encourage an applicant to buy or renew an insurance policy.

antireferral statutes Laws that forbid a physician from referring a patient to receive a service or supply in which the referring physician has a financial relationship to the supplier. Also known as *Stark I Regulations* and *Stark II Regulations.*

antitrust laws Federal and state statutes that prohibit institutional mergers and acquisitions, exclusive contracts, joint ventures, price discriminations, price fixing, monopolies, and business dealings in situations that may greatly reduce competition, which may lead to a detrimental effect on consumer welfare. In medical care, this concerns arrangements between specialists that render exclusive service contracts with their hospitals. The main federal antitrust acts are: Sherman Antitrust Act (1890), Clayton Act (1914), Federal Trade Commission Act (1914), and Robinson-Patman Act (1936).

any willing provider (AWP) laws Multiple state laws that establish policies for managed care agreements that require a provider network must enroll any provider who meets the network's plan provisions.

AOA See *American Osteopathic Association (AOA).*

AOE/COE See *arise out of employment and in the course of employment (AOE/COE).*

AP 1. See *anteroposterior (AP).* 2. HCPCS Level II modifier that may be used with CPT or HCPCS Level II codes indicating there was no determination of refractive state during an eye examination. Use of this modifier does not affect payment.

AP and L See *anteroposterior and lateral (AP and L).*

AP-DRG See *all patient diagnosis-related group (APDRG or AP-DRG).*

APA See *American Psychiatric Association (APA)* and *American Psychological Association (APA).*

APC system See *ambulatory payment classification (APC) system.*

APDRG See *all patient diagnosis-related group (APDRG or AP-DRG).*

APGs See *ambulatory patient groups (APGs).*

appeal 1. Request for a review of an insurance claim that has been underpaid or denied by an insurance company to receive additional payment. Such requests are made to the health plan by the patient who is represented by the physician or provider who submitted the original insurance claim. Appeals to self-insured plans are submitted to the employer or U.S. Department of Labor. In some cases, an appeal may be submitted to the Department of Insurance of the state where the plan is located. 2. Redetermination process whereby the provider and/or beneficiary (or representative) exercises the right to request a review of a contractor's decision to deny Medicare coverage or payment for a service in full or in part. Also called *postservice appeals.* See also *preservice appeal* and *expedited appeal.*

appeal process In the Medicare program, a course of action used by a patient (beneficiary) if he or she disagrees with any decision about the health care services received. Now referred to as *redetermination process.*

appeal review 1. Request process to reconsider a decision by an insurance plan after a first appeal. 2. In the Medicare program, the first step for an appeal is called redetermination (telephone, letter, or CMS-20027 Form) and the second step after a first appeal is called *reconsideration.*

appeal rights Right of an individual or provider to ask for a review of the case for a possible change in the decision.

appeals board In workers' compensation cases, this phrase refers to the Workers' Compensation Appeals Board (WCAB) of the Division of Workers' Compensation in each state.

appellant Individual who appeals a claim decision.

Appendix A Section of the CPT manual located near the back that is a comprehensive list of all the two-digit CPT modifiers and two-digit Level II HCPCS national modifiers with complete explanations for their use.

Appendix B Section of the CPT manual near the back that contains a complete list of additions, deletions, and revisions from the previous edition.

applicant 1. Person applying for insurance coverage. 2. Practitioner, provider, or supplier that is applying for a Medicare national provider number.

application for benefits See *application form.*

application form 1. Request form to be completed with pertinent data when applying for employment. This may be done in person, by telephone, or on the Internet. 2. Statement of information form that is completed and signed by an individual to obtain insurance coverage. The prospective insured is required to undergo a medical examination. The information supplied on this form and the results of the medical examination assist the insurance company in making a decision whether to accept or reject the risk. The application is usually made part of the policy.

appointment of health care agent See *power of attorney* and *durable power of attorney for health care.*

apportionment In workers' compensation cases, the process of determining if some portion of an injured worker's permanent disability is due to a cause other than the current injury. This is an estimate of the degree of either occupational or nonoccupational factors that may have contributed to the impairment. Apportionment applies only to permanent disability.

appraisal Professional evaluation to determine a property's insurable value or the amount of a loss.

appropriateness Term used by some health plans to define the proper setting of medical care for which the expected health benefits exceeds the expected negative outcome by sufficient margin to justify treatment. Also referred to as *appropriateness of care.*

appropriateness evaluation protocol (AEP) Nineteen criteria for admission under the prospective payment system, separated into two categories: severity of illness and intensity of illness. To allow a patient admission to an acute care facility, one criterion from each category must be met.

appropriateness of care See *appropriateness.*

approval See *preauthorization.* Also see *precertification* and *predetermination.*

approval wire Blue Cross and Blue Shield phrase that means the formal notice sent by a host plan from the home plan after the home plan has received the admission wire and verified membership information. This approval is given for a specific number of days and insurance contract benefits. See also *admission wire.*

approved amount See *approved charge.*

approved charge 1. Maximum dollar value the commercial private insurance company or managed care contract assigns to each procedure or service on which payment is based. Typically, a percent (e.g., 80%) of the allowed amount is paid by the insurance carrier. 2. Allowed amount based on the Medicare fee schedule or its transition rules, which may or may not be the same as the actual amount billed. The patient may or may not be responsible for the difference. Nonparticipating physician charges are subject to the limiting charge. 3. Also called the *allowed amount* or *approved amount.* See also *Medicare-approved amount, maximum allowable,* and *maximum allowable charge (MAC).*

approved health care facility 1. Medical facility authorized to provide medical services and specific health care services stated in managed care contracts. 2. Hospital authorized to treat and admit beneficiaries of the Medicare program. Also known as *approved health care hospital.*

approved health care hospital See *approved health care facility.*

approved health care program Medical program certified or endorsed to provide services to members of a managed care plan or beneficiaries of a federal program (e.g., Medicare, TRICARE).

approved services See *benefit package.*

APR See *average payment rate (APR)* and *adjusted payment rate (APR).*

APS See *Attending Physician's Statement (APS).*

APT See *admissions per 1000 (APT).*

AQ Modifier used by physicians who provide medical services in health professional shortage areas (HPSAs) that became effective January 1, 2006. Previously, two modifiers (QB and QU) distinguished between physicians providing HPSA services in rural areas and those providing HPSA services in urban areas. These are no longer used.

AR 1. HCPCS Level II modifier that may be used with CPT or HCPCS Level II codes indicating a physician scarcity area. Use of this modifier affects Medicare payment. 2. Abbreviation for accounts receivable. See *accounts receivable (AR).*

A/R transaction See *accounts receivable (A/R) transaction.*

arbitration Proceeding for settling a dispute in which disputes are given to a third party or panel of experts to hear two sides of the story and who has power to make a legal binding decision for both parties on the case.

area See *locality.*

Area Agency on Aging (AAA) Local (city or county) organization, funded under the federal Older Americans Act, that plans and coordinates various social and health service programs for persons 60 years of age or more. These needs include adult day care, skilled nursing care/therapy, transportation, personal care, respite care, and meals. The network of AAA offices consists of more than 600 approved agencies.

ARGUS Software program created by the Office of the Inspector General (OIG) that helps to access provider claims data and to limit the need for the OIG to send multiple requests to insurance carriers for claims information. It can assist in detection of aberrant billing practices of providers.

ARHCP See *Association of Registered Health Care Professionals (ARHCP).*

arise out of employment and in the course of employment (AOE/COE) In workers' compensation cases, a criterion for determining liability, or whether a claim is or is not compensable. AOE refers to how the activity of work led to the injury in question. It is one of the legal tests that must be met for a medical condition to be covered by workers' compensation insurance. COE refers to how the activity the employee was engaged in at the time of injury must grow out, or be incidental to, the employment.

arithmetic mean length of stay (AMLOS) In the Medicare program, the average number of days for a patient's DRG inpatient hospital stay. This figure is used to determine payment for outlier cases and to predict occupancy rates. To obtain this number, use this formula: total number of patient days divided by (÷) the total number of hospital admissions for a specific time period. It is also known as *average length of stay (ALOS).*

armed services disability Disability occurring or aggravated while the patient is in military service.

ARNP See *advanced registered nurse practitioner (ARNP).*

arrears Status of an insurance policy on which the monthly premiums have not been paid by a subscriber or member and are past due but which has a grace period that has not expired.

arrow (➲) Symbol used in the procedure code book titled *Current Procedural Terminology (CPT).* It is used to identify where to find additional reference material about a procedure code.

arson Willful, deliberate, and malicious act of setting fire to property.

ART See *Registered Health Information Technician (RHIT).*

AS 1. See *administrative simplification (AS).* 2. HCPCS Level II modifier that may be used with CPT or HCPCS Level II codes indicating services of an assistant at surgery. Use of this modifier affects Medicare payment. 3. See *assistant surgeon (AS).*

ASA See *American Society of Anesthesiologists (ASA).*

ASC See *Accredited Standards Committee (ASC X12); ambulatory surgery center (ASC).*

ASC payment group rate Payment received by an ambulatory surgery center (ASC) when a Medicare beneficiary has a covered surgical procedure performed in an ASC. ASC procedures are grouped into eight payment categories.

ASC surgical procedure Operative procedure performed in an ambulatory surgical center (ASC) and done as an outpatient.

ASC X12 See *Accredited Standards Committee X12 (ASC X12).*

ASCII Commonly pronounced "AS-key." See *American Standard Code for Information Interchange (ASCII).*

ASCs See *ambulatory surgery categories (ASCs).*

ASO See *administrative services only (ASO).*

ASO agreement See *administrative services only (ASO) agreement.*

ASR See *age/sex rates (ASR).*

assessment Systematic collection and review of data (test results, signs, symptoms) pertaining to an individual for either receiving health care services or to enter a health care setting.

assets 1. Anything owned that has exchange value, e.g., cash, federal treasury notes and bonds, property, data processing equipment, and investments. 2. Under Medicaid, property owned that the government takes under review when a patient applies for financial assistance. 3. Under Medicare Part D, the government counts cash or any property that can be turned into cash within 20 days, such as checking and savings accounts, certificates of deposit, IRAs, and 401(k)s, stocks, bonds, and similar items. It does not include a patient's primary home, or certain property related to burial expenses. 4. Treasury notes and bonds guaranteed by the federal government, owned properties, and cash held by the trust funds for investment purposes.

assigned claim Insurance claim form from a provider sent to the insurance company on which the provider agrees to accept the Medicare allowable amount as payment in full for the services and payment is sent directly to the provider of the service.

assigned risk Uncertainty (risk) that insurance underwriters do not want to insure but because of state laws are required to insure. For example, individuals who may be within a certain young age group, may have had an automobile accident, heart condition, diabetes, or hypertension. Most assigned risks are issued insurance through a system of proportional assignment chosen from a group of insurance companies. This is more commonly seen in casualty insurance.

assigned risk plan State-supervised automobile insurance plan that has been obtained through a proportional assignment from a group of insurance companies because the insured is unable to buy in the regular or voluntary market. Each driver in the plan is assigned to an insurance company. Cost of this insurance is higher than in the regular market.

assignee Individual to whom contract rights are transferred under an assignment.

assignment 1. Transfer of ownership rights in a life insurance policy or other type of contract from one individual to another. 2. Document that creates the transfer of ownership rights of a life insurance policy to go into effect. See also *absolute assignment* and *collateral assignment.* 3. Transfer, after an event insured against, of an individual's legal right to collect an amount payable under an insurance contract. 4. For Medicare, an agreement in which a patient assigns to the physician the right to receive payment from the fiscal intermediary. Under this agreement, the physician must agree to accept 80% of the allowed amount as payment in full, once the deductible has been met. 5. For TRICARE, providers who accept assignment agree to accept 75% or 80% of the TRICARE allowable charge as the full fee, collecting the deductible and 20% or 25% of the allowable charge from the patient. 6. In hospital billing, the assignment is inserted in Field 53 of the Uniform Bill (UB-04) inpatient hospital billing claim form. Also known as *assignment of benefits.*

assignment of benefits See *assignment.*

assignor Individual who transfers specific contract rights under an absolute or collateral assignment.

assistant-at-surgery See *assistant surgeon (AS).*

assistant surgeon (AS) Physician who gives assistance to another surgeon during the performance of an operation on a patient. Also called *assistant-at-surgery.*

assisted living Care for long-term, physical non-occupational activities of daily living (ADL), such as bathing, continence, dressing, eating, housekeeping, laundry, medications, mobility, transferring in and out of bed or a chair, using the toilet, and walking. These individuals want to remain independent and do not require constant care. In most cases, the "assisted living" residents pay a regular monthly rent. Then, they typically pay additional fees for the services they receive, such as hair cuts or pedicures.

assisted living center (ALC) Residences that provide help with the activities of daily living (ADLs) and that emphasize residents' privacy and choice. Residents typically have private locking rooms (only shared by choice) and bathrooms. Personal care services are available on a 24-hour-a-day basis, licensed as residential care facilities or as rest homes. The size of an ALC may range from 3 to 15 residents to as large as 600 to 800 residents. Also called *assisted living facility (ALF), adult foster care, domiciliary care,* or *residential care.*

assisted living facility (ALF) See *assisted living center (ALC).*

associated signs and symptoms Changes in normal bodily function or any indication of disease perceived by the patient that are documented in detail in the patient's medical record. These details are used to assist in establishing a diagnosis.

association 1. Group of individuals who unite together for business purposes. 2. In psychology, the connection of remembered feelings, emotions, sensations, thoughts, or perceptions with certain persons, ideas, or situations.

Association for Electronic Health Care Transactions (AFEHCT) Organization that promotes efficient, secure, and cost effective health information data exchanges in an open electronic environment using industry standards. Web site: www.afehct.org.

Association for Integrity of Healthcare Documentation (AIHD) Organization established in 1978 as part of an effort to achieve recognition for the medical transcription profession; formerly known as *American Association for Medical Transcription (AAMT).* Vision: To direct the evolution of the medical transcription profession. Mission: To advance and represent the profession of medical transcription through the promotion of quality health care documentation. Purpose: To set and uphold standards for education and practice in the field of medical transcription that ensure the highest level of accuracy, privacy, and security of health care documentation for the U.S. health care system to protect public health, increase patient safety, and improve quality of care for health care consumers. Goals and Objectives: Medical transcriptionists are provided the tools to ensure accuracy, privacy, and security of health care documentation to improve patient safety and quality of care through the following objectives: Participate in the development of health care documentation standards to protect consumer privacy and security of medical information; advocate for legislation and regulations that protect the public's health care information; set standards of education and practice for the medical transcription profession.

Association of Registered Health Care Professionals (ARHCP) Nationwide community of members that support medical providers practicing in the United States and advance their knowledge of important socioeconomic issues through continuing education, exchange of ideas between members, and certification programs that recognize personal educational achievements.

assuming company See *reinsurer.*

assumptions Values relating to future trends in certain key factors that affect the balance in the trust funds. Demographic assumptions include fertility, mortality, net immigration, marriage, divorce, retirement patterns, disability incidence and termination rates, and changes in the labor force. Economic assumptions include unemployment, average earnings, inflation, interest rates, and productivity. Also called *demographic assumptions.*

assurance Word that means "insurance" that is commonly used in Canada and Great Britain.

ASTM See *American Society for Testing and Materials (ASTM).*

AT HCPCS Level II modifier that may be used with CPT or HCPCS Level II codes indicating acute treatment services.

at risk contract Type of managed care contract between Medicare and a payer or a payer and a provider wherein patients receive care during the entire term of the contract even if actual costs exceed the payment established by the agreement.

ATD See *Aid to the (permanently) Disabled (ATD).*

attachment See *claim attachment.*

attained age Age of the insured as of the insured's last birthday.

attending physician Medical staff member who is legally and primarily responsible for the medical care and treatment given to a patient and who would normally be expected to certify and recertify the medical necessity of the number of services rendered for the patient's care while in the hospital. An attending physician who has a patient admitted to the hospital may be referred to as the admitting physician.

attending physician's statement (APS) Form that, when completed, provides the insurance company with information about the patient's injury or illness, diagnosis, and treatment. An APS form is completed when the insurance company requests information to decide whether to insure an individual or, if insured, when settling an insurance claim.

attrition rate Disenrollment from a health insurance plan expressed as a percentage of total membership. For example, a managed care plan with 40,000 members with a 2% attrition rate would need to gain 800 new members each month to retain the initial 40,000 covered lives.

AU HCPCS Level II modifier that may be used with CPT or HCPCS Level II codes indicating item(s) used with urological, ostomy, or tracheostomy supplies. Use of this modifier affects Medicare payment.

audiologist Individual who has a certificate of clinical competence from the American Speech and Hearing Association and has completed the equivalent educational requirements and work experience necessary for the certificate or has completed the academic program and is acquiring supervised work experience to qualify for the certificate.

audiology Research and clinical practice of the study of hearing disorders, examination of hearing, aural rehabilitation, and hearing observation.

audit 1. Formal, methodical examination or review done to inspect, analyze, and scrutinize the way something is being done (e.g., bookkeeping practices, medical record documentation, insurance claim filing) to determine operational efficiency. 2. In the Medicare program, a process to ensure that the fiscal intermediary reimburses providers based only on costs associated with patient care.

audit by request Type of audit of hospital patient records that occurs when a patient asks for an audit to verify hospital charges. Also see *defense audit* and *random internal audit.*

audit of provider Formal review for quality and quantity of medical services rendered and fees charged by a provider. Various methods used are: comparing patient records and insurance claim form data, patient questionnaire, review of hospital records, and pretreatment or posttreatment clinical examination of patients.

audit trail (audit log) Ongoing record of events or paper trail or path left by a transaction when it is processed. The software tracking system traces the history including the identity of the person who used the computer, when it was used, what patient information was accessed, medical record or billing number, and history of actions to computer files or programs. The Health Insurance Portability and Accountability Act (HIPAA) mandates this type of system for patients' medical information. See *HIPAA.*

auditor Professional who reviews and evaluates a provider's utilization, medical necessity of treatment provided, quality of care, and level of reimbursement.

augmentation Add to or increase a body site (e.g., plastic reconstruction procedure, implant, prosthesis, bone or soft tissue graft).

AUR See *ambulatory utilization review (AUR).*

authenticate 1. Verify authorship of a patient's medical record by signature, initials, or rubber stamp that data are accurate, complete, and final. 2. Verify or identify access privileges of a user or user device to an information system. 3. Process to certify that a document is genuine.

authoritative approval Method of type of approval that requires a determination that the service is likely to have a diagnostic or therapeutic benefit for patients for whom it is intended.

authoritative evidence Written medical or scientific conclusions demonstrating the medical effectiveness of a service produced by the following: controlled clinical trials, published in peer-reviewed medical or scientific journals; controlled clinical trials completed and accepted for publication in peer-reviewed medical or scientific journals; assessments initiated by the Centers for Medicare and Medicaid Services (CMS); evaluations or studies initiated by Medicare contractors; case studies published in peer-reviewed medical or scientific journals that present treatment protocols.

authorization 1. Under the HIPAA privacy rule, an individual's formal, written permission to use or disclose his or her personally identifiable health information for purposes other than treatment, payment, or health care operations. 2. Verbal or written agreement that a third-party payer will pay for professional services rendered. 3. Requirement in some health insurance plans to obtain permission for a service or procedure before it is done and to see whether the insurance program agrees it is medically necessary. Also called *preauthorization.* See also *precertification.* 4. Legal document giving an individual the right to act.

authorization form Under the Health Insurance Portability and Accountability Act (HIPAA), this is a document signed by the patient that is necessary for use and disclosure of protected health information (PHI) that is not included in any existing consent form agreements.

authorization number Approval number given to a provider who requests a specific service, treatment, test, or procedure. It does not guarantee payment if the insurance claim does not establish medical necessity and appropriateness of the care requested for a patient.

authorized official 1. Individual who is a direct owner of 5% or more of a provider (e.g., business partner, chairman of the board, chief financial officer, chief executive officer, president). 2. Person to whom the provider gives legal authority to be enrolled in the Medicare program. The authorized official can make changes or updates to the provider's status in the Medicare program and signs a statement that the provider will abide by the laws and regulations of Medicare.

authorized provider Physician, other individual authorized provider of care, hospital, or supplier who meets the licensing and certification requirements, practices within the scope of that license, and is approved by TRICARE to provide medical care and supplies.

authorized reinsurer See *admitted reinsurer.*

autologous bone marrow transplant (ABMT) Type of treatment for cancer in which the patient is his or her own bone marrow donor as compared with allogenic bone marrow transplant in which the donor is another individual.

automated claim review Claim evaluation and determination made using system logic (edits). Automated claim reviews never require the intervention of a human to make a claim determination.

automated claims payment Computerized claims processing system used in reimbursement of medical, dental, or disability insurance claims.

automated clearinghouse (ACH) Third-party administrator (TPA) that receives information from another entity, performs software edits, and redistributes the claims electronically to various insurance carriers in a standard transaction. Also known as *clearinghouse.*

automated eligibility verification system (AEVS) An interactive voice response system in the Medi-Cal program that allows providers to access recipient eligibility, clear share of cost, and/or reserve a Medi-Service.

automated Medicaid payment system (AMPS) Name of an insurance claim reimbursement method that uses computer technology in settling Medicaid claims.

automatic bill payment Bank service that permits payment by one check to a number of creditors or direct payment by the bank for specified recurring bills by monthly transfer of funds (e.g., payment of insurance premiums). See also *electronic funds transfer system (EFTS)* and *preauthorized payment.* Also called *bank check plan, check deposit billing, electronic funds transfer system (EFTS), check-o-matic, preauthorized checking,* or *preauthorized payment.*

automatic premium loan option Insurance plan choice that automatically pays any premium that is in default at the end of a grace period (usually 31 days). This payment is charged against the insurance policy as a loan, provided the premium is not in excess of the policy's cash surrender value on the due date of the premium.

automatic renewal clause Clause in a contract that automatically reestablishes the contract with the same terms for another stated period of time. See also *reinstatement.*

automatic reinstatement clause Clause in an insurance policy that provides for automatic restoration of the full face value of the policy after payment for a loss. Also called *reinstatement.*

automatic reinsurance Type of formal agreement between a reinsurer and a ceding insurer that automatically transfers the risks and their acceptance by the reinsurer. Also called *treaty.*

automatic stay Court order that goes into effect once a bankruptcy petition is filed; all other legal actions such as attachments and foreclosures are halted.

automobile Under Medicare Secondary Payer guidelines, this is defined as any self-propelled land vehicle of a type that must be registered and licensed in the state in which it is owned.

automobile insurance An automobile owner's protection against various risks such as bodily injury liability, medical, property damage, collision, comprehensive, and uninsured motorists.

automobile insurance premium discounts Some insurance companies reduce premium rates for drivers who have good driving records, have taken a driver education course, are between the ages of 50 and 74, car pool, buy homeowner's or renter's insurance from the same company, install antitheft prevention devices and receive antitheft prevention services, or drive cars with special safety features.

automobile policy See *automobile insurance.*

automobile premium Cost of automobile insurance coverage paid either monthly, quarterly, or annually to an insurance company that keeps the policy in force. Insurance companies base their premium rates on historical loss experience for similar risks.

AV HCPCS Level II modifier that may be used with CPT or HCPCS Level II codes indicating item(s) furnished with a prosthetic or orthotic device.

availability 1. One of the assessments made by The Joint Commission to see if the performance and location of medical services is available to meet the demands of an individual's and a community's needs. 2. Measurement in terms of type, volume, and location of the supply of health resources and services relative to the needs or demands of an individual or a community. Health care is available to an individual when he or she can obtain it at the time and place that he or she needs it, from appropriate personnel. Available is a function of the distribution of appropriate resources and services, as well as the willingness of the provider to serve the particular patient in need. See also *access* and *acceptability.*

available hours Regular, overtime, and holiday hours for which pay is earned and for which time is provided by an assigned employee to perform the medical work.

available time Hours worked in health care.

average community rate (ACR) See *adjusted community rate (ACR)*.

average daily census Count (enumeration) and demographics of hospital inpatients or members of a managed care plan. The census is given in a daily hospital admission and disposition report that shows patients gained and lost in census, changes in status, and numerical strengths of transient patients and boarders.

average daily patient load—bassinet (ADPL-BASS) Average number of live births in the hospital that are provided medical care daily during a specific report period. The formula is to divide the number of bassinet days during the period by the total number of days in the report period. See *bassinet day*.

average daily patient load—inpatient (ADPL-IP) Average number of hospital inpatients, excluding live births, who receive care daily during a specific period that is to be reported. This includes same-day admission/discharge patients. The formula is to divide the number of inpatient bed days during the period by the total number of days in the report period.

average daily patient load—total (ADPL-TOT) Average number of inpatients including live births that receive care daily during a specific period, which is to be put into a report. This includes same-day admission/discharge patients. The formula is to divide the sum of occupied bed days during the period by the total number of days in the report period.

average daily revenue (ADR) Formula for determining the ADR is performed by dividing revenue for a 3-month period ending on the date of the calculation by the number of days in the 3-month period.

average length of stay (ALOS) See *arithmetic mean length of stay (AMLOS)*.

average market yield Computation that is made on all marketable interest-bearing obligations of the United States. It is computed on the basis of market quota-tions as of the end of the calendar month immediately preceding the date of such issue.

average monthly earnings (AME) Formula for finding the AME is to divide the total earnings in a computation year by the number of months in those same years. This dollar amount (AME) is used to calculate a worker's monthly Social Security benefit.

average payment rate (APR) Amount of money the Centers for Medicare and Medicaid Services (CMS) could pay a health maintenance organization (HMO) for services given to Medicare beneficiaries under a risk contract.

average resources Relative volume and types of diagnostic, therapeutic, and hospital/facility bed services used in managing a particular illness.

average weekly wages (AWW) In workers' compensation cases, employee's ability to earn wages including tips, gratuities, and nonmonetary earnings, expressed as a weekly earnings amount. AWW is established by using earnings from up to the 12 months (52 weeks) prior to the injury and divided by the actual number of weeks used.

average wholesale price (AWP) 1. Pharmaceutical price based on common data and written in a pharmacy provider contract. 2. Average cost for a medicine charged to pharmacy providers by a pharmaceutical wholesaler supplier.

AVGs See *ambulatory visit groups (AVGs)*.

avoidable hospital condition Situation in which the patient's diagnosis for which he or she was hospitalized could have been avoided if ambulatory care was given in an immediate and efficient manner.

avulsion Ripping or tearing away of a part.

AW HCPCS Level II modifier that may be used with CPT or HCPCS Level II codes indicating item(s) used with a surgical dressing.

AWP 1. See *average wholesale price (AWP)*. 2. See *any willing provider (AWP) laws*.

AWW See *average weekly wages (AWW)*.

AX HCPCS Level II modifier that may be used with CPT or HCPCS Level II codes indicating item(s) used with dialysis services.

B

BA 1. See *business associate (BA)*. 2. HCPCS Level II modifier that may be used with CPT or HCPCS Level II codes indicating item(s) used with parenteral enteral nutrition (PEN) services.

baby boom Period from the end of World War II through the mid-1960s marked by unusually high birth rates.

baby group plan See *small group insurance plan*.

back charge Amount owed by an insured (policyholder) on a current billing statement for premium due on insurance that has lapsed.

back date Issuance of an insurance policy for an individual or a group that is effective on a month, day, and year earlier than the date of actual issue so that the premium rate will be lower. State law usually limits backdating to not more than 6 months. Also called *dating back*.

back-loaded policy Life insurance policy in which most of the expense charges occur when the policyholder gives up the policy or makes cash withdrawals from the policy. Generally, charges are highest in the beginning policy years and eliminated at the end of a certain number of years.

backloading System in which there is a higher accrual of pension benefits during a participant's later years of employment. This is designed to encourage long employment.

backlog Queue of insurance claims at the insurance company that have not been processed for payment (adjudicated) to the provider of medical services.

backup Duplicate data file; tape, CD-ROM, disk, or external hard disk used to record data; it may be used to complete or redo an operation if the primary equipment fails.

bad debts Accounts receivable considered uncollectible in a medical practice because of failure of patients to pay amounts owed. This does not include write-off accounts of indigent patients.

balance Amount owed on a credit transaction; also known as the *outstanding* or *unpaid balance*.

balance bill 1. In third-party payer cases, this is the amount the provider bills the patient after the insurance payment has been posted. This amount may be the copayment and deductible and also the difference between the physician's fee for medical services and the amount paid by the insurance company. 2. In Medicare cases, the participating physician accepts the Medicare-allowed amount and the patient may not be billed for the balance. The balance difference is not collected and an adjustment entry is posted to the patient's financial account. However, the patient is also responsible for the 20% copayment and deductible. Also called *excess charge*. 3. In some plans, this billing amount is limited to the difference between the insurance plan's allowable fee and the amount paid by the plan. Patients are responsible for copayments, coinsurance amounts, and deductibles.

balance billing Act of the provider of medical services to bill the patient for charges not paid by the insurance company. This is prohibited in the Medicare program and some managed care contracts if the physician has accepted assignment. See *balance bill*. Also called *excess charge*.

balance sheet 1. Financial accounting statement that shows the assets, liabilities, and equity of a medical practice. 2. Financial document that contains a tabulated list of the assets and liabilities of an insurance company as of a specific date.

Balanced Budget Act of 1997 (BBA) Federal legislation signed and passed on August 5, 1997, that changes sections of the Social Security Act. Its purpose is to reduce spending, balance the federal budget, and fight fraud and abuse. It introduced provisions and improvements to protect program integrity such as permanent exclusion for those convicted of three health care–related crimes on or after the date of enactment and mandated prospective payment systems for outpatient and home health services. Sometimes the Balanced Budget Act of 1997 is informally pronounced as "bubba."

Balanced Budget and Emergency Deficit Control Act of 1985 See *Gramm-Rudman-Hollings Act*.

BAMC See *Board of Advanced Medical Coding (BAMC)*.

band grading To group life insurance policies according to death benefit amounts for the intent of calculating loading.

bank check plan See *electronic funds transfer system (EFTS)*, *automatic bill payment*, and *preauthorized payment*.

bankruptcy Condition under which a person or corporation is declared unable to pay debts.

baptismal certificate Religious record of an individual's birth or baptism that is used to establish age in certain situations.

BAR See *billing and accounts receivable (BAR)*.

barium enema Suspension of barium sulfate injected into the lower bowel to render it radiopaque, usually followed by injection of air to inflate the bowel and increase definition for the purposes of identifying disorders or early signs of cancer.

base capitation Specific dollar amount per member per month (PMPM) in a managed care plan that covers medical costs. Usually this excludes administrative costs, mental health services, pharmacy, and substance abuse services.

base charge Specific dollar amount from the Medicare fee schedule that is allowed for a participating provider according to the specialty. Commonly referred to as *participating provider's fee*.

base estimate Updated approximation of the most recent historical year.

base payment amount Dollars and cents amount that is established for one unit as applied to a service rendered or product furnished. This unit (sometimes called a *conversion factor*) is then used to convert various services/procedures into fee-schedule payment amounts by multiplying the relative value unit by the conversion factor (base payment amount). It establishes the level of the payment rates in the payment system.

base plan Basic health insurance plan that gives limited first-dollar hospital, surgical, or medical benefits as compared with major medical benefit plans that provide comprehensive hospital, surgical, and medical coverage.

base rate Dollar amount assigned to a hospital that assists in adjusting diagnosis-related group (DRG) payment. The base rate takes into account the hospital's geographic location, status (urban, rural, teaching), and local labor costs.

base unit Value that is determined by taking fees, work, and cost of a group of services or procedures to develop a relative value scale for payment. Also referred to as *basic value*.

base year costs Medicare phrase that means the amount a hospital actually spends to provide care in a prior time period. Usually the base year is the fiscal year that ends on or after September 30, 20XX, and before September 30, 20XX, of the next year.

base years For Social Security benefits, wage earner's years after 1950 up to the year of entitlement to retirement or disability insurance benefits. For a survivor's claim, the base years include the year of the worker's death.

basic and major medical program Insurance plan that combines basic benefits with major medical benefits. Usually this insurance coverage has no front-end deductible and benefits begin with the first dollar of expense incurred by the patient for a covered benefit. Sometimes basic benefits are referred to as "first-dollar" benefits.

basic benefits Base health services listed in an individual's health insurance plan plus coverage required under applicable federal and state regulations. Also called *basic medical benefits*.

basic compensation Wages paid to an employee excluding overtime, bonuses, and other types of additional compensation. It may or may not include commission income. This financial amount is a way of determining an employee's benefits and insurance contributions.

basic coverage 1. Insurance protection to offset hospital expenses for an individual. 2. Under Blue Cross and Blue Shield plans, this is coverage exclusive of major medical. 3. For Medicare beneficiaries, basic coverage is Medicare Part A and/or Part B exclusive of any supplemental coverage.

basic death benefit Death benefit in keeping with the terms of the original, basic contract of a life insurance policy, which is equivalent to the face amount. A basic death benefit does not include supplementary riders (e.g., accidental death benefit [ADB] rider). See also *death benefit* and *face amount*.

basic experience table See *basic mortality table*.

basic health services 1. Specific benefits that federally qualified health maintenance organizations (HMOs) must offer to enrollees, defined under Subpart A, 110.102 of the Federal HMO Regulations. 2. Minimum health services that should be available for adequate health care for a population.

basic life insurance Insurance policy that provides for payment of a specific dollar amount on the insured's death either to his or her estate or to a designated beneficiary so named.

basic medical benefits See *basic benefits*.

basic mortality table Statistical table without a safety margin that shows the death rate at each age, expressed as so many per thousand. Also called a *basic experience table*.

basic premium Premium for workers' compensation or life insurance that takes into consideration the following: an individual having an average expectation of loss, insurance company's administrative expenses, and insurance agent's commission. Also called *standard premium rate*.

basic value See *base unit*.

basket clause 1. In investing, a rule that allows insurance companies to invest a small percentage of their assets without statutory restrictions. 2. In accounting, a clause that permits life and health insurers to keep a specific amount of their assets as nonauthorized assets that are not restricted in the same way as authorized assets.

bassinet day Day in which a live birth occupies a bassinet in the hospital's newborn nursery and is continuous since birth at the time the census is done for a report. The status of the mother does not affect this.

batch Group of claims for different patients from one office submitted in one computer transmission.

batch balancing Process of comparing the number of documents that have been processed against a control total that has been estimated (e.g., an insurance company that issues 500 claims checks that are batch balanced against 500 insurance claims).

batch number Assigned numerals to each group of insurance claims processed for different patients from one office and submitted in one computer transmission. The batch number appears on the document (report) when payments are made for the batch.

batch processing Method used by a provider to group (collect) computerized transactions over a period of time and transmit them in a single operation either at night or in a time-delayed manner (e.g., daily insurance claims).

bathing Ability of an individual to wash oneself on a routine basis in the bathtub, shower, or by sponge bath. Also see *activities of daily living (ADLs)*.

BBA See *Balanced Budget Act of 1997 (BBA)*.

BCBSA See *Blue Cross and Blue Shield Association (BCBSA)*.

beaming Electronic, wireless method of transferring files from one computer to another computer or personal digital assistant device. The devices are pointed toward each other and selected files are transferred.

bearer See *payee*.

bed Place for sleeping or resting in a hospital or other inpatient medical facility. The size of a hospital is often referred to by its number of bed capacity. Licenses and certificates of need (CON) are granted for the numbers or types of beds such as extended care, obstetric, pediatric, and surgical.

bed, available Vacant, accessible bed that is obtainable to a patient.

bed capacity See *bed count*.

bed capacity, expanded Space that is available for patient beds in addition to the number of beds that can be occupied in hospital units.

bed conversion Changing a bed assigned for one type of care to a bed designated for another type of care such as converting an acute-care bed to a long-term care bed. See also *swing bed*.

bed count Total number of beds maintained by a hospital or inpatient health facility for a designated patient population. Also called *bed capacity* or *bed size*.

bed day, inpatient Day spent by a patient in an available bed at the hour (midnight) census is taken in the hospital, excluding bassinet days. This includes the patients admitted and discharged for same-day surgeries.

bed days per 1000 (bed days/1000) See *days per thousand (DPT)*.

bed, occupied by transient patient Hospital bed assigned as of midnight to a patient who is to be moved between medical facilities and who stops to stay over while en route to his or her destination before reaching the next facility.

bed, operating Hospital bed ready for the medical care of a patient that includes the space, equipment, and

staff. This excludes transient patient beds, bassinets, incubators, labor beds, and recovery beds.

bed, set up Hospital bed set up and ready for the medical care of a patient that includes space, equipment, medical material, and ancillary and support services but no available staff to operate.

bed size See *bed count*.

beds, licensed Number of hospital beds that are licensed and certified and capable of operating. This includes space, equipment, medical material, and ancillary and support services, but staff may not be available. Licensed beds equal the total of operating beds and set-up beds.

beginning balance Account balance at the beginning of a period that is an amount owed on a credit transaction. It is also known as *account balance carried forward*, *running balance*, or *outstanding* or *unpaid balance*.

behavior health care Examination and treatment of mental health, chemical dependency, forensic, mental retardation, developmental disabilities, and cognitive rehabilitation services provided in acute, long-term, and ambulatory care settings. Also called *behavioral health care*.

behavioral health care See *behavior health care*.

benchmark Sustained superior performance by a medical care provider, which can be used as a reference to raise the mainstream of care for Medicare beneficiaries. The relative definition of superior will vary from situation to situation. In many instances, an appropriate benchmark would be a provider that appears in the top 10% of all providers for more than a year. Factors that are looked at to determine what to benchmark are physician productivity, practice efficiency, revenue generation, coding performance, and collections. A practice management system can be used to generate reports on the most important factors at regular intervals.

benchmarking Continual comparison measurement of a medical practice to those of the toughest competitor to find and implement methods to improve the business. There are three types: *internal benchmarking*, *competitive benchmarking*, and *functional benchmarking*. Internal is when similar processes in the same organization are compared. Competitive is when an organization's processes are compared with the best medical practices within the industry. Functional refers to benchmarking a similar function or process in another industry (e.g., appointment scheduling).

beneficial occupancy date (BOD) Month, day, and year on which a health care facility is available to provide the services it was built for.

beneficiary 1. Individual entitled to receive insurance policy or government program health care benefits. Enrollees in the Medicare and Medicaid programs are commonly referred to as *beneficiaries*. Also known as *participant, subscriber, dependents, enrollee, recipient,* or *member*. 2. Dependents eligible for TRICARE or CHAMPVA benefits. 3. Person named in the insurance policy or pension plan to receive the proceeds at the death of the insured (policyholder). Types of beneficiaries are: *alternate beneficiary, contingent beneficiary, irrevocable beneficiary, primary beneficiary, revocable beneficiary, secondary beneficiary, successor beneficiary,* and *tertiary beneficiary.*

beneficiary appeal See *appeal.*

beneficiary declaration Separate written document after an insurance policy has been issued that designates the beneficiary.

beneficiary encrypted file Restricted public use file for which a completed Agreement for Release of the Centers for Medicaid and Medicaid Beneficiary Encrypted Files is required.

beneficiary impersonation Use of a lost, stolen, or fraudulently obtained Medicare or Medicaid identification card to unlawfully procure federal or state benefits.

beneficiary notification letter Letter required with the Centers for Medicaid and Medicaid Services (CMS) administrator's signature when Medicare beneficiaries are contacted to participate in a research project.

beneficiary of benefits See *beneficiary.*

benefit 1. Health care service that the insurance company agrees to pay to a claimant, assignee, or beneficiary under a health insurance policy or contract. 2. Amount of money an insurance company (payer) will pay for the medical care and services. See *covered expenses* or *coverage.* Also called the *policy benefit.*

benefit booklet See *benefit limitations* and *explanation of coverage (EOC).*

benefit contract See *benefit plan.*

benefit days 1. Total number of days that an insurance company will pay within a benefit period. 2. Under the Medicare program, the number of days that a beneficiary is entitled to receive payment for covered services with the exception of lifetime reserve days. Also see *lifetime reserve.*

benefit exhausted date Medicare phrase that refers to the date on which the beneficiary has used the maximum benefits for a current benefit period. This applies when a patient refuses to use or has used all of his or her lifetime reserve days. Under the Medicare program, a reserve of 60 days of inpatient hospital care is available over an individual's lifetime beyond the normal limit. Also see *lifetime reserve.*

benefit formula Method for establishing the amount of benefit payable under each contingency (unforeseen event) covered by a group insurance contract. The formula includes salary and job or years of employment at the time the benefit is paid.

benefit levels 1. Limit of benefits an individual is entitled to receive depending on the insurance policy. 2. In workers' compensation cases, benefit levels for an injured employee are set by state laws.

benefit limitations Insurance provision that restricts coverage regardless of medical necessity. Benefit limitations may be found in the explanation of coverage section of the insurance policy or in a booklet supplied by the insurance company. Also known as *benefit booklet, benefit plan summary, summary plan description*; also see *explanation of coverage (EOC).*

benefit maximum Highest dollar amount that an insurance company or managed care plan will pay for specified health care services. A benefit can be expressed either as a length of time (e.g., 60 days of semiprivate hospital room charges) or as a dollar amount (e.g., $1500 for a certain procedure).

benefit plan Insurance contract that provides hospital, surgical, medical, or other health coverage; also called *benefit contract.*

benefit plan summary See *explanation of coverage (EOC).*

benefit of survivorship Annuity payable to the annuitant for as long as the recipient is alive at the time the payment is due.

benefit package Covered medical services a managed care plan or government program offers to individuals or to groups. In addition to physician and hospital services, some insurance policies have coverage for acupuncture, alternative therapies, assisted living care, chiropractic care, dental, drugs, home nursing care, skilled nursing care, and vision care. Also called *approved services, benefit plan, benefits,* and *health benefits package.*

benefit payment schedule List of fees, sometimes with procedural code numbers of the services, and description of the services that an insurance plan will pay and are covered under the managed care plan or insurance policy. Also known as *schedule of benefits, table of allowances, fee schedule, fee allowance, fee maximum,* or *capped fee.*

benefit payments Amounts disbursed for covered services to beneficiaries after the deductible and coinsurance amounts have been deducted.

benefit period 1. Time period for which benefits are payable under an insurance contract without a new deductible requirement. These effective dates of coverage can be a designated 6-month period, calendar year, or a plan's anniversary date. Also called *spell of illness.* 2. Period of time for which payments for Medicare inpatient hospital benefits are available. A benefit period begins the first day an enrollee is given inpatient hospital care (nursing care or rehabilitation services) by a qualified provider and ends when the enrollee has not been an inpatient for 60 consecutive days. Patient must pay the hospital insurance deductible for each benefit period. 3. In workers' compensation cases, the maximum amount of time that benefits will be paid to the injured or ill person for the disability.

benefit plan See *benefit package* and *certificate of coverage (COC).*

benefit plan summary See *benefit limitations*.

Benefit Policy Manual (BP) See *Medicare Benefit Policy Manual (BP)*.

benefit products Phrase used by insurance companies and managed care companies that refers to the types of insurance plans they offer; also used as a synonym for *benefits*.

benefit provision Health care service explained in detail that the insurance company agrees to pay to a claimant, assignee, or beneficiary under a health insurance policy or contract.

benefit schedule Under a group insurance plan, a table that lists the amount of coverage given to each class of insured and may show earnings and job position. Also known as *benefit payment schedule, schedule of benefits, table of allowances, fee schedule, fee allowance, fee maximum*, or *capped fee*.

benefit verification letter Official document from the Social Security Administration that provides information on how much an individual receives in monthly Social Security benefits and/or Supplemental Security Income payments. A letter is normally issued after a request from a beneficiary or his or her authorized representative.

benefit waiting period Time period that must elapse before health insurance benefits are payable.

benefit year Twelve-month period used by employers for administration of health benefits. Most employers' benefit year is from January through December. However, a benefit year does not always coincide with a group's fiscal year. See *benefit period*.

benefits See *benefit package, benefit products*, and *Social Security benefits*.

benefits description Scope, terms, and conditions of coverage including any limitations associated with the plan provision of the service. Also called *benefits plan* and *benefit package*.

benefits identification card (BIC) Medi-Cal identification card.

Benefits Improvement and Protection Act (BIPA) of 2002 Federal legislation that made the Medicare appeals process easier to negotiate with clearly defined levels that address reasons for rejection based on complexity of the situation. Terminology for these levels is called "redetermination" or "reconsideration" and is no longer known as an appeal.

benefits plan See *benefits description*.

benign tumor Neoplasm (growth) that does not have the properties of invasion and metastasis and is usually surrounded by a fibrous capsule.

BIC See *benefits identification card (BIC)*.

bilateral procedure A surgical procedure performed on both sides of the body or organ.

bilateral surgery Situation when a surgical procedure is performed on both sides of the body or organ. A five-digit CPT code number is used with an attached

modifier -50 to list the procedure. If listing more than one modifier, place modifiers affecting reimbursement first, in descending order, followed by status modifiers.

bill To assign a fee for medical services and supplies provided by a provider that were rendered to the patient and to present an itemized statement of the charges.

bill cycle 1. Day of the month on which specific groups (Medicare, Medicaid, managed care, commercial payers) are scheduled to be billed. There are 30 bill-cycle days per month including weekends and holidays. 2. Day of the month on which specific accounts by alphabet, account number, insurance type, or date of first service are scheduled to be billed. Also see *cycle billing*.

bill frequency Rate of regularity that a subscriber or group is billed by the insurance company for premiums due. This may be monthly, quarterly, or annually.

billed-at-home See *direct pay*.

billed claims Insurance claims with fees and procedural and diagnostic code numbers submitted by the provider to the insurance plan for health care services or supplies provided to their enrolled members or insureds.

billed direct See *direct pay*.

biller Individual who completes and transmits insurance claim forms for professional services rendered to a patient by a health care provider or supplier to insurance carriers and/or fiscal agents for private, state, or federal programs.

billing 1. To send a statement for medical services rendered to the patient. 2. In Medicare fraud, to bill for services or supplies that were not provided. This includes billing for "no shows" (i.e., billing for a service not actually furnished because a patient failed to keep an appointment).

billing address Patient's or third-party payer's location (street, city, state, and zip code) to which a billing statement is sent.

billing and accounts receivable (BAR) Automated functions that address the procedures and processes of billing and accounts receivable.

billing and service specialist Individual designated to an insured group who handles collection of charges and subscriber correspondence and other clerical and administrative tasks.

billing limit In the Medicare program, the amount the physician can bill for a procedure and the maximum amount he or she can collect from the patient when the claim is taken unassigned. Formerly known as *maximum allowable actual charge (MAAC)*. See *limiting charge*.

billing manager Administrator or supervisor of the medical billing and collections department, which may or may not include diagnostic and procedural coding.

billing provider Provider (physician, clinic, group) who submits an insurance claim for reimbursement for services rendered to a patient.

billing service Company that charges a fee for billing patients, collecting on accounts, and submitting insurance claims to insurance plans for physicians and/or suppliers.

billing statement See *itemized billing statement.*

binding receipt See *temporary insurance agreement (TIA).*

biological father 1. Male who genetically fathered a child. 2. Male who genetically fathered an adoptee. See *birth father.*

biological mother Female who is genetically the mother of an adoptee. Also known as *birth mother.*

biologicals Drugs or vaccines made from a live product and used medically to diagnose, prevent, or treat a medical condition (e.g., flu, pneumonia injection).

biometric identifier Personal identification based on a physical characteristic and used for security purposes such as a fingerprint. Sometimes a personal identification number (PIN) may be used with the fingerprint sample to gain access to a computer or other system.

biopsy Removal and examination, usually microscopic, of tissue from the living body to establish a diagnosis.

birth certificate Original record maintained by a governmental entity including states, counties, parishes, cities, and/or boroughs that documents an individual's birth.

birth father 1. Male who genetically fathered a child. 2. Identifies the male who is biologically the parent of an adoptee. Also known as *biological father.* See *biological father.*

birth mother 1. Female who genetically births a child. 2. Identifies the female who gave birth to an adoptee. Also known as *biological mother, natural mother*, or *real mother.* See *biological mother.*

birthday law Legal state statute to determine coordination of benefits for primary and secondary carriers of dependent children covered under both parents' insurance plans. The health plan of the parent whose birthday (month and day, not year) falls earlier in the calendar year pays first, and the plan of the other person covering the dependent is the secondary payer. If both policyholders are born on the same day, the policy that has been in force the longest is the primary policy. Birth year has no relevance in this situation. Also called *birthday rule.*

birthday rule See *birthday law.*

birthing center Facility, other than a hospital's maternity department or physician's office, that is owned and operated by obstetricians or nurse midwives and located near a hospital. It is a less expensive alternative to hospitalization and mainly for low-risk deliveries. It provides a setting for labor, delivery, and immediate postpartum newborn care, as well as immediate care of newborn infants.

bit Binary digit, either a 1 or 0.

Black Lung Benefits Act See *Federal Coal Mine Health and Safety Act of 1969.*

Black Lung Program See *Federal Coal Mine Health and Safety Act of 1969.*

blanket authorization One-time release of confidential information form that because of the Health Insurance Portability and Accountability Act (HIPAA) is no longer used. Also see *authorization.*

blanket contract Comprehensive group insurance coverage through plans sponsored by professional associations for their members such as athletic teams.

blanket coverage 1. Health insurance benefits under a family subscriber contract for dependents whose names and ages are not stated on the insurance application form. 2. Insurance policy that covers several different properties at either a single location or in different locations. 3. Insurance contract that is issued to cover several individuals such as an athletic team.

blanket insurance See *group health plan.*

blanket medical expense Insurance provision that gives the insured a stated maximum in the policy for hospital and medical expenses without limits on individual types of medical expenses.

blanket position bond Insurance that provides coverage for all employees regardless of job title, in the event of a financial loss to the employer by the act of an employee.

blended payment rate Combination of federal and local area wage indexes that was used to phase in a prospective payment system.

blended rates Group mortality rates based partially on a group's experience and partially on manual rates. These rates are used to establish the right group insurance premium rates for intermediate-size groups.

blind mailing To send resume with cover letter to possible prospects that the individual does not know personally and that have not advertised for a job opening.

blogging See *blogs.*

blogs Online publications that allow anyone with Internet access to become an instant publisher. Content can range from personal thoughts (diary or journal) to news to analysis or political rants. Also known as *weblogs.* When physicians or health care workers participate, it is referred to as *medical blogging* or *medblogging.* Under HIPAA compliance regulations, patients' names and clinical information cannot be used in blog messages.

blood deductible Number of unreplaced pints of whole blood or units of packed red blood cells given to a Medicare patient that he or she is responsible for. A Medicare patient is responsible for paying for the first three pints of blood used in each calendar year unless they are replaced. This policy applies to Medicare Part A and Part B benefits. The Part A blood deductible is reduced to the extent that the blood deductible under Part B is satisfied.

blood, urea, nitrogen (BUN) Measure of the amount of urea in the blood, which is the major breakdown product of protein metabolism and is removed by the kidneys. It is determined by a blood test. During kidney failure, urea accumulates in proportion to the degree of kidney failure and to the amount of protein breakdown. Symptoms of uremia correspond roughly to the amount of urea in the blood.

Blue Cross Insurance programs that provide protection against the costs of hospital, surgical, and professional care. Most are nonprofit organizations and other managed care plans for their subscribers. Blue plans contract with the federal government as an administrative agency for federal health programs.

Blue Cross and Blue Shield Association (BCBSA) National organization (trade association) headquartered in Chicago that represents state and local Blue Cross and Blue Shield health plans and administers rules and regulations for regional Blue plans. BCBSA acts as the administrator for the Health Care Code Maintenance and helps maintain the HCPCS Level II code system. It is America's oldest and largest family of health benefits companies and the most recognized brands in the health insurance industry. In 1929 it began by assuring hospital care to Texas teachers and providing physician care to lumber and mine workers in the Pacific Northwest. Regional plans process claims for members who have plan coverage for hospital expenses, outpatient care, other institutional services, home care, dental benefits, and vision care. Most of the affiliated organizations have converted to for-profit status, have plans similar to private insurance companies, and operate in much the same way as other private insurance carriers. Blue Cross/Blue Shield may act as a Medicare fiscal intermediary in certain regions. A provider must be contracted with Blue Cross/Blue Shield to receive payment as a member physician.

Blue Cross logo Registered symbol of the Blue Cross and Blue Shield Association that is used to identify all Blue Cross plans. It depicts a blue Greek cross with the figure of a man in the heart of the cross and the words Blue Cross. Also see *Blue Shield logo.*

Blue Cross plan Corporation that administers a voluntary prepayment medical/surgical/hospital program in a specific region and operates under the membership standards of the Blue Cross and Blue Shield Association (BCBSA). Individuals or groups that join the plan are called *members* or *subscribers,* and providers of service that contract with the Blue plan are called *member physicians.* Also see *Blue Shield plan.*

Blue Shield Insurance programs that provide protection against the costs of hospital care, surgery, and other items of medical care. Most are nonprofit

organizations offering prepaid health care services for their subscribers.

Blue Shield logo Registered symbol of the Blue Cross and Blue Shield Association that is used to identify all Blue Shield plans. It depicts a caduceus that is the Greek healing symbol over a shield in blue that signifies protection. The Buffalo, New York, plan designed the logo in 1929 based on the U.S. Army Medical Corps insignia. Also see *Blue Cross logo.*

Blue Shield plan Corporation that administers a voluntary prepayment medical/surgical/hospital program in a specific region and operates under the membership standards of the Blue Cross and Blue Shield Association (BCBSA). Individuals or groups that join the plan are called *members* or *subscribers* and providers of service that contract with the Blue plan are called *member physicians.* Also see *Blue Cross plan.*

BO HCPCS Level II modifier that may be used with CPT or HCPCS Level II codes indicating oral administration of nutrition using no tube.

board and care home See *adult care home.*

board certification Certification in a medical specialty based on the physician's proof of experience and expertise. If a physician wishes to practice a specialty, board certification is not a requirement. A doctor who meets the criteria to apply for board certification is referred to as "board eligible." Also see *board eligible.*

board certified Statement issued by a medical specialty board or association verifying that a physician or other health professional meets professional standards after having passed an examination. Also called *boarded* or *diplomate.*

board eligible Description of a physician who is entitled and qualified and who meets the criteria to take the specialty board examination (e.g., has graduated from an approved medical school, has completed specific training, has practiced medicine for a designated time period). Also called *board prepared.*

Board of Advanced Medical Coding (BAMC) Professional organization of coders, clinicians, and compliance professionals dedicated to the evaluation, recognition, and advancement of professional medical coders within physician practice, facility, and postacute settings. BAMC offers certification as Advanced Coding Specialists (ACS) to physician and facility coders who successfully complete the qualifying examination. Website: www.advancedmedicalcoding.com

Board of Healing Arts See *physician licensing board.*

Board of Medical Examiners See *physician licensing board.*

Board of Medical Practice See *physician licensing board.*

Board of Trustees Board established by the Social Security Act to oversee the financial operations of the Federal Supplementary Medical Insurance Trust Fund. The Board is composed of six members, four of whom serve automatically by virtue of their positions in the federal government: the Secretary of the Treasury, who is the Managing Trustee; the Secretary of Labor; the Secretary of Health and Human Services; and the Commissioner of Social Security. The other two members are appointed by the President and confirmed by the Senate to serve as public representatives. The Administrator of the Centers for Medicare and Medicaid Services serves as Secretary of the Board of Trustees.

board prepared See *board eligible.*

boarded See *board certified.*

boarder Person who receives lodging, is not a patient, but needs to be near the patient.

boarder baby 1. Newborn infant who remains in the hospital nursery after discharge because the mother remains hospitalized. 2. Premature infant who is out of intensive care but needs observation or to reach developmental milestones.

BOD See *beneficial occupancy date (BOD).*

body record Body or data record that contains information on a single outcomes and assessment information set (OASIS-B1) patient assessment.

body section radiography See *tomography.*

bond 1. Certificate of debt that contains a promise to pay and issued either on the security of a mortgage, a deed of trust, or on the credit of the issuer. 2. Obligation (fidelity bond) of an insurance company to protect the insured against financial loss caused by dishonesty of a covered employee. It would pay the insured up to the limits of the policy for such a loss. 3. Certificate of ownership of a specified portion of a debt due by the federal government to holders, bearing a fixed rate of interest.

bonding An insurance contract by which, in return for a stated fee, a bonding agency guarantees payment of a certain sum to an employer in the event of a financial loss to the employer by the act of a specified employee or by some contingency over which the employer has no control.

bone mass measurements Radiologic or radioisotopic procedure or other procedure that identifies bone mass, detects bone loss, or determines bone quality.

bonus Payment a physician receives beyond any salary, fee-for-service payments, capitation, or returned withhold from a managed care plan. Bonuses and other compensation that are not based on referral or utilization levels (such as bonuses based solely on quality of care, patient satisfaction, or physician participation on a committee) are not considered in the calculation of substantial financial risk.

bonus payment Additional dollar amount paid by Medicare for services provided by physicians in health professional shortage areas (HPSAs).

book of business Insurance payer's list of clients and managed care and private insurance contracts.

bookkeeping Process used for posting (recording), summarizing, and allocating all business transactions to show a company's income and expense by analyzing and verifying posted entries. The purpose is for collecting amounts due and reporting the financial condition of the business at a future date.

Boren Amendment From 1980 to 1997, federal law directly linked Medicaid nursing home rates with minimum federal and state quality of care standards. As part of the Omnibus Reconciliation Act of 1980, the "Boren amendment" required that Medicaid nursing home rates be "reasonable and adequate to meet the costs which must be incurred by efficiently and economically operated facilities in order to provide care and services in conformity with applicable state and federal laws, regulations, and quality and safety standards" (Section 1902[a][13] of the Social Security Act). State Medicaid officials overwhelmingly came to oppose the amendment as impossible to operationalize, believing that they were forced by the courts to spend too much on nursing homes at the expense of other services. The federal Balanced Budget Act of 1997 repealed the Boren amendment, giving states far greater freedom in setting nursing home payment rates.

bounce E-mail message returned to the sender either due to incorrect address or because of a configuration problem on the receiver's end.

boutique medicine See *concierge care.*

BP 1. See *business partner.* 2. HCPCS Level II modifier that may be used with CPT or HCPCS Level II codes indicating that the Medicare beneficiary elected to purchase the item. 3. See *Medicare Benefit Policy Manual (BP).*

BR 1. HCPCS Level II modifier that may be used with CPT or HCPCS Level II codes indicating the Medicare beneficiary elected to rent the item. 2. Abbreviation for by report. See *by report (BR).*

braces { } Punctuation symbols used in the diagnostic code book titled *International Classification of Diseases, Ninth Revision, Clinical Modification (ICD-9-CM).* It is used to enclose a series of terms, each of which is modified by the statement appearing at the right of the brace in the descriptions of the diagnoses. This convention does not appear in ICD-10-CM.

brackets [ ] Punctuation symbols used in the diagnostic code book titled *International Classification of Diseases, Ninth Revision, Clinical Modification (ICD-9-CM).* Brackets are used to enclose synonyms, alternate wording, and explanatory phrases of the descriptions of the diagnoses. This convention does not appear in ICD-10-CM.

branch manager Administrative individual of a field (branch) office of an insurance company. Also called a *general manager.*

branch office distribution system Common method in which insurance companies use commissioned agents to sell and deliver individual insurance policies and the agents work out of a field office under contract to the insurance company. The branch manager, supervisors, and clerical personnel in the field office are employees of the insurance company.

brand name drugs Prescription drugs that are sold under a registered trademark (brand) name. Also known as *trade name*.

breach of confidential communication "Breach" means breaking or violation of a law or agreement. In the context of the medical office, it means the unauthorized release of confidential information about the patient to a third party.

break-even point Level of membership in a managed care plan at which the situation of total revenues and total expenses are equal and produce neither a net gain nor loss from operations.

break in service Length of time between the date an employee leaves a company and the date the employee resumes work for that company. For pension and employee benefit plans, a plan participant cannot be deprived of benefits that accumulate before a break in service unless the break is longer than (1) five years or (2) the amount of time that the participant has been employed when the break commences, whichever is greater.

brief history of present illness (HPI) 1. In procedural coding and determining the extent of brief history of present illness or problem, there are two types: problem focused or expanded problem focused. 2. See *history of present illness (HPI)*.

broker State-licensed sales and service representative who handles insurance for his or her clients and may represent and sell insurance of various types and for several companies. By law, a broker may be an agent to the insurer for certain purposes such as delivery of the policy or collection of the premium. Also called *licensed broker*.

broker of record Insurance broker who has been designated in writing by a client to provide certain insurance coverages and services.

brokerage distribution system Method of some insurance companies that rely on commissioned agents (brokers) who sell various types of insurance for several companies.

brokerage general agency See *brokerage shop*.

brokerage manager Salaried insurance company employee or independent agent who is responsible for appointing brokers for the insurance company and encouraging brokers to sell the products of a specific insurance company.

brokerage shop Insurance agency operated by an independent general agent who is under contract with several insurance companies. Also known as a *brokerage general agency*.

BU HCPCS Level II modifier that may be used with CPT or HCPCS Level II codes indicating the Medicare beneficiary is undecided on purchasing or renting the item.

BUBBA Sometimes the Balanced Budget Act of 1997 is informally pronounced as "bubba."

budget neutrality Under Medicare, adjustment of payment rates so that total costs are expected to remain the same as under the previous payment rules.

buffing A physician's justifying the transference of sick, high-cost patients to other physicians in a managed care plan.

bug An error in a computer software program.

BUI See *Bureau of Health Insurance (BUI)*.

bullet (•) 1. Alert symbol used in the diagnostic code book titled *International Classification of Diseases, Ninth Revision, Clinical Modification (ICD-9-CM)*. It is used to indicate a diagnostic code or line of text that indicates the description is new to that specific annual edition. 2. New code symbol used in the procedure code book titled *Current Procedural Terminology (CPT)*. It is used to identify a service or procedure code that is new to that specific annual edition. 3. When an audit is taking place, term used to indicate evaluation and management criteria for documenting services rendered. Also known as an *element*.

BUN See *blood, urea, nitrogen (BUN)*.

bundled 1. Collection of several types of health insurance policies under one payer. 2. Inclusive grouping of procedural codes related to medical services when submitting an insurance claim.

bundled billing Establishing a price for an all-inclusive package or global fee for all medical services needed for specific procedures. Bundled billing may include professional and institutional services that are high-cost or common procedures (e.g., coronary artery bypass graft, kidney transplant, maternity care).

bundled codes To group more than one component (service or procedure) provided in one day into one CPT code for submission on an insurance claim.

bundled insurance product Type of life insurance in which the mortality, investment, and expense factors used to calculate premium rates and cash values are not identified separately in the policy (e.g., traditional whole life insurance).

bundled rate See *flat fee-per-case*.

bundling 1. To group minor medical services or surgeries together with principal procedures when provided at the same time and submit them to the insurance company for reimbursement. 2. A payment method in which the insurance company or government program groups together the payment of the lesser service into the payment for the principal procedure to reimburse the provider of the medical service. Also called *global pricing* and *package pricing*. See *packaging*.

Bureau of Health Insurance (BUI) Agency within the Social Security Administration that administers the Medicare program. Actual operation of the program is carried out through arrangements with fiscal intermediaries and insurance carriers, who operate under contract with BHI/SSA and receive all policy guidance from the Centers for Medicare and Medicaid Services (CMS).

burglary insurance Type of business and personal insurance for loss of property due to theft or larceny.

burnout Occupational illness in which there is mental or physical energy depletion after a period of chronic, unrelieved, job-related stress. It is characterized sometimes by physical illness, perception of being tired, and being disgruntled with one's work.

burns See *rule of nines*.

business associate (BA) Person who, on behalf of the covered entity, performs or assists in the performance of a function or activity involving the use or disclosure of individually identifiable health information including claims processing or administration, data analysis, processing or administration, utilization review, quality assurance, billing service, benefit management, practice management, medical transcription service, and repricing.

business associate agreement Contract between the provider and a clearinghouse that submits the electronic claims on behalf of the provider.

business coalition Organization of several employers with a purpose of monitoring and communicating information on health care issues that affect employees. These employers form a cooperative to manage the benefits and expenditures and purchase group health care insurance coverage at a discounted price for their employees.

business consultant See *physician advisor (PA)*.

business-continuation insurance Type of business insurance that provides funds so that the remaining business partners can buy the business interest of a deceased or disabled partner.

business ethics Moral standards as they apply to certain business policies, institutions, and behavior.

business insurance Insurance that insures the business rather than an individual person.

business interruption insurance Insurance policy that covers a business owner from losses during a time when the business is not operating due to fire or other peril. The insurance provides reimbursement for salaries, taxes, rent, necessary continuing expenses, and net profits that the business would have earned during the interrupted period.

business life insurance Life insurance bought by a business on the life of a member of the company. It may be bought by partnerships to protect the surviving partners against loss caused by the death of a partner, or by a corporation to receive payment for loss caused by the death of a key employee.

business model Type of business organization or process.

business office personnel Employees carrying out the administrative duties in a medical practice such as office manager, billing manager, receptionist, collection specialist, health information or medical record employees, and medical coders.

business partner (BP) Owner that performs an activity on behalf of another owner of the business who is not part of the workforce.

business relationships Person or organization that assumes some of the responsibilities of another one. This phrase has been avoided in the final Health Insurance Portability and Accountability Act (HIPAA) rules so that a more specific meaning could be used for business associate.

buy-in National program in which the state enters into an agreement with the Bureau of Health Insurance, which is under the Social Security Administration and obtains supplementary medical insurance benefits for eligible participants. The state pays the monthly health insurance premium on behalf of the beneficiary.

buy-out settlement See *financial settlement*.

buy-sell agreement Contract made by partners of a business to buy the share of a disabled or deceased owner and which terms are established before the beginning of disability or death.

by report (BR) Documentation in the form of a report submitted with the claim when the notation BR follows the procedure code description. This term is sometimes seen in workers' compensation fee schedules.

byte The number of bits used to represent one character.

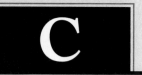

C See *comprehensive*.

C & R See *compromise and release (C and R)*.

C codes HCPCS codes that include device categories, new technology procedures, and drugs, biologicals, and radiopharmaceuticals that do not have other HCPCS assigned.

CA HCPCS Level II modifier that may be used with CPT or HCPCS Level II codes indicating the procedure is payable only in the inpatient setting but the patient was seen as an emergency (outpatient) and expired before admission to the facility as an inpatient.

CAAHEP See *Commission on Accreditation of Allied Health Education Programs (CAAHEP)*.

CAC See *Carrier Advisory Committee (CAC)* and *computer-assisted coding (CAC)*.

cadaveric transplant Surgical procedure of excising a kidney from a deceased individual and implanting it into a suitable recipient.

cafeteria plan 1. Managed care plan offered by an employer to his or her employees that allows them to select the type and amount of benefits from a "menu" of different options the employer offers such as health care, life insurance, vacation, and disability insurance. Some cafeteria plans give an employee a certain number of benefit "points," which can be used to purchase one or all of the benefits offered by the company. An employee who did not want to participate in a health plan could apply more points toward a 401(k) plan, life insurance, or any other benefit offered. Under some plans, the credits can be redeemed for cash. The employer pays for the plan with before-tax dollars. Also called *flexible benefit plan, flex plan*, or *flexible compensation*. 2. See *Section 125 of the Internal Revenue Code*.

CAH See *critical access hospital (CAH)*.

CAHPS See *consumer assessment of health plans survey (CAHPS)*.

CAL See *coverage analysis for laboratories (CAL)*.

calendar year (CY) Period of 1 year commencing on January 1 and ending on December 31.

calendar year deductible Common form of deductible under major medical and comprehensive medical expense insurance plans. Insureds may accumulate covered expenses for the purpose of satisfying the deductible for the entire 12-month period.

calendar year experience Occurrence or events developed on premium and incurred loss transactions that occur during the 12 calendar months beginning January 1, regardless of the effective dates of the insurance policies on which these transactions arose.

call center See *referral center*.

call share Physicians or providers on whom a medical practitioner depends for backup support during times that he or she is not available.

call share group Group of physicians with similar medical specialties who have joined together to give call share services.

callable Subject to redemption on notice (e.g., a bond).

CAM See *catchment area management (CAM)* and *complementary and alternative medicine (CAM)*.

cancelable contract See *cancelable policy*.

cancelable policy Individual health insurance policy that can be terminated at any time by the insurance company. Also called *cancelable contract*. See also *conditionally renewable*.

cancellation Termination of an insurance contract by either the insured or the insurance company before the contract matures or the end of its term period. This may occur for nonpayment of premiums.

cancer registrar Individual who captures a complete summary of the history, diagnosis, treatment, and disease status for every cancer patient. Registrars' work leads to better information that is used in the management of cancer and, ultimately, cures. Also see *National Cancer Registrars Association (NCRA)* and *Certified Tumor Registrar (CTR)*.

cap 1. Private insurance or managed care plan contract maximum amount (capital sum or principal amount) placed on the expenditure of money for a specific purpose (e.g., maximum benefit coverage). 2. Abbreviation for capitation.

CAP See *claims assistance professional (CAP)* and *capitation (cap or CAP)*.

cap rate See *capitation rate (cap rate)*.

capacity 1. Maximum amount of insurance an insurer or reinsurer is capable of underwriting for either one individual (single risk) or for all of its business. 2. Ability of a health care facility to provide necessary medical services.

capacity to contract Legal condition for both parties (insurance company and insured) to understand the insurance policy terms for a drawn-up agreement to be considered a valid contract.

capital gain Dollar amount profit that is made when stocks or bonds (securities) are sold. This is called a *realized gain*. An unrealized capital gain is when there has been an increase in the value of the stocks or bonds but they have not been sold.

capital stock Investment certificates that represent the amount of money or property contributed by shareholders invested to provide money for a corporation to do business and buy equipment.

capitated payment Annual fee paid by the insurance company to the physician, hospital facility, or network that provides health care to a patient.

capitation (cap or CAP) System of payment used by managed care plans in which physicians and hospitals are paid a fixed, per capita amount for each patient enrolled over a stated period of time (month or year), regardless of the type and number of services provided; reimbursement to the hospital on a per member per month (PMPM) basis to cover costs for the members of the plan.

capitation basis Method of compensation used by managed care plans in which a provider is paid either a flat amount per year per subscriber or a predetermined amount for each service. For the flat amount per year arrangement, the provider must treat the subscriber as often as needed during the year.

capitation rate (cap rate) 1. Providers and managed care plans negotiate a per member per month (PMPM) amount per enrollee to cover the expected cost of services to be provided to a member. The provider gives all contracted care and services to members for a prospective payment with retroactive adjustments, taking the risk that the capitation rate will cover all of the costs of care to the members. Although cap rates are usually fixed, they can be adjusted for the age or gender of members based on actuarial (statistical) projections of health care utilization. 2. Under Medicare guidelines, fixed amount the Centers for Medicare and Medicaid Services (CMS) pays to an approved managed care plan selected by an enrolled Medicare beneficiary.

capped fee See *fee schedule.*

capped rental item Durable medical equipment that costs more than $150 (e.g., nebulizers, manual wheelchairs) and is rented by the supplier to Medicare beneficiaries more than 25% of the time.

captive Insurer that is created and owned by one or more noninsurers to provide their owners with insurance coverage.

captive agent Individual who has agreed to sell insurance for only one company. Also called *exclusive agent.*

captive insurance company Insurance company formed and controlled by a separate company, whose purpose is to insure the risks of its owner(s) such as hospitals, physicians, companies that extend credit to customers, banks, and retailers. Also called *captive insurer.*

captive insurer See *captive insurance company.*

captured care Percentage of a provider's care to be given under an exclusive managed care and/or capitation contract.

cardiology Study of the anatomy, normal functions, disorders, and diseases of the heart.

care Providing to an individual hospital accommodations, comfort, diagnosis, and treatment of a condition and implying responsibility for services, equipment, supplies, and rehabilitation.

CARE See *Continuity Assessment Record and Evaluation (CARE).*

Care/Caid See *Medicare/Medicaid (Medi-Medi).* Also see *crossover patient.*

Care/Caid case See *Medicare/Medicaid (Medi-Medi).* Also see *crossover patient.*

care management See *case management.*

care mapping See *disease management.*

care plan See *plan of treatment.*

care plan oversight (CPO) services Continuous review and revision of a patient's complex care and treatment by the primary care physician. Usually these involve cases of children and adults under either the home health agency (HHA) or hospice benefit that have special health care needs and chronic medical conditions (e.g., Down syndrome patient).

care unit Department in a health care facility for treatment of a certain type of patient (e.g., obstetrical care unit).

career agent Full-time insurance company representative licensed by the state who sells insurance policies and services to the policyholder for the insurer and sends all or almost all of his or her business to that company. He or she may also act as a broker with other companies.

career average benefit formula Defined benefit formula in which the retirement benefit amount is based on the participant's compensation during the entire period of participation in the plan. Also called *career earnings benefit formula.* See also *defined benefit formula.*

career earnings benefit formula See *career average benefit formula.*

caregiver Individual who helps care for someone who is ill, disabled, or aged such as a relative or friend who volunteers to help. However, some people provide caregiving services for a cost.

carrier 1. Insurer, underwriter of risk. See *insurance carrier.* 2. See *fiscal agent (FA).* 3. See *fiscal intermediary (FI).* Also referred to as *contractor* or *insurer.* 4. Individual who harbors specific organisms but does not have any symptoms and who can infect and cause disease in other people. 5. Person who has a recessive gene and can transmit this to offspring.

Carrier Advisory Committee (CAC) Formal system for physicians to be informed of and participate in the development of local medical review policies (LMRPs) in an advisory capacity. This committee discusses methods to improve administrative policies that are within the insurance carrier's discretion.

carrier-direct system Direct electronic transmission of insurance claims by the physician to the insurance company.

carrier replacement (CR) One health insurance company replaces one or more other health insurance

C

carriers for a group client. This process allows merging and combining the experience and risk of the group.

carry-over provision Provision in some medical expense policies in which expenses incurred during the last 3 months of a benefit period or calendar year are used to satisfy the current benefit period's deductible and may also be used to satisfy any or all of the following benefit period's (or next year's) deductible.

carryover line Format used when a complete entry does not fit on one line and then drops down to the next line.

carve out 1. Medical service not included within the capitation rate as a benefit of a managed care contract and may be contracted for separately. For example, carve-out services might include vision and dental, sometimes called a *single-service plan (SSP)*. 2. Integrated plan of providing medical coverage to Medicare-eligible employees. See *Medicare carve-out*.

carve-out plan Insurance coverage for specific health care services available for purchase separately from the basic managed care plan. Also called *single-service plan (SSP)*. Also see *Medicare/employer supplemental insurance*.

case 1. A particular instance of injury or disease, as a *case* of leukemia; sometimes used incorrectly to designate the patient with the disease. 2. Entire plan of a group insurance policyholder.

case history Past and current clinical information that the physician wants to know about the patient. The case history becomes part of the patient's health record.

case managed See *case management*.

case management 1. Ongoing review of cases by clinical professionals to ensure the necessity of the clinical services given and most appropriate use of services to a patient. Typically, case managers are nurses or social workers. They may operate privately or may be employed by social service agencies or public programs. 2. Process that integrates and coordinates patient care in complex and high-cost cases. Sometimes a patient is referred to as *case managed*. 3. Process of developing a defined health care plan for a patient for better communication and to improve quality of care and reduce costs. Case management is sometimes a "carve out." See *carve out*. 4. In the Medicare program, an arrangement of services needed to give proper health care to a beneficiary; tracking of beneficiary's use of facilities and resources. Also known as *catastrophic case management, catastrophic claim management, large claim management,* or *medical case management*.

case manager 1. Clinical professional (nurse or social worker) who works with the patient and all those involved with the patient in coordinating a plan of medical necessity and appropriateness of health care. He or she reviews cases after a predetermined amount of time and certifies ongoing care. 2. Registered

or licensed vocational nurse assigned to a workers' compensation case to supervise the administration of medical or ancillary services provided to the patient.

case mix Distribution of patients into categories reflecting differences in severity of illness or resource consumption. These categories include age, medical diagnosis, severity of illness, or length of stay. A nursing home or hospital's actual case mix influences cost and scope of the services provided by the facility to the patient, and case mix reimbursement systems adjust payment rates accordingly.

case mix index (CMI) 1. Average relative weight of all cases treated at a facility or by a certain physician that reveals the clinical severity of a defined group in relation to other groups in the classification system. Formula: Divide the sum of the weights of diagnosis-related groups (DRGs) for patient discharged during a specified period by the total number of patients discharged. A low CMI may indicate DRG assignments that do not adequately reflect the resources used to treat Medicare patients. 2. In prospective payment systems, this is the comparison of a hospital's cost for its case mix to the national or regional average hospital cost for a similar case mix.

case mix index (CMI) formula Mathematical method used to determine the case mix index by taking the sum of all diagnosis-related groups' (DRGs') relative weights and dividing it by the number of Medicare cases.

case number 1. Numeric assigned by the insurance carrier (payer) to an insurance claim. When appealing a denied or rejected claim, it must appear on each page of the document that is submitted to the payer. 2. See *group number*.

case rate 1. In managed health care, an averaging after a flat rate is given to certain categories of procedures. 2. Package price for a specific procedure or diagnostic-related group (DRG). Also called *bundled rate* or *flat fee-per-case*.

case-rate capitation In managed health care, payment to specialists such as orthopedists, urologists, and oncologists based on either referral or episode of care of the patient. Also called *contract capitation*.

case summary card Form sent by an insurance company's home office to a branch office that condenses important information about a new case or a change in an existing case. Also known as an *abstract*.

case universe Database of billed insurance claims from which CMRI selects the specific review category samples.

cash-balance pension plan Type of defined benefit plan in which each person participating has an account that is credited with amounts that reflect the employer's contributions and reflect investment interest. The balance in the account is called the *participant's accrued benefit*. When the participant retires, he or she may receive the full account balance in a lump sum if the benefits are fully vested or may use the account balance to purchase an annuity.

cash basis Costs of the service when payment was made rather than when the service was performed.

cash claim Cash paid, draft redeemed or drawn, for settlement of a group insurance claim.

cash deductible See *deductible.*

cash flow In a medical practice, the amount of *actual* cash generated and available for use by the medical practice within a given period of time.

cash indemnity benefits Payment to the insured by the insurance company after submission of an insurance claim. The insured may assign these benefits directly to the provider. Payment may or may not fully cover the insured's total costs for the service.

cash or deferred arrangement (CODA) See *Section 401(k) plan.*

cash payment option Life insurance policy that has a dividend option under which the dividends are paid to the policyholder in cash.

cash premium Insurance premium paid by the insured and received by the insurance company as distinguished from premium earned.

cash premium accounting system Bookkeeping system used for industrial insurance in which the agent informs the home office of the amount collected for each policy. The home office updates the policy records by posting these collections and then prepares new route collection records.

cash refund option Life income option with a refund that specifies proceeds remaining on the death of the beneficiary will be paid in a lump sum to the contingent payee.

cash surrender value Amount of money (cash) in a life insurance policy (usually whole life) that is adjusted for factors such as policy loans or late premiums that the policyholder will receive if the policyholder cancels the coverage or surrenders the policy to the insurance company. See *cash value.* Also called *net cash value.*

cash surrender value option Nonforfeiture option in a life insurance policy that states if a policyholder discontinues premium payments, he or she can surrender the policy and receive the policy's cash surrender value. Also see *cash value.*

cash value 1. Amount of money in a life insurance policy before adjustment for factors such as policy loans or late premiums that the policyholder will receive if the policyholder allows the policy to lapse or cancels the coverage and surrenders the policy to the insurance company. This feature is usually in whole life and universal life policies. Also called *inside build-up* and *policy owner's equity.* 2. Amount available in cash on surrender or voluntary termination of a policy by its owner before it becomes payable by death or maturity. Also called *cash surrender value option.*

casualty insurance Type of insurance that covers loss or liability caused by an accident that includes injury to persons or damage to the property of others. It includes automobile liability insurance, aviation insurance, burglary and theft insurance, employees' liability insurance, bonding or forgery insurance, personal liability insurance, plate glass insurance, power plant insurance, public liability insurance, and workers' compensation. Also referred to as *property/casualty insurance.*

catastrophe Single incident or many related incidents that cause property loss to insureds.

catastrophe insurance policy Insurance that provides coverage for earthquake, flood, hailstorm, hurricane, nuclear accident, riot and civil commotion, tornado, and volcanic eruption. Some homeowners' policies cover some of these catastrophes.

catastrophic Term that refers to an illness that has the potential to financially ruin an individual or his or her family because of the high cost of medical care.

catastrophic cap Maximum dollar amount that an active-duty family member has to pay out of their pocket under TRICARE for covered medical services in any fiscal year or enrollment period.

catastrophic case Severe medical injury or prolonged illness where the total cost of treatment will exceed the amount specified in the managed care contract.

catastrophic case management Ongoing review of cases that involve patients who encounter catastrophic or very high medical expenses. Sometimes referred to as *large case management.* See *case management.*

catastrophic claim Request for health benefits coverage for a case of severe injury or prolonged illness where it is foreseen that there may be very high medical expenses involved.

catastrophic claim management See *case management.*

catastrophic coverage 1. Health benefit insurance policy that offers minimal coverage for medical expenses under a specific level such as $10,000 a year but gives coverage for severe and prolonged chronic illness or injury that may cause the patient difficult financial hardship. Generally there is no maximum amount of coverage for this type of plan, but there may be some coinsurance. 2. Under a Medicare Part D plan, the name for the step in which the plan pays nearly all of the patient's drug expenses until the end of the year, with no upper limit. The patient pays only a small share of the drug expenses (approximately 5%). Also called *catastrophic insurance, catastrophic health insurance, catastrophic plan,* or *major medical.*

catastrophic health care Medical services for a patient who has suffered a severe injury or has a long-term illness that may substantially diminish a family's income and resources.

catastrophic health insurance See *catastrophic coverage.*

catastrophic illness Severe injury or illness that has very large expenses and for which the patient must be treated long term.

catastrophic insurance See *catastrophic coverage.*

catastrophic limit Highest amount of money the patient must pay out of pocket during a certain period of time for specific covered charges. When obtaining health insurance, setting a maximum amount protects the insured.

catastrophic plan See *catastrophic coverage.*

catchment area 1. Specific geographic area in which a managed care plan enrolls its members. 2. In the TRICARE program, a certain region defined by ZIP codes that is approximately 40 miles in radius surrounding each U.S. military treatment facility. Also called *service area.*

catchment area management (CAM) System in which medical services planning and resource budgeting are based on the population in a specific geographic area in which a managed care plan enrolls its members.

categorical programs Federal health programs created to benefit a certain group of people (e.g., Medicare for elderly and some disabled individuals and Medicaid for the indigent).

categorically needy Classification in the Medicaid program of aged, blind, or disabled individuals or families and children who meet financial eligibility requirements for Aid to Families with Dependent Children, Supplemental Security Income, or an optional state supplement.

categories One of the divisions of the *Current Procedural Terminology (CPT)* code book. The book is divided into seven code sections and appendices. Within each of the main sections are subsections and categories divided according to anatomical body system, organ, or site; procedure or service; condition; and specialty.

category 1. Three-digit code that represents a single disease or a group of closely related conditions in the diagnostic code book titled *International Classification of Diseases, Ninth Revision, Clinical Modification (ICD-9-CM).* 2. Letter with two digits that represents a single disease or a group of closely related conditions in the diagnostic code book titled *International Classification of Diseases, Tenth Revision, Clinical Modification (ICD-10-CM).* Also referred to as *three-character category.*

category III CPT codes Procedure codes in the *Current Procedural Terminology (CPT)* code book that end with the letter "T." They are temporary codes for emerging technology, services, and procedures and must be used instead of a Category I unlisted code.

causal relation requirements Proof required by law in some states to show that the facts misrepresented in an insurance application were related to the loss insured against.

causation In a workers' compensation case, an alleged physical, chemical, or biological factor that contributed to the incidence or happening of a medical condition.

CAVK Acronym for computer-assisted video keratography. See *corneal topography.*

CB HCPCS Level II modifier that may be used with CPT or HCPCS Level II codes indicating a service is ordered by a renal dialysis facility (RDF) physician because of end-stage renal disease (ESRD), but service is not part of the composite rate and is separately reimbursable. The patient must be admitted to a Medicare Part A stay in the skilled nursing facility.

CC 1. Abbreviation for comorbid condition. See *comorbid condition (CC).* 2. Abbreviation for complications and comorbidities. See *complications and comorbidities (CC).* 3. HCPCS Level II modifier that may be used with CPT or HCPCS Level II codes indicating the insurance carrier changed the procedure code because an incorrect code was billed or because of an administrative reason. 4. Abbreviation for chief complaint. See *chief complaint (CC).* 5. Abbreviation for condition category. See *condition category (CC).* 6. Abbreviation for condition code. See *condition code (CC).*

CC plans See *coordinated care (CC) plans.*

CCAP See *Certified Claims Assistance Professional (CCAP).*

CCF See *congregate care facility (CCF).*

CCI Abbreviation for Correct Coding Initiative. See *Correct Coding Initiative (CCI),* also known as *National Correct Coding Initiative (NCCI).*

CCI edits See *Correct Coding Initiative (CCI) edits.*

CCN See *community care network (CCN)* and *claim control number (CCN).*

CCR See *cost to charge ratio (CCR)* and *continuity-of-care record (CCR).*

CCRC See *continuing care retirement community (CCRC).*

CCS See *Certified Coding Specialist (CCS).*

CCS-P See *Certified Coding Specialist–Physician (CCS-P).*

CCU See *coronary care unit (CCU)* and *critical care unit (CCU).*

CD HCPCS Level II modifier that may be used with CPT or HCPCS Level II codes indicating AMCC test for end-stage renal disease or MCP MD.

CDC 1. Acronym for claims distribution center. 2. See *Centers for Disease Control and Prevention (CDC).*

CDHP See *consumer-directed health plans (CDHP).*

CDM See *charge description master (CDM).*

CDR See *clinical data repository (CDR).*

CDSS See *clinical decision support system (CDSS).*

CDT-2005 See *Current Dental Terminology (CDT).*

CDW Acronym that means clinical data warehouse. See *clinical data repository (CDR)*.

CE 1. HCPCS Level II modifier that may be used with CPT or HCPCS Level II codes indicating medical necessity AMCC test separate reimbursement. 2. Abbreviation for covered entity. See *covered entity (CE)*. 3. Abbreviation for consultative examiner. See *consultative examiner (CE)*. 4. Abbreviation for continuing education. See *continuing education (CE)*.

CECP See *Certified Electronic Claims Professional (CECP)*.

cede To buy reinsurance; to effect reinsurance.

cedent See *ceding company*.

ceding company Insurance company that places reinsurance business of its original risk, all or part of those risks that it does not wish to retain in full, with a reinsuring company. Insurer that sells its policies directly to the public either through its own salaried employees or exclusive agents. Also called *ceding insurer* or referred to as *cedent*.

ceding insurer See *ceding company*.

celiac disease Ailment known as *gluten sensitive enteropathy (GSE)*, which is an inherited disorder marked by sensitivity to gluten, the component of wheat that makes flour smooth and elastic.

census Count (enumeration) and demographics of hospital inpatients or members of a managed care plan.

census data Statistical information that is used to establish insurance premium rates or benefits on individuals eligible for or insured under a group policy (e.g., age, sex, income, insurance classification, dependent status).

Center for Healthcare Information Management (CHIM) Health information technology industrial association.

center of excellence (COE) Health care facility or hospital that specializes in treating certain illnesses and has highly specialized product lines that are chosen by a provider for developing larger financial resources. COEs are developed for competitive reasons and may offer quality of care, larger volume of admissions, and cost-effective care. COEs are listed in the *Federal Register*.

Centers for Disease Control and Prevention (CDC) One of the 13 major operating components of the Department of Health and Human Services (DHHS), which is the principal agency in the U.S. government for protecting the health and safety of all Americans and for providing essential human services, especially for those people who are least able to help themselves. Founded in 1946 to control malaria and to prevent and control infectious and chronic diseases, injuries, workplace hazards, disabilities, and environmental health threats. CDC applies research and findings to improve people's daily lives and responds to health emergencies. CDC is committed to achieving true improvements in people's health. To do this, the agency is defining specific health impact goals to prioritize and focus its work and investments and measure progress. CDC maintains several code sets included in the HIPAA standards including the ICD-9-CM codes.

Centers for Medicare and Medicaid Services (CMS) Division of the Department of Health and Human Services (DHHS), formerly Health Care Financing Administration (HCFA). Develops and administers policies for the Medicare program and works with the states to manage the Medicaid program. Responsibilities include managing contractor claims payment, fiscal audit and/or overpayment prevention and recovery, and developing and monitoring payment safeguards necessary to detect and respond to payment errors or abusive patterns of service delivery. CMS sets standards for Medicare Part D insurance plans. CMS maintains the UB-92 institutional EMC format specifications, the professional EMC NSF specifications, and specifications for certifications and authorizations used by the Medicare and Medicaid programs. CMS maintains the HCPCS medical code set and the Medicare Remittance Advice Remark Codes administrative code set.

Centers for Medicare and Medicaid Services (CMS-1500) claim form Universal insurance claim form developed and approved by the American Medical Association Council on Medical Service and the Centers for Medicare and Medicaid Services, formerly the Health Care Financing Administration. It is used by physicians and other professionals to bill outpatient services and supplies to TRICARE, Medicare, and some Medicaid programs, as well as most private insurance carriers and managed care plans.

Centers for Medicare and Medicaid Services (CMS) Data Center User Form Form that is required for access to the CMS data center.

central processing unit (CPU) Brains of a computing device controlling the internal memory that directs the flow and processing of information.

CERT See *Comprehensive Error Rate Testing (CERT) Program*.

certain payment Insurance company payment that will be made under any circumstances and is not contingent on any predesignated condition.

certificate Statement that an insurance policy has been written for the benefit of one or more individuals. This document may be used in evidencing reinsurance between insurance companies.

certificate holder Insured individual of a group insurance policy that has been issued a certificate of insurance, which certifies that an insurance contract has been written.

This certification of insurance contains a summary of the coverage of the policy in general terms applicable to that member.

certificate membership benefit maximum Largest total payment limit that an insurance plan will generate for certain kinds of care that a member may receive while the certificate is valid.

certificate number Numeric or alphanumeric characters issued to an insured or member of an insurance plan and used for identification. It appears on an insured's health insurance identification card and is placed on insurance claim forms when submitting claims or when communicating with insurance companies. Also called *identification number (ID #)*.

certificate of assumption In assumption reinsurance, each policyholder is sent an official document (certificate) when the policy has been ceded about a notice of the assumption and information about the new insurer.

certificate of authority (COA) 1. State license to operate as a health maintenance organization (HMO). 2. Insurance company's document that grants authority to a particular agent or group of agents to act on behalf of the insurer. 3. Certificate issued by a state's insurance department that authorizes an insurance company to issue certain types of insurance in the state.

certificate of confidentiality Federal document that legally protects researchers from having to disclose information about research participants as a result of a subpoena or court order. It is for projects involving information of a sensitive nature that, if released, could harm participants. See *sensitive information.*

certificate of coverage (COC) Document given to an insured by the insurance company or any employer that offers a health plan. It describes the benefits in detail under the policy issued. It is required by state law. Also called *evidence of coverage (EOC), benefit plan, insurance policy, subscriber agreement, subscriber certificate,* and *subscriber contract.*

certificate of indebtedness 1. Document issued by an insurance company and given to the beneficiary of a life insurance policy that states a guaranteed minimum interest rate and the frequency of interest payments. 2. Short-term certification, 12 months or less, of a specific portion of debt due by the federal government to individual holders, bearing a fixed rate of interest.

certificate of insurance Document (statement or booklet) issued by an insurance company and given to a group or beneficiary of an insurance policy to verify that a group, individual (e.g., physician), or an institution is insured for an amount of coverage for a certain type of risk during a specific time period.

certificate of medical necessity (CMN) 1. Certification by a provider to an insurance carrier that a medical service or procedure is medically necessary because of the patient's condition. 2. Form required by

Medicare that allows the patient to use certain durable medical equipment prescribed by a physician or one of the physician's staff. 3. In Medicare fraud, to complete a CMN for patients not personally and professionally known by the physician.

certificate of merit Document that is required for an independent medical expert to review a patient's medical record and certify that a claim has merit before a formal medical liability lawsuit is filed.

certificate of need (CON) Document of approval issued by a state or government agency that legally allows an organization or health care institution to construct or modify a health care facility, incur a major capital expenditure, obtain expensive medical equipment, or offer a new or different health service. An investigation is done before receiving the CON to make sure the facility or service meets the needs of those for whom it is intended. Also referred to as *planning approval.*

certificate of waiver Document issued to a laboratory to perform only waived tests. These are simple examinations or procedures that use methodologies that are so easy and accurate that the likelihood of erroneous results is negligible and poses no reasonable risk of harm to the patient if the test is performed incorrectly.

certificate rider Amendment or supplement to the certificate of insurance.

certification 1. Statement issued by a board or association verifying that a person meets professional standards. 2. Hospital certification means that a hospital has passed a survey done by a state government agency. Although it is similar, it is not the same as being accredited. Certification is usually applied to individuals and accreditation to hospital facilities. Note that Medicare only covers care in hospitals that are certified or accredited. See *accreditation.* 3. Approval by an insurance payer's case manager to continue a patient's care for a certain number of days or visits. 4. In home health plan certification, the physician receives, reviews, adjusts treatment, documents the plan in coordination with the care of the home health agency, and then bills for this service. For subsequent plan adjustment, see *home health plan recertification.*

certification and recertification of service need Attestation by the patient's attending physician on admission and at stated intervals of the need for hospitalization and continued stay in the facility.

Certified Claims Assistance Professional (CCAP) Certification awarded to a person after appropriate training and passing a certification examination administered by the Alliance of Claims Assistance Professionals, Inc.

certified coding professional Individual who has obtained appropriate training, met experience prerequisites, and passed a national certification examination administered by a professional coding association.

C

Certified Coding Specialist (CCS) Title received by a person after appropriate training and successfully passing a national certification examination administered by the American Health Information Management Association for hospital-based coding.

Certified Coding Specialist–Physician (CCS-P) Title received by a person after appropriate training and passing a certification examination administered by the American Health Information Management Association (AHIMA) for physician-based coding.

Certified Electronic Claims Professional (CECP) Certification awarded to a person after appropriate training and passing a certification examination administered by the Alliance of Claims Assistance Professionals, Inc.

certified form Document used to guarantee insurance benefits.

Certified Health Consultant (CHC) Certification awarded to an individual who has successfully completed the CHC program. CHCs have a broad knowledge of the field of health care financing, act as consultants to purchasers of employee benefit packages, and are administrators of employee health care benefit programs.

Certified Health Consultant Program Certification program developed by the Blue Cross Blue Shield Association in 1978. It consists of a series of comprehensive examinations that test an individual's knowledge of health care financing such as health care economics, pricing, underwriting, financing, marketing, and selling. Besides passing each of the examinations, the individual must complete 2 weeks of residency training.

Certified Health Insurance Plan (CHIP) See *State Children's Health Insurance Program (SCHIP).* Formerly, CHIP was a government-sanctioned cooperative health coverage plan offering one or more basic benefit options with mandated employer, insurer, and provider participation.

certified mail Correspondence or documents sent by the U.S. post office and officially marked to whom sent, showing date and address of delivery. This type of mail service is used often by medical offices for collection purposes and important letters (e.g., relocation of a medical practice, closure, dismissal of a patient). When certified mail is received, the receiver must sign a receipt of delivery and the sender is provided with a receipt of the delivery. This receipt remains on file at the receiver's post office for 2 years.

Certified Medical Assistant (CMA) Title received by a person after appropriate training and passing a certification examination administered by the American Association of Medical Assistants, Inc.

Certified Medical Transcriptionist (CMT) Professional medical transcriptionist who has passed the written and practical examination offered by the Association for Integrity of Healthcare Documentation, formerly the American Association for Medical Transcription, and who participates in an ongoing program of continuing medical education to increase his or her knowledge of medicine and improve skills in medical transcription.

Certified Medical Billing Specialist (CMBS) Title received by a person after appropriate training and passing a certification examination administered either by the American Association of Medical Billers in Los Angeles or the Medical Association of Billers in Las Vegas.

Certified Nurse Administrator (CNA) Registered nurse (RN) who holds an administrative position at the nurse manager level or nurse executive level in a health care organization, is responsible for the proper allocation of available resources to provide efficient and effective nursing care, and who possesses evidence of certification by passing a nurse administration certification examination by the American Nurses Credentialing Center (ANCC).

Certified Nurse-Midwife (CNM) (as defined by the American College of Nurse-Midwives) "an individual educated in the two disciplines of nursing and midwifery, who possesses evidence of certification according to the requirements of the American College of Nurse-Midwives." This individual may be a registered professional nurse who is licensed in the state and legally authorized to practice as a CNM.

Certified Nursing Assistant (CNA) Individual trained and certified to help nurses by providing nonmedical assistance to patients such as help with bathing, dressing, and using the bathroom.

Certified Occupational Therapy Assistant (COTA) Title received by an individual after appropriate training and passing a certification examination by the National Board of Certification in Occupational Therapy, Inc.

Certified Ophthalmic Technician (COT) Title received by an individual after appropriate training and passing a certification examination by the Joint Commission on Allied Health Personnel in Ophthalmology (JCAHPO). JCAHPO also offers certification as an ophthalmic coding specialist.

Certified Professional Coder (CPC) Title received by a person after appropriate training and successfully passing a national certification examination administered by the American Academy of Professional Coders.

Certified Professional in Health Information Technology (CP Health IT) Certification provides professional training and certification for those responsible for planning, selecting, implementing, and managing electronic health records (EHR) and other health information technology (HIT). CPHIT designation indicates that the holder has mastered the common body of knowledge for an electronic health records professional and, in addition, has evidenced expertise in a variety of health information technology applications including CPOE and electronic prescribing.

certified provider Physician or other individual who meets certain quality standards for providing outpatient self-management training services and other Medicare-covered items and services.

Certified Registered Nurse Anesthetist (CRNA) Individual who, after completing basic educational and appropriate training requirements in nursing, is trained for an additional time (about 2 years) in the administration of anesthesia and passes a certification examination administered by the American Association of Nurse Anesthetists. CRNAs are licensed to give anesthesia under the direction of a physician.

Certified Respiratory Therapist (CRT) Title received by a person after appropriate training and by passing a certification examination administered by the National Board for Respiratory Care, Inc.

Certified Tumor Registrar (CTR) Professional certification received after passing a certification examination by the National Cancer Registrars Association, Inc. (NCRA). To maintain the CTR status, NCRA members and nonmembers are required to complete 20 hours of continuing education every 2 years.

CERTS See *claims and eligibility real-time software (CERTS).*

cession 1. A reinsurance. 2. In reinsurance, a property, parcel, or unit of insurance that an insurance company cedes to a reinsurer. 3. An amount ceded as reinsurance.

CF 1. Abbreviation for conversion factor. 2. HCPCS Level II modifier that may be used with CPT or HCPCS Level II codes indicating AMCC test, not composite rate.

CFR See *Code of Federal Regulations (CFR).*

CG HCPCS Level II modifier that may be used with CPT or HCPCS Level II codes indicating innovator drug dispensed.

chain of trust (COT) Term used in HIPAA security Notice of Proposed Rulemaking (NPRM) for a pattern of agreements that extend protection of health care data. Each covered entity that shares health care data with another entity requires that that entity provide protections comparable with those provided by the covered entity, and that that entity, in turn, requires that any other entities with which it shares the data satisfy the same requirements.

chain of trust agreement (CTA) Agreement that specifies what procedures and technologies are implemented between two or more parties who have the need to electronically exchange or share health care information. Also see *chain of trust (COT).*

CHAMPUS See *TRICARE.*

CHAMPUS maximum allowable charge (CMAC) Highest amount TRICARE will pay for a medical service.

CHAMPUS National Pricing System Database that allows retrieval of pricing information for a particular medical service or procedure within a specific geographic area.

CHAMPVA See *Civilian Health and Medical Program of the Department of Veterans Affairs (CHAMPVA).*

CHAMPVA claim form VA Form 10-7959A that must be completed and submitted by the provider to request payment for a medical service or procedure rendered to a beneficiary from the CHAMPVA program.

CHAMPVA identification card Insurance card issued to dependents of military veterans who are beneficiaries of the CHAMPVA government program (see Figure C-1). Essential information is included on front and back sides of the card.

change agent Individual whose efforts assist change in a group or organization.

change of condition provision Insurance article or clause specifying that for an insurance policy to become effective, all conditions stated in the application for insurance must be true at the time of delivery of the policy.

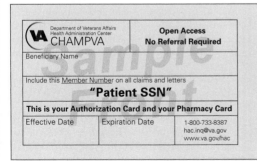

Figure C-1 CHAMPVA identification card.

change of occupation provision Article or clause in an individual health insurance policy that gives the insurer the right to adjust a policy's premium rate or benefits when the insured changes jobs or careers.

change of ownership (CHOW) Situation when a provider undergoes a change in the proprietorship of their medical practice. A Medicare provider is required to notify the Centers for Medicare and Medicaid Services of the identity of both old and new owners, effective date of change, how the new entity will be organized, and a seller's terminating cost report.

channeling Process of directing patients to certain providers and hospitals by a managed care plan, provider, or medical group (e.g., managed care plan that sends [channels] patients to providers within the plan's network).

chapter First major section in the Tabular List in the *International Classification of Diseases, Ninth Revision, Clinical Modification (ICD-9-CM)* code book. A chapter represents a body system or type of condition.

Chapter 7 bankruptcy See *straight petition in bankruptcy.*

Chapter 9 bankruptcy Type of bankruptcy case that is used for reorganization proceedings when a city or town is insolvent or unable to meet its debts. A plan is put into effect to adjust such debts.

Chapter 11 bankruptcy Type of bankruptcy case that is used for reorganization of a business enterprise when the company is unable to meet its debts but would like to continue business and would be unable to do so if creditors took away its assets.

Chapter 12 bankruptcy Type of bankruptcy case that is used for reorganization when a farmer is unable to meet his or her debts.

Chapter 13 bankruptcy Type of bankruptcy case that is designed to protect the wage earner from creditors while allowing the wage earner to make arrangements to repay a portion of his or her bills (about 70%) over a 3- or 5-year period. Also called *wage earner's bankruptcy.*

charge Dollar amount (fee) for a medical service or procedure given by a provider.

charge-based reimbursement Method of compensation in which institutional providers are paid for the actual incurred costs of covered medical services plus payment for bad debts, cost of charity cases, and a profit.

charge description list See *charge description master (CDM).*

charge description master (CDM) Computer program that is linked to various hospital departments and includes detailed charges for items and services provided to each patient such as procedure codes, procedure descriptions, service descriptions, fees, and revenue codes; also known as *charge master* and *master charge list.*

charge document See *multipurpose billing form.*

charge entry Process in which fees for medical services are posted into the patient's billing and collection financial account statement.

charge master See *charge description master (CDM).*

charge reduction In the Medicare program, the percentage difference between a provider's billed fee and the Medicare allowed charge.

charge slip See *multipurpose billing form.*

charges 1. Dollar amount a hospital bills an outlier case based on the itemized bill. 2. Dollar amount assigned for a medical service and billed by a health care provider to the patient's financial account statement. 3. In Medicare fraud, unbundling or exploded charges (e.g., to bill a multichannel set of laboratory tests to appear as if the individual tests had been performed).

charity allowance Discounted fee for medical services for indigent or medically indigent patients. See also *medically needy (MN).*

charity care Free or discounted fee for medical services provided to the poor or individuals unable to pay. Because some indigent patients are not eligible for federal or state programs, the costs covered by Medicaid are usually recorded separately from indigent care costs. See also *charity allowance; medically needy (MN).* Also called *indigent care* or *indigent medical care.*

chart See *medical record.*

chart note See *progress note.*

charts Group of patient medical records maintained by the physician. Each record documents the patient's treatment in progress notes, diagnostic and therapeutic procedures or tests and their results, findings and conclusions from special examinations, correspondence from other providers, specialists, or consultants, medications, surgical operations, and other reports pertinent to the patient's care.

CHC See *Certified Health Consultant (CHC)* or *community health center (CHC).*

CHDP See *Child Health and Disability Prevention Program (CHDP).*

cheat sheet Reference page developed by a medical practice that acts as a shortcut to locating diagnostic codes for conditions commonly seen by a physician specialist. See *encounter form.*

check deposit billing See *automatic bill payment, electronic funds transfer system (EFTS),* and *preauthorized payment.*

check-o-matic See *electronic funds transfer system (EFTS), automatic bill payment,* and *preauthorized payment.*

check voucher Document that accompanies an explanation of benefits from a third-party payer that may be detached and deposited in a bank account. Sometimes referred to as a *payment voucher.* Also see *explanation of benefits (EOB)* and *remittance advice (RA).*

CHEDDAR One of a standard style of charting (documenting) procedures for progress notes in patient's medical records. This acronym may be interpreted as follows: C = chief complaint stated by the patient as the main reason for seeing the doctor; usually a subjective statement. H = history of the present illness and includes social history and physical symptoms, as well as contributing factors. E = examination performed by the physician. D = details or list of complaints and problems. D = drugs and dosages of the current medications the patient is taking. A = assessment that includes the diagnosis process and the impression (diagnosis) made by the physician. R = return visit information or referral to specialists for additional tests. Also see *SOAP.*

chemical dependency See *substance abuse.*

cherry picking 1. Scheme to enroll in a managed care plan only those individuals who are healthy and excluding individuals who have existing health problems. 2. Situation in which a coder chooses the easier cases to code and leaves behind the more difficult ones. This situation also may occur with transcription, where one transcriptionist may skip a more difficult-to-understand dictator for the dictation of another physician who enunciates.

chief complaint (CC) Patient's statement describing symptoms, problems, or conditions as the reason for seeking health care services from a physician.

child For Social Security purposes includes the worker's biological child or any other child who can inherit intestate personal property under state law or who meets certain specific requirements under the Social Security Act: legally adopted child; equitably adopted child, stepchild, grandchild.

child conversion code Code that shows the length of time a dependent child has health insurance coverage under a family's membership (e.g., end of calendar year of limiting age, birth date).

Child Health and Disability Prevention Program (CHDP) A state health and disability prevention program for children.

Children's Health Insurance Program (CHIP) See *Children's Special Health Care Services (CSHCS).*

Children's Special Health Care Services (CSHCS) State child health program that operates with federal grant support under Titles V and XXI of the Social Security Act. In some states this program may be known as *Maternal and Child Health Program (MCHP), Children's Health Insurance Program (CHIP),* or *State Children's Health Insurance Program (SCHIP).*

CHIME See *College of Healthcare Information Management Executives (CHIME).*

CHIN See *community health information network (CHIN).*

CHIP Acronym for Children's Health Insurance Program; see *State Children's Health Insurance Program (SCHIP).*

chiropody See *Doctor of Podiatric Medicine (DPM)* and *podiatry.*

chiropractor Practitioner of chiropractic, a system of mechanical therapeutics based on the principles that the nervous system largely determines the state of health, and that disease results from abnormal nerve function and conformity. Treatment consists primarily of the adjustment or manipulation of parts of the body, especially the spinal column. Some chiropractors also use physiotherapy, nutritional supplementation, and other therapeutic modalities; radiography is used for diagnosis only. Chiropractors are licensed by all states. Their services are covered in some Medicaid programs. Manual manipulation of the spine is covered under Medicare when subluxation of the spine is demonstrated on x-ray. Also known as *Doctor of Chiropractic Medicine (DC).*

CHOW See *change of ownership (CHOW).*

chronic Refers to a medical condition that persists, continues, or recurs over a long period of time.

chronic care Medical care and treatment given to an individual whose health problem is of a long-term and continuing nature. Rehabilitation facilities, nursing homes, and mental hospitals may be considered chronic care facilities.

chronic illness Long-term or permanent illness that often results in some type of disability and may require a person to seek help with various activities (e.g., diabetes, arthritis).

chronic maintenance dialysis Kidney dialysis regularly furnished to an end-stage renal dialysis (ESRD) patient in a hospital-based independent (non–hospital-based) or home setting.

chronological resume A datasheet that outlines experience and education by dates.

church plan Religious organization or church that offers a health plan for its employees.

churning 1. Physicians seeing a high volume of patients more often than medically necessary, to increase revenue. This situation may be seen in fee-for-service or managed care environments. 2. Payment system based on performance and productivity of the provider of health care services.

CIF See *claims inquiry form (CIF).*

CIM See *National Coverage Determinations Manual (NCDM),* formerly named Coverage Issues Manual.

cineradiography Procedure in which an injection of a nontoxic radiopaque medium is given in order to produce movie camera images on a fluorescent screen to view various body structures.

circled bullet (⊙) Symbol used in the procedure code book titled *Current Procedural Terminology (CPT)* to indicate that conscious/moderate sedation is included for that specific procedural code number for billing and payment purposes.

CIS See *clinical information system (CIS).*

Civil Monetary Penalty Statute (CMPS) Fines and sanctions imposed on individuals or health care facilities by the Office of Inspector General (OIG) for noncompliance with Centers for Medicare and Medicaid Services (CMS) regulations. This includes fraud violations. These fines may be in addition to other criminal and civil penalties depending on the legal situation.

Civil Service Retirement System (CSRS) Program for federal employees hired before 1984.

Civilian Health and Medical Program of the Uniformed Services (CHAMPUS) See *TRICARE.*

Civilian Health and Medical Program of the Department of Veterans Affairs (CHAMPVA) Service benefit program similar to TRICARE, which is for veterans with total, permanent, service-connected disabilities or surviving spouses and dependents of veterans who died from service-connected disabilities. The Veterans Administration is now known as the *Department of Veterans Affairs.*

claim Formal request for payment (bill) sent to an insurance carrier or fiscal intermediary for a private insurance program, managed care plan, or a government program for medical services rendered to insureds or beneficiaries; also called *insurance claim.*

claim adjustment reason codes National administrative code set that identifies the reasons for any differences, or adjustments, between the original provider charge for a claim or service and the payer's payment for it. This code set is used in the X12 835 claim payment and remittance advice and the X12 837 claim transactions and is maintained by the Health Care Code Maintenance Committee.

claim administration department Section or division in a life and health insurance company that processes insurance claims. In this division, claim examiners review claims submitted by medical providers, policy owners, or beneficiaries; verify the validity of claims; and authorize payment of benefits to either the provider or beneficiary of each claim.

claim attachment Document with information, hard copy or electronic, related to a completed insurance claim that assists in validating the medical necessity or explains the medical service or procedure (e.g., operative report, discharge summary, invoice). When a claim attachment is included with a paper claim, Block 19 of the CMA-1500 insurance claim form is completed. When a claim is electronically transmitted, practice management and claims software include a data field that indicates that a paper claims attachment is included with the claim. Under the Health Insurance Portability and Accountability Act (HIPAA), electronic standards for claims attachments are being developed. Attachments may be structured (such as Certificates of Medical Necessity) or non-structured (such as an operative report). Though attachments may be submitted separately, it is common to say the attachment was "submitted with the claim."

claim audit Evaluation of insurance claims for duplicate medical services or billing that may be in excess of a normal pattern.

claim control number (CCN) Unique multidigit number assigned by the Medi-Cal fiscal intermediary on a Treatment Authorization Request and used for reference when processing the request.

claim cost control Insurance company's attempt to streamline operations to contain and direct claim payments so that insurance premium funds are used efficiently.

claim edits Electronic examination of transmitted insurance claims for errors, conflicting code entries, and a match of diagnosis to medical service(s) provided. Also called *edit check.* See *front-end edits.*

claim file Accumulation of information needed for payment or denial of an insurance claim.

claim form See *Health Insurance Claim Form (CMS-1500).*

claim fraud Intentional misrepresentation by either providers or patients to obtain services, payment for services, or claim program eligibility. In insurance claims, fraudulent practices are intentionally double billing for the same services, reporting diagnoses and procedures to maximize payments, billing for services that were not performed, and so on.

claim frequency rate In health insurance calculations, this is a value obtained from the expected percentage of insured individuals who will file claims and the number of claims they will file within a specific period of time. This rate is used to calculate average claim costs, which are used to establish premium rates.

claim investigation Process of obtaining insurance claim information to decide if a claim should be paid by the insurance company.

claim lag 1. Time period between the patient's encounter (incurred) date of the insurance claim and its submission to the third-party payer. 2. Time period between the incurred date of the insurance claim and its payment by the third-party payer.

claim list Data evidence of claims paid under an insurance plan or coverage for a specific time period. Such lists include identification of the insured, cause of the insurance claim, description of service, and amount paid.

claim manual Administrative guidelines documented in a book used by insurance claims adjusters to settle (adjudicate) claims for payment according to the insurance company's policies and procedures.

claim reference number (CRN) Number assigned to a Medicare insurance claim for processing by the fiscal intermediary.

claim representative See *adjuster.*

claim reserve In insurance, an estimate of the amount of money to set aside that will be needed to pay insurance claims. The claim department gathers information during the course of handling the claim to obtain this estimate. These data may include the extent to which the claim is covered by the policy, the effect of previously paid claims on the amount of coverage available to pay a current claim, and the effect of any applicable reinsurance coverage on the claim.

claim services only (CSO) agreement Type of contract in which the insurance company provides claims processing and bases its fee on the number of processed claims.

claim settlement See *adjudicate.*

claim status category codes National administrative code set that indicates the general category of the status of health care claims. This code set is used in the X12 277 claim status notification transaction and is maintained by the Health Care Code Maintenance Committee.

claim status codes National administrative code set that identifies the status of health care claims. This code set is used in the X12 277 claim status notification transaction and is maintained by the Health Care Code Maintenance Committee.

claimant Insured individual or beneficiary who makes a formal request for payment of insurance benefits because of illness or injury that meets the terms of an insurance contract. This individual could be a provider or legal representative of the insured who makes a claim to an insurance plan.

claims administrator See *adjuster* or *claims processor.*

claims and eligibility real-time software (CERTS) Computer software that allows Medi-Cal providers to electronically verify recipient eligibility, clear share of cost liability, reserve Medi-Services, perform Family PACT (planning, access, care, treatment) client eligibility transactions, and submit pharmacy or CMS-1500 claims using a personal computer.

claims assistance professional (CAP) Practitioner who works for the consumer and helps patients organize, complete, file, and negotiate health insurance claims of all types to obtain maximum benefits, as well as tell patients what checks to write to providers to eliminate overpayment.

claims examiner 1. In industrial cases, a representative of the insurer who investigates, evaluates, and negotiates the patient's insurance claim and acts for the company in the settlement of claims. 2. Individual employed by an insurance company who assists in settlement of claims by investigating claims, approving claims that are valid, and denying claims that are invalid or fraudulent. Some claims examiners are individuals who operate independently and are hired by insurance companies to adjust a specific loss. Also called *adjuster, claims processor, claims representative, claims administrator,* or *health insurance adjuster.*

claims inquiry form (CIF) A Medi-Cal form used for tracing a claim, resubmitting a claim after a denial, or when requesting an adjustment for underpaid or overpaid claims.

claims manager Insurance company's reimbursement director or executive administrator who supervises and oversees employees who process insurance claims for payment.

claims processor Employed representative of the insurance company who is responsible for handling insurance claims as they are received from patients and medical practices and who determines the dollar amount of a claim or debt. Also called *adjuster, claims examiner, claims representative, claims administrator,* or *health insurance adjuster.*

claims representative See *claims processor.*

claims review Audit by a peer review organization, insurance company, or other group of insurance claims submitted by a provider to validate payment or non-payment, eligibility, or establish medical necessity of care and appropriateness of services provided.

claims-review type of foundation A type of foundation that provides peer review by physicians to the numerous fiscal agents or carriers involved in its area.

claims reviewer Insurance company's reimbursement employee who analyzes insurance claims similar to an auditor who checks procedure and diagnostic codes, prior authorizations, insurance contract violations, and so on.

claims transfer See *crossover claim.*

class Groups or categories of individuals with similar characteristics and risks for the purpose of setting insurance rates or to determine the amount of coverage for which a person is eligible under an insurance policy.

class beneficiary designation Description that names several people as a group instead of naming each person individually (e.g., children of the insured).

class rate See *standard class rate (SCR).*

classification system Method that provides the basis for payment that identifies medical services that will be charged fees separately (e.g., diagnosis-related groups [DRGs] patient classification system used for inpatient hospital prospective payment system, Healthcare Common Procedure Coding System [HCPCS] used in the Medicare fee schedule for physicians).

clause See *provision.*

clean bill Type of hospital invoice (patient's financial accounting statement) assessed by someone auditing a hospital bill that has no errors. Also see *under bill* and *over bill.*

clean claim Completed insurance claim form submitted within the program time limit that contains all the necessary information without deficiencies so that it can be processed and paid promptly; a claim that passes all electronic claim edits and claim audits; or a claim that is subject to medical review but is submitted with complete data attached or forwarded simultaneously with electronic media claim records.

clean-up fund Lump-sum type of life insurance death benefit to assist in paying the insured's outstanding debts, funeral expenses, and related expenses—in other words, "cash" to clean up expenses.

clearinghouse Independent organization that receives electronically transmitted insurance claims from the physician's office, performs software edits, routes, and transmits the claims to various insurance carriers. Also see *health care clearinghouse.*

clerical error Minor omission or error in form or content on Medicare Part A or Part B claims, such as missing data items (provider number or date of service). Omissions do not include failure to bill for certain items or services or third-party payer errors.

clerical error provision Insurance policy condition that if a person is eligible and submits a written request for coverage, he or she will not be denied coverage if the policyholder fails to give proper notice to the insurance company because of a clerical error.

CLIA See *Clinical Laboratory Improvement Amendments (CLIA).*

client 1. Person who is the recipient of a professional service. 2. Recipient of health care. 3. Patient. 4. System (software running on a piece of hardware) that initiates the process or requests services in a client/server computing arrangement.

client/server system Computer configuration that allows several local area network–based workstations (clients) to share access to a more powerful server computer, as might be used in a health care management plan. Processes are divided between two systems (client and server) that work together to perform a task such as obtaining information from a database.

client service department See *customer service department.*

clinic Outpatient facility that provides medical services by a group of physicians practicing medicine together and assumes health care responsibility for ambulatory patients (e.g., physical therapy for rehabilitative purposes, diagnostic x-rays, laboratory tests, educational services).

clinic without walls (CWW) Corporation formed by several medical practices with administrative and contracting functions centralized. Physicians' offices have different locations, but all patient revenue is shared by the group. Sometimes called *group practice without walls.* See *group without walls (GWW).*

clinical 1. Pertaining to a clinic. 2. Pertaining to direct bedside medical or nursing care. 3. Pertaining to materials or equipment used in the care of a sick person. 4. Experience of students in training. 5. Pertaining to tasks connected with medical practice.

clinical breast exam Examination of a patient by a physician to check for breast cancer by feeling and inspection. It is not the same as a mammogram and is performed in a doctor's office during a Papanicolaou test and pelvic examination.

clinical data repository (CDR) Computer-based patient record (CPR) that contains a collection of clinical key data from several sources. These data may be monitored and analyzed and are retrievable. The data can be assembled into reports or used for help in decision making. They can also be part of an institutional information warehouse or community or state health information system. Sometimes referred to as a *data warehouse* or *clinical data warehouse (CDW).*

clinical decision support system (CDSS) Method used to provide clinical data to health care providers and clinicians with the use of embedded flags (e.g., alert to a case manager that a patient's eligibility for a specific medical service is almost used up). CDSS is a major functional requirement to support a clinical or critical pathway.

clinical evaluation In a workers' compensation case, collection of data by a physician for assessing the health of an individual for the purpose of creating a medical management plan and beginning a course of treatment.

clinical examples Medical cases that support clinical situations related to some evaluation and management services and shown in an appendix of the *Current Procedural Terminology* code book. These illustrations may be used as a tool in coding professional services for billing.

clinical information system (CIS) Computer system that maintains a database of actual patient information on active medical care and treatment. CIS may be used for supporting medical decisions. In expanded form, a CIS becomes an electronic health record system. Also called *clinical system.*

clinical laboratory Workplace where diagnostic tests and procedures are performed on specimens that are directly related to the care of patients such as blood, infectious materials, saliva, and tissues.

Clinical Laboratory Improvement Amendments (CLIA) Federal act established in 1988 that regulates laboratory certification and accreditation standards, quality control, proficiency testing, personnel standards, program administration, and safety measures for all freestanding laboratories including physician office laboratories (POLs). CLIA mandates that all laboratories have a CLIA certificate to receive payment from federal programs. Adopted by Medicare and Medicaid programs.

clinical medical assistant Person who, under the direction of a physician, performs various routine back office tasks in a hospital, clinic, or other health facility.

These duties may consist of assisting with the physical examinations, taking x-rays, performing electrocardiograms, taking vital signs, weighing patients, obtaining urine specimens, and other medical-related activities. Also see *administrative medical assistant.*

clinical note Memo or concise written communication about contact with a patient that includes the date seen; description of signs and symptoms, treatment, and drugs administered; the patient's reaction; and any changes in physical or emotional condition.

clinical outlier Cases that cannot adequately be assigned to an appropriate DRG owing to unique combinations of diagnoses and surgeries, very rare conditions, or other unique clinical reasons. Such cases are grouped together into clinical outlier DRGs and are therefore considered outliers. Also see *outlier.*

clinical pathology Study of disease by the use of laboratory tests and methods of body tissue and fluids.

clinical pathway Description of an activity or practice that may result in favorable outcomes for patients with a specific disease. A clinical pathway uses defined resources to keep costs down. It may be based on research, literature, or common practice. Also called *critical pathway, practice guideline,* or *treatment protocol.*

clinical performance measure This is a method or instrument to estimate or monitor the extent to which the actions of a health care practitioner or provider conform to practice guidelines, medical review criteria, or standards of quality.

clinical practice guidelines Reports written by experts who have carefully studied whether a treatment works and which patients are most likely to be helped by it.

clinical practice plan See *faculty practice plan (FPP).*

clinical privileges Right or permit to provide medical, dental, and other medical services to patients by a hospital facility within certain limits based on the physician's education, professional license, experience, competence, ability, health, and judgment. Also called *practice privileges.*

clinical protocols Written plans or guidelines that specify procedures to be followed in performing a specific examination, treating certain injuries, conducting research, providing medical care for a particular condition, and evaluating appropriateness of certain procedures. Also known as *medical protocols* or *protocols.*

clinical psychologist Health care professional that specializes in the diagnosis, treatment, and prevention of a wide range of personality, mental, and behavioral disorders. Generally, clinical psychologists are state licensed and may practice independently. Many insurance companies pay for their services. However, they do not treat physical causes of mental disease with drugs or other medical or surgical treatments because they are not licensed to practice medicine. Also see *psychologist.*

clinical service organization (CSO) Health care organization created by academic medical centers to integrate medical school, faculty practice plan, and hospital.

clinical social worker (CSW) Individual who has obtained a degree in social work, met the requirements of being supervised in clinical social work, and obtained state licensure or certification. A CSW provides psychotherapy or counseling in many types of health care settings. Also referred to as a *licensed clinical social worker (LCSW).*

clinical staff Employees in a medical practice who perform mainly clinical duties such as physician, physician assistant, clinical medical assistant, registered nurse, licensed practical nurse, nurse practitioner, and technicians.

clinical support personnel Members of the clinical staff in a medical practice who provide assistance to the physician such as physician assistant, nurse practitioner, registered nurse, licensed practical nurse, and technician.

clinical system See *clinical information system (CIS).*

clinical trials One of the final stages of a long and careful research process to help patients live longer, healthier lives. Clinical trials help doctors and researchers find better ways to prevent, diagnose, or treat diseases. They test new types of medical care such as how well a new cancer drug works and if it is safe. The trials may also be used to compare different treatments for the same condition to see which is better or to test new uses for treatments already employed.

clinician General term denoting a medical or dental practitioner who has hospital staff admission privileges and primary responsibility for care of inpatients.

cloning 1. When each entry in a patient's medical record is worded exactly alike or similar to the previous entries. 2. When medical documentation is worded exactly the same from patient to patient. Cloning is considered a misrepresentation of the medical necessity requirements for insurance coverage of medical services. If suspected or identified, the services will be denied and may result in recovery of any overpayments made.

closed access Managed care plan that requires enrollees to select a primary care physician (PCP) from the plan's approved panel of providers. The PCP acts as a gatekeeper and may refer the patient to a specialist when required.

close Conclusion of the sales presentation that leads to the signing of the insurance application.

closed adoption To take into one's own family by legal process and raise as one's own child, but the identifying information about the adoptive and birth families is not shared. The adoptive and birth families do not establish or maintain contact.

closed claim Status of an insurance claim when all benefits have been paid.

closed contract Insurance agreement in which rates and policy provisions cannot be changed between the policy owner and the insurer. Commercial insurance companies write closed contracts. Fraternal insurance companies are not permitted to write this type of insurance.

closed formulary List of drugs covered by a benefit plan in which the drugs on it are the only ones covered. Sometimes nonformulary drugs can be covered if authorization is obtained and if there is a good medical reason. See also *open formulary* and *restricted formulary.*

closed fracture Fracture of the bone with no skin wound.

closed grievance Decision that has been made and cannot be appealed or is not under appeal by the member of a managed care plan.

closed-model HMO See *closed panel program.*

closed panel program Form of health maintenance organization (HMO) that limits the patient's choice of personal physicians to those doctors practicing in the HMO group practice within the geographical location and/or facility. Such plans allow members to receive nonemergency medical services, but adhering to a closed panel is usually not applicable to emergency care. A physician must meet very narrow criteria in order to join a closed panel.

closed treatment Alignment of a fracture without the site opened for surgical intervention. Three treatment methods for closed fractures exist: without manipulation, with manipulation, and with or without traction.

closing That portion of the insurance sales presentation when a prospective applicant has made a purchase commitment for insurance coverage and signs the sales proposal or application form.

clustering Situation in which a provider bills for midlevel services for various patient encounters under the assumption that some visits will be a little higher and some will be a little lower (upcoding some services and downcoding other services).

CMA See *Certified Medical Assistant (CMA).*

CMAC See *CHAMPUS maximum allowable charge (CMAC).*

CMBS See *Certified Medical Billing Specialist (CMBS).*

CMC See *computer media claims (CMC).*

CME Acronym that means continuing medical education. See *continuing education (CE).*

CMHC See *community mental health center (CMHC).*

CMI See *case mix index (CMI).*

CMI formula See *case mix index (CMI) formula.*

CMM See *comprehensive major medical (CMM).*

CMM insurance See *comprehensive major medical (CMM) insurance.*

CMN See *certificate of medical necessity (CMN).*

CMP See *competitive medical plan (CMP).*

CMPS See *Civil Monetary Penalty Statute (CMPS).*

CMS See *Centers for Medicare and Medicaid Services (CMS).*

CMS agent Any individual or organization, public or private, with whom the Centers for Medicare and Medicaid Services (CMS) has a contractual arrangement to contribute to or participate in the Medicare survey and certification process. The state survey agency is the most common example of a CMS agent as established through the partnership role that the state agency (SA) plays in the survey process under the provisions of §1864 of the Act. A private physician serving a contractual consultant role with the SA or CMS regional office as part of a survey and certification activity is another example of a CMS agent.

CMS Data Center User Form See *Centers for Medicare and Medicaid Services (CMS) Data Center User Form.*

CMS directed improvement project Any project where Centers for Medicare and Medicaid Services (CMS) specifies the subject, size, space, data source, analytical techniques, educational intervention techniques, or impact measurement model. These projects may be developed by CMS in consultation with networks, the health care community, and other interested people.

CMS manual system See *Medicare Carriers Manual (MCM).*

CMSP See *County Medical Services Program (CMSP).*

CMS-1450 Medicare Uniform Institutional Provider Bill (insurance claim) form used for submission after hospital services have been provided to a patient. This is commonly known as the *Uniform Bill (UB-04) institutional claim form,* which replaces the Uniform Bill (UB-92) claim form. See *Uniform Bill (UB-04) claim form.*

CMS-1500 Health Insurance Claim Form, a uniform professional insurance claim form used for submission after medical services have been provided to a patient. See *Health Insurance Claim Form (CMS-1500).*

CMT See *Certified Medical Transcriptionist (CMT).*

CNA See *Certified Nurse Administrator (CNA)* and *Certified Nursing Assistant (CNA).*

CNM See *Certified Nurse-Midwife (CNM).*

COA See *certificate of authority (COA).*

coal miners Persons whose work is digging coal, a solid mineral, in a mine.

coalition Association of health care plan sponsors who join together to negotiate with insurance companies or other managed care plans and providers.

COB See *coordination of benefits (COB).*

COBA Acronym for coordination of benefits agreement; see *coordination of benefits contractor agreement identifiers (COBA IDs).*

COBC Acronym for coordination of benefits contractor (COBC); see *coordination of benefits contractor agreement identifiers (COBA IDs)*.

COBRA See *Consolidated Omnibus Reconciliation Act of 1985 (COBRA)*.

COC See *certificate of coverage (COC)*.

CODA Acronym for cash or deferred arrangement. See *Section 401 (k) plan*.

code creep See *upcoding*.

code edit Computer software function that performs online checking of CPT codes on an insurance claim to detect unbundling, splitting of codes, and other types of improper code submissions. Sometimes referred to as *code screening*.

code first Phrase used to identify the need for two ICD-9-CM diagnostic codes.

code first (the) underlying condition Phrase used in ICD-9-CM diagnostic coding that indicates the medical illness is the result of another underlying disease.

code modifier See *modifier*.

Code of Federal Regulations (CFR) Official compilation of federal rules and requirements.

code ranges Assortment of procedure code numbers that belong to the same general category that appear in the "Index," which is the last section of the annually published *Current Procedural Terminology* code book. Whenever more than one code applies to a given index entry, a code range is listed. If several nonsequential codes apply, they are separated by a comma:
Esophagus
    Reconstruction. 43300, 43310, 43313
If two or more sequential codes apply, they are separated by a hyphen:
Debridement
    Burns. 01951-01953, 16010-16030

code screening See *code edit*.

code set Under the Health Insurance Portability and Accountability Act (HIPAA), this is any set of codes used to encode data elements such as tables of terms, medical concepts, medical diagnostic codes, or medical procedure codes. This includes both the codes and their descriptions.

code set maintaining organization Under the Health Insurance Portability and Accountability Act (HIPAA), this is an organization that creates and maintains the code sets adopted by the Secretary for use in the transactions for which standards are adopted.

coder Trained individual who has obtained a skill in classifying medical data from patient records. A coder translates the written diagnoses, treatments, and procedures into numeric and alphanumeric codes for submission on insurance claims to insurance carriers for reimbursement. In medical office settings, the coder may extract these data from patient encounter forms and patient records.

codicil Separate document that is an addition to a will that may modify, add to, subtract from, or revoke certain provisions of a will.

coding 1. Process of translating written descriptions into numerical and alphanumerical codes. 2. Choosing codes from numerical and alphanumerical systems that identify and describe a patient's diagnosis, as well as medical, surgical, and diagnostic procedures and services such as ICD-9-CM, CPT, and HCPCS.

coding conventions Rules or principles for determining a diagnostic code when using diagnostic code books such as each space, typefaces, indentations, punctuation marks, instructional notes, abbreviations, cross-reference notes, and specific usage of the words *and, with,* and *due to*. These rules assist in the selection of correct codes for the diagnoses encountered. Also see *conventions*.

coding creep See *diagnostic creep*.

coding guidelines 1. Official policies published by the Centers for Medicare and Medicaid Services (CMS) that tell how procedure codes are to be assigned by providers when submitting insurance claims for patients who have received medical services. 2. Official rules for assigning ICD-9-CM diagnostic codes to patients' conditions of illnesses, injuries, and diseases.

coding rules Official code conventions used when selecting diagnostic and procedural code numbers for a patient who has received medical services by a provider.

coding specialist Expert in coding diagnoses and procedures using diagnostic and procedural code books.

coding specialist for payers (CSP) One type of certification earned by meeting the requirements of the American College of Medical Coding Specialists (ACMCS).

COE 1. Acronym for occurring in the "course of employment." An injury must occur in the course of employment to be compensable in workers' compensation. Thus the activity the employee was engaged in at the time of injury must grow out of, or be incidental to, the employment. 2. Abbreviation for center of excellence. See *center of excellence (COE)*.

cognitive Relevant to the mental processes of comprehension, judgment, memory, perception, and reasoning as compared with emotional and volitional processes.

cognitive impairment Deterioration or loss of intellectual capacity that requires continual supervision to protect the insured or others, as measured by clinical evidence and standardized tests that reliably measure impairment in the area of (1) short- or long-term memory; (2) orientation as to person, place, and time; or (3) deductive or abstract reasoning. Such loss in intellectual capacity can result from Alzheimer's disease or similar forms of senility or irreversible dementia.

cohort Population group that shares a common property, characteristic, or event such as a year of birth or year of marriage. The most common one is the birth cohort, a group of individuals born within a defined time period, usually a calendar year or a 5-year interval.

coinsurance 1. A cost-sharing requirement under a health insurance policy providing that the insured will assume a percentage of the costs for covered services. Also referred to as *coinsurance payment, copayment, cost sharing,* or *percentage participation.* 2. In the Medicare program, the amount that Medicare will not pay. The Medicare beneficiary or the beneficiary's supplemental insurance plan is responsible for the yearly cash deductible and the portion of the reasonable charges (20%). 3. In the Medicaid Qualified Medicare Beneficiary (MQMB) program, the amount of payment that is above the rate that Medicare pays for medical services. The state assumes responsibility for payment of this amount.

coinsurance maximum Dollar amount that a patient must pay in coinsurance expenses each year before an insurance plan will pay 100% of eligible expenses for the rest of the year. Also known as *out-of-pocket maximum.*

coinsurance payment Specific percentage of the fee the patient is responsible for paying the provider of the medical service or supply; also called *coinsurance.*

coinsurance provision 1. Clause in a health insurance contract that requires the insured to pay a specific percentage in excess of the deductible of all eligible medical expenses. 2. Clause in property insurance agreement whereby the property owner is to carry insurance up to an amount established with the provisions of the policy. This is a stated percentage of the value of the property.

COLA See *cost-of-living adjustment (COLA).*

COLI See *corporate-owned life insurance (COLI).*

collaborative decision making All those in a group contribute their input on what they want and why and how conflicts between different parties may be resolved to reach a final determination to a problem or project.

collateral Any possession such as an automobile, furniture, stocks, or bonds that secures or guarantees the discharge of an obligation.

collateral assignment Transfer of some ownership rights in an insurance contract from one individual to another, sometimes for a temporary period. An insurance policy can be assigned as collateral for a loan, in which case all transferred rights revert to the assignor when the loan is repaid. Also called *collateral loan.* See *absolute assignment* or *assignment.*

collateral dependents Individuals made eligible for dependent insurance coverage for a group policy by expanding the definition of dependent (e.g., parents, grandparents, brothers, sisters, or others that depend on the insured for the main part of their financial support).

collateral loan See *collateral assignment.*

collateral source rule Legal doctrine under torts that if an injured person receives proceeds for the injuries, the payment should not be deducted from the health or disability insurance (collateral source).

collection agency Professional business service employed by a medical practice or hospital facility as an agent to pursue and attempt to collect unpaid or past-due accounts owed by a debtor that arose from an expressed or implied agreement. Generally, a collection agency is paid by receiving an agreed-upon percentage of the amount collected.

collection agency business See *collection agency.*

collection ratio Relationship between the amount of money owed and the amount of money collected in reference to the doctor's accounts receivable.

collections employee Administrative member of the staff in a medical practice who is given the responsibility of collecting from patients and insurance companies payments due for medical services.

collective bargaining To negotiate between organized labor and employer(s) issues about salaries, work conditions, work hours, and health and welfare programs.

College of Healthcare Information Management Executives (CHIME) Association formed in 1992 with the dual objective of serving the professional development needs of health care chief information officers (CIOs) and advocating the more effective use of information management within health care. Its mission is to serve the professional needs of health care CIOs and to advance the strategic application of information technology in innovative ways aimed at improving the effectiveness of health care delivery. Its supporting goals are networking, education, career development, information access, partnership advancement, and advocacy.

collision insurance Optional automobile insurance coverage that pays for damages to the insured's car caused by a collision with another car or object or by rolling the car over. Frequently this type of insurance is required if an individual has taken out a car loan.

collusion In Medicare fraud, to participate in a scheme with others that might result in higher costs or charges to the Medicare program such as conspiracy between provider and beneficiary or between a supplier and a physician.

colon 1. One of the punctuation symbols used in the diagnostic code book titled *International Classification of Diseases, Ninth Revision, Clinical Modification (ICD-9-CM).* It is used in the Tabular List section of the

---

code book after an incomplete term that needs one or more of the essential modifiers that follow to make it assignable to a given category. 2. Portion of the intestines (large) extending from the cecum to the rectum.

colonoscopy Endoscopic examination of the colon to identify disorders (polyps) or early signs of cancer.

colorectal cancer screening Various medical procedures or tests to identify disorders or early signs of cancer of the gastrointestinal tract such as fecal occult blood test, sigmoidoscopy, colonoscopy, or barium enema.

combination clause Provision in a disability income contract that defines when total disability will no longer be based on the insured's inability to perform his or her occupation but on the insured's inability to perform any occupation.

combination code 1. A code from one section of the procedural code book combined with a code from another section that is used to completely describe a procedure performed. 2. In diagnostic coding, one code that is used to classify two related diagnoses.

combination company Life and health insurance company whose agents sell both industrial and ordinary life insurance products.

combination dental plan Dental insurance contract that features scheduled and nonscheduled plans. Combination plans cover preventive and diagnostic procedures on a nonscheduled basis and other dental services on a scheduled basis.

combination plan Retirement (pension) plan wherein part of the funding is allocated and part is unallocated. The allocated part of the employer's contribution is used to purchase annuities or life insurance contracts with cash values. The unallocated part is put into a conversion fund.

combination program Combination of state, employer self-insured, and commercial workers' compensation programs.

combination resume Datasheet that combines specific dates or work experience with educational skills.

comma One of the punctuation symbols used in the diagnostic code book titled *International Classification of Diseases, Ninth Revision, Clinical Modification (ICD-9-CM)*. It is used in the Tabular List section of the code book after an incomplete term that needs one or more of the essential modifiers that follow to make it assignable to a given category.

comment Public review and remarks on the merits or appropriateness of proposed or potential federal regulations provided in response to a notice of proposed rulemaking (NPRM), a notice of intent (NOI), or other federal regulatory notice. Anyone may submit comments and suggestions during this time. Also called *comment period.*

commercial carriers Private for-profit insurance companies that offer individual and group health insurance policies.

commercial general liability insurance (CGL) Insurance policy that covers all liability risks of a business that are not specifically excluded. Also referred to as *commercial lines* or *general liability insurance.*

commercial inspection report Written document by an organization that specializes in investigating and obtaining information on persons who apply for insurance, employment, or credit.

commercial lines Insurance products that are created for businesses versus personal lines products. Also called *commercial general liability insurance (CGL).*

commercial managed care organization (MCO) Health maintenance organization that is an eligible organization with a contract under §1876 or a Medicare+Choice organization; a provider-sponsored organization or any other private or public organization that meets the requirements of §1902(w). These MCOs provide comprehensive services to commercial and/or Medicare enrollees, as well as Medicaid enrollees.

commercial MCO See *commercial managed care organization (MCO).*

commercial plan Benefit package that an insurance company or managed care plan offers to employers as compared with a senior plan offered to Medicare beneficiaries.

commercial workers' compensation program Industrial insurance plan in which the employer purchases the policy that provides benefits to injured employees.

commission Amount of money paid to an insurance agent for selling and servicing an insurance policy. Usually a commission is calculated as a percentage of the premium.

Commission on Accreditation of Allied Health Education Programs (CAAHEP) Group that accredits proprietary, community college, or trade technical schools medical assisting program. Students who wish to sit for the Certified Medical Assisting (CMA) examination provided by the American Association of Medical Assistants (AAMA) should select a CAAHEP-approved school for his or her education as a medical assistant.

Commission on Professional and Hospital Activities (CPHA) Nonprofit, nongovernmental organization in Ann Arbor, Michigan, established in 1955, that collects, processes, and distributes data on hospital use for management, evaluation, and research purposes. Two main programs of CPHA are the Professional Activity Study (PAS) and the Medical Audit Program (MAP), which represents a continuing study of hospital practice. CPHA maintains the coding system for the international classification of diseases.

Commissioner of Insurance State official responsible for the enforcement of laws pertaining to insurance in the respective states. The commissioner's title, status in government, and responsibilities differ somewhat from state to state, but all states have an official with such responsibilities regardless of his or her title. Also known as *Insurance Commissioner, Superintendent of Insurance*, or *Director of Insurance*.

commissioner's method System for calculating modified net premiums and reserves for life insurance policies.

common accident provision 1. Clause in a medical expense insurance contract that states if two or more members of the same family are injured in the same accident, their combined medical expenses will be subject to one deductible. 2. Clause in voluntary group accidental death and dismemberment insurance plans that states the amount payable by the insurance company is limited to a maximum for all employees killed or injured in one accident.

common control Under the Health Insurance Portability and Accountability Act (HIPAA), this management exists if an entity has the power, directly or indirectly, significantly to influence or direct the actions or policies of another entity.

common data file Abstract of all recent insurance claims filed for a patient.

common disaster clause Provision in a life insurance policy that states that the primary beneficiary must survive the insured by a specific period such as 60 or 90 days to be eligible to receive the policy proceeds. Otherwise, the proceeds will be paid as if the primary beneficiary had died before the insured.

common ownership Under the Health Insurance Portability and Accountability Act (HIPAA) Subpart E, this relationship exists if an entity or entities possess an ownership or equity interest of 5% or more in another entity.

common pleas See *small claims court*.

common stock Securities such as stocks and bonds that represent an ownership interest in a corporation. Holders of common stock may elect directors and collect dividends. Common stocks are subordinate to bondholder claims, preferred stockholders, and general creditors.

common working file (CWF) System of nine regional sectors with databases that contain the total Medicare beneficiary histories developed by the Centers for Medicare and Medicaid Services (CMS) to improve claims processing. Medicare fiscal intermediaries access CWF databases for eligibility, utilization, Medicare Secondary Payer (MSP), and other claims information.

communicate To convey information about a debt either directly or indirectly to a debtor through any medium (telephone, letter, facsimile).

communication 1. Ability to receive, interpret, and express spoken, written, and nonverbal messages. 2. Delivery of a message by any process to facilitate the collection of a debt, either directly or indirectly, to or from any individual through any number of media (letter or telephone call).

communicator See *multipurpose billing form*.

community-based services Local or regional assistance or support designed to help older people remain independent and in their own homes. This can include senior centers, transportation, delivered meals or congregate meals site, visiting nurses or home health aides, adult day care, and homemaker services.

community care network (CCN) See *accountable health plan (AHP)*.

community health center (CHC) Ambulatory health care facility that provides programs and care to the indigent in a community. CHCs usually serve a catchment area that has scarce or nonexistent health services or a population with special health needs. These centers attempt to coordinate federal, state, and local resources in a single organization capable of delivering both health and related social services to a defined population. Although such a center may not directly provide all types of health care, it is usually responsible for arranging all medical services needed by its patient population. Also called *neighborhood health center*.

community health information network (CHIN) Integrated network of computers and telecommunication systems that links many providers, payers, employers, and other health care entities within a geographical region. This system permits sharing and communicating clinical, administrative, and financial information. Also called *community health information system*.

community health information system See *community health information network (CHIN)*.

community hospital Facility that gives health care to individuals within a specific locale.

community mental health center (CMHC) Facility that provides comprehensive, ambulatory outpatient mental health day services to individuals residing in a specific locale (catchment area). CMHC is defined in the community Mental Health Centers Act (Section 201), which specifies the services to be provided and requirements for the governance, organization, and operation of the centers. The CMHC Act provides for federal financial assistance for the construction, development, and initial operations of CMHCs and, on an ongoing basis, for the costs of their consultation and education services. Health care services may consist of counseling, education, evaluation, development of skills for daily living, vocational rehabilitation, and short-term stabilization services.

community-oriented primary care (COPC) Type of medical care that combines primary care with a community population-based approach by identifying and addressing community health problems.

community rating Method for determining premiums for a managed care health insurance plan wherein the

C

premium is based on the average cost of the actual or anticipated health services used by all subscribers in a certain geographical area. Use of this method helps spread the cost of illness evenly for all subscribers to the insurance plan. Individual characteristics of the insured are not considered. Sometimes called *pooled rate*. See also *pooling*.

community rating area (CRA) Defined geographical region for which each insurance company must determine a single set of health insurance premiums.

community rating by class (CRC) See *adjusted community rating (ACR)*.

commutation See *financial settlement*.

commutation rights In life insurance, the right of the beneficiary to receive in a lump sum the cash value of the remaining payments under an insurance option chosen by the insured.

comorbid condition (CC) Medical condition that coexists with the primary cause for hospitalization and affects the patient's treatment and length of stay.

comorbidity Underlying condition or other condition that exists along with the condition for which the patient is receiving treatment. Used in diagnostic-related group (DRG) reimbursement. Sometimes referred to as *comorbidity condition* or *concurrent condition*.

comorbidity condition See *comorbidity* and *concurrent condition*.

comp See *compensation (comp)*.

company code number See *group number*.

company retention method System of comparing costs of several types of life insurance policies such as the present value of premiums, cash values, and dividends. It is calculated by weighing each item each year by the probability that it will be paid. See also *cost comparison methods*.

comparability In the Medicaid program, this term means that each state provides the same (comparable) benefits for those eligible except for those benefits in Medicaid waiver programs and benefits for children through Early and Periodic Screening, Diagnosis, and Treatment (EPSDT) programs.

comparability provision Medicare guideline stating that reasonable charges for medical services cannot be greater than similar services billed to non-Medicare patients covered by private insurance or managed care plans.

comparative condition Patient's situation that is documented as "either/or" in the medical record. Conditions include illness, disease, injury, pregnancy, bodily defect or abnormality, mental illness, alcoholism, or drug or chemical dependence.

comparative performance report (CPR) Document that gives the annual comparison of a physician's services and procedures to those of another doctor in the same specialty and geographical location.

compendium Collected information that includes standards of strength, purity, and quality of drugs. Official compendia in the United States are the *United States Pharmacopoeia*, the *National Formulary*, the *Homeopathic Pharmacopoeia of the United States*, and their supplements.

compensable injury Any trauma suffered by an employee that arises out of employment (AOE) and occurs in the course of employment (COE). This includes any aggravation or acceleration, because of employment, of a preexisting physical or mental condition or pathology.

compensation (comp) 1. Monetary payment for work performed or services rendered. 2. Used variously to refer to the workers' compensation law, compensation benefits generally, or compensation payments.

compensatories See *compensatory damages*.

compensatory damages Monetary payment awarded in court for actual loss or injury to a person or property sufficient in the amount to indemnify the injured person for the loss suffered. Also called *compensatories*.

competent Individual able to understand and act sanely and reasonably.

competitive benchmarking See *benchmarking*.

competitive medical plan (CMP) 1. Established by the Tax Equity and Fiscal Responsibility Act (TEFRA). This is a state-licensed health plan similar to a health maintenance organization (HMO) that delivers comprehensive, coordinated services to voluntary enrolled members on a prepaid, capitated basis. 2. CMP status may be granted by the federal government for the enrollment of Medicare beneficiaries into managed care plans, without having to qualify as an HMO. CMPs with Medicare contracts offer Medicare beneficiaries all services covered by fee-for-service Medicare. Medicare pays these plans on a monthly basis for each Medicare beneficiary. Medicare beneficiaries get all Medicare-covered hospital and medical insurance benefits through the plan. The CMP may also collect a premium from each Medicare member enrolled in the plan.

competitive pricing Method that uses market information for establishing payment rates that reflect the costs of an efficient managed care plan or health care provider (e.g., competitive bidding that obtains information on costs through the process of bidding).

complaint Expression of dissatisfaction about a certain problem encountered by the member of a managed care plan, or about a decision by the insurance company. A complaint must include a request for action to resolve the problem or change the decision. Also see *grievance*.

complaint (of fraud or abuse) Statement, oral or written, alleging that a provider or beneficiary received a Medicare benefit of monetary value, directly or indirectly, overtly or covertly, in cash or in kind, to which he or she is not entitled under current Medicare law, regulations, or policy. Included are allegations of misrepresentation and violations of Medicare requirements applicable to persons or entities that bill for covered items and services.

complaint register List of consumer complaints created by the state insurance department. It may be used for enforcing unfair trade practice laws.

complementary program Supplementary medical insurance for individuals who participate in Medicare Parts A and B. Also known as *Medigap (MG) policy, gap fill, Medifill, Medicare supplement policy,* or *wraparound plan.*

complementary and alternative medicine (CAM) Group of diverse medical and health care systems, practices, and products that are not presently considered to be part of conventional medicine. It is therapy using complementary medicine together with conventional medicine (e.g., using aromatherapy to help lessen a patient's discomfort after major surgery) or conventional medicine in place of alternative medicine (e.g., use of a special diet to treat cancer instead of major surgery or chemotherapy). Also see *National Center for Complementary and Alternative Medicine (NCCAM).*

complete care organization (CCO) Hospital facilities and providers that work together to give medical care within a community.

complete past history (complete PH) See *past history.*

complete procedure 1. Comprehensive diagnostic service when a radiological procedure can be separated into a professional component performed by a physician and a technical component that is supplied by technical staff, equipment, overhead, and supplies. See also *separate procedure* to learn the difference between complete versus separate. 2. Main or large surgical procedure performed. See *partial procedure* to learn the difference between complete versus partial.

complete review of systems (complete ROS) See *review of systems (ROS).*

complete ROS See *review of systems (ROS).*

completed claim Formal request for payment transmitted to a third-party payer.

completion factor Monthly sum (factor) that is used to adjust incurred and paid insurance claims to expected incurred claims.

complex repair Physical restoration of damaged tissue when the wound requires more than layered closure as with scar revision, débridement (e.g., traumatic lacerations or avulsions), extensive undermining, stents, or retention sutures. Necessary preparation includes creation of a defect for repairs (e.g., excision of a scar requiring a complex repair) or the débridement of complicated lacerations or avulsions. Other examples are reconstructive surgery; complicated wound closure; skin grafting; intricate, unusual, and time-consuming

methods to get maximum function and cosmetic results; and creation of a defect by extending excisions.

complexity In reference to medical decision making, see *straightforward (SF), low complexity (LC), moderate complexity (MC),* and *high complexity (HC).*

compliance 1. To satisfy federal mandates under the Health Insurance Portability and Accountability Act (HIPAA) by ensuring the physician or facility provides and bills for services according to the laws, regulations, and guidelines that govern it. 2. Degree to which a patient follows a treatment program directed by a physician or health care provider.

compliance audits Formal, methodical examination or review done to ensure compliance with all laws, HIPAA regulations, and guidelines. This is accomplished by inspecting, analyzing, and scrutinizing the way something is being done (e.g., bookkeeping practices, medical record documentation, insurance claim filing, diagnostic and procedural code selection).

compliance committee Under HIPAA, those individuals in a facility or in a physician's medical practice that are assigned to help the compliance officer teach and comply with all laws, regulations, and guidelines related to health care.

compliance date Under HIPAA, the date a covered entity must comply with a standard, an implementation specification, a requirement, or a modification. This is usually 24 months after the effective date of the associated final rule for most entities, but 36 months after the effective date for small health plans. For future changes in the standards, the compliance date would be at least 180 days after the effective date but can be longer for small health plans and for complex changes.

compliance deadline Target date when a final rule developed by the Secretary of Health and Human Services to meet a specific law under the Health Insurance Portability and Accountability Act (HIPAA) becomes mandatory and is strictly enforced.

compliance guidance Document published by the Office of the Inspector General (OIG) to enable hospitals, home health care, nursing homes, third-party billing companies, and physician medical practices to establish compliance programs.

compliance monitoring Under the Health Insurance Portability and Accountability Act (HIPAA), to check provider and insurance company responsibilities in regard to the accuracy of procedure codes and verification of medical services provided to patients to prevent fraud and abuse.

compliance officer Individual overseeing a facility's or medical practice's compliance program who plans, implements, and monitors the program with a staff trained to perform activities that comply with the Health Insurance Portability and Accountability Act (HIPAA) rules.

compliance plan Auditing, monitoring, and staff training implemented to get rid of errors in coding, billing, and transmission of electronic claims for compliance with HIPAA guidelines.

compliance program A management plan adopted by a medical practice or facility that is composed of policies and procedures to accomplish uniformity, consistency, and conformity in medical recordkeeping that fulfills official HIPAA requirements. It fosters prevention of fraudulent activities by the development of internal controls.

complication Disease or condition arising during the course of, or as a result of, another disease, modifying medical care requirements; for diagnosis-related groups (DRGs), a condition that arises during the hospital stay that prolongs the length of stay by at least 1 day in approximately 75% of cases. Also known as *substantial complication.*

complications and comorbidities (CC) Key factors in establishing a diagnosis-related group (DRG). See *complication* and *comorbidity.*

component code 1. The portion of a service described before the semicolon (;) of a CPT comprehensive code, together with the portion of a service described by the indented (component) code. 2. Under the Correct Coding Initiative (CCI), a CCI file known as *component edits* lists pairs of codes considered an integral part of the main surgical service provided or a component of a more comprehensive procedure. When billing a Medicare case, a component code that follows a comprehensive code cannot be charged to Medicare if the comprehensive code is billed.

component code, column I In the Correct Coding Initiative (CCI) edits, the code that follows the column I code, which cannot be billed when the more comprehensive code is billed.

component coding Standardizing method that allows a physician to list a code, regardless of specialty, that specifically identifies whether the procedural component, the radiological component, or both aspects of the service was provided.

composite rate 1. Flat or standard rate charged to all enrollees of a managed care plan in a particular group regardless of whether they are enrolled for single or family coverage. 2. Phrase that describes the average unit cost per employee covered. 3. In the Medicare program, this system is one of two methods of payment for dialysis services rendered in the patient's home. Payment does not include the physician's professional services, separately billable laboratory services, and separately billable drugs.

comprehensive 1. Term used to describe a level of history and/or physical examination. 2. When an audit is taking place, term that indicates a general multisystem examination (eight or more organ systems or complete examination of a single organ system).

Comprehensive Alcohol Abuse and Alcoholism Prevention, Treatment and Rehabilitation Act Federal legislation in 1970 that protects the confidentiality of the identity, diagnosis, prognosis, or treatment of any patient for alcohol abuse.

comprehensive code 1. Single procedural code that describes or covers two or more CPT component codes that are bundled together as one unit. 2. Under the Correct Coding Initiative (CCI), a file known as *component edits* lists pairs of codes considered an integral part of the main surgical service provided. The comprehensive procedure is listed first and then behind it is a component code.

comprehensive code, column I In the Correct Coding Initiative (CCI) edits, a column I comprehensive code that represents the major procedure or service when billed with another code.

comprehensive/component edit One of two main types of Correct Coding Initiative (CCI) edits. This type of edit is applied to code combinations in which one of the codes is a component of the more comprehensive code. Note: Only the comprehensive code is paid. Also see *mutually exclusive edit.*

comprehensive coverage Insurance agreement that protects and covers all named hazards or perils within the general scope of one contract except those specifically excluded.

Comprehensive Error Rate Testing (CERT) Program One of two programs established by the Centers for Medicare and Medicaid Services (CMS) to monitor and report the accuracy of Medicare FFS payments: the Comprehensive Error Rate Testing (CERT) program and the Hospital Payment Monitoring Program (HPMP). The national error rate is calculated using a combination of data from the CERT contractor and HPMP with each component representing about 60% and 40% of the total Medicare FFS dollars paid. The CERT program measures the error rate for claims submitted to Carriers, Durable Medical Equipment Regional Carriers (DMERCs), and Fiscal Intermediaries (FIs). The HPMP measures the error rate for the quality improvement organizations (QIOs). Beginning in 2003, CMS elected to calculate a provider compliance error rate in addition to the paid claims error rate. The provider compliance error rate measures how well providers prepare Medicare FFS claims for submission. CMS calculates the Medicare Fee-For-Service error rate and estimate of improper claim payments using a methodology the OIG approved. The CERT methodology includes randomly selecting a sample of approximately 120,000 submitted claims, requesting medical records from providers who submitted the claims, and reviewing the claims and medical records for compliance with Medicare coverage, coding, and billing rules.

comprehensive examination In 1995 the American Medical Association (AMA) and Centers for Medicare and Medicaid Services (CMS) developed documentation guidelines for CPT evaluation and management services and modified them in 1997.
Comprehensive examination 1995 guidelines: a general multisystem examination or a complete examination of a single organ system. Comprehensive examination 1997 guidelines for multisystem examination: at least nine organ systems or body areas. For each system or area selected, all elements of the examination identified in a table by a bullet (•) should be performed, unless specific directions limit the content of the examination. For each area or system, documentation of at least two elements identified in a table by a bullet (•) is expected. The 1997 guidelines for a single organ system examination: performance of all elements identified in a table by a bullet (•), whether in a shaded or unshaded box. Documentation of every element in each shaded box and at least one element in each unshaded box is expected. See Figure C-2.

comprehensive health care clinic (CHCC) Medical facility that provides outpatient and ambulatory care services with a limited holding bed capacity.

comprehensive health planning (CHP) Health planning initiative of the Comprehensive Health Planning and Public Health Services Amendment of 1966 and replaced by the National Health Planning and Resources Development Act of 1974. It was intended to encompass all factors and programs affecting the health of people in the United States. Federal support for CHP was eliminated in 1986.

comprehensive history In 1995 the American Medical Association (AMA) and Centers for Medicare and Medicaid Services (CMS) developed documentation guidelines for CPT evaluation and management services and modified them in 1997. For a comprehensive history, medical documentation must include the chief complaint, an extended history of present illness (HPI), a complete review of systems (ROS), and complete past, family, and/or social history (PFSH).

comprehensive inpatient rehabilitation facility Facility that provides comprehensive rehabilitation services under the supervision of a physician to inpatients with physical disabilities. Services include physical therapy, occupational therapy, speech pathology, social or psychological services, and orthotics and prosthetics services.

comprehensive major medical (CMM) See *comprehensive major medical (CMM) insurance.*

comprehensive major medical (CMM) insurance Health insurance that combines the features and benefits of basic hospital, basic medical-surgical, and supplemental major medical benefits into one policy with coinsurance and a deductible. Sometimes called *comprehensive program, comprehensive medical care,* *comprehensive medical expense insurance,* and *comprehensive major medical (CMM).*

comprehensive managed care organization (MCO) Health maintenance organization that is an eligible organization with a contract under §1876 or a Medicare+Choice organization; a provider-sponsored organization, or any other private or public organization, that meets the requirements of §1902(w). These MCOs provide comprehensive services to commercial and/or Medicare enrollees, as well as Medicaid enrollees.

comprehensive MCO See *comprehensive managed care organization (MCO).*

comprehensive medical care See *comprehensive major medical (CMM) insurance.*

comprehensive medical expense insurance See *comprehensive major medical (CMM) insurance.*

comprehensive medical insurance See *comprehensive major medical (CMM) insurance.*

comprehensive medical-legal evaluation Assessment of an employee that results in the preparation of a narrative medical report prepared and performed by a qualified medical evaluator (QME) and agreed medical evaluator (AME), or the primary treating physician, to prove or disprove a contested workers' compensation claim.

comprehensive outpatient rehabilitation facility (CORF) Facility providing services such as physician's services related to administrative functions; physical therapy, occupational therapy, speech pathology services, and respiratory therapy; social and psychological services; and prosthetic and orthotic devices.

comprehensive perinatal services program (CPSP) Program that offers a wide range of services to pregnant Medi-Cal recipients.

comprehensive physical damage coverage Optional insurance that pays for damage to the insured's automobile caused by events other than collection or rolling the car over such as fire, theft, vandalism, flood, or hail. This type of insurance is frequently required if a person has taken out a car loan.

comprehensive program See *comprehensive major medical (CMM) insurance.*

comprehensive type of foundation A type of foundation that designs and sponsors prepaid health programs or sets minimum benefits of coverage.

compromise Under Medicare Secondary Payer guidelines, this is a settlement of differences by mutual consent or adjustment of matters in dispute by mutual concession; a negotiated settlement between parties who are in essentially equal bargaining positions, wherein neither party admits nor concedes that he or she is entitled to less than he or she desires, but accepts less to end the dispute.

compromise and release (C and R) Agreement or settlement arrived at, whether in or out of court, for settling a workers' compensation case after the patient

C

MULTIORGAN SYSTEM EXAMINATION REQUIREMENTS (SHADED)
CONTENT and DOCUMENTATION

Level of Exam	Perform and Document
Problem focused	One to five elements identified by a bullet.
Expanded Problem Focused	At least six elements identified by a bullet.
Detailed	At least twelve elements identified by a bullet.
Comprehensive	Perform all elements identified by a bullet; document every element in every shaded box and at least one element in every unshaded box.

Genitourinary		Genitourinary (continued)	
System/Body Area	**Elements of Examination**	**System/Body Area**	**Elements of Examination**
Constitutional	• Measurement of **any three of the following seven** vital signs: 1) sitting or standing blood pressure, 2) supine blood pressure, 3) pulse rate and regularity, 4) respiration, 5) temperature, 6) height, 7) weight (may be measured and recorded by ancillary staff) • General appearance of patient *e.g. development, nutrition, body habitus, deformities, attention to grooming*	Lymphatic	• Palpation of lymph nodes in neck, axillae, groin and/or other location
		Skin	• Inspection and/or palpation of skin and subcutaneous tissue *e.g. rashes, lesions, ulcers*
		Neurological/ psychiatric	Brief assessment of mental status including: • Orientation to time, place and person • Mood and affect *e.g. depression, anxiety, agitation*
Neck	• Examination of neck *e.g. masses, overall appearance, symmetry, tracheal position, crepitus* • Examination of thyroid *e.g. enlargement, tenderness, mass*	Skin	
		System/Body Area	**Elements of Examination**
		Constitutional	• Measurement of **any three of the following seven** vital signs: 1) sitting or standing blood pressure, 3) pulse rate and regularity, 4) respiration, 5) temperature, 6) height, 7) weight (may be measured and recorded by ancillary staff) • General appearance of patient *e.g. development, nutrition, body habitus, deformities, attention to grooming*
Respiratory	• Assessment of respiratory effect *e.g. intercostal retractions, use of accessory muscles, diaphragmatic movement* • Auscultation of lungs *e.g. breath sounds, adventitious sounds, rubs*		
Cardiovascular	• Auscultation of heart with notation of abnormal sounds and murmurs • Examination of peripheral vascular system by observation *e.g. swelling, varicosities* and palpation *e.g. pulses, temperature, edema, tenderness*	Eyes	• Inspection of conjuctivae and lids
		Ears, nose, mouth and throat	• Inspection of lips, teeth and gums • Examination of oropharynx *e.g. oral mucosa, hard and soft palates, tongue, tonsils, and posterior pharynx*
Chest (breasts)	See genitourinary (female)		
Gastrointestinal (abdomen)	⊙ Examination of abdomen with notation of presence of masses or tenderness • Examination for presence or absence of hernia • Examination of liver and spleen • Obtain stool sample for occult blood test when indicated	Neck	• Examination of thyroid *e.g. enlargement, tenderness, mass*
		Gastrointestinal (abdomen)	• Examination of liver and spleen • Examination of anus for condyloma and other lesions
		Lymphatic	• Palpation of lymph nodes in neck, axillae, groin and/or other location
Genitourinary (male)	• Inspection of anus and perineum Examination (with or without specimen collection for smears and cultures) of genitalia including: • Scrotum *e.g. lesions, cysts, rashes* • Epididymides *e.g. size, symmetry, masses* ⊙ Testes *e.g. size, symmetry, masses* • Urethral meatus *e.g. size, location, lesions, discharge* ⊙ Penis *e.g. lesions, presence or absence of foreskin, foreskin retractability, plaque, masses, scarring, deformities* Digital rectal examination including: ⊙ Prostate gland *e.g. size, symmetry, nodularity, tenderness* • Seminal vesicles *e.g. symmetry, tenderness, masses, enlargement* • Sphincter tone, presence of hemorrhoids, rectal masses	Extremities	• Inspection and palpation of digits and nails *e.g. clubbing, cyanosis, inflammation, petechiae, ischemia, infections, nodes*
		Skin	• Palpation of scalp and inspection of hair of scalp, eyebrows, face, chest, pubic area (when indicated) and extremities • Inspection and/or palpation of skin and subcutaneous tissue *e.g. rashes, lesions, ulcers, susceptibility in and presence of photo damage* in **eight of the following ten areas:** 1) head including face, 2) neck, 3) chest including breasts and axilla, 4) abdomen, 5) genitalia, groin, buttocks, 6) back, 7) right upper extremity, 8) left upper extremity, 9) right lower extremity, 10) left lower extremity Note: For the comprehensive level, the examination of all eight anatomic areas must be performed and documented. For the three lower levels of examination, each body area is counted separately. For example, inspection and/or palpation of the skin and subcutaneous tissue of the head and neck extremities constitutes two areas • Inspection of eccrine and apocrine glands of skin and subcutaneous tissue with identification and location of any hyperhidrosis, chromhidroses or bromhidrosis
Genitourinary (female) Includes at least seven of the eleven elements to the right identified by bullets:	• Inspection and palpation of breasts *e.g. masses or lumps, tenderness, symmetry, nipple discharge* • Digital rectal examination including sphincter tone, presence of hemorrhoids, rectal masses Pelvic examination (with or without specimen collection for smears and cultures) including: • External genitalia *e.g. general appearance, hair distribution, lesions* • Urethral meatus *e.g. size, location, lesions, prolapse* • Urethra *e.g. masses, tenderness, scarring* • Bladder *e.g. fullness, masses, tenderness* • Vagina *e.g. general appearance, estrogen effect, discharge, lesions, pelvic support, cystocele, rectocele* • Cervix *e.g. general appearance, lesions, discharge* • Uterus *e.g. size, contour, position, mobility, tenderness, descent or support* • Adnexa/parametria *e.g. masses, tenderness, organomegaly, nodularity* • Anus and perineum	Neurological/ psychiatric	Brief assessment of mental status including: • Orientation to time, place and person • Mood and affect *e.g. depression, anxiety, agitation*

Figure C-2 Review/Audit worksheet of a general multiorgan system physical examination that shows the details (elements) of examination for each body area/system.

has been declared permanent and stationary. This phrase is used both as a noun and as a verb.

computation years For Social Security benefits, years with highest earnings selected from the base years. Total earnings in the computation years are added together and divided by the number of months in those years to obtain the average monthly earnings (AME).

computer-assisted coding (CAC) Use of computer software that automatically generates a set of medical codes for review, validation, and use based on clinical documentation provided by health care practitioners. CAC uses two technology options: natural language processing (NLP) and structured input.

computer-assisted video keratography (CAVK) See *corneal topography.*

computer-based patient record (CPR) See *electronic medical record (EMR).*

Computer-based Patient Record Institute-Healthcare Open Systems and Trials Industry organization that promotes the use of health care information systems including electronic health care records.

computer billing Producing statements via a computer system.

computer data Information entered into a computer, retrieved from a computer, or transmitted to another computer.

computer matching agreement Any computerized comparison of two or more systems of records or a system of records of nonfederal records for the purpose of (1) establishments or verifying eligibility or compliance with law and regulations of applicants or recipients/beneficiaries or (2) recouping payments or overpayments.

computer media claims (CMC) System that permits submission of Medi-Cal claims via telecommunication through magnetic tape or diskette and modem.

computerized patient record (CPR) See *electronic medical record (EMR).*

computerized physician order entry (CPOE) Process of electronic entry that allows physicians to enter orders into a computer instead of handwriting them, thus reducing errors in communicating in the hospital setting.

computerized tomography (CT) Sophisticated radiological scanning device that creates a series of transverse images for detecting abnormalities.

CON See *certificate of need (CON).*

conciliation Informal meeting between the attorney for the workers' compensation insurance company and the employee and/or the employee's attorney. A conciliator is not an attorney and cannot grant the employee's request for benefits. It is the conciliator's job to determine if there is some way that the parties can reach an agreement and, if not, to assist in taking it to the next step to settle (resolve) the dispute.

concierge care System of medical care in which physicians either have patients pay for whatever services are received or charge patients annual membership fees entitling them to certain services (e.g., annual physical, medical screenings for certain diseases or illnesses, preventive care). Patients are given paperwork to submit claims to their insurance companies. This system is usually for well-to-do clientele, which is why it sometimes is referred to as *boutique medicine.* Physicians prefer that it be called *personalized, preventive care* or *fee-based medical care.*

conciliation court See *small claims court.*

concomitant operations Additional procedures completed during the same surgical session.

concurrent care Provision of similar services (e.g., hospital visits) to the same patient by more than one physician on the same day. Usually there is the presence of a separate physical disorder, but it is possible they may be providing care for the same diagnosis on the same day. When concurrent care is provided, the diagnosis must reflect the medical necessity of different specialties. Also called *concurrent medical care.*

concurrent coding Process in which employees trained in coding work directly on the hospital inpatient units and code medical care as it happens.

concurrent condition Disorder that coexists with the primary condition, complicating the treatment and management of the primary disorder. It may alter the course of treatment required or lengthen the expected recovery time of the primary condition. It is also referred to as *comorbidity* or *comorbidity condition.*

concurrent medical care See *concurrent care.*

concurrent payment audit Assessment and review that occurs at the time reimbursements are posted to financial records to evaluate the accuracy of payments received on the day of the audit.

concurrent review Evaluation of health care services to determine medical necessity and appropriateness of medical care during the time the services are being provided. It is done to encourage discharge of the patient from the hospital as soon as his or her medical condition no longer needs continued inpatient care. This may occur for inpatient, residential, partial hospitalization treatment, and outpatient care. The review is usually done at the time services are provided by a health care provider other than the one giving the care.

condition 1. Any illness, disease, injury, pregnancy, bodily defect or abnormality, mental illness, alcoholism, or drug or chemical dependence. 2. Part of an insurance policy that states the insured's obligation and those of the insurance company in order for the policy to be in effect.

condition category (CC) Wide-ranging sets of similar diseases clinically and cost comparable under the Centers for Medicare and Medicaid Services (CMS)

Hierarchical Condition Categories (HCC) Model for capitated payments to managed care organizations.

condition code (CC) Two-digit numeric code inserted in Fields 18 through 28 on the Uniform Bill (UB-04) insurance claim form to show that a condition applies and affects payment of the claim. Condition codes denote if coverage exists under another insurance, the illness or injury is employment related, the bill is an outlier, or medical necessity affects room assignment.

conditional contract Insurance agreement in which the insured's acceptance is considered uncertain during a specific time period and during which time the individual may cancel the agreement and receive a refund of the premium payments.

conditional fee See *contingency fee.*

conditional payment Reimbursement made by Medicare for services for which a third-party (primary payer) is responsible. The provider (physician) requests payment from the Medicare Secondary Payer because a lengthy processing delay (more than 120 days) by the third-party payer is expected. The provider must agree to send a refund or request for reconsideration from Medicare within 60 days of the third-party payer's payment.

conditional premium receipt Type of premium receipt given to the applicant on payment of the initial premium. The life insurance policy becomes effective before it is actually issued only on acceptance or approval of the application (i.e., the proposed insured is found to be insurable). Also called *conditional receipt.*

conditional primary payer status Circumstance in which Medicare is billed as the primary payer for a temporary period of time.

conditional receipt See *conditional premium receipt.*

conditionally renewable Insurance policy renewal provision that grants the insurer a limited right to refuse to renew a health insurance policy either to a stated date, at the end of a premium payment period, or at an advanced age.

conditions 1. Illnesses, diseases, injuries, pregnancies, bodily defects or abnormalities, mental illnesses, alcoholism, or drug or chemical dependencies. 2. Part of an insurance policy that states the insured's obligations and those of the insurance company in order for the policy to be in effect.

conditions of participation (COPs) Federal requirements that health care facilities must meet to be eligible to participate in the Medicare program and receive payments for medical services rendered to beneficiaries. These conditions include meeting a statutory definition of the particular institution or facility, conforming to state and local laws and having an acceptable utilization review plan. Surveys to determine whether facilities meet conditions of participation are made by the appropriate state health agency.

conference In a workers' compensation case, a meeting of the injured employee's attorney and the insurance company's lawyer before an administrative judge who will make a decision about an industrial claim in dispute.

confidential 1. Private information about one individual entrusted to another person that must be protected from unauthorized disclosure to any third party. 2. Information that may not be freely disclosed.

confidential communication Privileged communication that may be disclosed only with the patient's permission.

confidential health care information Private data that contain an individual's health care history, present complaints, signs and symptoms, condition, diagnosis, treatment, or evaluation. It may be oral or recorded in any form or medium (paper, microfilm, electronic).

confidential information Data recognized by an individual that should not be freely disclosed and must be protected for unauthorized disclosure to another entity; private information.

confidentiality State of treating privately or secretly, and not disclosing to other individuals or for public knowledge the patient's conversations or medical records.

confinement See *hospital confinement.*

confining sickness Illness that requires an individual to either remain at home or be admitted to the hospital.

confirmation certificate Document issued to a beneficiary of a life insurance policy that states the amount of life insurance proceeds in a retained asset account, the account number, and the interest rate.

conflict of interest Incompatibility between one's private interests and one's business duties such as a relative of an incompetent patient who has wishes that are not in the patient's best interests or when a physician is contracted with a managed care plan in which he or she makes more profit if less medical care is given to patients.

congenital Anomaly or defect present since the time of birth.

congregate care facility (CCF) Housing complexes designed and created to meet the special accommodation, dietary, and health needs of the elderly, disabled, or mentally retarded.

congregate housing Individual apartments in which residents may receive some services such as a daily meal with other tenants. Buildings usually have some common areas such as a dining room and lounge and additional safety measures such as emergency call buttons. Such housing may be rent-subsidized, which is known as *Section 8 housing.*

connecting words Phrases or terms in ICD-9-CM diagnostic coding that indicate a relationship between the main term and the associated conditions or causes of a disease or illness.

conscious/moderate sedation (⊙) Symbol used in the procedure code book titled *Current Procedural Terminology (CPT)*. It precedes a procedure code and identifies when conscious sedation with or without analgesia is used with a procedure.

consent Verbal or written agreement that gives approval to some action, situation, or statement.

consent form Because of the Health Insurance Portability and Accountability Act (HIPAA), this document is not required before physicians use or disclose protected health information for treatment, payment, or routine health care operations of the patient. For other purposes, see *authorization form*.

conservation Insurance company or agent's efforts to prevent a policy from lapsing.

consideration In contracts, anything of value given by one individual to another to induce the other person to enter into the contract.

consideration clause Insurance policy section that states the reason an insurance company issues an insurance contract (i.e., the statements on the application and the payment of the insurance premium).

consistency edits Computer software screening system that identifies clinical, coding, billing, and data errors on insurance claims. Under the Medicare program, insurance claims must pass edits for all Medicare-required fields on both the Uniform Bill (UB-04) and CMS-1500 claim forms for payment.

Consolidated Omnibus Reconciliation Act of 1985 (COBRA) Federal law requiring employers to offer continuation of health insurance coverage for at least 18 months to employees and their beneficiaries after any of the following: the death of a spouse, their current position has been terminated, work hours are reduced, left job voluntarily, or getting a divorce. Employees may have to pay both their share and the employer's share of the premium. Generally, they may also have to pay an administrative fee. The law does not affect employers with fewer than 20 employees. However, some state laws may apply to employers with fewer than 20 employees. Legislation also includes protection for patients seeking emergency treatment in a hospital in that every hospital participating in the Medicare program must treat any patient in an emergency situation regardless of the patient's ability to pay and the patient does not have to be on Medicare.

consolidation Uniting health care facilities under the control of a few health care organizations through mergers, acquisitions, alliances, and formation of contractual networks. This process is related to integration. See *integration*.

constant pain In a workers' compensation case, pain approximately 90% to 100% of the time.

constant symptoms In workers' compensation cases, any indication of disease perceived by the patient (symptoms) that occur approximately 90% to 100% of the time.

constitutional signs and symptoms Vital signs (temperature, pulse, respiration, blood pressure) and an assessment of an individual's general well-being.

constructive delivery Physical delivery of an insurance policy either to the insured or to the insurance agent of the applicant.

consultant Individual who by training and experience has acquired special knowledge in a subject area (medical, dental, or other medical specialty) and is recognized by a peer group as an expert and provides professional advice or medical services on request.

consultation 1. Act of requesting advice from another physician or medical specialist about diagnosis or treatment of a patient. 2. In the Medicare program, services rendered by a physician (specialist, professional advisor, or qualified nonphysician practitioner) whose opinion or advice is requested by another physician, agency, or primary care provider in the evaluation or treatment of a patient's illness or a suspected problem. The consultant reviews the history, does an examination of the patient, and provides a written opinion to the requesting physician. 3. In coding procedures, this is a type of service provided by a physician whose opinion or advice regarding evaluation and/or management of a specific medical problem is requested by another physician or other appropriate source. A physician consultant may initiate diagnostic and/or therapeutic services at the same or subsequent visit. The written or verbal request for a consult and the medical reason for it may be made by a physician or other appropriate source and documented in the patient's medical record. The consultant's opinion and any services that were ordered or performed must also be documented in the patient's medical record and communicated by written report to the requesting physician or other appropriate source. Remember the 3R's for documentation for both physicians: written or verbal *request* and *medical reason*, *render* opinion and document findings, and *report* to requesting physician. Also called *medical consultation*.

consultative examiner (CE) A physician who is paid a fee to examine and/or test a person for disability under either the SSDI or SSI program.

consulting nurse Registered nurse (RN) trained to assess medical problems by telephone and advise patients where to obtain medical care, as well as what treatment to do at home for symptoms.

consulting physician Provider whose opinion or advice regarding evaluation and/or management of a specific problem is requested by another physician. This may involve either examining the patient or the patient's medical record.

consumer In the area of health care, an individual who may receive medical services, such as a patient or a member of a managed care plan. Also called *health care consumer*.

consumer assessment of health plans study (CAHPS) Annual national survey that releases information on Medicare beneficiaries' experiences and satisfaction with receiving care in managed care plans.

consumer-directed health plan (CDHP) Type of health insurance plan that places more control of health care into the consumer's hands. These plans have high deductibles that the patient must pay; thus it is important that the provider collect the deductible and coinsurance amounts. Also see *health reimbursement account (HRA)* and *health savings account (HSA).*

consumer health alliances Regional, private, nonprofit components of managed care systems that purchase health care benefit packages for small employers and individuals. They act as cooperatives between government and the public so that health plans in a region conform to federal benefits and quality standards and keep costs within a mandated budget. They enroll individuals, collect premiums, purchase enrollee's insurance from participating health plans, and enforce rules that manage health plan competition. Also referred to as *alliances, health insurance purchasing cooperatives (HIPCs), health insurance purchasing corporations, health alliances, regional health alliances, health plan purchasing cooperatives (HPPC),* or *purchasing group.*

consumer price index (CPI) Economic barometer used by the Department of Labor Statistics to measure the average change in prices over time in a fixed group of goods and services. In this report, all references to the CPI relate to the CPI for urban wage earners and clerical workers (CPI-W).

consumer report Communication of information that pertains to a consumer's credit standing, credit capacity, general reputation, or personal characteristics.

consumer reporting agency Organization that prepares consumer reports and provides them either for profit or on a nonprofit basis to other persons or organizations. Also called a *credit reporting agency.*

consumer self-report data Information collected through survey or focus groups. Surveys may include Medicaid beneficiaries currently or previously enrolled in a managed care organization (MCO) or prepaid health plan (PHP). The survey may be conducted by the state or a contractor to the state.

consumer survey data Information collected through a survey of those Medicaid beneficiaries who are enrolled in the program and have used the services. The survey may be conducted by the state or managed care entity (if the managed care entity reports the results to the state).

consumerism Theory or system to protect buyers against products that are inferior and advertising that is misleading.

consumption tax See *value added tax (VAT).*

contact lens Small, curved glass, or rigid gas-permeable or soft plastic ophthalmic corrective lens shaped to fit the individual's eye(s) either to correct refractive error or to enhance appearance. These lenses are prescribed by a physician or optometrist.

contaminated Presence of blood or other infectious materials on any item or surface.

contaminated laundry Dirty clothes that have been soiled with blood or other infectious materials or that may contain sharps.

contaminated sharps Any dirty or impure object that can penetrate the skin such as broken capillary tubes, broken glass, exposed ends of dental wires, needles, and scalpels.

contestable clause Policy stipulation that states conditions under which the insurance contract may be contested or voided such as misrepresentation in an insurance application, fraud, or material misstatement.

contestable period Time frame of usually 2 years in which an insurance company may investigate the validity of a life insurance application and cancel the policy.

context 1. In a medical problem, an entire situation, interrelated condition, environment, or other factors pertaining to a particular event. 2. Part of a sentence or paragraph that surrounds a specified word or passage and determines its exact meaning such as to quote a remark out of context.

continence Ability of an individual to control bowel and bladder functions and maintain a reasonable level of personal hygiene. Also see *activities of daily living (ADLs).*

contingencies Events that may or may not happen. Insurance companies base their premium rates and acceptability of risks on the probability that certain contingencies will or will not occur.

contingency 1. Event that may or may not occur. 2. Funds included in the trust fund to serve as a cushion in case actual expenditures are higher than those projected at the time financing was established. Because the financing is set prospectively, actual experience may be different from the estimates used in setting the financing. Also see *contingency fee.*

contingency fee Fee for an attorney's services only if the plaintiff's (patient's) lawsuit is successful or is favorably settled out of court. The fee is calculated as a percentage of the client's net recovery (e.g., 25% of the recovery if the case is settled and 35% if the case is won at trial). If no settlement, the attorney is not paid. Also called *contingent fee, contingency,* or *conditional fee.*

contingency margin Amount included in the actuarial rates to provide for changes in the contingency level in the trust fund. Positive margins increase the contingency level and negative margins decrease it.

contingency reserve Portion of funds that insurance companies separate from surplus funds to provide for unusual and unexpectedly large claim amounts for catastrophic losses.

contingent beneficiary Person or persons named in a life insurance policy to receive the proceeds in the event the original or primary beneficiary should die before the person whose life is insured. Also called *alternate beneficiary, secondary beneficiary,* or *successor beneficiary.*

contingent fee See *contingency fee.*

contingent liability Legal responsibility of individuals, corporations, or partnerships, for injuries or accidents caused by persons (other than employees) for whose actions or omissions the individuals, corporations, or partnerships are responsible.

contingent payee Individual who receives life insurance proceeds that are still payable under a settlement option at the time of the primary payee's death. Also called *successor payee.*

contingent payment Payment to be made only if a specific predesignated condition is met.

contingent renewal privilege Insurance policy provision that allows an insured to continue insurance coverage when specific conditions are fulfilled (e.g., continued full-time employment beyond age 65).

continued stay review Evaluation conducted by a hospital or managed care plan to determine if the current place of service is the most appropriate to give the level of care needed by the patient. Also called *utilization review (UR), utilization and management control,* and *medical review (UR).*

continuance tables Record or schedule that shows morbidity statistics indicating the distribution of insurance claims categorized by duration of illness or amount of expense of the claims.

continuation of coverage Insurance coverage that remains even though an employee has a termination of employment or becomes divorced. Continuation of coverage is required by and specified in the Consolidated Omnibus Reconciliation Act of 1985 (COBRA) legislation.

continuation of enrollment Managed care plan option that allows an enrollee to continue in the Medicare+Choice plan when he or she leaves the plan's service area to reside elsewhere, possibly permanently.

continuing care retirement community (CCRC) Self-sufficient community that provides residential services (meals, housekeeping, laundry) and housing to meet the needs of elderly individuals. There is usually a large lump-sum entrance fee and a monthly fee. CCRCs provide independent living, intermediate and skilled nursing care, personal care, and organized social and recreational activities designed for participation in community life. Licensed as nursing homes/residential care facilities or as homes for the aging.

continuing claim Insurance claim submitted for the same confinement or course of ongoing treatment for which a previous initial bill has been submitted. Such claims can be submitted every 30 or 60 days.

continuing education (CE) Formal education pursued by a working professional and intended to improve or maintain professional competence by obtaining current knowledge pertinent to the individual's specific health care career. Also called *continuing medical education.*

continuing medical education (CME) See *continuing education (CE).*

Continuity Assessment Record and Evaluation (CARE) Standardized data set created under the Deficit Reduction Act of 2005 and developed to unify and standardize federal assessment to improve continuity of care when patients transfer between providers and facilities. It is accessed through an Internet-based health and functional assessment instrument. This federal demonstration project will collect data until 2011.

continuity of care Continued treatment of a patient who is referred by one physician to another for the same condition.

continuity of care record (CCR) Subset of a patient's health record that provides a basic set of information from one incident of care to another episode of care.

continuity of coverage Health care contract in which benefits may be transferred from one plan to another without a lapse of coverage.

continuous ambulatory peritoneal dialysis Type of kidney dialysis where the patient's peritoneal membrane is used as the dialyzer. The patient dialyzes at home, using special supplies, but without the need for a machine.

continuous care Nursing care 24 hours a day during a period of crisis when the patient needs uninterrupted care to manage acute medical symptoms or needs emotional support as in a hospice case.

continuous coverage Insurance benefits that transfer from one health plan to another with no break in coverage or from one type of membership to another (e.g., from dependent to subscriber with a new subscriber identification number). Also called *continuity of coverage.*

continuous cycling peritoneal dialysis Type of kidney dialysis where the patient generally dialyzes at home and uses an automated peritoneal cycler for delivering dialysis exchanges.

continuous home care day In hospice cases, this is a day on which the patient is not in an inpatient facility and elects to receive nursing care on an uninterrupted basis at home. This type of care is furnished during brief periods of crisis and only as needed to maintain a terminally ill patient at home.

continuous-premium whole life insurance Type of whole life insurance that requires premiums payable until the death of the insured. Also called *straight life insurance* or *whole life insurance.*

continuous quality improvement (CQI) Process that continually monitors program performance. When a quality problem is identified, CQI develops a revised approach to that problem and monitors implementation and success of the revised approach. The process includes involvement at all stages by all organizations, which are affected by the problem and/or involved in implementing the revised approach. Sometimes called *total quality management (TQM)* and *quality improvement (QI)*.

continuum of care Medical care of all levels and intensity such as skilled nursing care and intermediate care provided to frail and chronically ill patients in a variety of settings (e.g., hospital facilities, nursing homes) over an extended period of time. Services also focus on the social, residential, rehabilitative, and supportive needs of individuals. Also see *episode of care (EOC)*.

contract 1. Legal enforceable agreement between the insurance carrier or managed care plan and the insured when relating to an insurance policy. 2. For workers' compensation cases, an agreement involving two or more parties in which each is obligated to the other to fulfill promises made. In industrial cases, the contract exists between the physician and the insurance carrier.

contract capitation See *case-rate capitation*.

contract group See *enrolled group*.

contract mix Distribution of types of enrollees who are dependents in insurance health plans (i.e., individual [single] coverage, husband and wife, family, subscriber and spouse, or subscriber and children). This is used to determine average insurance contract size.

contract month One month within an insurance contract period. This phrase is used by insurance companies and managed care plans to describe utilization or market share stated in terms of the number of subscriber contracts per month.

contract number Numerical identification assigned by an insurance plan to each employer or individual plan. Contract numbers help to identify benefits of specific health insurance plans.

contract of adhesion Legal agreement prepared by an insurance company that must be either accepted or rejected completely by the other party (insured), without negotiations between the parties to the agreement. Insurance contracts are contracts of adhesion.

contract of indemnity Type of agreement in which the amount of benefit paid is based on the actual amount of financial loss that is determined at the time of the loss. Many hospital expense insurance contracts are contracts of indemnity.

contract provider Entity that has a contractual agreement with a health insurance plan to give services to the plan's members. Such entities include ambulatory surgical centers, dentists, extended care facilities, home health care agencies, hospitals, pharmacists, physicians, and skilled nursing facilities. Also called *cooperating provider*.

contract rate See *premium rate*.

contract type See *coverage type*.

contract year Twelve consecutive months starting with the beginning date of coverage; this period may not always coincide with a calendar year.

contracted discount rate See *discounted fee-for-service (discounted FFS)*.

contracted services Those covered insurance benefits provided by the physician that are consistent with the physician's training, licensor, and scope of practice.

contracting hospital Facility that has a legal agreement with a managed care plan to provide specific hospital services to members of the plan.

contractor 1. See *insurance carrier*. 2. See *fiscal agent*. 3. See *fiscal intermediary*. 4. See *durable medical equipment regional carrier (DMERC)*. 5. See *regional home health intermediary (RHHI)*. 6. See *program safeguard contractor (PSC)*. Also known as *insurer* or *carrier*.

contractor policy Policy developed by Centers for Medicare and Medicaid Services (CMS) contractors (fiscal intermediary or carrier, affiliated contractor, provider service carrier) and used to make coverage and coding determinations. It is developed when there is an absence of national coverage policy for a service or all of the uses of a service; there is a need to interpret national coverage policy; or there is a need for local coding rules.

contractual adjustment Difference between the allowed amount and the billed amount that is credited to an account as agreed upon in the insurance contract with the provider of service.

contractual adjustment arrangement System of making hospital payments through a formal agreement with an insurance payer to accept for a patient or group of patients a discounted amount instead of actual fees as full payment for medical services.

contractual allowance Legal agreement between a provider and third-party payers such as Medicare or Medicaid to provide medical services for a predetermined fee; often used in a discounted fee arrangement. Also called *purchase discount*. See also *disallowance*.

contrast material See *contrast medium*.

contrast medium Substance that is injected into the body, introduced via catheter, or swallowed to allow radiographic images of internal structures that would normally be difficult to see on x-ray films. Also called *contrast material*.

contribution 1. Full or partial payment amount by an insurance company under an insurance contract that may be one or two or more contracts that cover the same loss. 2. A part of the insurance premium that is paid by either the policyholder or the insured or both. 3. Act of contributing.

contribution base See *maximum tax base*.

contribution limit Maximum yearly contribution legally permitted to a participant's account in a defined benefit pension plan (DBPP). This may include employer and employee contributions and forfeitures that have been reallocated from other participants' accounts. The contribution limit is set under Section 415 of the Internal Revenue Code.

contribution requirements Dollar amount an employer must pay for the cost of health insurance coverage for employees or employees and dependents.

contribution to surplus Income that results when a mutual insurance company makes more money than it needs to pay for the cost of providing insurance.

contributions See *payroll taxes.*

contributory elements Parts of documentation that confirm the selection of procedure codes for evaluation and management (E/M) services but may not be of sufficient quantity to make a change in code selection. An exception is if counseling or coordination of care requires more than half the intraservice time for the encounter, then time is used to determine the code selection when billing.

contributory group insurance Group insurance plan in which the insured pays a portion of the cost of the group insurance coverage.

contributory negligence Action of an individual that helps to bring about another's negligent act.

contributory plan or program 1. Health insurance payment system in which part of the premium is paid by the employer or local union and part by the employee through monthly or periodic payroll deductions. 2. Any pension or employee benefit plan in which participants make contributions to the plan from their own monies.

control number Unique multidigit number assigned to a submitted insurance claim by the insurance company and used to track claims in a carrier's computer system.

control plan Blue Cross and Blue Shield phrase that refers to a Blue plan that has sold a health insurance plan to a company with employees in other states and arranged for other Blue plans in the other locations to provide the same benefits. The control plan has the primary responsibility in administering the groups served by more than one Blue plan.

controller Officer in charge of the funds of an insurance company or an organization.

controversy Disputed differences of opinion.

convalescent care See *extended care.*

convention blank Annual statement form that all insurance companies complete and submit annually to their state's insurance regulators.

conventional group insurance See *indemnity plan.*

conventions 1. Rules or principles for determining a diagnostic code when using diagnostic code books such as each space, typefaces, indentations, punctuation marks, instructional notes, abbreviations, cross-reference notes, and specific usage of the words *and, with,* and *due to.* These rules assist in the selection of correct codes for the diagnoses encountered. Also

called *coding conventions.* 2. Space-saving rule used in the "Index," which is the last section of the annually published *Current Procedural Terminology* code book. For example:

> Knee
>   Incision (of)

In this example, the word in parentheses (of) does not appear in the Index, but it is inferred. As another example:

> Pancreas
>   Anesthesia (for procedures on)

In this example, because there is no such entity as pancreas anesthesia, the words in parentheses are inferred (i.e., anesthesia for procedures on the pancreas).

conversion See *conversion plan* and *conversion privilege.*

conversion clause Provision in a group insurance policy that allows the insured to convert to an individual insurance policy if and when the group coverage is ever terminated.

conversion factor (CF) 1. The dollars and cents amount that is established for one unit as applied to a service rendered. This unit is then used to convert various services/procedures into fee-schedule payment amounts by multiplying the relative value unit by the conversion factor. 2. National multiplier used to convert the relative value units for each procedure into dollar amounts. The CF is announced annually by the Centers for Medicare and Medicaid Services (CMS) for all services paid under the resource-based relative value scale (RBRVS) Medicare Fee Schedule. Sometimes called *conversion number* or *national conversion factor.*

conversion factor update Annual percentage change to the Medicare Fee Schedule conversion factor. It is determined by the Congress or the default formula under Volume Performance Standards.

conversion fund Fund in which unallocated employer contributions are made to a combination plan. Also called *side fund.*

conversion member Individual whose employment has been terminated and is no longer a member of the employer's group insurance plan but is still able to continue his or her insurance benefits because of eligibility under the Consolidated Omnibus Reconciliation Act of 1985 (COBRA).

conversion number See *conversion factor (CF).*

conversion plan Group health plan that permits a member to change his or her insurance coverage (different benefits and rates) to an individual contract without a physical examination. This situation may occur at termination of employment. Also known as *conversion privilege* or *conversion.*

conversion privilege 1. Right of an individual covered by a group insurance policy to convert to coverage under an individual insurance policy. This can occur when a person leaves the group, benefits are downgraded or terminated for a specific class, or when the group policy is terminated. 2. Right to change insurance coverage in specific situations from one type of policy to another (e.g., individual term insurance to individual whole life insurance). Also known as *conversion.*

convert Act of transferring group insurance coverage to an individual insurance policy.

convertible bond Type of investment that permits the owner to change it into a specific number of shares of stock.

convertible term insurance Type of term insurance in which the policyholder is allowed to change the term insurance policy to a whole life policy without giving evidence of insurability. The premium amount is based on the age of the insured at the time of the conversion.

cooperating parties Associations that maintain and update the *International Classification of Diseases, Ninth Revision, Clinical Modification (ICD-9-CM).* They are the American Hospital Association (AHA), American Health Information Management Association (AHIMA), Centers for Medicare and Medicaid Services (CMS), and National Center for Health Statistics (NCHS).

cooperating provider See *contract provider.*

cooperative payment See *copayment (copay).*

cooperative care Term used when a patient is seen by a civilian physician or hospital for services cost-shared by TRICARE.

coordinated care (CC) plans Prepaid health care plans that meet federal legal standards for managed care plans (e.g., health maintenance organizations, provider-sponsored organizations, preferred provider organizations, or other types of network plans [except network medical savings account plans]). They incorporate cost containment and emphasize preventive care to members of the plans. Also referred to as *managed care plans.*

coordination of benefits (COB) 1. Provision in a group health insurance policy in which two insurance carriers work together and coordinate the payment of insurance benefits so that there is no duplication of benefits paid between the primary insurance carrier and the secondary insurance carrier. The purpose of this provision is to ensure that an insured's benefits from all insurance companies do not exceed 100% of allowable medical expenses. 2. In Medicare, the process of determining which plan or insurance policy will pay first if two health plans or insurance policies cover the same benefits, which is called a *crossover claim.* If one of the plans is a Medicare health plan, federal law may decide who pays first.

coordination of benefits contractor agreement identifiers (COBA IDs) Five-digit identification numbers (55000 to 59999) of insurers of Medicare supplemental (Medigap) plans that are issued for automatic crossover of Medicare claims. As of October 1, 2007, they replaced the traditional Medigap claim-based identifiers. Also referred to as *coordination of benefits agreement (COBA)* and *coordination of benefits contractor (COBC).*

coordination period Time frame when an individual's employer group health plan will pay first on the medical services and Medicare will pay second. If the employer group health plan does not pay 100% of the medical bills during the coordination period, Medicare may pay the remaining costs.

copay See *copayment (copay).*

copayment (copay) 1. Specific dollar amount to be collected when services are received. For example, the patient might pay out of pocket $10 for each prescription received and the plan would pay the remaining cost of the drug. This cost-sharing arrangement is sometimes referred to as *coinsurance and deductible, cooperative payment,* and *cost sharing.* However, coinsurance has a slightly different meaning under some programs (see *coinsurance*). 2. Under the Medicare program, it is considered fraud to routinely waiver copayments and deductibles, regardless of need. 3. In the Medicaid program, a dollar amount that an individual must pay at each office visit for receiving medical and child care services. Different copayment amounts may be set for each patient type and certain medical procedures. Child care copayments are based on gross annual income, number in the home, and number needing child care. Note: If a health plan integrates the copayment into the membership fee, then do not collect copays from the patients (members) of the plan.

COPC See *community-oriented primary care (COPC).*

COPs See *conditions of participation (COPs).*

core groups See *anchor group.*

CORF See *comprehensive outpatient rehabilitation facility (CORF).*

corneal mapping See *corneal topography.*

corneal topography Computer-assisted test of the cornea of the eye in which a special instrument projects a series of concentric light rings on the cornea creating a color map of the corneal surface and a cross-section profile. It is used to find subtle corneal surface irregularities associated with a large number of corneal disease states; also known as *computer-assisted video keratography (CAVK)* and *corneal mapping.*

coronary care unit (CCU) Department within a hospital facility dedicated to patients who have suffered heart attacks, strokes, or other serious or complex cardiopulmonary problems.

coroner Elected or appointed public official who investigates and provides official opinions about the cause and circumstance of deaths that occur in a specific legal jurisdiction or territory, especially a death that may have occurred from unnatural causes. See also *medical examiner (ME).*

corporate integrity agreement Agreed settlement between a provider and the Office of the Inspector General (OIG) as a result of an investigation for health care fraud and abuse violations of the False Claims Act. The provider must meet certain government-imposed requirements (such as annual audits) and follow the guidelines of this government-mandated compliance program.

corporate-owned life insurance (COLI) Life insurance policy that an employer or a trust can purchase on a group of employees, which is considered a tax-advantaged asset. The employer or trust can be named as the beneficiary of the policy.

corporation An entity or group of individuals who obtain a state charter that gives certain legal rights to conduct business.

Correct Coding Council See *National Correct Coding Council (NCCC)*.

Correct Coding Initiative (CCI) Federal legislation implemented in 1996 that attempts to eliminate unbundling or other inappropriate reporting of procedural codes for professional medical services rendered to patients. The quarterly updated code list identifies services considered either an integral part of a comprehensive code or mutually exclusive of it. Also known as *National Correct Coding Initiative (NCCI)*.

Correct Coding Initiative (CCI) edits Procedure/ service code edits annually published to guide providers in appropriate choice of code(s) to submit for Medicare Part B insurance claims. There are two main types: comprehensive/component edits and mutually exclusive edits.

correction To fix an error by adding data to a patient's existing chart or progress note by including the date, data, and signature of the individual making the correction.

correctional institution Penal facility, jail, reformatory, detention center, work farm, halfway house, or residential community program center operated by, or under contract to, the United States, a state, a territory, a political subdivision of a state or territory, or an Indian tribe, for the confinement or rehabilitation of persons charged with or convicted of a criminal offense or other persons held in lawful custody (i.e., juvenile offenders, aliens awaiting deportation, persons committed to mental institutions through the criminal justice system, witnesses, or others awaiting charges or trial).

correctionist See *medical editor (ME)*.

correspondence All documented communication that relates to the handling of an insurance claim (e.g., medical reports, test results, chart notes, electronic messages).

corridor 1. Required difference between a universal life insurance policy's death benefit and the policy's cash value. This difference is a specific percentage according to the insured's age. If a policy's cash value exceeds the required percentage of the death benefit (intrudes on the corridor), the policy is considered an investment contract instead of an insurance contract. Also called *TEFRA corridor*. 2. In reinsurance, an amount of insurance that is in excess of the ceding company's retention limit but is less than the reinsurer's minimum cession.

corridor deductible In a managed care plan, the amount that a member must pay before plan benefits are accessible.

cosmetic surgery Elective operation of cutaneous or underlying tissues performed to improve appearance and correct a structural defect or to remove a scar, birthmark, or normal evidence of aging. Most health insurance plans do not pay for it unless disfigurement resulted from an accident or catastrophic event. Cosmetic surgery is differentiated from reconstructive surgery, which insurance programs feature as a benefit. Also called *aesthetic surgery*. See *reconstructive surgery*.

cost accountant Individual whose work is to inspect, keep, or adjust financial accounts. When a patient is denied certain treatment, it may be the result of the cost accountant determining that treatment was not cost-effective and thus unnecessary.

cost-based health maintenance organization (HMO) Type of managed care organization (MCO) that will pay for all of the enrollees' (members') medical care costs in return for a monthly premium, plus any applicable deductible or copayment. The HMO will pay for all hospital costs (generally referred to as *Part A*) and physician costs (generally referred to as *Part B*) that it has arranged for and ordered. Like a health care prepayment plan (HCPP), except for out-of-area emergency services, if a Medicare member (enrollee) chooses to obtain services that have not been arranged by the HMO, he or she is liable for any applicable deductible and coinsurance amounts, with the balance to be paid by the regional Medicare fiscal intermediary and/or carrier.

cost-based HMO See *cost-based health maintenance organization (HMO)*.

cost-based reimbursement Insurance payment that is based on the cost of health care services in which allowable costs are determined by the insurer. This method is used by some insurance plans or programs but is being replaced by prospective payment. Also called *cost-related reimbursement*.

cost-benefit analysis Evaluation method that measures the insurance program's economic benefits to the program's medical care over a period of time expressed in dollar amounts. This is done to see if future health care costs can be reduced and earnings increased because of improved health of the members of a health plan.

cost center Department to which a revenue or expense is allocated.

cost comparison methods Various formulas that insurance companies use to show prospective insurance applicants the cost of different insurance policies.

cost containment Ongoing process used by government programs and managed care plans to keep costs within a certain budget and reduce expenditures. Types of cost curtailing activities include reducing administrative costs, controlling use of health care services, limiting demand for medical services, and managing other situations that add to higher costs. Various strategies used to keep costs down are capitation, disease management, preventive care, and wellness programs.

cost contract Arrangement between a managed care plan and Centers for Medicare and Medicaid Services (CMS), under which the health plan provides health services and is reimbursed its costs. The beneficiary can use providers outside the plan's provider network.

cost effectiveness Efficiency and competence of an insurance plan or program in achieving given intervention outcomes in relation to the program or plan costs. For example, the production of services with the least possible cost or treatment of a medical condition with the least expensive level of care that obtains the desired health outcome of the patient. Also called *cost efficiency*.

cost efficiency See *cost effectiveness*.

cost index Method used to compare the costs of similar plans of life insurance. Policies with smaller index numbers are usually a better buy than comparable policies with larger index numbers.

cost-of-living adjustment (COLA) To increase monthly benefits in disability income benefit, pension benefit, or life income benefit to make up for a change in the cost of living. Also known as *cost of living rider*.

cost-of-living rider See *cost-of-living adjustment (COLA)*.

cost of practice index In the Medicare program, this is a measurement of the differences across geographical areas of the cost of operating a medical practice.

cost outlier Typical case that has an extraordinarily high or extremely low cost when compared with most discharges classified to the same diagnosis-related group (DRG).

cost outlier review Review by a professional review organization (PRO) for the necessity of a patient's hospital admission and to determine whether all services rendered were medically necessary. Cost outlier cases are recognized only if the case is not eligible for day outlier status.

cost per gross add (CPGA) Average amount of money a company spends to acquire one new customer.

cost plus 1. Health insurance funding in which the insurance carrier does not assume an underwriting risk. The group that is insured pays the costs of benefits (incurred claims), pays administrative costs, and contributes to the insurance carrier's contingency reserve fund. 2. System of payment for inpatient hospitalization in which total operating costs and certain allowable capital costs are used in determining the per diem (per day) rate. When the amount of payment from a payer becomes insufficient or when uncompensated services are given, providers go to cost shifting and charge extra to the payers who do not exercise strict cost controls. This system is a typical means for providing uncompensated care to the uninsured.

cost plus reimbursement Payment system in which providers receive payment based on their actual costs plus a profit. This system is usually seen in fee-for-service (FFS) plans.

cost rate Ratio of the cost (or outgo, expenditures, or disbursements) of the program on an incurred basis during a given year to the taxable payroll for the year. In this context, the outgo is defined to exclude benefit payments and administrative costs for those uninsured persons for whom payments are reimbursed from the general fund of the U.S. Treasury and for voluntary enrollees, who pay a premium to be enrolled.

cost reimbursement System of payment by insurance plans to providers based on their actual incurred costs.

cost-related reimbursement See *cost-based reimbursement*.

cost report Annual information document that all institutions and providers participating in the Medicare program must generate. It analyzes the direct and indirect costs of providing care to Medicare patients and the payments received during a certain period of time. The purpose is to make a proper determination of amounts payable under the Medicare program.

cost sharing 1. Portion of payment of health expenses that the insured or beneficiary must pay including the deductible, copayment, coinsurance, and balance bill, thus sharing the costs with the insurance plan. 2. Under TRICARE, the portion of the allowable charge (20% or 25%) after the deductible has been met that the patient is responsible for. The most common types of cost sharing are *coinsurance* and *copayment*.

cost shifting 1. Practice of a provider to charge a higher fee to patients with private health insurance plans to make up for underpayment of fees for patients under Medicare, Medicaid, or managed care plans. 2. Practice of a provider charging a group of one managed care plan more than another for the same procedure. One reason this may occur is that one group may have large discounts from the provider or not adequately reimburse the provider for expenses. To make up for the shortage in revenue, the provider may charge another managed care group more.

cost to charge ratio (CCR) Method in which a hospital facility is paid for outpatient services by Medicare based on the hospital's last audited cost report.

COT See *chain of trust (COT)* or *Certified Ophthalmic Technician (COT)*.

COTA See *Certified Occupational Therapy Assistant (COTA).*

counsel Legal advisor (attorney, lawyer).

counseling Discussion between the physician and a patient, family, or both concerning the diagnosis, recommended studies or tests, treatment options, risks, benefits of treatment, patient and family education, and so on. See also *E/M counseling* and *psychiatric counseling.*

counter check Blank check in which the name of the bank and account number is filled in with ink or typed by the maker.

counteroffer Proposal that is slightly changed in response to an original offering that was not satisfactory.

countersignature Signature of a licensed insurance agent or representative on an insurance policy that is necessary to validate or authenticate the contract or document that has been signed by another person.

County Medical Services Program (CMSP) County program for medical services in the Medi-Cal program.

course of employment (COE) See *COE.*

courtesy adjustment Credit entry posted to a patient's account for a debt that has been determined to be uncollectible. In the Medicare program, the difference between the amount charged and the approved amount.

cover letter Letter of introduction prepared to accompany a resume when seeking a job.

coverage 1. Section in the insurance policy stating the medical conditions that may or may not be a benefit paid by the insurance company. 2. Benefits the patient receives from an insurance plan (e.g., medical services and procedures, medical supplies). It may include surgery or medical treatment of illnesses or injuries, emergency department care, and hospital services. 3. Under a Medicare Part D plan, the prescription drug costs that are paid by the insurance plan are the patient's benefits, or coverage. Also called *covered expenses* or *covered services.* 4. Amount of insurance an individual has.

coverage analysis for laboratories (CAL) Abbreviated process for making changes to the coding component of the negotiated laboratory National Coverage Determinations (NCDs). The process is used for adjusting the list of covered or noncovered diagnostic codes and coding guidance in the NCDs when there is a question regarding whether the code flows from the narrative indications in the NCD. A tracking sheet is posted after opening a CAL, and a 30-day public comment period follows. A decision memorandum that announces and explains the decision is posted after the comment period. Changes are adopted in the next available quarterly update of the laboratory edit module.

coverage basis Medicare+Choice plan charge schedule used to base the maximum dollar coverage or coinsurance level for a service category (e.g., a $500 annual coverage limit for a prescription drug benefit may be based on a Published Retailed Price schedule, or 20% coinsurance for durable medical equipment benefit may be based on a Medicare fee-for-service fee schedule).

coverage category Type of medical service in which insurance coverage is either fully covered, limited, restricted, or not provided in an insurance plan (e.g., dental or vision benefits).

coverage code Numerical or alphanumeric identifier of any special insurance policy benefits. Sometimes coverage codes appear on a patient's insurance identification card.

coverage decision Determination by a health plan or insurance company whether to pay for or provide a medical service for specific clinical manifestations.

coverage decision memorandum See *national coverage analyses (NCA) decision memorandum.*

coverage effective date Month, day, and year on which a group's or individual's health insurance coverage starts. Also called *enrollment date.*

coverage gap Under a Medicare Part D plan, the step in which the patient pays all of the expenses for eligible drugs, until he or she has spent $3850. This step is sometimes referred to as the *doughnut hole,* also spelled *donut hole.*

Coverage Issues Manual (CIM) See *National Coverage Determinations Manual (NCDM).*

coverage sequence Illness or injury described in a health insurance plan that may limit insurance coverage on a procedure.

coverage type Several varieties (contract types) of health insurance benefit plans exist:

1. Individual coverage is a plan in which only one person has been accepted into the health plan. Maternity care and obstetrical services are included as benefits, but routine newborn services are not included.

2. Family coverage is for the subscriber and the spouse who have been accepted into the health plan. Maternity care, obstetrical services, and routine newborn services may be included as benefits.

3. Family coverage with dependents is a plan that covers maternity care, obstetrical services, and routine newborn services to the subscriber but not to the children.

4. Family coverage is a plan in which the subscriber, spouse, and subscriber's or spouse's enrolled dependents who are his or her children are in the health plan. Maternity care, obstetrical services, and routine newborn services are benefits to the subscriber or the subscriber's spouse but not to the children.

A *significant other* rather than spouse is a newer change to the coverage terminology. Also known as *contract type.*

covered benefit Medically necessary health care service or item that is included in a health insurance plan and that is paid for either partially or fully. Some medically necessary services may not be a benefit of an insurance policy (e.g., custodial care may be necessary but not covered). Also called *covered services.*

covered charges Dollar amounts for medical services and supplies that the insurance plan will pay either partially or fully because they are covered benefits.

covered drug Medication that a health insurance plan will pay a pharmacy when the drug is dispensed to a member or subscriber of the plan.

covered earnings Employment income covered by the hospital insurance (HI) program.

covered employment All employment and self-employment creditable for Social Security purposes, except in a few employment situations (e.g., religious orders under a vow of poverty, foreign affiliates of American employers), or the employer must elect state and local government coverage. However, as of July 1991 coverage became mandatory for state and local employees who do not participate in a public employee retirement system. All new state and local employees have been covered by Social Security since April 1986 except ministers or self-employed members of certain religious groups who can opt out of coverage. Covered employment for hospital insurance includes all federal employees, whereas covered employment for the Old Age, Survivors, and Disability Insurance (OASDI) Program includes some, but not all, federal employees.

covered entity (CE) 1. Under the Health Insurance Portability and Accountability Act (HIPAA), this is a health plan, clearinghouse, or health provider who transmits health information and financial and administrative transactions in electronic form in connection with a HIPAA transaction. 2. From the perspective of the medical transcription service owner or independent contractor, the covered entity is the client. The CE is responsible for the protection of health information and, if there is a violation, can request documentation from its business associates to prove their compliance.

covered expenses Defined health care charges that an insurer will consider for payment as listed in the terms of an insurance policy or contract. Also called *covered services* or *coverage.*

covered function Under the Health Insurance Portability and Accountability Act (HIPAA), this phrase refers to the tasks (functions) of a covered entity, the performance of which makes the entity a health plan, health care provider, or health care clearinghouse.

covered lives Total of insured members of a managed care plan or individual or group insurance plan.

covered person Individual who is an insured, enrolled participant, member, or enrolled dependent entitled to benefits under a health insurance policy or managed care plan; also referred to as *policyholder, subscriber,* or *employee.*

covered services 1. Specific health care services and supplies for which the insurance plan or federal or state program will provide reimbursement for covered persons under the terms of the plan; these consist of a combination of mandatory and optional services stated in each plan. 2. Services for which supplemental medical insurance (SMI) pays, as defined and limited by statute. Covered services include most physician services, care in outpatient departments of hospitals, diagnostic tests, durable medical equipment, ambulance services, and other health services that are not covered by the hospital insurance program. Also called *coverage* or *covered expenses.*

covered worker Person who has earnings creditable for Social Security purposes on the basis of services for wages in covered employment and/or on the basis of income from covered self-employment. The number of hospital insurance covered workers is slightly larger than the number of Old Age, Survivors, and Disability Insurance (OASDI)–covered workers because of different coverage status for federal employment.

CPC See *Certified Professional Coder (CPC).*

CPGA See *cost per gross add (CPGA).*

CP Health IT See *Certified Professional in Health Information Technology (CP Health IT).*

CPHA See *Commission on Professional Hospital Activities (CPHA).*

CPI See *consumer price index (CPI).*

CPO See *care plan oversight (CPO) services.*

CPOE See *computerized physician order entry (CPOE).*

CPR 1. See *comparative performance report (CPR).* 2. See *electronic medical record (computer-based patient record).* 3. See *computer-based patient record (CPR).* 4. Clinically this abbreviation may be translated as cardiopulmonary resuscitation. 5. See *customary, prevailing, and reasonable (CPR) charge.*

CPSP See *comprehensive perinatal services program (CPSP).*

CPT See *Current Procedural Terminology (CPT).*

CPT-4 *Current Procedural Terminology, Fourth Edition,* code reference book. See *Current Procedural Terminology (CPT).*

CPT code Description of a procedure with a five-digit code number to identify professional services (see Box C-1). The codes are maintained (published annually) and copyrighted by the American Medical Association (AMA).

CPT modifier Two-character code that may follow a five-digit CPT code to indicate a service or procedure has been altered in some way from the stated CPT or HCPCS Level II description but not sufficient to change the basic definition of the service.

CPU See *central processing unit (CPU).*

CQI See *continuous quality improvement (CQI).*

CR See *carrier replacement (CR).*

CRA See *community rating area (CRA).*

CRC Abbreviation for community rating by class. See *adjusted community rating (ACR).*

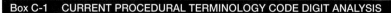

Box C-1   CURRENT PROCEDURAL TERMINOLOGY CODE DIGIT ANALYSIS

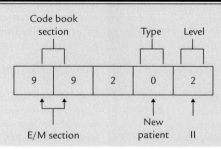

credential University degree, postgraduate training and education, licensure and/or board certification that indicates a person or institution has obtained professional status in a specific field of health care.

credential verification organization (CVO) Association that validates a health care professional's background, licensing, and schooling, and follows continuing education and other measures of professional performance.

credentialing 1. Generic term that refers to either licensing or certification. 2. Act of reviewing and evaluating qualifications such as education, training, experience, medical degrees, licensure, other credentials, malpractice, and any disciplinary record of a medical provider for quality assurance for the purpose of granting hospital staff membership to give patient care services. Periodically, a check of the status of staff qualifications is done and is referred to as *recredentialing*. 3. Process by which a managed care plan endorses that a physician is competent to render medical services to members of the plan. Also see *economic credentialing*.

credibility Percentage weight given to an insured group's past claim history. It is done to set the premium for future expected claims or to determine claim charges for experience refund purposes.

credibility factor See *credibility percentage*.

credibility percentage Amount of credit given to a group's actual insurance claims experience in establishing a projection of future claims or in calculating a dividend. Also called *credibility factor*.

credit 1. From the Latin *credere*, meaning "to believe" or "to trust"; trust in regard to financial obligation. 2. Accounting; entry reflecting payment by a debtor (patient) of a sum received on his or her account.

credit card Card issued by an organization and devised for the purpose of obtaining money, property, labor, or services on credit.

credit insurance Insurance coverage that will pay off an outstanding loan if the policyholder dies or makes loan payments if the policyholder becomes disabled.

credit life insurance Type of decreasing term insurance calculated to pay the balance due on a loan, installment purchase, or other obligation, in case the borrower dies before the loan is repaid. Another form is credit group life insurance for insuring lives of a group of persons who are in debt to a creditor.

credit reporting agency See *consumer reporting agency*.

creditable coverage 1. Any previous health insurance coverage that can be used to shorten the preexisting condition waiting period. See also *preexisting condition*. 2. Under a Medicare Part D plan, a prescription drug coverage from another private insurance plan (Medigap and employer plans) that meets certain Medicare standards. When a patient is enrolled in a drug plan that gives prescription drug coverage, the plan tells the patient that coverage is equal to or better than the standard model and it is considered creditable coverage. Also called *creditable prescription drug coverage*.

creditable prescription drug coverage See *creditable coverage*.

creditor 1. Person to whom money is owed either directly or indirectly. 2. Individual who offers or extends credit creating a debt or to whom a debt is owed.

credits Represent insurance underwriting factors that have a favorable effect on an individual's mortality rating. Credits are assigned negative values.

credits, Social Security Word used to count toward eligibility for future Social Security benefits. Individuals work and pay taxes and earn credits. A maximum of four credits can be earned each year. Most people need 40 credits to qualify for benefits. Younger people need fewer credits to qualify for disability or survivors' benefits. Work credits were formerly called *quarters of coverage*.

criteria 1. Expected levels of achievement or specifications against which performance can be assessed. 2. Guidelines or standards of medical care that compare the necessity, appropriateness, or quality of medical services.

critical access hospital (CAH) Freestanding hospital emergency department that gives limited inpatient care to stabilize a patient before discharge or transfer to an essential access community hospital (EACH) for extensive treatment. This was established as part of the Balanced Budget Act of 1997 (BBA) Medicare Rural Hospital Flexibility Program to replace the Essential Access Community and Rural Primary Care Hospital Programs.

critical care Intensive care provided in a variety of settings for acute life-threatening conditions that requires constant bedside attention by a physician.

critical care unit (CCU) Area or section within a hospital facility with special equipment designed for treatment of patients with sudden, life-threatening conditions such as intensive care unit (ICU), medical intensive care unit (MICU), surgical intensive care unit (SICU), pediatric intensive care unit (PICU), neonatal intensive care unit (NICU), coronary care unit (CCU), and the burn unit.

critical pathways See *clinical pathway* and *practice guidelines.*

CRN See *claim reference number (CRN).*

CRNA See *Certified Registered Nurse Anesthetist (CRNA).*

crop-hail insurance Insurance protection for growing agricultural crops against damage as a result of hail or other named perils.

crossover claim Bill for services rendered to a patient receiving benefits simultaneously from Medicare and Medicaid or from Medicare and a Medigap supplemental plan. Medicare pays first and then determines the amounts of unmet Medicare deductible and coinsurance to be paid by the secondary insurance carrier. The claim is automatically transferred (electronically) to the secondary insurance carrier for additional payment; also known as *claims transfer.*

crossover patient Beneficiary who has both Medicare and Medicaid coverage. Sometimes referred to as a *Medi-Medi* or *Care/Caid case.*

cross purchase Arrangement of buy-sell arrangements made by business owners while living, which in the event of an owner's death, binds the shareholders or partners to purchase the deceased's interests in the business.

cross purchase agreement Buy-sell contract that is often funded with life insurance policies owned by each business principal on the lives of all other business principals.

cross-selling To sell both property and casualty and life and health insurance and other financial services products to the same client or customer.

crosswalk 1. Cross-reference of CPT codes with ICD-9-CM, anesthesia, dental, or HCPCS Level II codes. Also known as *data mapping.* 2. Cross-reference connection between discontinued CPT codes and new codes that replace them. Also called *visit crosswalk.* 3. Mapping to locate the corresponding diagnosis between an ICD-9-CM code set and an ICD-10-CM code set.

crosswalking When a new test is determined to be similar to an existing test, multiple existing test codes, or a portion of an existing test code, the new test code is then assigned the related existing local fee schedule amounts and resulting national limitation amount. In some instances, a test may only equate to a portion of a test and, in those instances, payment at an appropriate percentage of the payment for the existing test is assigned.

CRT See *Certified Respiratory Therapist (CRT).*

CSHCS See *Children's Special Health Care Services (CSHCS).*

CSO See *clinical service organization (CSO).*

CSO agreement See *claim services only (CSO) agreement.*

CSP See *coding specialist for payers (CSP).*

CSRS See *Civil Service Retirement System (CSRS).*

CSW See *clinical social worker (CSW).*

CT See *computerized tomography (CT).*

CTA See *chain of trust agreement (CTA).*

CTR See *Certified Tumor Registrar (CTR).*

cumulative approach Another method for establishing a conversion factor under the Volume Performance Standard system. It brings actual spending in line with targeting spending and also recovers any surpluses or shortfalls in spending from 2 years before Medicare updates in the fee schedule are made.

cumulative injury In workers' compensation cases, that occurring as repetitive mentally or physically traumatic activities extending over a period of time, the combined effect of which causes any disability the need for medical treatment.

current assumption whole life insurance Type of whole life insurance in which premium rates and cash values vary depending on the insurer's assumptions about mortality, investment, and expense factors. A client can choose favorable changes in assumptions that result in a lower premium or a higher cash value for the policy. The premium will not increase above the rate guaranteed when the policy was purchased. Also called *interest-sensitive whole life insurance.*

Current Dental Terminology (CDT) Medical code set maintained and copyrighted by the American Dental Association (ADA) for use by the dental profession in Health Insurance Portability and Accountability Act (HIPAA) transactions. More commonly referred to as *CDT-2005.*

current disbursement Payment of premiums and benefits as they become due. Also referred to as *pay-as-you-go plan.*

Current Procedural Terminology (CPT) Reference book using a five-digit numerical system to identify codes and describe medical, surgical, and diagnostic procedures and services established, maintained, and copyrighted by the American Medical Association. It has been selected for use under the Health Insurance Portability and Accountability Act (HIPAA) for non-institutional and nondental professional transactions. This code system is used by physicians and outpatient facilities to identify the type and level of service given to each patient when submitting insurance claims to insurance companies for payment. In the Medicare program, this system is referred to as *Level 1 codes*.

current settlement option rates These rates reflect the interest rates currently earned by the insurance company.

current year Present insurance plan contract year.

curriculum vitae Summary or résumé that documents an individual's credentials, education, work experience, special accomplishments, and professional activities.

curtailment Amendment to a pension plan that reduces the plan's benefits or employer's contributions. Curtailment types include a reduction of expected years of future service of present employees and elimination of accrual of defined benefits for future services of a large number of employees.

custodial care Services and care of a nonmedical nature to assist a patient in the activities of daily living (ADLs) on a long-term basis, usually for convalescent and chronically ill persons. This type of care includes acting as a companion and help in bathing, dressing, eating, preparation of special diets, supervision over self-administration of medications, using the toilet, and walking. Custodial care may or may not be a benefit of an insurance plan. In most cases, Medicare does not pay for custodial care but the Medicare home health benefit does pay for some personal care services.

custodial care facility Setting of care or institution that provides room, board, and other personal assistance services usually on a long-term basis and does not include a medical component.

custodial parent 1. Divorced parent the child lives with who bears the responsibility of the child's medical expenses unless the divorce decree states otherwise. 2. Adoptive parent who becomes the legal parent of a child who was not born to him or her such as stepparent or relative and who bears the responsibility of the child's medical expenses.

custodian See *custodian of records*.

custodian of records Employee who is legally responsible and has charge and custody of the care and handling for all the patient's medical records in a hospital facility or physician's medical practice. Electronically stored information has four levels of custodianship such as primary or direct custodian (e.g., staff nurse), data owner or steward (e.g., radiologist, pathologist, accountant), business associate and third party (e.g., claims clearinghouse, Internet service provider), and official record and system custodian (e.g., health information management department). Also called *custodian*.

customary charge See *customary fee*.

customary fee 1. Amount that a physician usually charges the majority of his or her patients. 2. Either the average fee charged for a specific procedure by all comparable physicians in the same geographical area or the 90th percentile of all the fees charged for a specific procedure by comparable physicians in the same geographical area.

customary, prevailing, and reasonable (CPR) charge From 1965 a method for determining an approved charge for a specific service for a physician before the implementation of the Medicare Fee Schedule in 1992. The approved charge is the lowest of the following three charges: the physician's actual charge for the service, the physician's customary charge for the service, and the charges made by each physician in the same geographical location. Currently, Medicare payment is based on a resource-based relative value scale (RBRVS) and not on CPR charges.

customer service department Division in a life and health insurance company that provides help to the company's agents, policyholders, and beneficiaries. Types of service include supplying answers to requests for information, interpreting policy language, answering questions about insurance policy coverage, and making changes requested by the policyholder. This department also sends premium notices and collects premium payments, processes policy loans, dividends, and so on. Also called *client service department, policy administration department, policy owner service department,* and *service and claim department.*

cutback Reduction in the amount or type of insurance for an individual who attains a certain age (i.e., 65 or 70) or condition (i.e., retirement).

CVO See *credential verification organization (CVO)*.

CWF See *common working file (CWF)*.

CWW See *clinic without walls (CWW)*.

CY Abbreviation for calendar year.

cybercrime Use of a computer to commit a crime such as medical identity theft.

cycle billing System of billing accounts at spaced intervals during the month based on breakdown of accounts by alphabet, account number, insurance type, or date of first service. This relieves the pressure of having to get all the statements or insurance claims out at one time and allows continuous cash flow throughout the month. Also called *cyclical billing.*

cyclical billing See *cycle billing.*

D

D codes HCPCS Level II alphanumerical codes that begin with the letter D and are used to report dental services and procedures. The final Health Insurance Portability and Accountability Act (HIPAA) transactions and code sets rule states that these D-codes will be dropped from the HCPCS and *Current Dental Terminology (CDT)* codes will be used to identify all dental procedures.

daily accounts receivable journal Summary of chronological financial transactions posted to patients' financial accounts (ledgers) on a specific day. Also called a *day sheet* or *daily log*.

daily benefit Maximum daily amount paid by a health insurance hospital or major medical plan for inpatient room and board charges.

daily hospital service charge Inpatient hospital fee every day that includes room and care, nursing, meals, linen, other services, and administrative costs.

daily log See *daily accounts receivable journal* and *day sheet*.

data In the health care setting, this is a collection of letters, numbers, dates, symbols, graphic images, and words about individuals and their medical conditions.

data aggregation Under the Health Insurance Portability and Accountability Act (HIPAA), combining protected health information by a business associate together with the protected health information received by the business associate in its capacity as a business associate of another covered entity.

data codes Digital coding system for data in a computer, such as American Standard Code for Information Interchange (ASCII, pronounced "asskey") and Extended Binary Coded Decimal Interchange Code (EBCDIC, pronounced "IB-sa-dik").

data condition 1. Explanation of the situation when specific information is required. 2. Under the Health Insurance Portability and Accountability Act (HIPAA), the data elements and code sets that encompass a transaction but are not related to the format.

data content Under the Health Insurance Portability and Accountability Act (HIPAA), these are all the data elements and code sets inherent to a transaction, and not related to the format of the transaction.

data council Board or committee in the Department of Health and Human Services that is responsible for overseeing implementation of the administrative simplification provisions of the Health Insurance Portability and Accountability Act (HIPAA).

data dictionary Document or system that characterizes the data content of a system.

data element Under Health Insurance Portability and Accountability Act (HIPAA), this is the smallest named unit of information in a transaction.

data integrity 1. Accuracy, consistency, comprehensiveness, and timeliness (currency) of medical information maintained by a computer system. 2. Principle of security to keep data from modification or corruption either intentionally or accidentally.

Data Interchange Standards Association Body that provides administrative services to X12 and several other standards-related groups.

data mapping 1. Method of matching one set of data elements or individual code values to the nearest equivalents in another set. Also known as *crosswalk*. 2. Systematized Nomenclature of Human and Veterinary Medicine (SNOMED International), Volumes I through IV are used to compare terminology context or classification description principles with the *International Classification of Diseases, Ninth Revision, Clinical Modification (ICD-9-CM)* system. This process of linking content from one terminology or classification scheme to another is called *mapping*. Also see *crosswalk* and *crosswalking*.

data mart Organized, well-planned, and searchable database system for a business department within an organization that draws information from a data warehouse (clinical data repository) to meet certain needs of users.

data model Conceptual model of the information needed to support a business function or process.

data quality manager Individual who ensures the quality of health information by doing quality reliability and validity checks. He or she develops reports and advises clinicians on identifying critical indicators.

data quality management Administrative process that guarantees the accuracy and comprehensiveness of a facility's information during data collection, application, warehousing, and analysis.

data resource manager Individual who uses computer-based health record systems, databases, and clinical data repositories to make sure the facility's information systems are suitable for those that provide and manage patient services and that the organization's data resources are secure, accessible, accurate, and reliable.

data security Electronic protection of computer-based information from unauthorized alteration or intentional or accidental destruction. Also, it is the process of controlling access and maintaining confidentiality when entering, storing, processing, and communicating information.

data segment Under HIPAA, a set of data elements of which there are two types, information segments or control segments. An information segment is used to convey information on the provider, payer, or services rendered. A control segment carries information necessary to the transmission and reception of a transaction.

data use agreement Legal binding agreement that the Centers for Medicare and Medicaid Services (CMS) requires to obtain identifiable data. It also delineates the confidentiality requirements of the Privacy Act of 1974 security safeguards and CMS's data use policy and procedures.

data use checklist Form used to provide pertinent information about the data request and identifies the identifiable data being processed.

data warehouse See *clinical data repository (CDR)*.

database Collection of data stored in a computer system for many applications. In the health care industry, the information may be used by insurance carriers for payment of claims, negotiating contracts, and tracking the use and cost of medical services.

date of employment Month, day, and year when an employee began work at a job. Often this date is the start of health insurance or workers' compensation coverage.

date of filing Day of the mailing (as evidenced by the postmark) or hand delivery of materials, unless otherwise defined. Also called *date of submission*.

date of injury (DOI) 1. Month, day, and year that the incident or exposure occurred. 2. In workers' compensation, months, day, and year the employee first suffered disability from an accident or exposure by present or previous employment. Many times, the date of injury may be the last day worked. When completing the CMS-1500, the date of injury is inserted in Block 14 of the paper claim form.

date of issue Date on which the insurance application is approved and the policy is issued by the insurance company. Life insurance policies sometimes provide suicide and incontestability clauses measured from the date of issue.

date of policy Month, day, and year that usually appears on the front page of an insurance policy as to when the policy became effective.

date of receipt Month, day, and year on the return voucher of "return receipt requested" certified or registered U.S. post office mail, unless otherwise defined.

date of service (DOS) 1. Month, day, and year that a professional service is rendered or a supply item is given to a patient by a provider. This date is entered on the patient's encounter form and charted in the patient's medical record along with documentation by the provider detailing the services and/or supplies provided, chief complaint, examination, and when the patient should return for an appointment. 2. When an insurance claim is manually submitted, the date of service is inserted in Block 24A of the CMS-1500 insurance claim form. This indicates the date on which health care services were provided to the insured. More than one date of service may be listed on a claim. Also called *service date*.

date of submission See *date of filing*.

dating back See *back date*.

DAW Acronym that means dispense as written and relates to a prescription note from a physician to a pharmacist. It infers that the brand name of the drug be given instead of a generic drug.

day outlier review Review of potential day outliers (short or unusually long length of hospital stay) to determine the necessity of admission and number of days before the day outlier threshold is reached, as well as the number of days beyond the threshold. The day outlier is no longer used. The peer review organization determined the certification of additional days. Under the Medicare program, this is known as the *Quality Improvement Organization (QIO)*. Also see *outlier*.

day sheet Register for recording daily business transactions (charges, payments, adjustments). Also called *daily log*, *accounts receivable (AR) journal*, and *daily accounts receivable journal*.

day surgery See *ambulatory care facility* and *free-standing surgical center*.

days of stay See *length of stay (LOS)*.

days per thousand (DPT) Utilization measurement of the number of days of inpatient, outpatient, residential, or partial hospitalization used in a year per 1000 health plan members. The formula is calculated as the # of days/member months × 1000 members × # of months. Also called *bed days per 1000* and *visits per 1000*.

DBPP See *defined benefit pension plan (DBPP)*.

DC 1. Abbreviation for Doctor of Chiropractic Medicine. See *Doctor of Chiropractic Medicine (DC)*. 2. Abbreviation for discharge. See *discharge (DC)*. 3. Abbreviation for dual choice provision. See *dual choice (DC) provision*.

DCA See *deferred compensation administrator (DCA)*.

DCGs See *diagnostic cost groups (DCGs)*.

DCI See *duplicate coverage inquiry (DCI) form*.

DD See *developmental disability (DD)*.

DDS 1. Abbreviation for Doctor of Dental Surgery. See *Doctor of Dental Surgery (DDS)*. 2. Abbreviation for Disability Determination Services. See *Disability Determination Services (DDS)*.

de facto standard Principle that is not official but has been accepted in an industry through long-time or common widespread usage.

deactivate Action taken by the Medicare administrative contractor that renders a provider's billing number inactive or ineffective for claims processing. The provider is notified and given a reason for this situation.

death benefit Amount of money payable to a designated beneficiary after the person insured (policyholder) under a life insurance policy dies. See also *basic death benefit* and *face amount.*

death claim Formal request for payment by the beneficiary under the terms of a life insurance policy after the policyholder of a life insurance policy dies. Certain death forms giving due proof of the death and establishing the beneficiary's rights to such insurance proceeds must be filed with the company. This is called a *death claim.*

death spiral Process in which health insurance premium rates continuously increase for individuals or small groups eventually making the insurance unaffordable. It may be due to the fact that healthier and younger employees choose managed care plans, leaving less healthy individuals in experience-rated indemnity plans. Other factors that may add to the problem are contribution strategies used by employers and pricing techniques of a plan.

debenture Bond that is not secured by any type of asset but only backed by the general credit of the issuing corporation.

debit 1. In accounting, this is an increase in assets or a reduction in liabilities or capital. It is the opposite of credit and an accounting entry is posted on the left side of the financial ledger. 2. In insurance, debits represent underwriting factors that have an unfavorable effect on an individual's mortality rating. This term is used in a numerical rating system.

debit card Card permitting bank customers to withdraw from any affiliated automated teller machine (ATM) and to make cashless purchases from funds on deposit without incurring revolving finance charges for credit.

debt Legal obligation to pay money. This may arise from a consumer credit transaction or rental purchase agreement.

debt collection Act of an individual who regularly engages in collecting money owed or any persons who sell or offer to sell forms for collection of money owed.

debt collector Individual who regularly engages in debt collection for themselves, an employer, or others and includes persons who sell or offer to sell forms represented to be a collection system.

debtor Person owing money that is obligated on a debt.

debtor-creditor groups Group composed of lending institutions such as banks, credit unions, savings and loan associations, finance companies, retail merchants, and credit card companies and their debtors.

debug To remove errors from a software program or the computer itself.

DEC See *decubitus (DEC).*

decapitation Insufficient payment by a managed care plan in which physicians and hospitals are paid a fixed, per capita amount for each patient enrolled over a stated period of time, regardless of the type and number of services provided; inadequate reimbursement to the hospital on a per-member/per-month basis to cover costs for the members of the plan.

DeCC See *Dental Content Committee (DeCC).*

decedent Individual who has died.

declaration Section in a property or liability insurance policy that lists the name and address of the policyholder, property insured, location and description, policy period, amount of insurance, premium, and additional information given by the insured.

declaration of readiness (DOR) to proceed In workers' compensation cases, a formal statement that a legal party is ready to proceed to hearing on issues and lists efforts made to resolve the issues.

declination Act of an insurance company's refusal (rejection) to insure a person after evaluating the insurance application, usually for reasons of the health or occupation of the applicant.

decrease in coverage Reduction of insurance benefits by the insurance company.

decreasing term insurance Type of term life insurance in which the amount of death benefit (coverage) decreases from the date the policy comes into force to the date the policy expires.

decrement Gradual diminution in the number of participants in a pension plan due to retirement, disability, death, or termination.

decubitus (DEC) 1. Recumbent or horizontal position, as lateral decubitus, lying on one side. 2. Decubitus ulcer (bedsore).

dedicated telephone line Telephone line with the sole purpose of transmission of insurance claims to a specific insurance carrier.

deductible 1. Specific dollar amount that must be paid either monthly, quarterly, or annually by the insured or a specified amount of time that must elapse before a medical insurance plan or government program begins covering health care costs. For the majority of plans, this amount must be paid each calendar or fiscal year. These amounts can change from year to year. 2. In Medicare Part D, some plans have an annual deductible and many plans have no deductible amount. Sometimes referred to as *cash deductible.* In Medicare, to routinely waiver copayments and deductibles, regardless of need, is considered a fraudulent practice.

deductible carry-over credit Medical service charges that were incurred during the last 3 months of a year that may be applied to the deductible and which may be carried over to the next year of insurance coverage and benefits.

deductible expenses Expenditures that the Internal Revenue Service has declared as those that can be deducted when computing an individual or joint annual income tax return.

deemed Providers are "deemed" when they know, before providing services, that the patient is in a private fee-for-service insurance plan, and they agree to give the patient care. Providers who are deemed agree to follow the patient's plan's terms and conditions of payment for the services given.

deemed status Designation that a Medicare+Choice organization has been reviewed and determined "fully accredited" by a Centers for Medicare and Medicaid Services (CMS)–approved accrediting organization for those standards within the deeming categories that the accrediting organization has the authority to deem.

deemed wage credits See *noncontributory wage credits*.

deemer clause Law that if an insurance policy is filed with an insurance department that it is considered approved after a specific period of time unless the Insurance Commission gives a disapproval notice.

deeming authority Power granted by the Centers for Medicare and Medicaid Services (CMS) to accrediting organizations to determine, on CMS's behalf, whether a Medicare+Choice evaluated by the accrediting organization is in compliance with corresponding Medicare regulations.

DEERS See *Defense Enrollment Eligibility Reporting System (DEERS)*.

DEF One of the abbreviation symbols used in the diagnostic code book titled *International Classification of Diseases, Ninth Revision, Clinical Modification (ICD-9-CM)*. It indicates a definition of disease or procedural term in the descriptions of the diagnoses.

defendant Individual who is sued or must answer to any lawsuit filed in the court.

defense audit Type of audit of hospital patient records that occurs when the insurance company requests a review of the patient's records to verify charges. The insurance auditor may or may not meet with a hospital auditor, depending on the circumstances. Also see *audit by request* and *random internal audit*.

Defense Enrollment Eligibility Reporting System (DEERS) Electronic database used to verify beneficiary eligibility for those individuals in the TRICARE programs.

defensive medicine Physician's policies and procedures such as complete documentation, overuse of tests, increased hospital admissions, or extended hospital stays that are done on each patient to guard against the risk of malpractice lawsuits or to provide a defense in case such a lawsuit occurs.

deferral date Month, day, and year after the first anniversary of a group insurance policy to which the insurance company puts off the payment of the policy's first renewal premium. This might be done so that the full year's experience assists the insurance company in calculating a new premium rate.

deferred annuity 1. Stipulation in an annuity contract that provides for income payments to begin at some future date such as a specific number of years or at a specified age. 2. Annuity contract in which premiums are accumulated at interest but the annuity payment period is postponed (deferred) for one or more periods.

deferred care Needed health care (medical or dental) that is delayed because the patient does not have insurance or is not able to pay for services.

deferred compensation Rescheduling of an employee's compensation to some future age or date. The employee agrees to receive payment at a later date for work performed before that date, for the purpose of retirement only or to provide a death benefit to the beneficiary of a pension plan.

deferred compensation administrator (DCA) Type of company that provides administrative and other services through a variety of situations such as retirement planning administration, third-party administration, self-insured plans, compensation planning, salary survey administration, and workers' compensation claims administration.

deferred compensation plan Type of plan created by an employer that gives benefits to employees at a later date or after their retirement. The money is not taxed until the later date, usually at retirement, when income is reduced and the deferred funds can then be taxed at a lower rate.

deferred group annuity Type of group annuity contract that provides for the purchase each year of a paid-up deferred annuity for each member of the group, the total amount received by the member at retirement being the sum of these deferred annuities.

deferred life annuity Type of plan that provides a series of payments only if a designated person is alive.

deferred nonemergency care Health care (medical or dental) that can be delayed without risk to the patient's physical condition such as eye refraction, immunizations, and dental prophylaxis).

deferred premium arrangement Agreement between the insurance company and the policyholder (company or business) to extend a group insurance policy's grace period permanently by either 30, 60, or 90 days. This allows the policyholder to use the deferred premium amounts for the length of time by which the grace period is extended. Such an arrangement is usually granted to companies with excellent credit ratings. Also called a *premium-delay arrangement*.

deferred premiums Premiums that are due after a policy's statement date but before the next policy anniversary.

deficiency In relation to a nursing home, finding that it failed to meet one or more federal or state requirements.

Deficit Reduction Act of 1984 (DEFRA84) Provisions of DEFRA make Medicare Secondary Payer for spouses age 65 through 69 of employed individuals of any age younger than 70 who are covered by an employer group health plan (EGHP).

Deficit Reduction Act of 2005 (DEFRA05 or DRA) Federal legislation effective January 1, 2007, that controls federal spending on entitlement programs such as Medicare and Medicaid. It transformed compliance programs from voluntary to mandatory, made certain employee handbook content and policies mandatory for recipients of $5 million or more in Medicaid reimbursement, encouraged states to adopt statutes that parallel the federal False Claims Act, and made available additional federal resources to combat fraud and abuse in Medicare and Medicaid programs.

defined benefit formula Calculation used to establish periodic payment amounts for each participant on retirement in this pension plan. It is based on the number of years of participation in the plan.

defined benefit pension plan (DBPP) Retirement plan that pays set monthly benefits to the participant on retirement. The amount is based on the retiree's age, tenure, and former wages and is calculated by using a certain formula. A DBPP is backed by the Pension Benefit Guaranty Corporation, a government agency that pays worker pension benefits, to set limits, in the event of a plan insolvency.

defined contribution formula Calculation used to establish the amount of money that is to be deposited into a pension plan each year for each participant. Contributions are based on a certain percentage of the participant's compensation.

defined contribution plan Retirement plan that states the amount of yearly contributions that the plan sponsor will make on behalf of a plan participant such as a 401(k), Keogh, or individual retirement account (IRA). This type of plan does not guarantee a certain amount of retirement benefits. A participant's benefits when retired are based on the amount that was contributed to the participant's account plus any investment earnings. Under a defined contribution plan, the employee directs the investment of his or her retirement savings. These kinds of plans are not covered by the Pension Benefit Guaranty Corporation.

DEFRA05 See *Deficit Reduction Act of 2005 (DEFRA05 or DRA)*.

DEFRA84 See *Deficit Reduction Act of 1984 (DEFRA84)*.

dehydration 1. Serious physiological condition in which the body's loss of fluid is more than the body's intake of fluid. 2. Rendering a substance free from water.

deinstitutionalization Change in the location and focus of mental health care and treatment for medically and socially dependent individuals from an institutional to a community setting.

delay clause See *survivorship clause*.

delayed payment clause Provision in a life insurance policy that means the beneficiary must outlive the insured by a specific amount of time to receive the death benefit.

delegated official Individual who is given legal authority by an authorized official of the provider to make changes to the organization's status in the Medicare program (e.g., change of address or new location for the practice) or to notify the provider to follow the regulations and Medicare program guidelines.

deleted claim Insurance claim that has been canceled, deleted, or voided by a Medicare fiscal intermediary for the following reasons: CMS-1500 (08-05) or current CMS-1450 is not used, itemized charges are not provided, more than six line items are submitted on the CMS-1500 (08-05) claim form, patient's address is missing, internal clerical error was made, Certificate of Medical Necessity (CMN) was not with the Part B claim or was incomplete or invalid, and name of the store is not on the receipt that includes the price of the item.

delinquent account Dollar amount that is overdue from a patient who has received medical services.

delinquent claim Insurance claim submitted to an insurance company, for which payment is overdue. See *pending claim*.

delinquent payment Dollar amount for which reimbursement is overdue.

delinquent premium Dollar amount due to the insurance company for an insurance policy premium that has not been paid by the end of the grace period. This sum may be due monthly, quarterly, or annually.

demand Amount of services and procedures required from a health care system by a specific population of patients.

demand bill Invoices sent to the Medicare administrative contractor for medical review and payment determination at the request of the beneficiary because the patient disputes the provider's opinion that the bill will not be paid by Medicare.

demand management This phrase is used in managed care and is a technique or process used to match patient needs with a quality, cost-efficient atmosphere and at the same time influencing self-care to members, which lowers their needs for services and results in lower costs of care.

demand-side rationing Phrase that refers to obstacles in getting medical care by patients who do not have the income to pay for health care services or obtain medical insurance.

demographic assumptions See *assumptions*.

demographic data Information that describes the characteristics of enrollee populations within a managed care entity. Demographic data includes but is not limited to age, sex, race/ethnicity, and primary language.

demographic information Data that describe specific characteristics about a patient such as name, address, date of birth, sex, and Social Security number. These data are usually obtained when the patient is either admitted to the hospital or seen for the first visit in a physician's office.

D

demographic rating Type of community rating that takes into consideration several statistical characteristics (e.g., age, geographic area, industry, sex of the population).

demographics Pertaining to statistical descriptions including distribution, density, and vital statistics of populations such as age, births, deaths, marital status, income, and unemployment.

demonstrations Projects and contracts that Centers for Medicare and Medicaid Services (CMS) has signed with various health care organizations. These contracts allow CMS to test various or specific attributes such as payment methodologies, preventive care, and social care and to determine if such projects/pilots should be continued or expanded to meet the health care needs of the nation. Demonstrations are used to evaluate the effects and impact of various health care initiatives and the cost implications to the public.

demutualization Process of converting a stock insurance company to a mutual insurance company.

denial In the Medicare program, electronic and paper insurance claims may be rejected (formally denied) because the medical service was not covered, medical necessity was not met, the service was bundled with other services, the diagnosis was not covered, the claim was payable only in certain locations (e.g., outpatient only), prior approval was not obtained, or so on.

denial code Alpha, numerical, or alphanumerical system used by insurance companies to explain partial or complete denials of insurance claims. Denial codes usually appear on documents such as explanation of benefits (EOBs).

denial of benefits 1. Rejection of a medical service due to insurance coverage policy or insurance program issues. 2. Rejection of all or part of an insurance claim. Application of contractual copayments and deductibles is not considered a denial of a claim. 3. Official Medicare decision that services will not be approved for payment. This may be due to a decision that the service is not an approved service, not being provided in the proper setting for the level of care, not provided by an approved participating provider, or not medically necessary.

denied claim Medical claim submitted to an insurance company in which payment has been rejected due to a technical error or because of medical coverage policy issues. Also called *denied paper claim* or *denied electronic claim.*

denied electronic claim See *denied claim.*

denied paper claim See *denied claim.*

dental care 1. Optional benefit offered by commercial insurance or managed care plans. Dental benefits may be combined with a health insurance plan or may be a separate policy with a different insurance company. 2. Insurance coverage for basic dental services such as cleanings, cavity repair, and necessary dental surgery including preventive care. Most dental plans do not cover the cost of orthodontia.

dental care, adjunctive This type of dental care includes dental and oral tissue examination and diagnosis at the request of a physician (MD). It is provided after the physician's examination and is done to help improve the systemic condition of the whole body and not just one area.

dental care, emergency Dental care performed to relieve oral pain, eliminate acute infection, control a life-threatening oral condition, or treat an injury to the teeth, jaws, or associated facial structures.

dental care, preventive Dental care that promotes oral health and prevents oral disease and injury.

dental clinic Outpatient facility that provides dental services by a group of dentists practicing together and assumes dental care responsibility for patients (e.g., examination of teeth and gums, cleaning of teeth, diagnostic x-rays for caries, educational services for prevention of diseases of the teeth and gums).

Dental Content Committee (DeCC) Organization endorsed by the American Dental Association that maintains the data content specifications for dental billing. Under the Health Insurance Portability and Accountability Act (HIPAA), this committee acts as a consultant for all transactions affecting dental health care services.

dental maintenance organization Managed care plan similar to a health maintenance organization (HMO) that provides only dental care.

dental plan 1. Optional insurance offered by commercial insurance or managed care plans that provides payment of expenses for dental care. Dental benefits may be combined with a health insurance plan or may be a separate policy with a different insurance company. 2. Insurance coverage for dental services and supplies including preventive care.

dental service Care of teeth and gums that includes preventive care, diagnostic x-rays of teeth and gums, and treatment to promote, maintain, or restore dental health. Ancillary services might be teeth whitening procedures, straightening and realigning teeth with braces, and so on.

dental treatment facility (DTF) See *dental clinic.*

dental treatment room (DTR) Examination and treatment room in a dental facility that includes a dental chair, dental unit, dental light, and wash basin where clinical dental procedures are performed.

dentist State-licensed individual who specializes in dental surgical procedures (DDS) or dental medicine (DMD). See *Doctor of Dental Surgery (DDS)* and *Doctor of Dental Medicine (DMD).*

dentist consultant State-licensed dentist who advises insurance companies as to the appropriateness of dental treatment.

deny See *denial of benefits.*

department number Numerical code used to indicate business sections in an employer company. Usually this is used when billing is produced through each business section.

Department of Business and Professional Regulation See *physician licensing board.*

Department of Defense (DOD) Department of the government that manages the TRICARE program.

Department of Health, Education, and Welfare (HEW) See *Department of Health and Human Services (DHHS or HHS).*

Department of Health and Human Services (DHHS or HHS) Cabinet-level federal agency that manages certain divisions of the federal government responsible for health and human services (welfare) and administers federal regulations. HHS oversees the Centers for Medicare and Medicaid Services (CMS), Food and Drug Administration (FDA), Public Health Service, and other related departments. It plays an active role in investigating health insurance fraud and abuse. Formerly called *Department of Health, Education, and Welfare (HEW).*

Department of Health Services (DHS) Medi-Cal is administered by this state department, which is a department of the California State Human Relations Agency.

Department of Industrial Accidents (DIA) In workers' compensation, a state body that administers the workers' compensation system and provides prompt and fair compensation to victims of occupational injuries and illness and sees that medical treatment to injured workers is provided in a timely manner while balancing the needs of employers to contain workers' compensation insurance costs. DIA also provides dispute resolution of workers' compensation cases through due process and adjudication. In some states, this is called *Department of Industrial Relations (DIR).*

Department of Industrial Relations (DIR) See *Department of Industrial Accidents (DIA).*

Department of Insurance (DOI) See *state insurance commission.*

Department of Justice (DOJ) Government body that investigates and prosecutes health insurance fraud and abuse.

Department of Labor (DOL) Cabinet-level department of the Executive Branch that administers the Black Lung health and disability program for coal miners.

Department, The The Department of Health and Human Services (HHS).

Department of Veterans Affairs (VA) Government department that administers and manages programs for veterans of the armed services; formerly known as the *Veterans Administration.*

dependent See *dependents.*

dependent age limitation Age when insurance coverage stops for a dependent child who is covered under a family insurance contract or plan.

dependent-care spending account Benefit that allows employees to set aside a portion of their wages, before taxes are taken out, to pay for certain dependent-care expenses such as child care or elder care, over-the-counter medically related items, and health premiums. Funds are taken out of an employee's wages through payroll deductions and put into an account controlled by a plan administrator. The employee submits proof of qualified expenses to the plan administrator, who will reimburse the employee from the employee's account. Employees have to estimate expenses carefully because any unused money at the end of the year is forfeited. Also known as a *tax saver* or *flexible spending account (FSA).*

dependent life insurance Group life insurance that covers the spouse, children, or other dependents of the group member. Generally it is sold in small amounts mainly to cover funeral expenses.

dependents Spouse and children of the insured. Under some insurance policies, parents, other family members, and domestic partners may be covered as dependents.

deposit administration contract Mechanism to fund a retirement plan in which the plan sponsor puts the plan assets in an insurance company's general account. At the time of the employee's retirement, the insurer withdraws sufficient funds from the general account to buy an annuity for the plan participant. This type of contract protects the plan sponsor from investment loss and guarantees minimum investment returns.

deposit administration group annuity Type of group annuity contract that provides for the accumulation of contributions in an undivided fund out of which annuities are purchased as the individual members of the group retire.

deposit-only bank account Type of bank account that provides protection against cyber thieves because it has a block or filter that enables it to only accept electronic deposits. Sometimes called *zero-balance account (ZBA).* See also *electronic funds transfer (EFT) system.*

deposit premium 1. Amount that is paid by a prospective insurance policyholder when an application is made for an insurance policy. It is usually the first month's estimated premium and is applied toward the actual premium when a statement is sent to the insured. 2. Funds left on deposit with the insurance company for plans subject to premium adjustment. Also called *premium deposits.*

deposit term life insurance Type of level term insurance that needs a larger premium payment in the first year than the amount of annual premiums in subsequent years. This higher first-year premium is called a *deposit.* If the insured dies, double the deposit is added to the death benefit. If the insured lives, double the deposit is returned. If the policy lapses, the insured forfeits the deposit and receives no refund.

deposition Process of taking a witness's sworn testimony out of court; usually done by an attorney. It is a chance for the opposing attorney to ask the witness whatever he or she wants to know, to fill in some blanks, finish preparing the case, evaluate the witness' testifying style, and determine how to approach the witness at trial.

derelict Failing in one's duty.

derivative file Subset from an original identifiable file.

dermatology Study of anatomy and physiology of skin, hair, and nails and the diagnosis and treatment of their diseases and disorders.

derogatory remark Statement, written or oral, giving an unfavorable or negative opinion of another individual or situation.

DES See *diethylstilbestrol (DES)*.

descriptor Text defining a code in a code set.

designated beneficiary Individual, other than the insured, who is to receive the proceeds on the death of the insured under a life insurance policy.

designated code set Medical code set or an administrative code set that Health and Human Services (HHS) has designated for use in one or more of the Health Insurance Portability and Accountability Act (HIPAA) standards.

Designated Data Content Committee (Designated DCC) Organization that Health and Human Services (HHS) has designated for oversight of the business data content of one or more of the Health Insurance Portability and Accountability Act (HIPAA)-mandated transaction standards.

Designated DCC See *Designated Data Content Committee (Designated DCC)*.

designated health services (DHS) Under federal Stark II laws, there are 11 types of health care services that a physician is prohibited from referring if he or she has a financial relationship. These services include clinical laboratory, physical therapy (including speech-language pathology services), occupational therapy, radiology (including magnetic resonance imaging, computerized axial tomography scans, and ultrasound), radiation therapy services and supplies, durable medical equipment and supplies, parenteral and enteral nutrients, equipment and supplies, prosthetics, orthotics and prosthetic devices and supplies, home health services, outpatient prescription drugs, and inpatient and outpatient hospital services.

designated hospital Facility under contract with a managed care plan to provide medical services to members of the plan. In an emergency situation, a member can save money by using a designated hospital instead of one that is not designated in the plan.

designated mental health provider Facility or physician hired by a health plan to provide mental health and substance abuse services.

designated mental health worker Individual or location authorized by a managed care plan to give mental health and substance abuse care to the plan's members.

designated record set (DRS) Under the Health Insurance Portability and Accountability Act (HIPAA), a group of records maintained by or for a covered entity that is (1) the medical records and billing records about individuals maintained by or for a covered health care provider; (2) the enrollment, payment, claims adjudication, and case or medical management record systems maintained by or for a health plan; or (3) used, in whole or in part, by or for the covered entity to make decisions about individuals.

designated standard Standard that Health and Human Services (HHS) has designated for use under the authority provided by the Health Insurance Portability and Accountability Act (HIPAA).

Designated Standard Maintenance Organization (DSMO) Association chosen by the Secretary of the United States Department of Health and Human Services to maintain standards adopted under Subpart 1 of 45 Code of Federal Regulations Part 162. A DSMO may receive and process requests for adopting a new standard or modifying an adopted standard.

detailed (D) A term used to describe a level of history and/or physical examination.

detailed examination 1995 guidelines Extended examination of the affected body areas or other symptomatic or related organ systems.

detailed history 1995 guidelines Documentation must include the chief complaint, an extended history of presenting illness (HPI), an extended review of systems (ROS), and a pertinent past, family, and/or social history (PFSH).

determination Decision made to either pay in full, pay in part, or deny a claim.

determination letter Communication from the Internal Revenue Service (IRS) stating whether the design of the pension plan meets the criteria to be a qualified plan.

development needed procedures See *questionable covered procedures*.

developmental disability (DD) Pathological condition (mental retardation or a related condition) that begins to develop before 18 years of age. This chronic disability results in impaired intellectual functioning and/or deficiencies in necessary physical skills used in daily living activities.

deviated rate In group creditor insurance, a premium rate for a contributory plan that is higher than the prima facie rate. It is based on the group's actual claims experience. An insurance company can charge a deviated rate only after the prima facie rate has been in effect for a specific period of time and only after being granted permission by the state insurance commissioner.

DG See *documentation guidelines (DG)*.

DHHS See *Department of Health and Human Services (DHHS or HHS)*.

DHS 1. Abbreviation for designated health services. See *designated health services (DHS)*. 2. Abbreviation for Department of Health Services. See *Department of Health Services (DHS)*.

DIA See *Department of Industrial Accidents (DIA)*.

diabetes mellitus Complex disorder of carbohydrate, fat, and protein metabolism that is primarily a result of a deficiency or complete lack of insulin secretion by the cells of the pancreas or resistance to insulin. There are two types as shown in Table D-1.

diabetes self-management training Program that educates patients in taking care of themselves because they have diabetes mellitus. It includes education about treatment, diet, and exercise.

diabetic durable medical equipment Purchased or rented ambulatory items such as glucose meters and insulin infusion pumps, prescribed by a health care provider for use in managing a patient's diabetes, as covered by the Medicare program.

diagnosis 1. Identification of a disease, syndrome, or condition by scientific evaluation of history, physical signs, symptoms, tests, and procedures. Diagnosis includes the technical description of the disease or condition and its cause, as well as the proper diagnostic code from the *International Classification of Diseases, Ninth Revision, Clinical Modification (ICD-9-CM)* code book. 2. In Medicare fraud, misrepresenting the diagnosis for the patient to justify the service provided or equipment furnished.

diagnosis code See *diagnostic code*.

diagnosis-related groups (DRGs) Patient classification system that categorizes patients who are medically related with respect to principal diagnosis, presence of a surgical procedure, age, presence or absence of significant complications, treatment, and who are statistically similar in length of hospital stay. Medicare

hospital insurance payments are based on fixed dollar amounts for a principal diagnosis as listed in DRGs regardless of the amount of charges accrued. See *all patient diagnosis-related group (APDRG or AP-DRG)* and *inpatient prospective payment system (IPPS)*.

diagnostic Medical service performed such as biopsy, thyroid function test, or radiographic procedure to establish the cause of the patient's complaints and symptoms.

diagnostic admission Registration of a patient either as an inpatient or outpatient primarily for diagnostic purposes in a health care facility.

Diagnostic and Statistical Manual of Mental Disorders, Fourth Edition (DSM-IV) Book published by the American Psychiatric Association that lists diagnostic criteria and terminology that is widely accepted as the preferred language of mental health clinicians and researchers.

Diagnostic and Statistical Manual of Mental Disorders, Fourth Edition, Text Revision (DSM-IV-TR) Diagnostic code book used by mental health clinicians as the system for substance abuse and mental health patients.

diagnostic code 1. Numerical three-, four-, or five-digit code located in the *International Classification of Diseases, Ninth Revision, Clinical Modification (ICD-9-CM)* code book and assigned to a patient's medical condition, symptoms, or reason for the encounter as documented in the patient's medical record. 2. Up to seven-digit code located in the *International Classification of Diseases, Tenth Revision, Clinical Modification (ICD-10-CM)*. The code is assigned to a patient's medical condition, symptoms, or reason for the encounter that is documented in the patient's medical record (see Figure D-1, *A*). 3. When the physician's office or an outpatient hospital is billing, the primary diagnosis code(s) is inserted in Block 21 of the CMS-1500 insurance claim form. For inpatient hospital billing, the principal diagnosis code is inserted in Field 66 and subsequent diagnosis codes in Fields 67 through 75 of the UB-04 insurance claim form. See Figure D-1, *B*.

Table D-1   FEATURES OF TYPE I AND TYPE II DIABETES

Type I Diabetes	Type II Diabetes
Insulin-dependent diabetes mellitus	Non–insulin-dependent diabetes mellitus
Patients must be treated with insulin	Patients may be treated with insulin
Insulin levels are very low	Insulin levels may be high, "normal," or low
Ketosis prone	Non–ketosis prone
Patients are usually lean	Patients are usually obese
Usually "juvenile onset" (peak onset at early puberty)	Usually "adult onset," although occasionally seen in children
Often little family history of diabetes mellitus	Often strong family history of diabetes mellitus

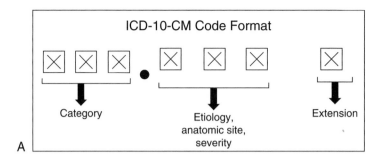

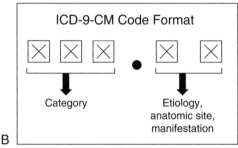

Figure D-1 Diagnostic codes.

diagnostic cost groups (DCGs) System of Medicare reimbursement for HMOs with risk contracts in which enrollees are classified into various DCGs on the basis of each beneficiary's prior 12-month hospitalization history.

diagnostic creep Coding that is inappropriately altered to obtain a higher payment rate. Also known as *coding creep*, *DRG creep*, or *upcoding*.

diagnostic examination Procedures used to find the nature and underlying cause of an illness, disease, or condition.

diagnostic laboratory services Mechanical or machine laboratory tests that are necessary to identify a disease, syndrome, or condition (e.g., electrocardiograph, electroencephalograph, complete blood count, urinalysis).

diagnostic services Procedures, tests, and examination (scientific evaluation of history, physical signs, symptoms) done on a patient to identify a disease, syndrome, or condition.

diagnostic test Procedure performed that provides information about a known problem or looks for disease after an illness is suspected.

diagnostic x-ray services Radiographic and other related studies and procedures performed to identify a disease, syndrome, or injury including portable x-ray services.

dialysate Solution used in dialysis to remove excess fluids and waste products from the blood. Also called *dialysate fluid*.

dialysate fluid See *dialysate*.

dialysis 1. Process by which dissolved substances are removed from a patient's body by diffusion from one fluid compartment to another across a semi-permeable membrane. The two types of dialysis that are in common use are hemodialysis and peritoneal dialysis. 2. Treatment that cleans the blood when the kidneys do not work. It gets rid of harmful wastes and extra salt and fluids that build up in the body. It also helps maintain blood pressure and appropriate fluid levels. Dialysis treatments help the patient feel better and live longer but are not a cure for permanent kidney failure.

dialysis center Hospital unit that is approved to furnish the full spectrum of diagnostic, therapeutic, and rehabilitative services required for the care of the end-stage renal disease (ESRD) dialysis patients (including inpatient dialysis) furnished directly or under arrangement.

dialysis facility Unit (hospital based or freestanding) that is approved to furnish dialysis services directly to end-stage renal disease (ESRD) patients.

dialysis station Portion of the dialysis patient treatment area that accommodates the equipment necessary to provide a hemodialysis or peritoneal dialysis treatment. This station must have sufficient area to house a chair or bed, the dialysis equipment, and emergency equipment if needed. Provision for privacy is ordinarily supplied by drapes or screens.

diethylstilbestrol (DES) Drug given to pregnant women from the early 1940s until 1971 to help with common problems during pregnancy. The drug has been linked to cancer of the cervix or vagina in women whose mothers took the drug while pregnant.

digital 1. Pertaining to fingers or toes. 2. Of or relating to the technology of computers and data communications wherein all information is encoded as bits of 1s or 0s (binary digits) that represent electrical on or off signals and can be stored in computer memory.

digital certificate Electronic credential that establishes one's identity.

digital fax claim Insurance claim sent to the insurance carrier via facsimile but never printed on paper. The fax is encoded with an electronic signal via an optical code reader and electronically entered into the claims processing system.

digital imaging and communications in medicine Standard for communicating images such as x-rays in a digitized form. This standard could become part of the Health Insurance Portability and Accountability Act (HIPAA) claim attachments standards.

digital rectal examination (DRE) Clinical examination of an individual's prostate for nodules or other abnormalities.

digital signature 1. In an electronic document, a signature that consists of lines of text or a text box stating the signer's name, date/time, and a statement indicating a signature has been attached from within a software application. 2. Electronically encrypted certification called *public key infrastructure* that is added to electronic documents to verify the identity of the signer. It is mandated in the Health Information Portability and Accountability Act for electronic prescriptions and other online documents.

dingy claim Insurance claim that cannot be processed due to the type of software program used to transmit the claim; it may be incompatible with the receiving system.

diplomate See *board certified.*

direct billing Standard traditional type of bill from an insurance company that is sent to the insured to notify him or her that the monthly, quarterly, or annual premium is due.

direct care Under the TRICARE program, medical care given in a military treatment facility. Also called *in-house care.*

direct claim payment System in which members of an insurance plan transact claims straight to the payer instead of submitting claims through an employer.

direct contract model Health plan that contracts straight to private practice physicians or provider groups in a locale rather than through an intermediary or managed care company (e.g., open panel health maintenance organization [HMO]).

direct contracting See *direct contract model.*

direct cost Dollar value that is related to a given object or specific service (e.g., medical equipment or medical supplies).

direct costs See *out-of-pocket expenses (OOPs).*

direct data entry Under the Health Insurance Portability and Accountability Act (HIPAA), this is the access of data directly into the computer through machine-readable source documents or through the use of online terminals that is immediately transmitted into a health plan's computer.

direct deposit Monies electronically sent to an account in a financial institution (i.e., bank, trust company, savings and loan association, brokerage agency, or credit union).

direct insurer See *direct writer.*

direct pay 1. System of billing members or subscribers of insurance policies for the premium payments, and they pay directly to their health plans. Direct pay rates are usually higher than group rates. Also called *billed direct* or *billed-at-home.* 2. Phrase used when the patient pays straight to the physician or health care provider for medical services rendered.

direct payment subscriber Individual enrolled in a managed care plan who pays premiums to the plan instead of through a group. Usually, payment is higher and benefits are not as wide ranging as the subscriber enrolled and paying as a member of the group.

direct placement Sale of a whole issue of bonds or stock to one or two large institutional clients without them being offered publicly.

direct premiums Property or casualty insurance premiums that are collected by the insurance company from the insured, before reinsurance is ceded to, or accepted from, another company.

direct referral Simplified authorization request form completed and signed by physician and handed to the patient at the time of referral.

direct response distribution system Method used in insurance to generate sales such as advertisements, telephone solicitations, and mailings. Insurance agents do not visit consumers to produce sales.

direct response marketing Method of selling insurance products directly to the consumer, which includes direct mail and advertising in print, radio, television, or by telephone without the use of insurance agents.

direct supervision In an office setting, direction and management of a medical procedure given by the physician. The doctor must be present in the office suite and available to give assistance and instruction during the performance of the procedure. The doctor does not need to be present in the room when the procedure is performed. Some medical procedures require direct supervision to bill for a specific level of service. This level of supervision is required when billing for "incident-to" services in an office setting. Also see *general supervision* and *personal supervision.*

direct treatment relationship Treatment association between a patient and a provider that is not an indirect treatment relationship. For example, a radiologist or a pathologist would be considered to have indirect treatment relationships with patients because they provide diagnostic services requested by other providers and furnish results to the patient through the direct treating physician.

direct writer Insurer that sells its policies directly to the public either through its own salaried employees or exclusive agents. Also called *direct insurer* or *direct-writing company*.

direct-writing company See *direct writer*.

directors and officers liability Type of insurance that covers directors and officers of a company for negligent acts or omissions or misleading statements that may result in a libel suit against the company.

Director of Insurance See *Commissioner of Insurance*.

dirty claim Claim submitted with errors or one that requires manual processing to resolve problems or is rejected or denied for payment.

disability 1. Impairment, loss of function (mental, physical, social), and inability to work either temporarily or permanently due to an injury or sickness. There are varying types (functional, occupational, learning); degrees (partial, total); and durations (short-term or long-term temporary, total, permanent) of disability. 2. For Social Security purposes, the inability to engage in substantial gainful activity by reason of any medically determinable physical or mental impairment that can be expected to result in death or to last for a continuous period of not less than 12 months. Special rules apply for workers aged 55 or older whose disability is based on blindness. The law generally requires that a person be disabled continuously for 5 months before he or she can qualify for a disabled worker cash benefit. An additional 24 months is necessary to qualify under Medicare. 3. In workers' compensation cases, a condition that renders the insured employee incapable of performing one or more of the duties required by his or her regular occupation. 4. In disability insurance, the definition of disability is variable. Some policies pay benefits if the individual cannot return to the exact occupation he or she had before. Some pay only if the individual cannot do any job for which he or she is reasonably qualified. Some policies pay if the person has been disabled by an accident and not by illness. Some policies have several tests to determine whether the insured is disabled according to the policy.

disability assessment See *functional capacity evaluation (FCE)*.

disability benefits 1. Payments for loss of income to an insured who is not able to work because of total and/or permanent disability for a covered injury or illness. Also called *disability compensation*. 2. Optional feature to a life insurance policy that provides for a waiver of premium and in some policies payment of monthly income if proof can be furnished that the insured has become totally and permanently disabled. 3. For Social Security disability, benefits are payable to people under full retirement age who have enough Social Security credits and who have a severe medical impairment (physical or mental) that is expected to prevent them from doing substantial work for a year or more or who have a condition that is expected to result in death.

disability buy-out insurance Type of disability insurance that gives funds to a business or professional partnership so that the business interest of a totally disabled partner may be bought if the disability is long term or permanent.

disability compensation See *disability benefits*.

Disability Determination Services (DDS) A state Social Security division office that assesses a case for disability benefits.

disability income benefits Payments for loss of income under a group life (permanent and total disability income), short-term disability income, or long-term disability income insurance contract.

disability income insurance Type of insurance that provides monthly payments to replace income when the insured is unable to work as a result of illness, injury, or disease—not as a result of a work-related accident or condition. Sometimes called *loss of time insurance, nonoccupational insurance*, or *disability insurance*.

disability insurance 1. See *disability income insurance*. Also known as *nonoccupational insurance* or *loss of time insurance*. 2. See *Old-Age, Survivors, and Disability Insurance (OASDI) Program*.

disability table 1. Statistical chart that shows the probabilities of becoming disabled at each age. 2. Tabulation of the number of individuals who continue to be disabled at each age and the length of disability.

disabled For purposes of enrollment under Medicare, individuals younger than 65 years of age who have been entitled to disability benefits under the Social Security Act or the railroad retirement system for at least 24 months are considered disabled and are entitled to Medicare.

disabled beneficiary See *disabled enrollee*.

disabled enrollee Individual younger than age 65 who has been entitled to disability benefits under Title II of the Social Security Act or the Railroad Retirement system for at least 2 years and who is enrolled in the supplemental medical insurance (SMI) program.

disabled life annuity Series of payments, each of which is conditional on a person being alive and still disabled.

disabled life reserve Funds set aside for payment of currently recognized or future claims on lives of disabled insureds.

disallowance Provider's fee that is above an insurance plan's fee ceiling (maximum allowable) and which the insurance company does not recognize for payment. Also referred to as *disallowed amount, nonallowed amount*, or *contractual disallowance*.

disallowed amount See *disallowance*.

discharge (DC) When related to the health care setting, this refers to the patient's formal release from the hospital as an inpatient or if a patient voluntarily departs the hospital. Types of discharge are discharge by death, discharge by transfer, and discharge to home. The discharge hour is inserted in Field 16 and patient discharge status is entered in Field 17 of the Uniform Bill (UB-04) inpatient hospital billing claim form.

discharge date Month, day, and year that the patient is formally released from the hospital or skilled nursing facility (e.g., patient left against medical advice, patient released to home, patient transferred to a skilled nursing facility or acute care hospital, patient expired).

discharge days See *length of stay (LOS)*.

discharge diagnosis One or more of the diagnoses listed after all the information from tests and observation have been obtained during the present course of a patient's hospital stay. This identification is given at the time of hospital discharge.

discharge management codes Procedure codes 99238 and 99239 indicate the provider takes full responsibility for the patient's entire hospital stay.

discharge plan Projected treatment plan by the primary care physician or discharging provider for the patient involving subsequent health care after formal release from the hospital as an inpatient. This may include home care, transfer to another facility, postoperative follow-up office visit, medication administration, and so on. Discharge plans are a requirement of the Medicare program and The Joint Commission for all hospital patients. Also called *discharge planning*.

discharge planning See *discharge plan*.

discharge provision Clause in an insurance contract about a small estates law that releases an insurance company from liability if it pays the proceeds to the deceased insured's estate.

discharge status 1. Disposition of the patient at the time of hospital discharge. This may be documented as patient left against medical advice, patient released to home, patient transferred to a skilled nursing facility or acute care hospital, or patient expired. 2. The patient discharge status is entered in Field 17 of the Uniform Bill (UB-04) inpatient hospital billing claim form.

discharge summary Report prepared by the patient's attending physician at the conclusion of a patient's hospital stay that summarizes the diagnosis, treatment, and results and outlines any further treatment after discharge. Also see *abstract* and *discharge plan*.

discharge transfer Formal reassignment of an inpatient to another facility for further health care.

discharged—not final billed (DNFB) balance Financial account balances of patients' records that remain uncoded after the bill-hold period expires or claims that have not passed the edits and have not yet been corrected.

disclaimer In managed care plans, this is a form used when a patient presents for services without a referral to a specialist. It may also be used when a patient accesses services of a primary care provider (PCP) who is not the patient's designated PCP or is not in the PCP's call share group. The patient is asked to sign this form to indicate an understanding that he or she may be financially responsible for charges incurred during the visit.

disclose Access, release, transfer, or otherwise divulge health information to any internal or external user of the data.

disclosure Release or divulgence of information by an entity to persons or organizations outside of that entity.

disclosure and use Under the Health Insurance Portability and Accountability Act (HIPAA), disclosure is when a patient's medical information is released to an individual or entity outside of the medical practice's organization and use is when information is shared within the medical office to facilitate patient treatment.

disclosure history Under the Health Insurance Portability and Accountability Act (HIPAA), a log that lists the individuals and companies that have received personal health information (PHI) for use that is unrelated to treatment and payment. Items to be documented must include date of disclosure, name of entity that received the PHI, brief description of the PHI disclosed, and brief statement of the purpose of the disclosure.

discount 1. Reduction of a normal charge based on a specific amount of money or a percentage of the charge. 2. In a managed care plan's contract with a provider, the discount is the percentage deducted during settlement of the claim from the allowed amount.

discount drug list Record of certain drugs and their proper dosages that shows the drugs the pharmaceutical company will sell at a reduced cost.

discounted fee-for-service (discounted FFS) Type of fee-for-service payment in which a managed care plan negotiates a discounted fee with a provider that is less than the usual or customary fee. It may be a fixed amount per service or a percentage discount. Physicians may be attracted to such negotiations because they represent a way to increase the volume of patients seen or reduce the chance of losing volume. Also called *contracted discount rate*.

discounted FFS See *discounted fee-for-service (discounted FFS)*.

discrepancy notice (DN) Formal statement that a managed care plan sends to a physician or hospital facility that indicates an inconsistency between their data about the disposition of a patient such as group number or difference in claim amount.

discretionary spending Outlays of funds subject to the federal appropriations process.

D

disease management Coordinated program that follows specific diseases or conditions and their treatments and introduces treatment to get the best outcome, prevent recurrence, and reduce the cost of care. Such programs exist for individuals who have asthma, diabetes, depression, and lipid disorders. Pharmaceutical companies work with physicians who maintain databases of drugs used to treat these diseases and conditions. Sometimes called *disease state management, outcomes management, population-based care, population-based care management,* or *care mapping.*

disease prevention See *preventive care.*

disease state management (DSM) Overseeing a patient's entire condition or disease state rather than treatment to individual components of a disease in isolation. Achievement of beneficial outcomes and cost effectiveness are emphasized. The patient's overall condition is treated carefully analyzing side effects and cost of treatment.

disenroll 1. Process in which a patient ends his or her health care coverage with a health plan. Generally this is now allowed unless a patient has been with a plan for at least 6 to 12 months. 2. In the Medicare program, a beneficiary may disenroll at the beginning of any given month if notice is given by a certain preceding deadline during the previous month.

disenrollment 1. Member's voluntary cancellation of membership in a managed care plan. 2. Involuntary disenrollment may occur because of a member's change in employment.

disfigurement Abnormal color, shape, or structure of a body part that if visible may cause social rejection and/ or poor self-image, causing a change in lifestyle and behavior.

disintermediation Process of removing funds from a financial intermediary so that it will earn a higher yield with another financial intermediary.

diskectomy Excision of the intervertebral disk material.

dismemberment Amputation or accidental loss of a limb or a portion of it.

dispensing fee Cost for filling a prescription for a drug, eyeglasses, or hearing aids.

disposition Physician's description of the patient's status and destination at discharge (e.g., discharged to home or self-care [routine discharge], left against medical advice, discharged to another short-term or long-term hospital, expired). These data may be used for quality assurance purposes. Also known as *disposition of patient.*

disposition of patient See *disposition.*

DISPRO share See *disproportionate (DISPRO) share* or *disproportionate share hospital (DSH).*

disproportionate (DISPRO) share Program that gives added payment to hospital facilities that serve an unequally large share of low-income patients. This assists in compensating for lost revenues in serving needy populations. Such facilities receive Medicaid funds if they provide care for a high volume of low-income patients.

disproportionate share hospital (DSH) Hospital facility with an unequally large share of low-income patients. Under Medicaid, states augment payment to these hospitals. Under a Prospective Payment System, Medicare inpatient hospital payments are also adjusted for this added burden.

disputed medical fact In workers' compensation cases, a medical issue in disagreement or with a difference of opinion, such as an objection to a medical determination made by a treating physician concerning the employee's medical condition, cause of the condition, or treatment for the condition. Other issues might be the existence, nature, duration, or extent of temporary or permanent disability caused by the employee's medical condition or the employee's medical eligibility for rehabilitation services.

distress termination To close a pension plan that does not have sufficient funds to cover the benefits to which the plan's participants are entitled.

distribution Separation of all prospective or presently insureds in group insurance plans by age, sex, location, income, status of dependency, and benefits for the purpose of computing premium rates.

distribution channels Various ways health plans and medical services are delivered such as insurance agents and brokers, pharmacies, pharmaceutical companies for drugs, and physicians.

distribution expenses Overhead costs in making insurance products available to the general public such as insurance agent compensation, group sales representatives' salaries, postage, printing, and telecommunications for direct response marketing.

distribution list See *list service (listserv).*

distribution system An insurance company's network of organizations and individuals who perform all the marketing activities to convey an insurance product from an insurer to the consumers.

divestiture Act of a medical supplier to sell part or all of its assets either by court order or voluntarily.

dividend 1. Refund of excess premium paid to the owner of an individual participating life insurance policy. It reflects the difference between the premium charged and actual experience. Also called *policy dividend* or *policy owner dividend.* 2. Part of a group insurance premium that is returned to a group policyholder that has a better claims experience than had been projected when the premium was calculated. Also called *experience rating refund, experience refund,* and *retroactive rate reduction.* 3. In a mutual or participating company, it is quarterly or annual payments by a business to a stockholder. Dividends paid in cash are called *cash dividends.* Dividends paid with shares of stock are called *stock dividends.*

dividend accumulations Policy dividend funds left on deposit with the insurer. Also called *dividend credits*.

dividend addition Amount of paid-up life insurance purchased with a policy dividend and added to the face value amount of the policy. This is an option written into the life insurance policy. Also called *paid-up additions*.

dividend credits See *dividend accumulations*.

dividend expenses Amount of money that it costs the insurance company to maintain each policy in force for the current year.

dividend interest rate Sum of money that accumulates and that represents the actual rate earned on an insurer's present investments. The dividend interest rate is used to calculate policy owner dividends.

dividend options Several choices that participating life insurance policy owners can choose to indicate how they want to receive their share of the insurance company's divisible surplus including accumulation at interest option, additional term insurance option, automatic dividend option, cash payment option, dividend accumulations, enhancement type policy, paid-up additions, and premium reduction option.

dividend rate of mortality Death (mortality) rate presently experienced by the insurance company on the insurance policies it has sold. The insurer chooses the rate of mortality for a given age in calculating the policy owner's dividends.

divisible surplus Portion of an insurance company's earnings available for distribution to owners of the company's participating policies.

DMD See *Doctor of Dental Medicine (DMD)*.

DME See *durable medical equipment (DME)*.

DME number See *durable medical equipment (DME) number*.

DMEPOS Commonly used acronym that may be translated as durable medical equipment, prosthetics, orthotics, and supplies.

DMERC Commonly used acronym that may be translated as durable medical equipment regional carrier. See *durable medical equipment regional carrier (DMERC)*.

DN See *discrepancy notice (DN)*.

DNFB See *discharged—not final billed (DNFB) balance*.

DNS See *no show*.

DO See *Doctor of Osteopathy (DO or MD)*.

DOB Abbreviation for date of birth.

docking pay Deducting part of an employee's wages for a particular reason.

Doctor of Chiropractic Medicine (DC) Individual trained in chiropractic medicine who may use diagnostic and therapeutic methods of chiropractic medicine. He or she is trained in adjustment and therapeutic manipulation of the spine and parts of the body and radiography for the purpose of diagnosis. Also called *chiropractor*.

Doctor of Dental Medicine (DMD) State-licensed individual, commonly called a *dentist*, who is trained and educated in a dental program and practices the prevention and treatment of diseases of the teeth and surrounding oral tissues.

Doctor of Dental Surgery (DDS) 1. State-licensed individual who specializes in surgical procedures involving the teeth and surrounding oral tissues. Operative dental surgeon restores teeth that have been damaged. Oral and maxillofacial surgeons specialize in surgical reconstruction of facial malformations caused by diseases of or trauma to mouth, face, head, or neck. Exodontists limit their practice to surgical removal of teeth. Oral surgeons specialize in surgical removal of teeth and surrounding oral tissues. 2. Under the Medicare program, a dentist for purposes of reimbursement is paid only with respect to surgery related to the jaw or any structure contiguous to the jaw or the reduction of any fracture of the jaw or facial bone.

Doctor of Medicine (MD) Health professional who has completed an approved course of study at an approved medical school, has satisfactorily passed the National Board of Examination, has done hospital internship or residency, and has obtained a state license to practice. Some physicians may elect to further train in a specialty such as allergy, cardiology, dermatology, or orthopedic surgery.

Doctor of Naturopathy (ND) Individual who has received training using a system of health care that does not employ drugs and has many varieties of therapies such as heat, massage, exercise, fresh food, hydrotherapy, and herbal medicine.

Doctor of Optometry (OD) Individual who has received training and is educated in the testing and correction of vision problems. He or she has obtained a degree of Doctor of Optometry (OD) after completion of 3 years of college followed by 4 years in an approved college of optometry and passing a state examination and receiving a license. Also called *optometrist*.

Doctor of Osteopathy (DO or MD) Physician trained in osteopathic medicine who may use diagnostic and therapeutic methods of standard medicine and is trained in therapeutic manipulation of the spine. License to perform medicine and surgery is required in all states. A DO may use the initials MD after their name in some states, and he or she is eligible for reimbursement by Medicare and Medicaid for professional services given to patients. Also called *osteopath, medical doctor*, or *MD*.

Doctor of Podiatric Medicine (DPM) Doctor trained in the examination, diagnosis, treatment, and prevention of diseases, conditions, and malfunctions affecting the human foot and its related structures. Podiatrists may use medical, surgical, or other means of therapy. Specialties of podiatric medicine consist of podiatric orthopedics, podiatric public health, and podiatric surgery. Formerly known as *chiropody*. Also called *podiatrist*.

Doctor of Veterinary Medicine (DVM) Individual trained in veterinary medicine, which pertains to the diseases and other disorders of domestic animals. He or she may use diagnostic and therapeutic methods of veterinary medicine and surgery.

Doctor's Final (or Monthly) Report and Bill See *Final Report*.

Doctor's First Report of Occupational Injury or Illness See *First Report of Injury*.

doctrine of reasonable expectations Rule or theory used by some courts that supports policy owners' and beneficiaries' rational expectations even though this is not stated in the policy. It means that the actual language of the insurance contract may not be the controlling factor if the insured could reasonably have expected something other than what the insurance contract states because of the circumstances of the case. Also known as *reasonable-expectation doctrine*.

documentation 1. Detailed chronological recording of pertinent facts and observations about a patient's health as seen in chart notes and medical reports, such as the patient's condition, treatment, and progress. These entries are required in the medical record to support charges submitted to third-party payers, as well as prescription refills, telephone calls, and other pertinent data. 2. Act of creating records to substantiate the performance of an action (e.g., financial records). 3. Claim forms, written communications, telecommunications, explanation of benefit documents, notes, transactions, and work papers that are relevant to a claim.

documentation guidelines (DG) In auditing of medical records, criteria used when preparing and evaluating documentation and physician performance by defining services and counting the items documented.

documents Forms and papers such as birth certificates, marriage certificates, W2 forms, tax returns, and deeds. These may be used by individuals applying for federal benefits.

DOD See *Department of Defense (DOD)*.

DOI 1. Abbreviation for Department of Insurance. See *Department of Insurance (DOI)*. 2. Abbreviation for date of injury. See *date of injury (DOI)*.

DOJ See *Department of Justice (DOJ)*.

DOL See *Department of Labor (DOL)*.

dollar limits The dollar amount of benefits that can be paid per month or over the life of an insurance policy.

domain manager Individual who must have knowledge of health information management, coding, laboratory, and pharmacy and works closely with product managers, operations staff, and quality control.

domestic carrier Insurance company in a specific state that has its head office (domiciled) in that state. Also called *domestic insurer*.

domestic company Insurance carrier that is incorporated under the laws of the state in which it is doing business.

domestic corporation Company incorporated under the laws of the state.

domestic insurer See *domestic carrier*.

domicile 1. Location of the permanent home or legal residence of an individual and, if absent, the individual has the intention of returning to. 2. Jurisdiction and site where a business or corporation maintains its headquarters and conducts its corporate affairs.

domiciled company Insurance carrier whose head office is in the same state as the individual referring to it.

domiciliary care See *adult foster care (AFC)* and *assisted living center (ALC)*.

donor Person who gives or contributes living tissue to be used in another body (e.g., blood for transfusion or a kidney for organ transplantation).

donut hole See *coverage gap* and *doughnut hole*.

DOR See *declaration of readiness (DOR) to proceed*.

DOS See *date of service (DOS)*.

double billing See *duplicate claims*.

double dipping Practice in which one piece of data in a patient record is counted as two data points when calculating an evaluation and management level of service for the code. This procedure may be considered either controversial, accepted, or rejected by third-party payers.

double high flux hemodiafiltration See *hemodiafiltration*.

double indemnity Feature in some life and disability insurance policies that provides for twice the face amount of the policy to be paid if death results to the insured from accidental causes.

doughnut hole Also spelled *donut hole*. Another name for the step in a Medicare Part D plan in which the patient pays all of the expenses for eligible drugs until he or she has spent $3850. Also referred to as *coverage gap* or *The gap*.

down time Period during which a computer, communications line, or other device is malfunctioning or not operating correctly because of mechanical or electronic problems.

downcode Reduce the value and procedure code of an insurance claim when the documentation supports a higher level of service billed by a provider.

downcoding 1. Coding system used by the physician's office does not match the coding system used by the insurance company receiving the claim. The insurance company computer system converts the procedure code submitted to the closest code in use, which is usually down one level from the submitted code, generating decreased payment. Sometimes downcoding may occur when the diagnosis code does not support the level of care. 2. Selecting procedure codes at a lower level than the medical service requires or documentation supports. Also called *undercoding*. Also see *penalized claim*.

download To transmit or receive a data or graphic file from one computer to another.

downscale To apply the correct commission scale to the insurance premiums received in order to compute the commissions due.

DPM See *Doctor of Podiatric Medicine (DPM)*.

DPR See *drug price review (DPR)*.

DPT See *days per thousand (DPT)*.

DRA See *Deficit Reduction Act of 2005 (DEFRA05 or DRA)*.

draft book claim payment Type of insurance claim adjudication (settlement) in which the insurance company authorizes the policyholder (insured) to settle claims and to issue payment on behalf of the insurer.

draft standard for trial use Archaic term for any X12 standard that has been approved since the most recent release of X12 American National Standards. The current equivalent term is X12 standard.

DRE See *digital rectal examination (DRE)*.

dread disease policy See *limited coverage policy*.

dressing Ability of an individual to put on and take off all garments and medically necessary braces or artificial limbs, if worn. Also see *activities of daily living (ADLs)*.

DRG See *diagnosis-related groups (DRGs)* and *all patient diagnosis-related group (APDRG or AP-DRG)*.

DRG coding Diagnosis-related group categories that are used by hospital facilities on discharge billing.

DRG creep See *diagnostic creep (DRG creep)*.

DRG grouper Computer software program that assigns diagnosis-related groups (DRGs) by abstracting data (i.e., patient's age, sex, principal diagnosis, principal procedures performed, and discharge status) to assign appropriate DRGs to discharged patients.

DRG payment rate Reimbursement amount a hospital receives for a Medicare patient who is assigned to a diagnosis-related group (DRG) that considers the wage rates in the hospital's region and the cost related to the DRG.

DRG weight Index number that reflects the resource spending associated with each diagnosis-related group.

DRGs See *diagnosis-related groups (DRGs)*.

drinking criticism Insurance underwriting phrase for evidence of alcohol abuse or alcoholism.

DRS See *designated record set (DRS)*.

drug formulary List of prescribed drugs recommended by a managed care plan and dispensed by participating pharmacies to members of the plan. It is periodically reviewed and modified. See the three types—open, closed, and restricted formularies for information. See *formulary*.

drug maintenance list See *adjusted drug benefit list*.

drug price review (DPR) Weekly update of drug prices at average wholesale price (AWP) that is from the *American Druggist Blue Book*. See *maximum allowable cost list*.

drug provider Entity licensed to dispense prescription drugs such as pharmacy (pharmacist), physician, or other licensed health care professional.

drug tiers Option introduced in the Medicare prescription drug plan that allows each plan to group different drug types together (i.e., generic, brand, preferred brand). Tiers could be used to describe drug groups that are based on classes of drugs. If the tier option is used, the plan should provide clarification on the drug types covered under the tier in the prescription drug plan notes section.

drug use evaluation (DUE) Same as drug utilization review except it is qualitative. See *drug utilization review (DUR)*.

drug utilization review (DUR) Evaluation of prescription drug use and prescribing patterns by physicians to establish the appropriateness of drug treatment. DUR may be done for individual patients, an entire insured group, for current, past, or future usage. Medication costs may be reduced by substituting generic for brand name drugs and use of a drug formulary.

DSH See *disproportionate share hospital (DSH)*.

DSM See *disease state management (DSM)*.

DSM-IV-TR See *Diagnostic and Statistical Manual of Mental Disorders, Fourth Edition, Text Revision (DSM-IV-TR)*.

DSMO See *Designated Standard Maintenance Organization (DSMO)*.

DTF See *dental treatment facility (DTF)*.

DTR See *dental treatment room (DTR)*.

dual choice (DC) See *dual-choice (DC) provision*.

dual-choice (DC) provision Part of the Health Maintenance Organization (HMO) Act of 1973 in which employers must meet specific specifications to offer health insurance through a federally qualified HMO as an alternative to a traditional health insurance plan. Also referred to as *dual choice*.

dual coverage See *duplication of benefits*.

dual eligible Individual who receives medical and/or disability benefits from both Medicare and Medicaid programs. Formerly called *Medicare/Medicaid (Medi-Medi)*. Also see *Medicare/Medicaid (Medi-Medi)*.

dual option program Insurance plan that allows an individual the opportunity to choose between joining a managed care plan or a traditional health insurance plan (e.g., indemnity insurance or a managed care organization).

dual registration Insurance sales representative who is licensed and registered with more than one broker.

DUE See *drug use evaluation (DUE)*.

due and uncollected premium Insurance premium that is due an insurance company and has not been received as of a certain date.

due and unpaid claims Incurred insurance claims that are due but not paid by the insurance company as of a specific date.

due care Legal phrase used in cases dealing with a defendant's negligence that implies that a person has not been negligent or violated the law in regard to the case in question. It calls attention to the degree of care that a competent person engaged in the same business or endeavor would exercise under similar circumstances. Also called *reasonable care, ordinary care, adequate care,* and *proper care.*

due date Month, day, and year when payment of a premium should be received by the insurance company.

dues Payment needed to maintain membership in a professional association.

dummy application Insurance application that is completed by the employer for an employee who is temporarily not available. The application is submitted unsigned to the insurance company. The health plan's group processing division includes this dummy application to verify group eligibility, estimate the enrollment percentage, and verify rates based on final enrollment. If necessary, modifications to the application are made when the employee returns to work.

dun message Messages or phrases to inform or remind a patient about a delinquent account, usually printed on monthly billing statements. They can appear as a handwritten note or a brightly colored adhesive label.

duplicate claims 1. Practice of billing for the same medical service more than once. In the Medicare program, a physician who repeatedly submits duplicate claims may be removed from the electronic billing network. 2. Resubmission of identical insurance claims with no changes. Duplicate claims are considered fraudulent. Also called *double billing.*

duplicate coverage inquiry (DCI) form Query form completed to an insurance company or medical provider to find out where there is other health insurance coverage under another plan. Such inquiries are made for the purpose of coordination of benefits between the two or more plans.

duplication of benefits See *duplication of coverage.*

duplication of coverage Insurance coverage of an insured under two or more policies who collects, or may collect, payments for the same hospital, or medical expenses from more than one insurer. Also known as *dual coverage, duplication of benefits,* or *multiple coverage.*

DUR See *drug utilization review (DUR).*

durable medical equipment (DME) 1. Billing phrase to Medicare and Medicaid fiscal intermediaries to specify medical supplies, devices, and equipment (e.g., crutches, urinary catheters, ostomy supplies, surgical dressings) for reimbursement. 2. Purchased or rented items such as a walker, seat lift equipment, wheelchairs, a hospital bed, and other medically neces-

sary equipment prescribed by a health care provider to be used in a patient's home and which are covered by the Medicare program. DME is paid under both Medicare Part B and Part A for home health services. Also called *home medical equipment.*

durable medical equipment (DME) number Group or individual provider number used when submitting bills for specific medical supplies, devices, and equipment to the Medicare fiscal intermediary for reimbursement.

durable medical equipment, prosthetics, orthotics, and supplies (DMEPOS) See *DMEPOS.*

durable medical equipment regional carrier (DMERC) Four contracted regional carriers (private companies) that contract with Medicare to process and pay insurance claims for durable medical equipment such as orthotics, prosthetics, and supplies. Providers are required to obtain supplier numbers and disclose ownership before submitting claims. Also called *contractor* and *durable medical equipment regional contractor (DMERC).*

durable medical equipment regional carrier advisory process (DAP) Formal method of obtaining comments about regional medical review policy development and revision and to discuss and improve administrative policies within the durable medical equipment regional contractor's discretion. These workgroups may consist of physicians, clinicians, Medicare beneficiaries, suppliers, and manufacturers who are able to give input.

durable power of attorney for health care Document that voluntarily designates a competent individual to make health care decisions if the patient becomes disabled or incapacitated and loses ability and cannot make decisions for treatment including the final decision about stopping treatment. Also see *power of attorney.* This type of advance directive also may be called a *health care proxy* or *appointment of health care agent.*

duration Length of time for each happening or occurrence of a medical problem or symptom.

duration of inpatient hospitalization See *length of stay (LOS).*

duty to warn Legal or ethical obligation to release confidential information on a patient when it is necessary to warn an individual who is in imminent danger from that patient (e.g., risk of acquiring a disease as a result of a relationship with the patient). The duty to warn is a legal mandate in many states.

DVM See *Doctor of Veterinary Medicine (DVM).*

DX Abbreviation for diagnosis or diagnosis code.

E

E&M See *EM, E/M*, and *evaluation and management (E&M)*.

E & M codes See *evaluation and management (E/M) codes*.

E&O insurance See *error and omissions (E&O) insurance*.

E code Numeric designation preceded by the letter "E" that is a classification of *International Classification of Diseases, Ninth Revision, Clinical Modification (ICD-9-CM)* coding for external causes of injury rather than disease. E codes are also used in coding adverse reactions to medications and should not be used as a principal diagnosis because the insurance carrier will reject the claim. Their use identifies causes of injury and poisoning and can be important in obtaining payment from insurance payers. The index for the E codes is located in Volume 2, following the Table of Drugs and Chemicals. Also known as the *Supplementary Classification of External Causes of Injury and Poisoning (E800-E999)*.

E1 HCPCS Level II modifier that may be used with CPT or HCPCS Level II codes and a procedure or service to the upper left eyelid. Use of this modifier does not affect reimbursement, but if not used may delay payment.

E2 HCPCS Level II modifier that may be used with CPT or HCPCS Level II codes and identifies a procedure or service to the lower left eyelid. Use of this modifier does not affect reimbursement, but if not used may delay payment.

E3 HCPCS Level II modifier that may be used with CPT or HCPCS Level II codes and identifies a procedure or service to the upper right eyelid. Use of this modifier does not affect reimbursement, but if not used may delay payment.

E4 HCPCS Level II modifier that may be used with CPT or HCPCS Level II codes and identifies a procedure or service to the lower right eyelid. Use of this modifier does not affect reimbursement, but if not used may delay payment.

EACH See *essential access community hospital (EACH)*.

eating Ability of an individual to get nourishment into the body by any means once it has been prepared and made available. Also see *activities of daily living (ADLs)*.

EAP See *employee assistance program (EAP)*.

earnings record Chronological history of the amount a worker earns each year during his or her working lifetime. For Social Security, credits earned remain on an individual's Social Security record even when changing jobs or during a period with no earnings.

e-care Use of electronic mail and the telephone to answer patients' questions, prevent unnecessary office visits, and consult online with other physicians. Insurers may or may not reimburse providers for e-care using CPT code 0074T for online medical evaluation. Physicians who offer this service have patients either prepay an annual fee for unlimited online messaging or pay a predetermined amount for each e-visit (fee-for-service model).

e-commerce Any transaction done using the Internet, such as purchasing medical supplies, books, and products and services and transmitting prescriptions and insurance claims. Many pharmacies will not accept electronic prescriptions, and transmission to pharmacies is illegal in some states.

e-discovery See *electronic discovery (e-discovery)*.

e-health Conducting health-related and health-care related transactions and communication via the Internet. This may include e-mail messages, consumers' putting their personal medical records on the Web, providers allowing patients to access their medical records, websites that give information on diseases and methods of treating them, and buying health-related products and services.

e-health information management (eHIM) Phrase that describes any and all transactions in which health care information is accessed, processed, stored, and transferred using electronic technologies.

e-mail See *electronic mail (e-mail)*.

e-mailing list See *list service (listserv)*.

e-signature Act of attaching a signature by electronic means. The e-signature process involves authentication of the signer's identity, a signature process according to system design and software instructions, binding of the signature to the document, and nonalterability after the signature has been affixed to the document. Types of e-signatures are (1) simple, electronic image of a person's signature; (2) digital signature—a more complex, technology-specific electronic signature that uses a level of authentication to verify that the person sending the information actually owns the signature; this type of signature is similar to a public key infrastructure and uses the exchange of keys (i.e., digital certificates and encryption algorithms) for authentication; and (3) the "click here if you agree" section of online click-through forms.

e-visit See *electronic visit (e-visit)*.

early retirement age Age stated in a pension plan that is before the normal retirement age but allows the plan participant to receive pension benefit. However, benefits received early are reduced from the amount that would have been received at normal retirement age.

Early and Periodic Screening, Diagnosis, and Treatment (EPSDT) Program Program that covers screening and diagnostic services to determine physical or mental defects in recipients younger than 21 years of age and health care, treatment, and other measures to correct or ameliorate any defects and chronic conditions discovered. In New York, this is called the *Child Health Assurance Program (CHAP)*.

earned income Money derived from personal services (i.e., salary, wages, commissions, or fees).

earned premiums Portion of a premium that pays for the protection that the insurance company has already provided on a policy; the expired part of the policy period.

earnings All wages from employment and net earnings from self-employment, whether or not taxable or covered.

earthquake coverage See *catastrophe insurance policy*.

EBM See *evidence-based medicine (EBM)*.

EBT See *electronic benefit transfer (EBT)* and *electronic funds transfer (EFT)*.

EC See *electronic commerce (EC)*.

ECF See *extended care facility (ECF)*.

economic assumptions Values relating to future trends in certain key factors that affect the balance in the trust funds. Economic assumptions include unemployment, average earnings, inflation, interest rates, and productivity. Also see *assumptions*.

economic credentialing 1. Process by which a managed care plan takes a physician's economic behavior into account and endorses that a physician is competent to render medical services to members of the plan. A physician's economic review might include tests ordered, hospital bed days, and outcomes. See also *provider profiling*. 2. Related to a hospital setting, it enables a hospital to obtain control over economic factors that affect the quality of medical care and range of medical services that a hospital can provide. 3. Analysis of claims and benefits data to identify cost, use, and quality of care by physicians, health care facilities, and allied health providers.

economic loss Total financial loss as a result of the death or disability of the wage earner or from destruction of property.

economic stabilization program Legislative program during the early 1970s that limited price increases.

ECP See *electronic claims processor (ECP)*.

ECRM See *electronic content and records management (ECRM)*.

ECS See *electronic claim submission (ECS)*.

ED See *emergency department (ED)*.

EDI See *electronic data interchange (EDI)*.

EDI translator Computer software program that accepts electronic data interchange (EDI) transmitted files and converts the data into another format, or converts a non-EDI file into an EDI format for transmission.

EDIFACT See *Electronic Data Interchange for Administration, Commerce and Transport (EDIFACT)*.

edit Software computer logic within an insurance claims processing system that selects certain claims, evaluates or compares information on the selected claims or other accessible source, and depending on the evaluation, takes action on the claims such as pay in full, pay in part, or suspend for manual review.

edit check Electronic examination of transmitted insurance claims for errors, conflicting code entries, and a match of diagnosis to medical service(s) provided. Also called *claim edits*. See *front-end edits*.

EDM See *electronic document management (EDM)*.

effective date 1. Under the Health Insurance Portability and Accountability Act (HIPAA), this is the month, day, and year that a final rule is effective, which is usually 60 days after it is published in the *Federal Register*. 2. In insurance, the month, day, and year on which the membership, insurance coverage, or rate becomes effective.

effectiveness Gross health benefits given by a medical service for typical patients in community medical practice settings.

efficacy Effectiveness of a drug or medical treatment or procedure to produce a certain result under ideal conditions, usually in controlled, expert settings with carefully selected patients. If a medical service results in a health benefit, then it is considered efficacious (effective).

efficient Activities performed effectively with minimum of waste or unnecessary effort, or producing a high ratio of results to resources.

EFT See *electronic funds transfer (EFT)*.

EGHP See *employer group health plan (EGHP)*.

eHIM See *e-health information management (eHIM)*.

EHO See *emerging healthcare organizations (EHO)*.

EHR See *electronic health record (EHR)*.

EIN See *employer identification number (EIN)*.

EJ HCPCS Level II modifier that may be used with CPT or HCPCS Level II codes and identifies a single treatment for subsequent claim for therapy (e.g., erythropoietin [EPO], sodium hyaluronate, infliximab).

eldercare Public, private, formal, and informal programs and support systems, government laws, and finding ways to meet the needs of the aged including housing, home care, pensions, Social Security, long-term care, health insurance, and elder law.

election Individual's decision to join or leave the Medicare plan or a Medicare+Choice plan.

election period 1. Under the Consolidated Omnibus Reconciliation Act (COBRA), 60-day length of time after an employee has been notified he or she may accept or decline health insurance coverage when their current position has been terminated. 2. Time when an eligible person may choose to join or leave the Medicare plan or a Medicare+Choice plan. A patient may join and leave Medicare health plans in four types of election periods: annual election period, initial coverage election period, special election period, and open enrollment period.

elective See *elective admission*.

elective abortion Induced termination of pregnancy before the fetus has developed enough to live if born and considered necessary by the woman carrying it and done at her request.

elective admission Inpatient or outpatient booking of a patient to a facility whose condition allows adequate time to schedule admission. Formal acceptance may be dependent on when the accommodations become available.

elective care Medical service or procedure that is optional and could be scheduled such as surgery for cosmetic reasons, sterilization surgery, or elective abortion.

elective contributions In an employee's retirement plan, cash or deferred dollar amount put into an employee's Section 401(k) plan by the employer. Contributions are made using before-tax dollars that are obtained through a voluntary reduction of the employee's salary. The employee pays taxes when the funds are paid out at retirement time, making it a tax-deferred system. Also called *elective deferrals*.

elective deferrals See *elective contributions*.

elective surgery Surgical procedure that may be scheduled in advance, is not an emergency, and is discretionary on the part of the physician and patient. Generally, elective surgery is required and may be major surgery.

electrodiagnostic (EDX) coding Procedure codes related to nerve conduction studies, needle electromyography, and neuromuscular junction testing. Because bundling rules may affect payment, these tests must be comprehensively and accurately documented. Also see *electrodiagnostic (EDX) medicine*.

electrodiagnostic (EDX) medicine Medical tests that include nerve conduction studies, needle electromyography, and neuromuscular junction testing for diagnosing motor neuron diseases, myopathies, radiculopathies, plexopathies, neuropathies, and neuromuscular junction disorders (e.g., myasthenia gravis and myasthenic syndrome). EDX studies are used to evaluate tumors involving an extremity, the spinal cord, or the peripheral nervous system.

electronic benefits transfer (EBT) See *electronic funds transfer (EFT)*.

electronic claim Insurance claim submitted to the insurance carrier by a provider of medical services or electronic media claim (EMC) vendor transmitted via a central processing unit (CPU), tape, diskette, direct data entry, direct wire, dial-in telephone, digital fax, or personal computer download or upload.

electronic claims processor (ECP) Individual who converts insurance claims to standardized electronic format and transmits electronic insurance claims data to the insurance carrier or clearinghouse to help the physician receive payment. Sometimes referred to as *electronic claims professional*.

electronic claims professional See *electronic claims processor (ECP)*.

electronic claim submission (ECS) Insurance claims prepared on a computer and submitted via modem (telephone lines) to the insurance carrier's computer system. Also called *electronic media claims (EMC)*.

electronic commerce (EC) Electronic transmission of business information.

electronic content and records management (ECRM) Merging of electronic content management and electronic records management functionality.

electronic data interchange (EDI) Process by which understandable data items are sent back and forth via computer linkages between two or more entities that function alternatively as sender and receiver. Common examples for medical billing that use the X12 format are insurance claims, quality assurance reviews, utilization data, and certifications. See also *Accredited Standards Committee X12 (ASC X12)*.

Electronic Data Interchange for Administration, Commerce and Transport (EDIFACT) United Nations rules for EDIFACT comprise a set of internationally agreed on standards, directories, and guidelines for computer-to-computer electronic interchange of data. It provides a forum and basis for development of international standards.

electronic discovery (e-discovery) To gather and use evidence in legal proceedings that complement traditional methods such as photocopies, printouts, and digital images of patient medical records.

electronic document management (EDM) Handling of a document in an electronic format by capturing, indexing, and storing it.

Electronic Fund Transfer Act (EFTA) Federal regulation that limits the consumers' liability if there has been an unauthorized use of an automatic teller machine (ATM) card, debit card, or other electronic banking device. Consumers are only covered by a $50 liability limit if they notify their financial institution within 2 business days of discovering a problem of unauthorized use of their debit card. If notification is delayed, the liability can jump to $500.

electronic funds transfer (EFT) system 1. Paperless computerized system enabling funds to be debited, credited, or transferred to a provider's financial institution, eliminating the need for personal handling of checks (e.g., from an insurance company's account directly to the accounts receivable of the physician's medical practice). Some insurance companies are using this system for Medicaid and Medicare payments. 2. Simple method of paying monthly insurance premiums in which the insured prearranges with his or her bank to automatically transfer payments to the insurance company's account from his or her checking account. See also *automatic bill payment* and *preauthorized payment*. Also called *automatic bill payment, bank check plan, check-o-matic, check deposit billing, preauthorized checking,* or *preauthorized payment*. See also *deposit-only bank accounts*.

electronic health record (EHR) Collection of medical information about the past, present, and future of a patient that resides in a centralized electronic system and is interoperable. This system receives, stores, transmits, retrieves, and links data for giving health care services from many information systems such as laboratory, radiology, pathology, and financial services. See also *electronic medical record (EMR)*.

Electronic Healthcare Network Accreditation Commission Organization that tests transactions for consistency with the Health Insurance Portability and Accountability Act (HIPAA) requirements and that accredits health care clearinghouses.

electronic mail (e-mail) Transmitting, receiving, storing, and forwarding of text, voice messages, attachments, or images by computer from one person to another or from one person to a defined group or all users on a system.

electronic media Under the Health Insurance Portability and Accountability Act (HIPAA), mode of electronic transmission that includes Internet (online mode—wide open), extranet or private network using Internet technology to link business parties, leased phone or dial-up phone lines including fax modems (speaking over phone is not considered an electronic transmission), and transmissions that are physically moved from one location to another using magnetic tape, disk, or compact disk media.

electronic media claims (EMC) Phrase that refers to a flat file format used to transmit or transport insurance claims, eliminating mailroom processing and manual data entry such as the 192-byte UB-92 Institutional EMC format and the 320-byte Professional EMC National Standard Format (NSF). In federal programs, payment is released when time requirements are satisfied, resulting in a faster cash flow turnaround for providers.

electronic media questionnaire Process that large employers can use to complete their requirements for supplying IRS/SSA/HCFA (Internal Revenue Service/Social Security Administration/Health Care Financing Administration) data match information electronically.

electronic medical record (EMR) Electronic depository or linked access to patient databases that contains patient care information that can be sent within only one health care organization. This allows health care entities to share data, improve quality of medical care, and quicken insurance claim processing. Also known as *computer-based patient record (CPR), online medical record, paperless patient chart,* and *computerized patient record (CPR)*. See also *electronic health record (EHR)*.

electronic payment posting Insurance company (payer) automatically posts a payment to the medical practice management system after transmitting an automatic deposit into the medical practice's bank account.

electronic records management (ERM) Handling of electronic medical records according to legal, regulatory, and operational requirements.

electronic remittance advice (ERA) Online transaction or electronic summarized statement about the status of an insurance claim with explanation of the payment for one or more beneficiaries. It is equivalent to the paper summarized statement called a *Medicare remittance notice (MRN)*. It is often referred to as *ANSI 835* or *Health Care Claim Payment/Advice (835)*. Also called *electronic remittance notice (ERN)*.

electronic remittance notice (ERN) See *electronic remittance advice (ERA)*.

electronic remittance voucher Electronic explanation of benefits that is transmitted to the medical practice when an insurance company (payer) transmits an electronic payment that is automatically deposited in the medical practice's bank account.

electronic signature Method of authenticating documents by either insertion of a facsimile of a person's actual handwritten signature, typed name, mark, symbol, or code that is affixed electronically to the end of a document. Electronic signatures are subject to federal and state laws. Some state laws permit their use in place of a pen-and-ink signature. Electronic signatures are not designed to be secure.

electronic submission Transmission of dental insurance claims for adjudication or eligibility transactions via modem (telephone lines). See *electronic claim submission (ECS)*.

electronic visit (e-visit) Communication via electronic mail (e-mail) of a patient with a physician for the purpose of health treatment/care (e.g., medication assessment or laboratory results). Some insurance plans allow some coverage for e-visits. The timeline is that usually an e-mail is answered before the end of the next business day.

element 1. Number of items necessary for coding an evaluation and management (E/M) service. 2. When an audit is taking place, term used to indicate E/M criteria for documenting services rendered. Also known as a *bullet*.

eligibility 1. Qualifying factors that must be met before a patient receives benefits (medical services) under a specified insurance plan, government program, or managed care plan. 2. Refers to the process whereby an individual is determined to be eligible for health care coverage through the Medicaid program. Eligibility is determined by the State. Eligibility data are collected and managed by the State or by its fiscal agent. In some managed care waiver programs, eligibility records are updated by an enrollment broker who assists the individual in choosing a managed care plan in which to enroll.

eligibility date Month, day, and year an individual and/or spouse and dependents become eligible for benefits under an insurance plan or date he or she may apply for insurance.

eligibility for coverage In group health insurance, the conditions that an individual must meet to obtain coverage such as age, employment status, and continued employment.

eligibility guarantee Promise of payment to the medical provider for services rendered to a member of an insurance plan who later is discovered to be ineligible for benefits.

eligibility—Medicare Part A An individual is eligible for premium-free (no cost) Medicare Part A (hospital insurance) if he or she is 65 or older and receiving, or eligible for, retirement benefits from Social Security or the Railroad Retirement Board, or is younger than 65 and has received Railroad Retirement disability benefits for the prescribed time and meets the Social Security Act disability requirements, or had Medicare-covered government employment, or is younger than 65 and has end-stage renal disease (ESRD). If an individual is not eligible for premium-free Medicare Part A, he or she can buy Part A by paying monthly premium if he or she is 65 or older and enrolled in Part B, a resident of the United States, and either a citizen or an alien lawfully admitted for permanent residence who has lived in the United States continuously during the 5 years before the month in which they apply.

eligibility—Medicare Part B An individual is automatically eligible for Part B if he or she is eligible for premium-free Part A. They are also eligible for Part B if they are not eligible for premium-free Part A but are age 65 or older and a resident of the United States or a citizen or an alien lawfully admitted for permanent residence. In this case, they must have lived in the United States continuously during the 5 years immediately before the month during which he or she enrolls in Part B.

eligibility period Time (usually 31 days) that follows the eligibility date during which a member of an insured group can apply for insurance.

eligibility requirements Insurance underwriting conditions that must be met by an insurance applicant with the purpose of becoming insured.

eligibility verification 1. Procedure performed by a provider or health facility of checking and confirming

that a patient is a member of an insurance plan and that the member identification number is correct. 2. Process of an insurance company to validate that a patient is a member of a plan and the authorization of payment for a medical service before it is rendered. Also called *insurance verification* or *verification*.

eligibility verification confirmation (EVC) Reference number on a printout from the Medi-Cal point of service device that verifies an inquiry was received and eligibility information was transmitted.

eligibility waiting period In group health insurance, the length of time an employee must be employed by an employer before he or she is eligible for insurance coverage. Also called *probationary period.*

eligible Qualified to receive health insurance or government program benefits.

eligible dependents Individuals who are permitted to apply and maintain membership in a health insurance plan (i.e., spouse and children of the insured). Under some insurance policies, parents, other family members, and domestic partners may be insured as dependents.

eligible drugs Medications that are covered by a prescription drug plan. In a Medicare Part D plan, drugs that qualify are listed on the plan's formulary.

eligible employee Employed worker who qualifies for health insurance plan benefits as one who is insured.

eligible expenses Specific medical services and supplies for which the insurance plan or federal or state program will pay for covered persons under the terms of the plan.

eligible groups Individuals allowed insurance under a group policy such as individual employer groups, multiple employer groups, labor union groups, credit-debtor groups, and certain association groups.

eligible individual See *eligible person.*

eligible medical expenses Types of medical care expenses that an insurance plan covers.

eligible members Individuals in a group who qualify for a group insurance plan, or in a family who qualify for a family insurance plan.

eligible person 1. Individual who qualifies and is permitted to apply and maintain membership in a health insurance plan. 2. Individual who was covered under a group health plan and who may qualify to purchase an individual insurance policy regardless of previous health problems.

elimination period See *waiting period (WP).*

ELOS See *estimated length of stay (ELOS).*

EM HCPCS Level II modifier that may be used with CPT or HCPCS Level II codes indicating emergency reserve supplies for end-stage renal disease (ESRD). This is for supplies dispensed to patients on home dialysis.

E/M Acronym that means evaluation and management services described and coded in the *Current Procedural Terminology (CPT)* code book.

E/M codes See *evaluation and management (E/M) codes.*

E/M counseling Discussion with a patient and/or family concerning treatment, results of diagnostic studies, recommended management, prognosis, and education of the disease process.

E/M section See *evaluation and management (E/M) section.*

E/M service components See *evaluation and management service components.*

emancipated minor Person younger than 18 years of age who lives independently, is totally self-supporting, and possesses decision-making rights. See *age of majority, mature minor,* and *minor.*

embezzlement Willful act by an employee of taking possession of an employer's money.

EMC See *electronic media claims (EMC).*

emergency (EMG) Sudden and unexpected medical condition, or the worsening of a condition, that poses a threat to life, limb, or sight and requires immediate medical treatment to alleviate suffering (e.g., shortness of breath, chest pain, drug overdose). In most managed care plans, the only time a person can be hospitalized without precertification is when there is an emergent situation. Also referred to as *medical emergency.*

emergency admission Inpatient hospital or facility acceptance of a patient who requires immediate medical or psychiatric care because of life-threatening, serious, and possibly disabling conditions.

emergency care Health care services provided to prevent serious impairment of bodily functions or serious dysfunction to any body organ or part. Advanced life support may be required. Not all care provided in an emergency department of a hospital can be termed "emergency care."

emergency center Free-standing health facility that is not hospital affiliated and provides short-term care. It usually is open 24-hours a day, 7 days a week and handles minor medical emergencies or services and procedures that need urgent treatment. Also called *emergi-center, free-standing emergency medical service center, free-standing urgent care center, episodic acute care center, urgent care center, urgi-center.*

emergency department (ED) Hospital outpatient facility available 24 hours a day that gives medical services to patients for emergent medical and surgical conditions that need immediate attention but for which the patient will not be admitted to that facility or transferred to another facility. Also called *emergency room (ER).*

emergency medical condition Serious medical condition that has symptoms of such a severe nature that if the patient does not receive immediate medical attention, it would place the health of the person, or a fetus in the case of a pregnant woman, in jeopardy.

emergency medical screening examination Inspection and/or testing of the patient and taking of a medical history to discover the nature and extent of an emergency medical condition (e.g., cardiovascular accident, heart attack, poisoning, loss of consciousness, or respiration difficulty).

emergency medical services (EMS) See *emergency services.*

emergency medical technician (EMT) Individual who provides vital attention as he or she performs prehospital care and transports the sick or injured to a medical facility. EMTs are dispatched to the scene by a 911 operator and work with police and fire department personnel. They determine the nature and extent of the patient's condition while trying to ascertain whether the patient has preexisting medical problems. Some paramedics are trained to treat patients with minor injuries on the scene of an accident or at their home without transporting them to a medical facility. Emergency treatment for more complicated problems is carried out under the direction of medical doctors by radio preceding or during transport. At the medical facility, EMTs and paramedics help transfer patients to the emergency department, report their observations and actions to emergency department staff, and may provide additional emergency treatment. If a transported patient had a contagious disease, EMTs and paramedics decontaminate the interior of the ambulance and report cases to the proper authorities. In addition, paramedics may administer drugs orally and intravenously, interpret electrocardiograms (ECGs), perform endotracheal intubations, and use monitors and other complex equipment. Formal training and certification is necessary to become an EMT or paramedic. A high school diploma is typically required to enter a formal training program. Some programs offer an associate degree along with the formal EMT training. All 50 states have a certification procedure. In most states and the District of Columbia, registration with the NREMT is required at some or all levels of certification. Other states administer their own certification examination or provide the option of taking the National Registry of Emergency Medical Technicians examination. To maintain certification, EMTs and paramedics must reregister, usually every 2 years. Also see *first responder, EMT basic* (EMT-1), *EMT intermediate* (EMT-2 and EMT-3), and *EMT paramedic* (EMT-4).

Emergency Medical Treatment and Active Labor Act (EMTALA) Requires any Medicare-participating hospital that operates a hospital emergency department to provide an appropriate medical screening examination to any patient who requests such an examination. If the hospital determines that the patient has an emergency medical condition, it must either stabilize the patient's condition or arrange for a transfer. However, the hospital may only transfer the patient if the medical benefits of the transfer outweigh the risks or if the patient requests the transfer. This is also known as the "anti-dumping law."

emergency medicine Branch of medicine that deals with the diagnosis and treatment of diseases and injuries that result from trauma or sudden illness. Generally these cases are seen in a hospital emergency department.

emergency outpatient Patient admitted for diagnosis and treatment of a condition that needs immediate attention but who will not be admitted to that facility or transferred to another facility.

emergency room (ER) See *emergency department (ED)*.

emergency services Medical services provided to patients for conditions arising, often unexpectedly, and that need immediate medical attention such as an acute illness or injury. These services are given in a hospital emergency department 24 hours a day. The Joint Commission accreditation manual lists three levels: I, II, and III. Also see *Level I emergency service, Level II emergency service*, and *Level III emergency service*.

emergency treatment In workers' compensation cases, medical treatment required by an injured employee immediately after an industrial injury or illness, which if delayed, could decrease the likelihood of maximum recovery.

emergent care Treatment for a medical condition or symptom (e.g., pruritus from poison oak or poison ivy or severe pain) that arises, often unexpectedly, and needs immediate attention.

emergent condition Any physical state of a patient that needs immediate medical care, is possibly life threatening, and may be harmful if treatment is postponed.

emergi-center See *emergency center*.

emerging healthcare organization (EHO) Hospital or other provider that is affiliating or partnering.

EMG See *emergency (EMG)*.

employability In workers' compensation cases, the ability of an individual to perform a job and meet the conditions of employment as defined by the employer.

employee 1. Person who performs a service for someone else under employment or contract for hire. A contract can be expressed or implied or oral or written. 2. Under Medicare Secondary Payer guidelines, this is defined as an individual who is working for an employer or an individual who, although not actually working for an employer, is receiving from an employer payments that are subject to Federal Insurance Contributions Act (FICA) taxes or would be subject to FICA taxes except that the employer is exempt from those taxes under the Internal Revenue Code (IRC).

employee assistance program (EAP) Occupational health service program for employees, their family members, and employers to assist with personal or financial problems (e.g., family or marital issues, on-the-job stress, legal problems, child care, substance abuse).

employee benefits Any type of indirect compensation besides an employee's salary and wage that is available through his or her employment. Also called *fringe benefits*. These benefits may include group health insurance, group life insurance, and a pension plan.

employee benefits consultant Individual who specializes in selling and servicing employee benefit plans. He or she may also assist the employer in changing a benefit program. Usually they are paid through commissions from the insurance company or by the policyholder.

employee census Data that relates to insured persons in a group insurance policy such as age, sex, occupation, earnings, and status of dependency.

employee contribution See *percentage contribution*.

employee life insurance Term life group insurance policy for employees of an employer.

employee-pay-all plan Group insurance plan in which the employees pay all of the premium.

Employee Retirement Income Security Act (ERISA) Federal legislation enacted in 1974 that protects pension rights of employees, prohibits states from applying specific mandates to self-insured group health benefit plans, and shields self-insured employers from paying premium taxes, which insurance companies and managed care plans must do. Additional ERISA provisions require that health plans provide a description of the benefits of the plan, identify the persons responsible for operating the plan, explain the arrangements for funding and amending the plan, provide an explanation of benefits (EOB) when a claim is denied, and provide information on members' rights of appeal if a claim has been denied. The Department of Labor administers the law. Also called the *Pension Reform Act*.

employee-selected physician In workers' compensation cases, a physician or medical facility chosen by the employee more than 30 days from the date of when the injury is reported.

employee's cost basis In a retirement plan, an amount that is subtracted from the total amount of distribution to the plan to determine the amount of the distribution subject to federal tax. Cost basis is the amount on which an employee has already been taxed. It includes the amount of nondeductible contributions made to the plan by the participant, cost of plan-provided life insurance reported as taxable income by the participant, and amount of employer contributions previously taxed as income to the participant.

employee stock ownership plan (ESOP) Qualified employee-benefit plan that invests some or all plan assets in employer stock. Under ERISA, an ESOP is a qualified stock bonus plan or a combination qualified stock bonus plan and defined contribution pension plan that invests in employer securities. The employer's contributions are tax deductible for the employer and tax deferred for the employee.

E

employer 1. In workers' compensation, an employer includes any person or entity that engages the services of a person. It includes an individual employer, partnership, legal representative of a deceased employer, or a corporation. It also includes the state and every state agency, every country, every city, and all public and quasi-public corporations and agencies. 2. Under Medicare Secondary Payer guidelines, in addition to individuals (including self-employed persons) and organizations engaged in a trade or business, other entities exempt from income tax such as religious, charitable, and educational institutions. Included are the governments of the United States, the individual states, Puerto Rico, the Virgin Islands, Guam, American Samoa, the Northern Mariana Islands, the District of Columbia, and foreign governments.

employer bulletin board service Electronic bulletin board service offered by the coordination of benefits (COB) contractor. Employers who have to report on fewer than 500 workers can fulfill their requirements under the Internal Revenue Service/Social Security Administration/Health Care Financing Administration (IRS/SSA/HCFA) data match law by downloading a questionnaire entry application from the bulletin board. The information will be processed through several logic and consistency edits. Once the employer has completed the information, he or she will return the completed file through the bulletin board.

employer coalition Employers who partner together to administer and manage their health insurance plan and also make purchases at discounted rates for the benefit of the members.

employer group Group of employees who are eligible for health care benefits extended through a benefits plan provider. A contract is drawn up and an employee-employer relationship must exist. Groups that would not qualify include social clubs and independent contractors.

employer group health plan (EGHP) 1. Group health plan paid for by the employer of 20 or more employees for medical benefits. It may be a federal employee health benefits program, employee pay all plan, multi-employer group health plan with at least one employer with 20 or more employees, or any plan in which the beneficiary is enrolled because of their employment or his or her spouse's employment. 2. Under Medicare Secondary Payer guidelines, any health plan that is offered or contributed to by an employer, and that provides medical care, directly or through other methods such as insurance or reimbursement, to current or former employees and/or their families. It includes the federal employees' health benefits program but not TRICARE. 3. Private group health plan paid for by the employer that covers an individual who is age 65 or older and has Medicare as the secondary payer.

employer identification number (EIN) An employer's or company's federal tax identification number issued by the Internal Revenue Service for income tax purposes (e.g., physician's EIN). This is sometimes referred to as a *federal identification number, employer identifier,* or *tax identification number (TIN).*

employer identifier See *employer identification number (EIN).*

employer liability Employer is responsible for the acts of his or her employees while they are working.

employer number See *group number.*

employer's bill of rights Employer's legal right to be advised of all aspects of a workers' compensation claim that affect an employer's premium, which includes a premium reimbursement provision.

employer's liability insurance Liability insurance that protects an employer against any claims for damages that are the result of injuries to employees while they are working. Workers' compensation insurance insures the employer against liability under state compensation laws. Employer's liability insurance gives protection in cases that are not covered by the compensation law.

employer mandate In insurance, some states have laws that require employers to pay part of their employees' health insurance plan or provide a standard benefits package of insurance to all employees and their dependents. Prior to 1995, employer mandate related to federally qualified health maintenance organizations (HMOs) and an employer was required to offer at least one HMO plan to their employees.

employer self-insured program See *self-insurance.*

employer-sponsored health insurance plan Health insurance plan that an employer pays all or part of the premium for his or her employees and their dependents.

employment agency Business organization that refers job applicants to potential employers.

employment related Injury or illness that occurs while a person is working.

EMR See *electronic medical record (EMR).*

EMS See *emergency medical services (EMS).*

EMT See *emergency medical technician (EMT).*

EMT basic Also known as *EMT-1,* represents the first component of the emergency medical technician system. An EMT-1 is trained to care for patients at the scene of an accident and while transporting patients by ambulance to the hospital under medical direction. The EMT-1 has the emergency skills to assess a patient's condition and manage respiratory, cardiac, and trauma emergencies. Also see *emergency medical technician (EMT).*

EMT intermediate Also known as *EMT-2* and *EMT-3* and has more advanced emergency medical training that allows the administration of intravenous fluids, the use of manual defibrillators to give life-saving shocks to a stopped heart, and the application of advanced airway techniques and equipment to assist patients experiencing respiratory emergencies. Also see *emergency medical technician (EMT)*.

EMT paramedic Also known as *EMT-4* and provides the most extensive prehospital care in an emergency situation. Also see *emergency medical technician (EMT)*.

EMTALA See *Emergency Medical Treatment and Active Labor Act (EMTALA)*.

enabling services Ancillary services that help patients to access medical care (e.g., shuttle transportation or translator services).

encoder Add-on software to practice management systems that can reduce the time it takes to build or review insurance claims before batch transmission to the carrier. It takes codes entered by a coder, and by using a series of built-in prompts it enables him or her to code more accurately and specifically. The encoder bases its code selection on clinical documentation and can generate diagnostic and/or procedural codes. The prompts perform such tasks as resequencing codes by priority, verifying the relationship between grouped codes, and suggesting additional related codes not originally entered by the coder. Two types of encoder systems exist: logic based and dictionary driven.

encoder dictionary-driven system Method used in encoder software in which a coder enters a keyword that brings up a menu of either diagnostic or procedural codes from which a coder can choose.

encoder logic-based system Method used in encoder software in which a coder enters a keyword that generates a series of prompts or questions that ends with a suggested diagnostic or procedural code.

encounter 1. Face-to-face meeting and communication of a provider and a patient for the diagnosis and treatment of a disease or injury. This may occur in an office, home, or hospital facility setting. 2. One contact or episode of service to a patient. Also known as a *visit*.

encounter data Detailed information about individual medical services, regarding how a patient was treated, that are provided to a capitated managed care plan by the provider. The level of detail about each medical service reported is similar to that of a standard insurance claim form. Encounter data are also sometimes referred to as *shadow claims*.

encounter fee Dollar amount that is charged to a managed care plan member by a provider when medical service is provided in a preferred provider hospital emergency department or in the office of the preferred provider. A schedule of benefits or fee schedule in the managed care contract lists the amount of the fee for each type of medical service along with the procedural code.

encounter form All-encompassing billing form personalized to the practice of the physician. It is considered a financial record source document that is used to record the patient's diagnosis, any services given to the patient during the current visit, and related service fees. It may be used when a patient submits an insurance claim; also called *charge slip, cheat sheet, communicator, fee ticket, multipurpose billing form, patient service slip, routing form, superbill,* and *transaction slip.* See *multipurpose billing form* and *cheat sheet.*

encounter record At one time considered a buzz word for "claim."

encounters In managed care plans, a report of capitated services, submitted for statistical purposes only. No reimbursement is made from this information.

encryption To assign a code to represent data. This is done for the purpose of security to protect the confidentiality of information. The only key to unlock the data is held by the user who is authorized to receive the data.

end-of-life planning Verbal or written information about a Medicare patient's ability to prepare an advance directive when an injury or illness causes inability of the individual to make health care decisions. It also involves whether or not the physician is willing to follow the individual's wishes as expressed in an advance directive.

end-stage renal disease (ESRD) Chronic, advanced kidney disease that needs renal dialysis or a kidney transplant to prevent imminent death. Individuals who have chronic kidney disease requiring dialysis or kidney transplant are considered to have ESRD. To qualify for Medicare coverage, an individual must be fully or currently insured under Social Security or the railroad retirement system or be the dependent of an insured person. Eligibility for Medicare coverage begins with the third month after the beginning of a course of renal dialysis. Coverage may begin sooner if the patient participates in a self-care dialysis training program or receives a kidney transplant without dialysis.

end-stage renal disease (ESRD) network Group of private organizations that makes sure the patient is getting the best possible care. ESRD networks also keep the facility aware of important issues about kidney dialysis and transplants.

end-stage renal disease (ESRD) treatment facility Facility, other than a hospital, that provides dialysis treatment, maintenance, and/or training to patients or caregivers on an ambulatory or home-care basis.

endocrinology Branch of medicine that studies the anatomical, physiological, and pathological characteristics of the endocrine system and the treatment of diseases of the ductless glands (adrenals, ovaries, pancreas, parathyroids, pituitary, testes, and thyroid). It is a subspecialty of internal medicine.

endorsement 1. Provision in written form added to an insurance policy that alters its terms. It may also be in the form of a rider. A valid endorsement must be signed by an executive of the insurance company and attached to it as part of the policy. Also known as *rider* or *amendment*. 2. In licensure, the recognition by one jurisdiction of a license given by another jurisdiction, when the standards required by the licensing jurisdiction are equal or higher than those of the endorsing jurisdiction.

endorsement method Procedure of changing the beneficiary of a life insurance policy. It may be done in one of two ways: (1) The policyholder sends the policy to the insurance company and the insurer attaches an endorsement with the name of the new beneficiary to the policy, or (2) the policyholder requests a change in writing or by telephone and the insurance company sends an endorsement with the change to the policyholder.

endoscopy Insertion of a flexible fiberoptic tube, referred to as a *scope*, through a small incision into a body cavity or into a natural body orifice (opening) such as the ears, nose, mouth, vagina, urethra, or anus. An endoscopy may be diagnostic, performed for the purpose of visualization and determination of the disease process, or it may be surgical including procedures such as incisions, repairs, and excisions.

endowment insurance 1. Type of life insurance that pays a specific sum of money on the death of the insured within a covered period or at the end of the covered period if the person is still alive. If the insured dies before the maturity date, payment is made to a beneficiary of the policy. 2. A type of life insurance policy in which the cash value and face value are equal to each other at the policy's maturity date.

end station 1. Computer that is connected to a network, which can include PCs, workstations, and minicomputers. 2. Work station.

engineering controls System component or element that removes hazards from the workplace (e.g., sharps containers, self-sheathing needles, no-splash Vacutainer tops).

enhanced benefits Additional, mandatory, and optional supplemental insurance benefits.

enhancement type policy Life insurance policy in which part of each dividend provides paid-up additions, and the other part gives 1-year term insurance to produce a predetermined total death benefit.

enroll To join a health insurance plan.

enrolled actuary Pension actuary who meets the standards of and is enrolled by the federal agency known as the *Joint Board for the Enrollment of Actuaries*.

enrolled dependents Eligible individuals under a member's family coverage who have applied and been accepted for membership in a health insurance plan (i.e., spouse and children of the insured). Under some insurance policies, parents, other family members, and domestic partners may be insured as dependents.

enrolled group Individuals with the same employer or members of an association who are enrolled together in an insurance health plan. Also called *contract group*.

enrolled patient See *enrollee*.

enrollee 1. Person eligible for service as either a subscriber or a dependent of an insurance plan. 2. Individual or employer who becomes a member or subscribes to a health insurance plan or program. Also called *beneficiary, enrolled patient, insured, member, policyholder, policy owner*, or *subscriber*.

enrollee hotlines Toll-free telephone lines, usually staffed by the State or enrollment broker, that beneficiaries may call when they encounter a problem with their managed care organization. The people who staff hotlines are knowledgeable about program policies and may plan an "intake and triage" role or may assist in resolving the problem.

enrollment 1. Total number of members or subscribers in a managed care plan at a given time. 2. Conversion of an eligible group into managed care plan membership. Some group plans have conditions of the minimum size or minimum percentage of a group that must enroll before insurance coverage is available. See also *open enrollment period*. 3. Process by which an individual becomes a subscriber for coverage in a health plan. 4. Process by which a Medicaid-eligible person becomes a member of a managed care plan. Enrollment data refer to the managed care plan's information on Medicaid-eligible individuals who are plan members. The managed care plan gets its enrollment data from the Medicaid program's eligibility system. 5. Information confirming that an individual is enrolled in a health insurance plan.

enrollment area Geographical area in which subscribers must reside to be eligible for enrollment in a managed care plan.

enrollment card 1. Signed document by an employee that indicates his or her desire in becoming a member of a group insurance plan. 2. In contributory insurance plans, enrollment cards authorize an employer to deduct the employee's contributions from his or her wages.

enrollment date Month, day, and year on which a group's or individual's health insurance coverage starts. Also called *coverage effective date*.

enrollment fee Amount the beneficiary must pay every year to get a Medicare-approved drug discount card.

enrollment/Part A During four time periods an individual can enroll in Medicare Part A: initial enrollment period (IEP), general enrollment period (GEP), special enrollment period (SEP), and transfer enrollment period (TEP).

enrollment period 1. Time in which individuals may apply for life insurance or health insurance. 2. Time in which individuals may choose either to re-enroll in an existing managed care plan or change to a competitor's plan. See also *open enrollment period, federal open enrollment*, and *group enrollment period*. 3. Specified time when an individual can sign up for Medicare benefits. The period for general enrollment is January 1 through March 31 of each year for Medicare supplementary insurance. 4. Certain period of time when an individual can join a Medicare health plan if it is open and accepting new Medicare members. If a health plan chooses to be open, it must allow all eligible people with Medicare to join.

enrollment regulations Recruitment rules of an insurance plan for establishing eligibility.

ENT See *otolaryngologist.*

enterprise liability Type of insurance plan wherein the medical liability is shifted from physicians to a health plan (e.g., health maintenance organization [HMO]). Any negligent injury to a patient under the HMO relieves individual providers of all personal liability for the injury. 2. Liability placed on each member of an industry responsible for the manufacture of a harmful or defective product. The distribution of liability is allotted by each manufacturer's share of the market. Also termed *industry-wide liability.*

enterprisewide network Computer network that connects every computer in every location of a business or corporation and runs the company's applications such as an integrated health care delivery system to tie together multiple delivery sites.

entire contract provision Life insurance policy that states that the policy, along with a copy of the application for insurance, represents the whole agreement between the insurance company and the policyholder.

entitlement State of meeting all of the requirements for a specific Medicare benefit; the date of entitlement begins at age 65 for most beneficiaries.

entitlement program Benefit that an individual has a right or a claim to (e.g., veterans' pensions).

entity assets Resources or material goods that the reporting entity has authority to use in its operations (i.e., management has the authority to decide how funds are used, or management is legally obligated to use funds to meet entity obligations).

entity plan Type of buy-sell insurance agreement in which the business entity assumes the obligation of buying a deceased owner's interest in the business.

entrance age Age up to which the insurance company will sell a policy. Entrance ages vary from one company to another, and some policies can be bought at any age.

environmental services Hospital services done for the safety, sanitation, and efficiency of operating a facility (e.g., housekeeping, laundry, maintenance, waste disposal).

EOB See *explanation of benefits (EOB).*

EOC 1. Abbreviation for episode of care. See *episode of care (EOC).* 2. Abbreviation for evidence of coverage. See *evidence of coverage (EOC).* 3. Abbreviation for explanation of coverage. See *explanation of coverage (EOC).*

EOI See *evidence of insurability (EOI).*

EOM Abbreviation for end of month.

EOMB See *Explanation of Medicare Benefits (EOMB).* This acronym also means explanation of Medicaid benefits or explanation of member benefits.

EOY Abbreviation for end of year.

EP HCPCS Level II modifier that may be used with CPT or HCPCS Level II codes indicating a service provided as part of the Medicaid Early and Periodic Screening, Diagnosis, and Treatment (EPSDT) Program.

EPF See *expanded problem focused (EPF).*

EPG See *episodic payment group (EPG).*

episode 1. Incident that is unusual or distinctive from everyday life such as an episode of illness or a trauma. 2. Sixty-day unit of payment for home health (HH) prospective payment system (PPS).

episode of care (EOC) 1. One or more medical services received by the patient during a specified time frame for a specific disease by a facility or provider. 2. Term coined by Lovelace Health Systems in 1993 when it began the Lovelace Episodes of Care Program. It means all services provided to a patient with a specific medical problem within a specified period of time. This system was introduced to improve treatment of complex, high-cost, and chronic diseases to enhance cost-effectiveness and patient satisfaction. Also called an *episode of hospital care.* See also *continuum of care.*

episode of hospital care See *episode of care (EOC).*

episodic acute care center See *emergency center.*

episodic payment group (EPG) Classification system that groups care given to a patient over time based on services, procedures, and diagnoses that are related to an episode of treatment so that a single payment may be made for the entire episode of care. Also known as *episodic treatment group (ETG).*

episodic treatment group (ETG) See *episodic payment group (EPG).*

EPMPY Abbreviation for encounters per member per year.

EPO See *exclusive provider organization (EPO).*

eponym Name of a disease, anatomical structure, operation, or procedure, usually derived from the name of a place or person who discovered or described it first or a patient first diagnosed with the condition or treated by the procedure (see Table E-1).

EPSDT See *Early and Periodic Screening, Diagnosis, and Treatment (EPSDT) Program.*

Table E-1	EPONYMS
Eponym	Comparable Medical Term
Buerger's disease	Thromboangiitis obliterans
Graves' disease	Exophthalmic goiter
Wilkes' syndrome	Myasthenia gravis

EQRO See *External Quality Review Organization (EQRO)*.

equitable assignment Type of written notice or act that does not fully meet the requirements of a legal assignment but is valid and enforced by the courts in the interest of fairness and justice.

equity Interest or value of an individual or business that is in excess of its liabilities.

equity-based insurance Life insurance in which the cash value and benefit level change according to how the investments in the portfolio perform. Equity investments (corporate stock) are those in which investors gain part ownership in a corporation.

equity pension Retirement fund that provides benefits that vary depending on the investments in the portfolio. It is meant to provide retirees with benefits that increase as inflation rises.

equivalency review Process that Centers for Medicare and Medicaid Services (CMS) employs to compare an accreditation organization's standards, processes, and enforcement activities to the comparable CMS requirements, processes, and enforcement activities.

equivalent single payment One payment that stands for several payments because it is equal to the value of the other payments.

equivocal suicide Type of suicide in which there is doubt as to whether it was intentional or not.

ER Abbreviation for emergency room. See *emergency department (ED)*.

ERA See *electronic remittance advice (ERA)*.

ergonomic Science and technology that seeks to fit the anatomical and physical needs of the worker to the workplace.

ERISA See *Employee Retirement Income Security Act (ERISA)*.

ERM See *electronic records management (ERM)*.

ERN See *electronic remittance advice (ERA)*.

error and omissions (E&O) insurance Type of insurance coverage for liability arising from a negligent act or mistake committed by an individual when doing professional work that may harm a client. It is usually purchased by those who are insurance agents and independent contractors who work as medical transcriptionists, medical billers, and medical coders.

error-edit feature Computer software element for insurance claims processing that edits claims for errors.

escheat laws State statutes under which unclaimed interest or financial values including life insurance benefits return (escheat) to the state because no designated beneficiary or heir can be located. Also called *unclaimed property statutes*. See also *unclaimed benefits*.

ESOP See *employee stock ownership plan (ESOP)*. Also see *leveraged employee stock ownership plan (LESOP)*.

escort services See *transportation services*.

ESRD See *end-stage renal disease (ESRD)*.

ESRD eligibility requirements To qualify for Medicare under the renal provision, a person must have end-stage renal disease (ESRD) and either be entitled to a monthly insurance benefit under Title II of the Act (or an annuity under the Railroad Retirement Act), be fully or currently insured under Social Security (railroad work may count), or be the spouse or dependent child of a person who meets at least one of the two last requirements. There is no minimum age for eligibility under the renal disease provision. An Application for Health Insurance Benefits under Medicare for Individuals with Chronic Renal Disease, Form CMS-43 (effective October 1, 1978) must be filed.

ESRD facility See *end-stage renal disease (ESRD) treatment facility*.

ESRD network All Medicare-approved end-stage renal disease (ESRD) facilities in a designated geographic area specified by the Centers for Medicare and Medicaid Services (CMS).

ESRD network organization Administrative governing body of the end-stage renal disease (ESRD) network and liaison to the federal government.

ESRD patient Person with irreversible and permanent kidney failure who requires a regular course of dialysis or kidney transplantation to maintain life.

ESRD services Type of care or service furnished to an end-stage renal disease (ESRD) patient. Such types of care are transplantation; dialysis; outpatient dialysis; staff-assisted dialysis; home dialysis; and self-dialysis and home dialysis training.

essential access community hospital (EACH) Rural hospital that has at least 75 beads and provides backup services to rural primary care hospitals for referred patients. In 1989 Congress created EACHs in only a few states (Public Law 101-239).

essential community providers Providers such as community health centers that have traditionally served low-income populations.

established patient Evaluation and management guidelines in *Current Procedural Terminology (CPT)* code book define an established patient as an individual who has received professional services from the physician or another physician of the same specialty who belongs to the same group practice, within the past 3 years.

estate administrator One who takes possession of the assets of a decedent, pays the expenses of administration and the claims of creditors, and disposes of the balance of an estate in accordance with the statutes governing the distribution of decedents' estates.

estate claim Assertion of a right to assets or money from the estate of a deceased person. Each state has different time limits on filing a claim within a number of months from the date of death or date of publication of death. Also, each state has a different person or place where the claim should be filed such as court of probate, estate executor, or commissioner.

estate executor One who takes possession of the assets of a decedent, pays the expenses of administration and claims of creditors, and disposes of the balance of an estate in accordance with the decedent's will.

estate planning Program or plan to prepare an individual's estate on death. It is done to provide and conserve funds and assets that are to be given to heirs after death of the individual. Estate planning involves accountants, attorneys, trust officers of banks, insurance agents, and an estate administrator to carry out the wishes of the deceased.

estate planning department See *advanced underwriting department.*

estate recovery Under the Medicaid program, recovery of financial assistance from certain deceased Medicaid recipients' estates up to the amount spent by the state for all Medicaid services (e.g., nursing facilities, intermediate care facilities for mentally retarded, home and community-based services, hospitals, prescription drug services). Federal law mandates that each state have an estate recovery program.

estimated length of stay (ELOS) Average number of days of hospitalization required for a specific illness or procedure. These data are based on previous histories of patients who have been hospitalized for the same condition or procedure.

ET HCPCS Level II modifier that may be used with CPT or HCPCS Level II codes indicating an emergency treatment.

ETG See *episodic treatment group (ETG).*

ethical issue Subject or matter that involves the core or basic values of practice.

ethics Standards of conduct generally accepted as a moral guide for behavior by which an insurance billing or coding specialist may determine the appropriateness of his or her conduct in a relationship with patients, the physician, coworkers, the government, and insurance companies.

ethics of care Moral approach based on the action that best supports the relationships of the parties involved.

etiology Cause of a disease; the study of the cause of a disease.

etiquette Customs, rules of conduct, courtesy, and manners of the medical profession.

euthanasia 1. Easy and painless death. 2. Act or method of causing death of an individual who is suffering from an incurable disease or condition (e.g., administering a lethal drug or withholding of treatment).

evaluation Act of careful appraisal or study to determine the significance or worth of the data collected.

evaluation and management (E&M) Name of a section from a book titled *Current Procedural Terminology (CPT)* that is used to obtain codes for billing medical

procedures and services. See *evaluation and management (E/M) section.*

evaluation and management (E/M) codes Five-digit procedural codes that appear in the *Current Procedural Terminology (CPT)* code book published annually and copyrighted by the American Medical Association (AMA). These codes describe the assessment and management of a patient's medical care and are used for encounters by providers for billing services performed in the outpatient and inpatient settings (e.g., consultations, critical care visits, office visit, hospital visits, emergency department care). E/M codes begin with 99201 and end with 99499.

evaluation and management (E/M) section Division of the *Current Procedural Terminology (CPT)* code book that contains information about medical services (e.g., physician's office visits, hospital visits, home visits, consultations).

evaluation and management (E/M) services Nontechnical services provided by a physician in a variety of settings (e.g., physician's office, hospital, patient's home) to evaluate the patient and manage the patient's condition; previously referred to as *office, hospital,* or *home visits.* Such services consist of taking a patient's history, performing a physical examination, and cognitive medical decision-making.

evaluation and management service components Three key components for evaluating and determining the correct level of evaluation and management (E/M) for selection of procedural codes for the purpose of billing. These components consist of history, examination, and medical decision-making.

EVC See *eligibility verification confirmation (EVC).*

evergreen contracts Managed care plan agreements that renew automatically after the first year has been completed.

evidence Signs or indications that something is true or not true (e.g., physicians can use published studies as evidence that a treatment works or does not work).

evidence-based medicine (EBM) Type of practice of medicine in which the doctor finds, assesses, and uses methods of diagnosis and treatment based on the best available evidence, current research, and clinical expertise together with the requirements and desires of the patient.

evidence of coverage (EOC) See *explanation of coverage (EOC).*

evidence of funding Proof that sufficient funds are available for completion of the project. Usually a copy of the face sheet of the grant, contract, or cooperative agreement is sufficient.

evidence of good health See *evidence of insurability (EOI).*

evidence of insurability (EOI) Written statement of an individual's physical condition that would affect eligibility for insurance coverage. This proof is usually necessary for those who do not enroll during an open enrollment period. Also called *evidence of good health*.

Ex See *examination (Ex)*.

ex parte communication 1. Contact by, or on behalf of, one party, without the knowledge of the opposing party. 2. In a workers' compensation case, this means that neither party may have communication with a judge, arbitrator, agreed medical evaluator (AME), or qualified medical evaluator (QME) without knowledge of the other party.

examination (Ex) 1. See *physical examination (PE or PX)*. 2. Audit of an insurer's records, transactions, methods, and assets by a state insurance department or by internal or external auditors or accountants.

exceptions See *exclusion(s)*.

excess amounts Group life or disability insurance that is presented to a specific category of insureds for enrollment that is more than normally allowed. This is based on the total number for the case.

excess benefits Medical insurance coverage that has a high maximum amount of benefits and is usually for supplementing older, low-limit major medical health insurance. It has a high deductible.

excess charge See *balance billing*.

excess insurance 1. Insurance policy or bond that covers the insured against certain hazards. It applies only to loss or damage in excess of a stated amount. 2. Portion of a line that exceeds the insurance company's net line or retention. 3. Insurance policy that pays over the primary amount of coverage.

excess interest Difference between the minimum rate of interest that is guaranteed on dividends left with the company and the interest actually credited.

excess risk Provision in an insurance policy designed to cut off the insurance company's loss at a certain point. It may be an aggregate payable under the policy, maximum payable for any one disability, or the like. See *stop loss*.

excess-surplus lines See *surplus lines*.

exchange program System that lets a proposed insured who is replacing a policy to obtain a new policy with little or no evidence of insurability if this was recently established by the company that issued the original policy.

excluded service Benefit not covered by Medicare such as routine physical examination, eye examination, foot care, eyeglasses, hearing aids, immunizations not related to injury or immediate risk of infection, cosmetic surgery not related to an illness or injury, custodial care, personal comfort items, and procedure not reasonable and necessary for diagnosing and treating an illness or injury.

Excludes 1 Word with number that is one of the conventions used in the diagnostic code book titled *International Classification of Diseases, Tenth Revision, Clinical Modification (ICD-10-CM)*. This indicates that the code excluded should never be used at the same time as the code above the Excludes 1 note. An Excludes 1 is when two conditions cannot occur together (e.g., congenital form versus acquired form of a condition). A note instructs the reader to go to another code for the excluded condition. This convention does not appear in the former ICD-9-CM code books.

Excludes 2 Word with number that is one of the conventions used in the diagnostic code book titled *International Classification of Diseases, Tenth Revision, Clinical Modification (ICD-10-CM)*. This note represents "Not included here" and indicates that the condition excluded is not part of the condition represented by the code, but a patient may have both conditions at the same time. When an Excludes 2 note appears under a code, it is acceptable to use both the code and the excluded code together. This convention does not appear in the former ICD-9-CM code books.

excludes notes Term (excludes) used in the *International Classification of Diseases, Ninth Revision, Clinical Modification (ICD-9-CM)* Tabular List, Volume 1, that refers to terms or conditions that are not included within the diagnostic code. These notes may further direct the coder to the correct diagnostic code assignment.

exclusion(s) 1. Provisions written into the insurance contract denying coverage or limiting the scope of coverage. They may be specific hazards, perils, or conditions. In connection with a preexisting condition, it means that the policy will not pay benefits arising from that condition. 2. Department of Health and Human Services (DHHS) and Office of the Inspector General (OIG) penalty imposed on a provider that prohibits the individual from billing Medicare or other government programs. 3. In the Medicare program, services not covered such as eye examinations, foot care, eyeglasses, hearing aids, cosmetic surgery, custodial care, and personal comfort items. Medical practices are required to make patients aware of their financial responsibility for noncovered services through waiver of liability statements. Also called *exceptions*.

exclusion endorsement See *waiver*.

exclusion list Office of the Inspector General (OIG) record of providers, individuals, and entities that are excluded from Medicare reimbursement. It includes identifying information about the sanctioned party, specialty, notice date, sanction period, and sections of the Social Security Act used in arriving at the determination to impose a sanction. It is titled List of Excluded Individuals/Entities (LEIE) and may be found at http://oig.hhs.gov/fraud/exclusions.asp. Also called *sanctioned provider list*.

exclusion note "Excludes" notation that lists a disease or condition with a diagnostic code that indicates it cannot be used when assigning a code from the *International Classification of Diseases, Ninth Revision,*

Clinical Modification (ICD-9-CM), Tabular List, Volume 1.

exclusion rider See *impairment rider*.

exclusive agent Insurance agent who works for one insurance company and is not permitted to sell products of other companies. He or she may be salaried or work on a commission basis. Also known as *captive agent*.

exclusive provider organization (EPO) Type of managed health care plan that combines features of HMOs and PPOs. It is referred to as *exclusive* because it is offered to large employers who agree not to contract with any other plan. EPOs are regulated under state health insurance laws. Such plans are for large clinics to participate in and combine fee-for-service PPO and HMO benefits.

exclusive territory Under the general agency distribution system, a region in which no person other than the general agent is allowed to sell the insurance company's products.

exclusivity 1. Sole right to render a service or benefit. The provider or group may provide certain services and does not have to share the right with other providers or groups. 2. Clause sometimes found in managed care contracts that prohibits contracting with other plans.

exclusivity clause Section in a contract that forbids physicians from contracting with more than one managed care plan (e.g., health maintenance organization, preferred provider organization).

exculpatory statute State law in community-property states that lets an insurance company pay proceeds of a life insurance policy in accordance with the terms of that policy without fear of double liability.

execution clause Section of an insurance contract that is signed by the insurer indicating that the insurance company has entered into a contract and is bound by its terms.

executor Person named in a will to carry out the provisions and directions of the will after the death of the testator (person who makes a will).

exempt employees Certain class of employees who are not subject to overtime wages and time limits for work under the Federal Labor Standards Act.

exoneration statutes Laws that excuse the insurance company from liability if an individual claims insurance policy proceeds that the insurance company has already paid to a third party and without knowledge of any conflicting claim.

expanded problem focused (EPF) A phrase used to describe a level of history and/or physical examination.

expanded problem focused examination 1995 guidelines Limited examination of the affected body area or organ system and other symptomatic or related organ systems.

expanded problem focused history Phrase used when the physician has documented the patient's chief complaint giving a brief history of the present illness and has completed a problem pertinent system review.

expanded problem focused history 1997 guidelines Documentation must include the chief complaint, a brief history of the presenting illness (HPI), and a problem pertinent review of systems (ROS).

expanded problem focused multisystem examination 1997 guidelines Performance and documentation of at least six elements identified in a table by a bullet (•) in one or more organ system(s) or body areas(s).

expanded problem focused single organ system examination 1997 guidelines Performance and documentation of at least six elements identified in a table by a bullet (•) whether in a shaded or unshaded box.

expansion Growth of a health insurance plan's network either geographically or in the amount of hospital facilities and providers added.

expectation of life See *life expectancy*.

expected incurred claims Total dollar amount of insurance claims within a specific period of time that are predicted to be paid.

expected mortality Deaths that are anticipated to occur to a certain group in a specific time based on the statistical figures in the mortality table. It is usually shown as a ratio of expected death insurance claim payments to premiums.

expedited appeal 1. Medicare+Choice organization's second look at whether it will provide a health service. A beneficiary may receive a fast decision within 72 hours when life, health, or ability to regain function may be jeopardized. 2. Appeal for medical service, thought by the physician, to be urgent.

expedited organization determination Fast decision from the Medicare+Choice organization about whether it will provide health service. A beneficiary may receive a quick determination within 72 hours if life, health, and ability to regain function may be jeopardized.

expenditure 1. Issuance of checks, disbursement of cash, or electronic transfer of funds made to liquidate an expense regardless of the fiscal year the service was provided or the expense was incurred. 2. When used in the discussion of the Medicaid program, expenditures refer to funds spent as reported by the states. Also called *outlay*.

expenditure limit Maximum level of spending for the health sector or certain categories of services. It is usually established by the government through rate setting or premium limits.

expense Funds spent or incurred providing goods, rendering services or carrying out other mission-related activities during a period. Expenses are computed using accrual accounting techniques that recognize costs when incurred and revenues when earned and include the effect of accounts receivables and accounts payable on determining annual income.

expense loading Practice in setting a rate that stands for the amount added to the pure premium required for the expenses of the insurance company such as administrative costs.

expense ratio Percentage that shows the relationship of expenses to earned premiums. This proportion is obtained by using a formula of dividing the premiums into the expenses. It shows the percentage of the premium that is used to pay the overhead costs such as costs of acquiring, writing, commissions, marketing, and servicing by the insurance company.

experience Classified statistical loss record of an insured, class of coverage, or usage of health plan benefits by subscribers or members. It is usually documented as a percentage or ratio (e.g., relationship of premium to claims for benefits).

experience analysis Statistical examination of insurance experience for any part of the group business such as a line or a territory; any group of cases, coverages, or benefits; or any single case, coverage, or benefit. The study may include single or multiple experience periods, past and future trends, and various descriptive statistics.

experience period Time period of usually 12 months in which premium and insurance claim records are gathered for a rate review. Also referred to as a *review period*.

experience-rated premium Insurance premium based on the experience rating. This is periodically adjusted in line with actual insurance claims or utilization experience.

experience rating Classification of rates from a group or subgroup of subscribers, members, or beneficiaries from previous insurance claims history to establish current insurance premium rates. Two types of experience rating are *prospective* and *retrospective*. In prospective rating, the premium includes anticipated costs of medical services, plus a margin for higher-than-expected claims, expenses, and profit. In retrospective rating, the insurer may refund some or all of the difference between claims expenses and paid premiums after the coverage period ends. Also called *community rating*.

experience rating refund See *experience refund* and *dividend*.

experience refund Insurance premium returned by an insurance company to a group policyholder because the financial experience of the group has been more than the premiums collected from that which was anticipated. Also called *dividend, experience rating refund, premium refund*, and *retroactive rate reduction*.

experience-related premium rates Insurance premium rates for group insurance coverage based, wholly or partially, on the past claims of the group.

experimental Any treatment, procedure, equipment, drug, drug usage, device, or supply not generally accepted as standard care in the practice of medicine. This includes services or supplies requiring federal or government approval not granted at the time services were rendered. Also called *investigative*. See *experimental care*.

experimental care 1. Medical care that has not yet been accepted as standard care in the practice of medicine. 2. Any medical care that needs federal or other governmental agency approval that was not given at the time the care was provided. Also called *investigative care*.

experimental medical procedures See *experimental procedures*.

experimental procedures Medical services, supplies, treatments, or drug therapies still in a trial stage, determined by the insurance plan not to be generally accepted as standard care in the practice of medicine, and not effective in treating the illness for which their use is intended. Also called *unproved procedures*.

experimental underwriting Insurance company that accepts certain types of risks considered uninsurable according to the insurer's normal underwriting guidelines.

explanation of benefits (EOB) A document or voucher detailing services billed and describing payment determinations that is sent to the insured and provider. It is known in Medicare, Medicaid, and some other programs as a *remittance advice (RA)*; formerly known as *Explanation of Medicare Benefits (EOMB)*. In the TRICARE program, it is called a *summary payment voucher*. A payment check is usually attached or a part of the EOB. The EOB should include details of the claim(s) submitted, payment(s), deductible status, and each insured's responsibility to the provider. See also *electronic remittance notice (ERN), remittance advice (RA)*, and *Medicare remittance notice (MRN)*.

explanation of coverage (EOC) Insurance booklet or section in the insurance policy that summarizes provisions (benefits and coverages) under an insurance policy. Also called a *benefit booklet, benefit plan summary*, or *summary plan description*.

Explanation of Medicare Benefits (EOMB) See *remittance advice (RA)*.

explanatory notes Additional information about items referenced by footnotes or symbols on an explanation of benefits (EOB) document.

exposure 1. State of being subject to the possibility of loss. 2. Number of insurance contracts subject to the chance of loss over a certain amount of time. This may be measured by participation in a group, ratio of female lives to total lives, ratio of male lives to total lives, or amounts at risk. 3. Condition of being subjected to extremes of weather or radiation, which may have a harmful effect.

express authority Permission and authorization that an individual or an insurance company gives to an insurance agent.

expressed contract Verbal or written agreement.

extend To carry forward the balance of an individual ledger.

extended benefits 1. Insurance coverage of more than basic health plans. 2. Insurance policy provision that extends coverage for a certain time period after termination of benefits. Also called *extended insurance*. 3. Allows medical coverage to continue past termination of employment. See also *Consolidated Omnibus Reconciliation Act of 1985 (COBRA)*.

extended care Long-term inpatient care in a skilled nursing facility (SNF) or convalescent or nursing home, rather than a hospital. Frequently patients who are recovering after hospitalization are sent to SNF. Also known as *convalescent care*.

extended care benefit Insurance policy provision that covers room and board charges in an extended care facility (ECF). It is stated similar to that for hospital room and board.

extended care facility (ECF) This phrase is no longer used. In 1972 when the Social Security statute was amended, a new phrase was introduced, "skilled nursing facility." See *skilled nursing facility (SNF)*.

extended care services Alternate name for *skilled nursing facility services*.

extended death benefit Insurance policy provision in a group life contract stating that if the insured is totally and continuously disabled, then from the date the insured ceases paying premiums until the date of his or her death, the insurance company will pay the amount of insurance at the date of stoppage of premium payments provided that death occurs within 1 year of the date of cessation of premium payments and before the insured's sixty-fifth birthday.

extended history of present illness (HPI) 1997 guidelines Medical record documentation that describes at least four elements of the present illness or describes the status of at least three chronic and/or inactive conditions.

extended insurance See *extended benefits*.

extended payment agreement Contract in which buyer and seller agree as to terms of payment of a debt.

extended review of systems (ROS) 1997 guidelines Documented report of an inquiry about the body system(s) directly related to the problems identified in the history of present illness (HPI) and a limited number (two to nine) of additional body systems.

extended term insurance Type of insurance available as a nonforfeiture option. It provides the original amount of insurance for a limited period of time. Also called *extended term insurance option*.

extended term insurance option See *extended term insurance*.

extension of benefits See *extended benefits*.

external audit Review done after claims of medical and financial records have been submitted by an insurance company or Medicare representative to investigate suspected fraudulent and abusive billing practices (retrospective review).

external disclosure Release, transfer, or divulging of confidential information beyond the boundaries of the provider health care organization or other entity that collected the data.

external fixation Method of using metal pins and an attaching mechanism to hold together the fragments of a fractured bone or for temporary treatment of acute or chronic bone deformity.

External Quality Review Organization (EQRO) 1. Federal regulations require states to use an EQRO to review the care provided by capitated managed care entities. EQROs may be a quality improvement organization (QIO) program, another entity that meets peer review organization requirements, or a private accreditation body. 2. Organization with which a state contracts to evaluate the care provided to Medicaid-managed eligibles. Typically, the EQRO is a peer review organization. It may conduct focused medical record reviews targeted at a specific clinical condition or broader analyses on quality. Although most EQRO contractors rely on medical records as the primary source of information, they may also use eligibility data and claims/encounter data to conduct specific analyses.

extirpate To surgically remove foreign body, organ, or unwanted tissue from the body.

extra medical provider Provider who participates in TRICARE Extra's preferred provider network.

extra-percentage tables method System or plan for rating substandard insurance risks in which each substandard class is charged a premium rate that is a certain percentage above the standard premium rate.

extraterritorial A review done after claims of medical and financial records have been submitted by an insurance company or Medicare representative to investigate suspected fraudulent and abusive billing practices (retrospective review).

EY HCPCS Level II modifier that may be used with CPT or HCPCS Level II codes indicating there was no physician's order for the item or service.

F

F & A See *findings and award (F & A)*.

F & O See *findings and order (F & O)*.

F1 HCPCS Level II modifier that may be used with CPT or HCPCS Level II codes and that identifies a service or procedure to the second digit of the left hand.

F2 HCPCS Level II modifier that may be used with CPT or HCPCS Level II codes and that identifies a service or procedure to the third digit of the left hand.

F3 HCPCS Level II modifier that may be used with CPT or HCPCS Level II codes and that identifies a service or procedure to the fourth digit of the left hand.

F4 HCPCS Level II modifier that may be used with CPT or HCPCS Level II codes and that identifies a service or procedure to the fifth digit of the left hand.

F5 HCPCS Level II modifier that may be used with CPT or HCPCS Level II codes and that identifies a service or procedure to the thumb of the right hand.

F6 HCPCS Level II modifier that may be used with CPT or HCPCS Level II codes and that identifies a service or procedure to the second digit of the right hand.

F7 HCPCS Level II modifier that may be used with CPT or HCPCS Level II codes and that identifies a service or procedure to the third digit of the right hand.

F8 HCPCS Level II modifier that may be used with CPT or HCPCS Level II codes and that identifies a service or procedure to the fourth digit of the right hand.

F9 HCPCS Level II modifier that may be used with CPT or HCPCS Level II codes and that identifies a service or procedure to the fifth digit of the right hand.

FA 1. HCPCS Level II modifier that may be used with CPT or HCPCS Level II codes and that identifies a service or procedure to the thumb of the left hand. 2. See *fiscal agent (FA)*.

face amount Dollar amount in a life insurance policy that is payable at the time of death of the insured or in an annuity when the contract reaches maturity. It does not include additional dollar amounts payable under other special provisions, accidental death, or policy dividends. Also called *face value*. See also *basic death benefit* and *death benefit*.

face page Generally the first page of an insurance policy that includes the name and age of the insured, name of the policy owner (if different from the insured), amount of premium, policy number, date of issuance of policy, and signatures of the insurance company officials.

face sheet First part of a patient's hospital health record that contains the patient's identification, demographics, date of admission, insurance coverage or payment source, referral data, hospital stay dates, attending physician information, discharge information, name of responsible party, emergency contact, and patient's diagnoses.

face-to-face time Documented minutes and hours spent face to face with a patient or a patient's family in an office or outpatient place of service. It is a component of evaluation and management codes.

face value See *face amount*.

FACF See *frequency-adjusted conversion factor (FACF)*.

facility Building location, equipment, and supplies for delivery of patient medical care (e.g., inpatient and outpatient hospital, acute or long-term care, intermediate or skilled nursing facilities).

facility charge Some managed care plans may vary cost shares for services based on place of treatment—in effect, charging a cost for the facility in which the service is received.

Facility Coding Specialist (FCS) One type of certification earned by meeting the requirements of the American College of Medical Coding Specialists (ACMCS).

facility-of-payment clause Insurance contract rule or section of a life insurance policy that allows the managed care payer or insurance company to reimburse someone other than the member or provider (e.g., designated beneficiary or estate of the insured). This clause allows the insurance company to pay benefits to the beneficiary in a timely manner.

facility practice expense One of three components in the formula used to find out the relative value of physician services paid under the resource-based relative value scale (RBRVS). Facility practice expense corresponds to the physician's direct and indirect costs associated with each service provided in a hospital, ambulatory surgery center (ASC), or skilled nursing facility (SNF).

facility provider number Number assigned to a facility (e.g., hospital, laboratory, radiology office, nursing facility) to be used by the facility to bill for services, or by the performing physician to report services done at that location.

facility specific Method of establishing insurance rates based on facility expenditures on items specific to patient care. It pays different rates to providers that deliver the same type of service.

facing triangles (▶◀) Symbol used in the procedure code book titled *Current Procedural Terminology (CPT)* to indicate new or revised text, other than the procedure descriptors, that is new to or revised for that specific annual edition.

facsimile Electronic process for transmitting written and graphic matter over telephone lines.

fact-oriented V codes Diagnostic codes that do not describe a problem or a service but state a fact. Generally these codes do not represent an outpatient primary or inpatient principal diagnosis.

factor table Statistical record used by insurance underwriters to establish the net worth of an insurance applicant. It shows the dollar amount to multiply with the applicant's annual income to obtain the maximum allowable amount of insurance.

factored rating See *adjusted community rating (ACR)*.

facultative reinsurance Type of reinsurance of an individual risk at the option (the "faculty" either to accept or reject) of the insurance company requiring reinsurance.

faculty practice plan (FPP) Policies and procedures in a document that state the manner in which patient services are delivered by a teaching program or medical school faculty physicians, the method of obtaining payment, and the disposition of the funds obtained for the services. Also known as *clinical practice plan* and *medical practice plan*.

Fair and Accurate Credit Transactions (FACT) Act Federal legislation (Public Law 108-159) enacted on December 4, 2003, that established medical privacy provisions as part of consumer credit law. This bill amended the Fair Credit Reporting Act (FCRA) to include improved medical privacy protections and protections against identity theft.

Fair Credit Billing Act (FCBA) Federal regulations that apply to open-end credit accounts such as credit cards and revolving charge accounts for department store accounts. It gives consumers the right to dispute charges on their credit card accounts and either withhold payment or ask for a refund because of a billing error. It also allows consumers to dispute charges if they are dissatisfied with the quality of the merchandise received. The federal law limits the consumer's responsibility for unauthorized charges to $50.

Fair Credit Reporting Act (FCRA) United States federal or state law that regulates the keeping and protecting of consumer credit reports by credit reporting agencies (e.g., acting fairly, impartially, and confidentially). It allows the consumer to see and correct his or her credit report. The federal FCRA was enacted in 1970.

fair hearing In the Medicare program, this stage of appeal of a claim has been renamed and is now called *reconsideration*. See *reconsideration*.

fair plans Insurance pools that sell property insurance to individuals who cannot purchase it in the volunteer marketplace because of their high exposure to risks that they may have no control over.

False Claims Act (FCA) Federal legislation that regulates civil action for filing of a false or inaccurate claim for payment, knowingly using a false record or statement to obtain payment on a false or fraudulent claim paid by the government, and conspiring to defraud the government by getting a false or fraudulent claim allowed or paid. Under this act, any person who knowingly presents or causes to be presented a false or fraudulent claim to the government for payment or approval is liable. This law covers all types of government payments, not just medical insurance claims.

false negatives Occur when the patient's medical record contains evidence of a service that does not exist in the encounter data. This is the most common problem in partially or fully managed care capitated plans because the provider does not need to submit an encounter in order to receive payment for the service and therefore may have a weaker incentive to conform to data collection standards.

false positives Occur when the encounter data contain evidence of a medical service that is not documented in the patient's medical record. If we assume that the medical record contains complete information on the patient's medical history, a false positive may be considered a fraudulent service. In a fully managed care capitated environment, however, the provider would receive no additional reimbursement for the submission of a false-positive encounter.

Family and Medical Leave Act of 1993 (FMLA) Federal law requires that covered employers must grant an eligible employee up to a total of 12 workweeks of unpaid leave during any 12-month period for one or more of the following reasons:
- For the birth and care of the newborn child of the employee
- For placement with the employee of a son or daughter for adoption or foster care
- To care for an immediate family member (spouse, child, or parent) with a serious health condition
- To take medical leave when the employee is unable to work because of a serious health condition

family benefit Rider or provision in a life insurance policy that provides term insurance coverage on the insured's dependents (e.g., spouse, children).

family deductible 1. Specific dollar amount that must be paid either monthly, quarterly, or annually by an individual, covered family member or a specified amount of time that must elapse before a medical insurance plan or government program begins covering health care costs. For the majority of plans, this amount must be incurred each calendar or fiscal year before insurance benefits will be reimbursed. 2. One deductible that when fulfilled relieves a family of satisfying a deductible for each individual family member.

F

family history (FH) Review of medical events in the patient's family including diseases that may be hereditary or contagious and conditions that place the patient at risk. Documented review of two or all three past, family, and/or social history (PFSH) areas, depending on the category of evaluation and management (E/M) service that may be performed. All three areas are required for comprehensive assessments.

family income insurance Special individual insurance policy that combines whole life insurance with decreasing term insurance. The whole life insurance part of the agreement is paid as a lump sum on the death of the insured. The decreasing term part of the policy gives an income for a predetermined period to assist in supporting the insured's family.

family income policy Life insurance policy that combines whole life and decreasing term insurance. In this type of agreement, the beneficiary is paid during a specific period of time if the insured dies before the end of the period specified and in addition receives the face amount of the policy either at the end of the specified period or after death of the insured.

family insurance policy One life insurance contract that gives coverage to all members of a family. Generally this is whole life insurance on the wage earner, whole life or term insurance on the spouse, and smaller amounts of term insurance on the children including automatic insurance with no premium increase for children born after the policy is issued.

family member Under Medicare Secondary Payer guidelines, a person enrolled in a group health plan based on another person's enrollment (e.g., spouse, adopted child, stepchild, parent, sibling).

family membership Health insurance plan that covers a subscriber or member and one or more dependents.

family policy Life insurance contract that insures all or several family members. Usually the husband is under a whole life arrangement and the rest of the family is under term insurance, as well as those born after issuance of the policy.

family practice physician See *family practitioner (FP)*.

family practitioner (FP) Medical doctor (MD) of the specialty of family medicine. He or she has usually completed a residency program in the specialty of family practice. Services may include internal medicine, pediatrics, and some surgical procedures. See *general practitioner*. Also called *family practice physician*.

FAR See *Federal Acquisition Regulation (FAR)*.

FASB See *Financial Accounting Standards Board (FASB)*.

favorable selection System in a managed care plan of choosing insurance subscribers or covered lives based on statistical data that show use of medical services in a particular population group to be lower than estimated or anticipated. See also *cherry picking*.

FBI See *Federal Bureau of Investigation (FBI)*.

FCA See *False Claims Act (FCA)*.

FCE See *functional capacity evaluation (FCE)*.

FCRA See *Fair Credit Reporting Act (FCRA)*.

FCS See *Facility Coding Specialist (FCS)*.

FDA See *Food and Drug Administration (FDA)*.

FECA See *Federal Employees' Compensation Act (FECA)*.

fecal occult blood test (FOBT) Guaiac-based test for peroxidase activity that the patient completes by taking samples from two different sites of three consecutive stools. CPT codes 82270 through 82274 and HCPCS codes G0107 and G0328 apply to this test.

Federal Acquisition Regulation (FAR) System established for the codification and publication of uniform policies and procedures for acquisition by all executive government agencies.

Federal Bureau of Investigation (FBI) Government agency that investigates and prosecutes federal offenses and criminal activities. It plays an active role in investigating health insurance fraud and abuse related to federal or private health insurance programs. It has direct access to Medicare administrative contractor data and other records.

Federal Coal Mine Health and Safety Act of 1969 Federal workers' compensation plan administered by the U.S. Department of Labor (DOL). This act, also referred to as the *Black Lung Benefits Act*, became effective on May 7, 1941. Services for Medicare patients with diagnoses related to black lung are billed to the DOL for reimbursement. Also known as the *Black Lung Program*.

Federal Drug Abuse Prevention, Treatment, and Rehabilitation Act Federal legislation that protects the confidentiality of the identity, diagnosis, prognosis, and treatment of any patient for drug abuse.

Federal Emergency Management Agency (FEMA) Agency headquartered in Washington, DC, that became part of the U.S. Department of Homeland Security (DHS) on March 1, 2003. FEMA's continuing mission within the new department is to lead the effort to prepare the nation for all hazards and effectively manage federal response and recovery efforts following any national incident. FEMA also initiates proactive mitigation activities, trains first responders, and manages the National Flood Insurance Program.

Federal Employee Health Benefits Acquisition Regulations (FEHBAR) Government legislation for acquiring health services by federal agencies and subcontractors.

Federal Employee Health Benefits Program (FEHBP) Group health insurance program for government employees that provides medical services and hospital benefits. It is the largest employer-sponsored contributory health insurance program in the world. In some states, referred to as *Federal Employee Program (FEP)*.

Federal Employee Health Benefits Acquisition Regulations (FEHBARS) Federal regulations for obtaining health services used by government agencies and subcontractors.

Federal Employee Program (FEP) See *Federal Employee Health Benefits Program (FEHBP)*.

Federal Employees' Compensation Act (FECA) Act instituted in 1908 providing benefits for on-the-job injuries or occupational illness to all federal civilian workers.

Federal Employees Retirement System (FERS) Program for federal employees hired after 1984 or those hired before 1984 who switched from CSRS to FERS.

Federal False Claims Act (FCA) See *False Claims Act (FCA)*.

federal flood insurance See *catastrophe insurance policy*.

federal general revenues Government tax from individual and business income taxes that are not reserved for any particular use.

federal identification number See *employer identification number (EIN)*.

Federal Insurance Administration (FIA) Administers the National Flood Insurance Program that provides insurance coverage for events that are not covered by traditional homeowners' policies. By partnering with private insurance companies, FIA makes insurance available to many people who would otherwise be unprotected.

Federal Insurance Contributions Act (FICA) Government law that imposes Social Security taxes on employers and employees under the Internal Revenue Code (IRC). These taxes provide for the Old Age, Survivors, Health and Disability Insurance (OASHDI) and health insurance programs. Covered workers and their employers pay the tax in equal amounts. Frequently referred to as *Social Security*.

Federal Insurance Contributions Act (FICA) payroll tax Medicare's share of FICA is used to fund the Health Insurance Trust Fund. In fiscal year 1995, employers and employees each contributed 1:45% of taxable wages, with no limitations, to the Health Insurance Trust Fund.

Federal Labor Standards Act (FLSA) Establishes minimum wage, overtime pay, recordkeeping, and child labor standards affecting full-time and part-time workers in the private sector and in federal, state, and local governments.

Federal Managers' Financial Integrity Act Program that identifies management inefficiencies and areas vulnerable to fraud and abuse and to correct such weaknesses with improved internal controls.

Federal Medicaid Managed Care Waiver Program Plan that may be used by states to obtain permission to institute managed care programs for their Medicaid or other categorically eligible beneficiaries.

Federal Medical Assistance Percentage (FMAP) Percentage of federal funds that are available to a state to give Medicaid services. FMAP is annually calculated using a formula that provides a higher federal matching rate to states with lower per capita income.

The federal share of Medicaid administrative costs is a flat 50% and is not based on a per capita income formula.

federal open enrollment Federal regulations mandate that managed care plans that service federal employees must have an annual open enrollment period of at least 30 days. This allows subscribers either to enroll in, re-enroll, or transfer between health insurance plans. See also *open enrollment period, open enrollment*, and *group enrollment period*.

federal qualification Status (federal classification) defined by the Tax Equity and Fiscal Responsibility Act (TEFRA) that lets a federally qualified health maintenance organization (HMO) or a competitive medical plan (CMP) participate in specific Medicare cost and risk contracts and also receive federal grants and loans. A managed care organization must be a federally qualified or state plan defined to participate in the Medicaid managed care program.

Federal Register Official daily publication of the federal government that is available online via the Internet. An important function of the *Federal Register* is its inclusion of proposed changes (e.g., final rules, legal notices and regulations, mandated standards, documents that have general applicability and legal effect) from all federal agencies, as well as executive orders and other presidential documents. HCPCS Level II and ICD-9-CM code standards appear online updated annually for the Medicare program.

federally qualified health center (FQHC) 1. Facility located in a medically underserved area that provides Medicare beneficiaries preventive primary medical care under the general supervision of a physician. 2. Health center that has been approved by the government for a program to give low-cost health care. Medicare pays for some health services in FQHCs that are not usually covered such as preventive care. FQHCs include community health centers, tribal health clinics, migrant health services, and health centers for the homeless. Also called *federally qualified health clinic (FQHC)*.

federally qualified health clinic (FQHC) See *federally qualified health center (FQHC)*.

federally qualified health maintenance organization (FQHMO) Health maintenance organization that applies and meets the requirements of the Centers for Medicare and Medicaid Services (CMS) guidelines for Medicare reimbursement as set forth in the Health Maintenance Organization Act of 1973. Staff, group, and independent practice association (IPA) model HMOs are eligible for federal qualification under the federal HMO law. Network model HMOs are usually not eligible for qualification. FQHMOs are eligible for selection by a company of more than 25 employees and the company must offer two types (i.e., one IPA and one group or staff model HMO). This is known as the "dual choice mandate" of the HMO law. FQHMOs are eligible to contract with Medicare to be reimbursed on a per capita basis for an amount equal to 95% of its estimated cost for total health care services to that person during the year.

fee Dollar amount for professional services rendered to a patient by a provider.

fee allowance See *fee schedule.*

fee disclosure Communication of medical charges with a patient by a provider or office manager before medical services and treatment are rendered.

fee-for-service equivalency Quantitative measure of the difference between the amount a physician receives from a managed care capitation system compared with fee-for-service payment.

fee-for-service (FFS) reimbursement 1. Method of payment in which the patient pays the physician for each professional service or procedure performed from an established schedule of fees. 2. Condition when the third-party payer pays the full fee for medical services. 3. In managed care plans, reimbursement for professional services on a service-by-service basis rather than by the capitation method. FFS reimbursement may involve either discounted or undiscounted rates. 4. Plan or primary care case management (PCCM) is paid for providing services to enrollees solely through fee-for-service payments plus a case management fee.

fee freeze To fix prices at a given level or place for a specific period of time.

fee maximum See *fee schedule.*

fee schedule 1. Listing in an insurance policy of procedure code numbers with charges or pre-established allowances for specific medical services and procedures. Also called *table of allowances, fee allowance, fee maximum, benefit payment schedule, benefit schedule, schedule of allowances, schedule of benefits,* or *capped fee.* 2. Record of procedure code numbers and services with dollar amounts, or payment amounts by a payer that could be percentages of billed charges, flat rates, or maximum allowable amounts set down by the managed care plan. 3. Annually published Medicare fee schedule (MFS) with procedure codes in the *Federal Register;* applies to surgeries, clinical laboratory tests, radiological procedures, and durable medical equipment. The fees shown are the maximum dollar amounts Medicare will allow for each service rendered for a beneficiary. MFS is based on the calculation of several components including relative value unit (RVU), which is based on three factors: the physician's work, overhead expenses, and malpractice insurance. Also called *schedule.* See also *relative value studies (RVS).*

fee schedule basis See *capitation basis.*

fee-screen year Specified period of time, usually 12 months, in which supplementary medical insurance–recognized fees pertain. The fee-screen year period has changed over the history of the Medicare program.

fee simple Highest and best estate, by which an owner is entitled to the entire property without limitations or conditions, as are his or her heirs.

fee ticket See *multipurpose billing form.*

FEHBAR See *Federal Employee Health Benefits Acquisition Regulations (FEHBAR).*

FEHBP See *Federal Employee Health Benefits Program (FEHBP).*

FEHBP members Federal workers who are members of the Federal Employee Health Benefits Program.

FEIN See *employer identification number (EIN).*

FEMA See *Federal Emergency Management Agency (FEMA).*

FEP See *Federal Employee Program (FEP).*

FERS See *Federal Employees Retirement System (FERS).*

FFS See *fee-for-service (FFS) reimbursement.*

FH See *family history (FH).*

FI See *fiscal intermediary (FI).*

FIA See *Federal Insurance Administration (FIA).*

FICA See *Federal Insurance Contributions Act (FICA).*

fiduciary Individual in a position of trust with regard to the affairs of another, who has a duty to act primarily for the benefit of the other, with respect to a particular undertaking. For example, when an insurance company manages pension funds, the insurance company is acting as a fiduciary.

field force Insurance agents who work out of an insurance company's local or regional field offices and not at the home office.

field offices Insurance company's local or regional sales offices.

field underwriter See *agent.*

field underwriting First step in the risk selection process in which an insurance agent puts together information about the proposed insured and puts this information on an application form so that the home office underwriter can make an underwriting evaluation and decision.

FIFO Acronym that means first in, first out. It is a queuing system in which the next item to be acquired is the oldest item (or first item) in the queue.

fifth digit ✓5ᵗʰ Symbol used in the diagnostic code book titled *International Classification of Diseases, Ninth Revision, Clinical Modification (ICD-9-CM)* . It is used to indicate that a fifth digit is required for coding to indicate the highest level of specificity. Also see *fourth and fifth digits.*

fifth dividend option Also called *additional insurance option.* See *additional term insurance option.*

file A collection of related data stored under a single title.

file number See *group number.*

file protection Process in a computer system that is designed to safeguard against unauthorized access of an electronic file.

filing In insurance, to submit a proposed policy form to get it approved by the insurance department of the jurisdiction where it will be issued.

filing claims See *claim.*

FIM See *functional independence measure (FIM).*

final average benefit formula Formula in a defined benefit retirement plan in which the retirement benefit amount is obtained based on the participant's average wages during a specific period (usually 3 to 5 years before retirement). Also known as *final earnings benefit formula.*

final earnings benefit formula See *final average benefit formula.*

Final Report In temporary disability workers' compensation cases, the last report submitted by a physician to the insurance company stating the patient is able to return to work. In permanent disability workers' compensation cases, the last report indicating permanent disability of the patient. Also called *Doctor's Final (or Monthly) Report and Bill.*

final rule Official release of a requirement or guideline created by the Secretary of Health and Human Services (HHS) to meet a specific law. When a final rule is officially released, entities may begin to use the rule. After a period of implementation, then a compliance deadline is mandated.

financial accounting record Individual financial account that has service fees, payments, adjustments, and balances posted. Also called *account, financial record, ledger, ledger card,* or *patient account ledger.*

Financial Accounting Standards Board (FASB) Designated organization in the private sector for establishing standards of financial accounting and reporting that govern the preparation of financial reports. Founded in 1973, FASB is part of a structure that is independent of all other business and professional organizations. Before the present structure was created, financial accounting and reporting standards were established first by the Committee on Accounting Procedure of the American Institute of Certified Public Accountants (1936-1959) and then by the Accounting Principles Board, also a part of the AICPA (1959-1973). Pronouncements of those predecessor bodies remain in force unless amended or superseded by the FASB. The Board is officially recognized as authoritative by the Securities and Exchange Commission (Financial Reporting Release No. 1, Section 101 and reaffirmed in its April 2003 Policy Statement) and the American Institute of Certified Public Accountants (Rule 203, Rules of Professional Conduct, as amended May 1973 and May 1979). Such standards are essential to the efficient functioning of the economy because investors, creditors, auditors, and others rely on credible, transparent, and comparable financial information.

financial class Individual's income or ability to pay a debt.

financial data Information about the financial status of managed care entities (e.g., medical loss ratio).

financial hardship discount Reduction of the balance due on a patient's financial account because of his or her financial status. A hardship waiver can vary from 25% to 100% of the bill and must be documented before a decision is made in these cases. Current guidelines on poverty income are used to determine eligibility for uncompensated services under the Hill-Burton program, the Community Services Block Grant program, and the Head Start program. Physicians may choose to follow these guidelines to direct patients to government-sponsored programs, obtain public assistance, and determine who is eligible for a hardship waiver. The physician may elect to collect the third-party payer's portion of the bill and adjust off the patient portion of the charge. A written policy about what qualifies a patient for a financial hardship discount must be created because it may be construed as discriminatory if not given to other patients consistently.

financial institution Government agency or privately owned entity that collects funds from the public to put in stocks, bonds, money market accounts, bank deposits, or loans. There are depository institutions (banks, savings and loan associations, savings banks, and credit unions) and nondepository institutions (insurance companies and pension plans).

financial interchange Provisions of the Railroad Retirement Act for transfers between the trust funds and the Social Security Equivalent Benefit Account of the Railroad Retirement program. It places each trust fund in the same position as if railroad employment had always been covered under Social Security.

financial intermediary Financial institution such as a bank, savings and loan association, or credit union that takes in deposits from the public and makes loans to individuals who need credit.

financial limitation Under the Medicare program, economic restrictions for outpatient rehabilitation services became effective after July 1, 2003. These affect physical therapy, occupational therapy, and speech-language pathology insurance claims submitted by physicians, nurse practitioners, clinical nurse specialists, physician's assistants, physical therapists, occupational therapists, and speech-language pathologists.

financial planning Investment service that reviews an individual's or family's economic picture and then determines a course of action to obtain financial goals within a certain period of time. This can include budgeting, planned accumulation of income through various investments, risk analysis, minimizing taxes, and estate planning. Also called *total-needs programming.*

financial policy statement Document signed by patients stating liability in paying for medical services received. This protects the physician's right to collect payment for professional services provided to patients.

financial record See *account, financial accounting record, ledger card,* and *ledger.*

financial responsibility Liability for payment of a patient's medical bill to the provider of service.

financial responsibility clause In automobile insurance, a provision in the policy stating that the insured has the minimum amount of liability insurance coverage required by the state's financial responsibility law. Each state has some form of financial responsibility law.

financial responsible party Individual who accepts liability for payment of the patient's bill to the provider of service.

financial settlement 1. Lump sum dollar amount paid by an insurance company to a disabled insured who has disability insurance to pay off an obligation. 2. Payment of a lump-sum benefit to an insurance plan participant. Also known as *buy-out settlement, commutation,* or *settlement.*

findings and award (F & A) In workers' compensation when settling a temporary or permanent disability case, this is the final determination and monetary settlement of the referee or appeals board.

findings and order (F & O) In workers' compensation, this is usually a phrase used in connection with a "take nothing" decision against the applicant (injured worker).

fine Punishment established by law to pay a sum of money that is imposed on an individual who has committed an act of wrongdoing.

fire insurance Insurance coverage that protects property against loss caused by fire and lightning.

first aid Immediate initial care of an illness or minor injury (scratches, cuts, burns, splinters) before treatment by medically trained personnel.

first-dollar coverage Type of insurance (hospital or surgical) policy that pays for the full value of each service up to the insured amount. The insured does not pay a deductible, but there may be copayments.

first pass Insurance claim that is being processed to be paid, rejected, or denied without being suspended for any reason. Also called *pass through.*

First Report of Injury In workers' compensation cases, a written statement of the initial contact of the physician with the injured worker. Each state has a different time frame when this report should be submitted to the workers' compensation insurance carrier. Also called *First Treatment Medical Report* and *Doctor's First Report of Occupational Injury or Illness (form)* or *preliminary report.*

first responder Individual who uses a limited amount of equipment to perform initial assessment and intervention and is trained to assist other emergency

medical services (EMS) providers. For example, at the scene of a cardiac arrest, the first responder would be expected to notify EMS (if not already notified) and initiate cardiopulmonary resuscitation (CPR) with an oral airway and a barrier device. Many firefighters, police officers, and other emergency workers have this level of training.

First Treatment Medical Report See *First Report of Injury.*

first-year commission Amount of money paid to an insurance agent that is based on an insurance policy's first annual premium.

fiscal agent (FA) See *Medicare administrative contractor (MAC).*

fiscal carrier See *fiscal intermediary (FI).*

fiscal intermediary (FI) 1. For Medicare, see *Medicare administrative contractor (MAC).* 2. For TRICARE and CHAMPVA, the insurance company that handles the claims for care received within a region of the United States and services specific states. Also see *TRICARE regions.*

fiscal soundness State in a managed care organization that has enough operating funds on hand, or in reserve, to cover all expenses associated with services for which it has taken on a financial risk.

fiscal year (FY) 1. Any continuous 12-month period used by insurance companies and the government as an accounting period. 2. In the Medicare and TRICARE programs, the federal government's fiscal year is from October 1 to September 30.

501(c)(9) trust Type of trust that a self-insured group can establish to fund its group insurance plan. Contributions to a 501(c)(9) trust and investment gains are deductible when computing federal income tax reports. Also called a *voluntary employees' beneficiary association (VEBA).*

five- and six-character subclassification In the *International Classification of Diseases, Tenth Revision, Clinical Modification (ICD-10-CM),* a letter and two digits followed by a period or decimal point and up to three numbers that give more information on the description of a condition.

fixation Use of internal and/or external hardware (e.g., pins, rods, plates, wires) to keep a bone in place; also referred to as *instrumentation.*

fixed amount option Settlement option in a life insurance policy wherein the insurance company uses policy proceeds plus interest to pay the beneficiary either annually or semiannually until the proceeds plus interest are all gone. Also called *fixed payment option.*

fixed capital assets Net worth of hospital or other health facilities and other resources.

fixed costs Expenses that do not change with fluctuations in number of members or use of medical services in a managed care plan.

fixed payment option See *fixed amount option.*

fixed period option Settlement option in a life insurance policy wherein the insurance company uses policy proceeds plus interest to pay the beneficiary either annually or semiannually for a specific period of time.

FL See *form locator (FL)*.

flame E-mail message that is interpreted as being hostile.

flare-up In workers' compensation cases, this phrase is sometimes used to refer to a recurrence of an industrial injury or illness and refers specifically to the symptoms that are considered to be related to the natural course of the previous injury or illness and not to a new injury from current employment.

flat amount formula Mathematical method used to determine the retirement benefit for participants in a defined benefit pension plan (DBPP). This type of formula gives the same monthly or annual benefit amount to each retiree (e.g., $700 per month).

flat extra premium method System for rating substandard insurance risks that is used when the extra risk is constant. Usually it is a specific extra premium for each $1,000 of insurance coverage.

flat fee-per-case Payment of one fee to a provider to cover all services related to a patient's treatment based on diagnosis (episode of care) or presenting problems. Also called *bundled rate* or *case rate*.

flat file Computer phrase that refers to a stand-alone data file that does not have any predefined linkages to locations of data in other files; a type of file in a relational database. However, the term is sometimes used to refer to a type of file that has no relational capability, which is exactly the opposite.

flat percentage of earnings formula Mathematical method used to determine the retirement benefit for participants in a defined benefit pension plan (DBPP). This type of formula gives each participant a specific percentage of preretirement compensation (e.g., 65%). The amount that is paid using this formula is dependent on how compensation is defined.

flat rate Method of payment in which all providers that render the same medical service are paid at the same rate. Also called *uniform rate*.

flex plan See *cafeteria plan* and *flexible benefit plan*.

flexible benefit option See *flexible benefit plan*.

flexible benefit plan Managed care plan offered by an employer to his or her employees that allows them to select the type and amount of benefits from among options the employer offers. It also allows employees to make contributions required for their choice of benefits with before-tax dollars. Also called *cafeteria plan, flexible benefit option, flex plan,* or *flexible compensation*.

flexible compensation See *flexible benefit plan* and *cafeteria plan*.

flexible premium annuity Type of deferred annuity investment contract that gives the buyer the ability to vary the amount of each premium payment to the insurance company during the accumulation period.

flexible premium life insurance See *indeterminate premium life insurance*.

flexible spending account (FSA) See *dependent-care spending account*.

floater policy Insurance policy for movable property that covers it wherever loss may occur (e.g., tourist's baggage).

flood insurance See *catastrophe insurance policy*.

floor time Documented minutes and hours spent working on behalf of an inpatient while the provider is physically present on the patient's floor or unit. It includes face-to-face time but is not limited to face-to-face time (e.g., at the bedside). It is a component of evaluation and management CPT codes. Also called *unit time*. Unit/floor time applies to hospital observation services, inpatient hospital care, initial and follow-up hospital consultations, and nursing facility visits.

FMAP See *Federal Medical Assistance Percentage (FMAP)*.

FMC See *foundation for medical care (FMC)*.

FMG See *foreign medical graduate (FMG)*.

FMLA See *Family and Medical Leave Act of 1993 (FMLA)*.

FMR See *focused medical review (FMR)*.

FOBT See *fecal occult blood test (FOBT)*.

focused medical review (FMR) Analysis of national data by Centers for Medicare and Medicaid Services (CMS) of Medicare insurance claims to locate the greatest risk of inappropriate program payment. This gathering of data is done to reduce the number of non-covered claims or unnecessary services. CMS provides its findings to the fiscal intermediaries who develop their review policies to identify abuse and overutilization of services.

focused studies State-required studies that examine a specific aspect of health care (such as prenatal care) for a defined point in time. These projects are usually based on information extracted from medical records or managed care organizations' data (enrollment files, encounter or claims data). State staff, External Quality Review Organization (EQRO) staff, managed care organization (MCO) staff, or more than one of these entities may perform such studies at the discretion of the state.

FOIA See *Freedom of Information Act (FOIA)*.

follow-up file Reminder method used to track pending or resubmitted insurance claims and to telephone or send inquiries about nonpayment. Also called a *suspense, tickler file,* or *tracing file*. Also see *tracing file* or *tickler file*.

follow-up medical-legal evaluation In a workers' compensation case, an evaluation done within 1 year following a comprehensive medical-legal examination performed by a qualified medical evaluator, agreed medical evaluator, or primary treating physician of the same injury or injuries.

Food and Drug Administration (FDA) Federal agency that protects public health by investigating and testing for the safety, effectiveness, and security of human and veterinary drugs, biological products, medical devices, national food supply, cosmetics, and radiation-emitting objects that are sold in the United States.

Food Stamp Act of 1977 Required all household members to disclose Social Security numbers to verify that they were eligible to participate in the food stamp program.

foreign carrier Insurance company domiciled in another state or, in some states, an insurance company domiciled in a foreign country.

foreign company Insurance company organized or incorporated doing business under the laws of some other state of the United States, such as a company organized under the laws of New York doing business in Missouri. This corporation is a foreign company in Missouri. Technically, an insurance company chartered in a foreign country is called an *alien company*, whereas a company chartered in another state than that in which it is doing business is referred to as a *foreign company*.

foreign corporation Insurance company incorporated under the laws of another state other than the one where it does business. A bank chartered in Pennsylvania but owning a loan production office in California is a foreign corporation in California. Also called *out-of-state corporation*. See also *foreign company*.

foreign insurer See *foreign company*.

foreign medical graduate (FMG) Physician who graduated from a medical school outside of the United States.

foreseeability Capability of an insured individual to know beforehand or have possible anticipation that injury would be the result of a specific act or an absent act.

forfeiture Unvested amount of money remaining in a retirement plan when a participant is terminated and the employee withdraws the amount vested. When this type of situation occurs, a forfeiture must either be used to reduce the plan sponsor's future plan contributions or be reallocated to the other participants.

form locator (FL) Field positions 1 through 81 on the Uniform Bill (UB-04) paper or electronic claim form for specific billing and coding information. Every FL accepts a certain number of characters, alphabetic or numeric and symbols or spaces. For some insurance carriers, FLs may be required, preferred, or optional, depending on the data.

formal referral Authorization request (telephone, fax, or completed form) required by the managed care organization contract to determine medical necessity and grant permission before services being rendered or procedures performed.

format 1. Organization or appearance of data. 2. Under the Health Insurance Portability and Accountability Act (HIPAA), this relates to those data elements that provide or control the enveloping or hierarchical structure, or assist in identifying data content of a transaction.

formulary 1. List of drugs shown in therapeutic or disease categories. 2. In some insurance plans, managed care plans, or Medicare Part D plans, providers are limited to prescribing medications to members from a list of drugs and dispensed through pharmacies participating in the plan. Most plans' formularies include the most common drugs prescribed for seniors. Also called *drug formulary, preferred-drug list (PDL)*, or *select drug list*.

formulary drugs List of prescribed medications recommended by a managed care plan and dispensed by participating pharmacies to members (enrollees) of the plan. It is periodically reviewed and modified. See the three types—open, closed, and restricted formularies—for information. See *formulary* and *drug formulary*.

foundation for medical care (FMC) Organization of physicians sponsored by a state or local medical association concerned with the development and delivery of medical services and the cost of health care. Two types of FMCs exist: (1) comprehensive type of foundation, which designs and sponsors prepaid health programs or sets minimum benefits of coverage; and (2) claims-review type of foundation, which provides evaluation of the quality and efficiency of services by a panel of physicians to the numerous fiscal agents or carriers involved in its area including the ones processing Medicare and Medicaid. Also called *foundation* or *medical foundation*.

401(k) Defined-contribution pension plan that involves employer (plan sponsor) and employee contributions. The employer establishes and administers the plan, advises employees of how much can be contributed by the employee, how much of that contribution will be matched by the employer (if any), and what the investment choices are. Employees' contributions are deducted from their pretax pay, reducing their taxable income. Employees then direct the investment of their money by choosing among the investment options offered by the employer.

four-character subcategory In the *International Classification of Diseases, Tenth Revision, Clinical Modification (ICD-10-CM)*, a letter with two digits followed by a period or decimal point and one number that gives more information on the description of a condition.

fourth and fifth digits Numerical characters in the *International Classification of Diseases, Ninth Revision, Clinical Modification (ICD-9-CM)* code book after three digits that gives additional specific information about the diagnosis or procedure to be coded. Under Medicare guidelines, some diagnostic and procedure codes require fourth or fifth digits to pass insurance claims processing edits for reimbursement.

fourth digit ✓4ᵗʰ Symbol used in the diagnostic code book titled *International Classification of Diseases, Ninth Revision, Clinical Modification (ICD-9-CM)*. It is used to indicate that a fourth digit is required for coding to indicate the highest level of specificity.

FP 1. HCPCS Level II modifier that may be used with CPT or HCPCS Level II codes indicating a service provided is part of a family planning program. 2. Abbreviation for family practitioner. See *family practitioner (FP)*.

FPP See *faculty practice plan (FPP)*.

FQHC See *federally qualified health center (FQHC)*.

FQHMO See *federally qualified health maintenance organization (FQHMO)*.

FR See *Federal Register*.

fractional premiums Insurance premiums that are paid in installments (fractions of the annual premium) such as semiannually, quarterly, or monthly.

fracture manipulation Manual stretching or applying pressure or traction to realign a broken bone; also referred to as a *reduction*.

fragmentation See *unbundling*.

frail elderly provision See *home and community care for the functionally disabled*.

franchise, blanket, or employee life plan See *wholesale life insurance*.

franchise insurance Accident and health insurance contracts sold to individuals of a common employer in which the employer collects and remits the premiums to the insurer. Usually the premiums are deducted from the payroll.

fraternal benefit society Professional organization that provides social and insurance benefits to its members.

fraternal insurance Cooperative type of insurance protection plan given to members of a professional association or fraternal benefit society usually on a nonprofit basis.

fraud 1. An intentional misrepresentation of the facts to deceive or mislead another. 2. In a health care setting, the intentional deception or misrepresentation that an individual knows, or should know, to be false, or does not believe to be true, and makes, knowing the deception could result in some unauthorized benefit to himself or some other person(s). In addition, fraud may be committed by either providers or patients to obtain services, payment for services, or claim program eligibility. 3. In insurance claims, some fraudulent practices are intentionally double billing for the same services, reporting diagnoses and procedures to maximize payments, billing for services that were not performed, altering claim forms for higher reimbursement, soliciting or receiving kickbacks or bribes, using another person's Medicare card, and falsely representing services provided. 4. Lying or intentional misrepresentation by insurance company managers, employees, agents, or brokers for their own gain.

fraudulent claim Type of insurance claim when a claimant intentionally uses false information to obtain medical services or payment for services from his or her insurance company.

fraudulent misrepresentation False statement to get an insurance company to provide insurance coverage for an applicant. Fraudulent misrepresentation gives an insurance company grounds to terminate a policy at any time.

free choice Insurance provision that allows the insured to choose any licensed health care provider for medical services.

free examination period Specific amount of time after delivery of an insurance policy by the agent during which the policy owner may look the policy over and return it to the insurance company for a complete refund of the first premium payment. Usually, complete insurance coverage is provided during this time period. Also called *10-day free look*.

free flap Section of tissue is detached from its base but its arterial and venous components are reattached. CPT codes include 15756 to 15758.

free look Period of time, usually 30 days, when an individual can try out a Medigap policy. During that time, if the individual changes his or her mind about keeping the policy, it can be cancelled and any money paid is refunded.

free-standing emergency medical service center See *emergency center*.

free-standing surgical center Health care facility for handling surgical procedures that do not need overnight hospital care. Also called *ambulatory care facility, ambulatory surgical center, clinic, day surgery, outpatient facility, primary care center*, or *urgent care center*.

free-standing urgent care center See *emergency center*.

freedom of choice 1. In the Medicaid program, the principle that a state ensures that Medicaid beneficiaries are free to obtain medical care from any provider. 2. In private health plans, refers to ability of members or subscribers to go to whomever they want for medical services without being referred.

Freedom of Information Act (FOIA) Federal law that any person has a right, enforceable in court, of access of federal agency records, except to the extent that such records, or portions thereof, are protected from disclosure by one of nine exemptions or by one of three special law enforcement record exclusions. Requests must be submitted in writing. FOIA applies only to records of the executive branch of the federal government, not to those of Congress or the federal courts, and does not apply to state governments, local governments, or private groups.

freelance To work for several clients as an independent, self-employed individual.

frequency-adjusted conversion factor (FACF) Dollar amount for one base unit that is obtained when converting a provider's fee schedule that is not based on the resource-based relative value scale (RBRVS) to one that is based on it, using current fees and the number of times the service is provided (frequency). By using a FACF, it is possible to develop an RBRVS fee schedule that produces the same amount of income that was generated under the non-RBRVS fee schedule.

frequency distribution Exhaustive list of possible outcomes for a variable, and the associated probability of each outcome. The sum of the probabilities of all possible outcomes from a frequency distribution is 100%.

frequent pain In a workers' compensation case, pain approximately 75% of the time.

FRG See *functional related group (FRG)*.

fringe benefits See *employee benefits*.

front-end edits Electronic check of transmitted insurance claims to screen the incoming data or claims before they enter a system for errors, conflicting code entries, and a match of diagnosis to medical service(s) provided. This electronic examination has the capability to accept or reject each transaction or claim based on whether or not it complies with the checks. Also called *claim edits* and *edit check*.

front-loaded policy Universal life insurance policy in which the majority of the expense charges are deductions from each premium payment. These deductions continue throughout the premium payment period.

frontal Position of the face forward.

FSA Abbreviation that means flexible spending account. See *dependent-care spending account*.

FTE See *full-time employee (FTE)*; see *full-time equivalent (FTE)*.

FUL See *full capitation (FUL)*.

full capitation (FUL) 1. Managed care plan is paid for providing services to enrollees solely through capitation. 2. Financial arrangement in which a plan or primary care case manager (PCCM) is paid for providing services to enrollees of a managed care plan through a combination of capitation and fee-for-service reimbursements.

full disability See *total disability*.

full disclosure in adoption To share relevant background information such as social, medical, and mental health with the adopting parents. There are no uniform guidelines for what constitutes full disclosure.

full-risk capitation See *global capitation*.

full-risk contract See *global capitation*.

full-service plan Health insurance plan that pays the actual cost in full instead of a specific maximum for each service. This is in cases where payment is based on usual, customary, and reasonable (UCR) fees.

full-time employee (FTE) In accounting, the equivalent of one individual working full-time (30 hours or more per week). This includes the wages, benefits, deductions (i.e., Social Security, disability insurance, state and federal income taxes) and other costs.

full-time equivalent (FTE) In relation to employment, the equivalent of one individual working full-time for a certain period. This can be made up of several part-time individuals or one full-time person.

fully accredited Designation that all the elements within all the accreditation standards for which the accreditation organization has been approved by the Centers for Medicare and Medicaid Services have been surveyed and fully met or have otherwise been determined to be acceptable without significant adverse findings, recommendations, required actions, or corrective actions.

fully capitated See *global capitation*.

fully contributory Situation in which those insured under a group policy pay the complete cost of their insurance.

fully insured Insurance plan method of funding in which the insurance company assumes all risk and the insured group bears none. Usually, premiums are higher in this type of plan.

functional benchmarking See *benchmarking*.

functional capacity evaluation (FCE) Test that assesses both the ability to perform a task and the structural design limits of the person who is actually doing the task. FCE focuses on work activities (in an effort to reduce the potential for injury) such as sitting, standing, walking, reaching, lifting, and bending. This standardized evaluation is also commonly referred to as a *physical capacity evaluation, work capacity evaluation*, or *disability assessment*.

functional capacity testing Standardized and validated advanced level of testing to determine safe job match for return to work, to assess the level of reasonable accommodations necessary to reinstate an injured worker, and to assign the level of disability for permanent and partial impairment ratings. This testing is used for an injured worker who has achieved maximum medical improvement.

functional costs Operating costs such as claims administration expenses (CAE) and general office expenses (GOE) that are categorized by function.

functional independence measure (FIM) Scoring system that measures the degree of functional self-sufficiency in patients going through the rehabilitation process.

functional limitation Individual's inability to perform specific movements due to some type of physical impairment.

functional overlay Emotional aspect of an organic disease. It is characterized by symptoms that continue long after clinical signs of the disease or disability have ended.

functional related group (FRG) Prospective payment system (PPS) used by rehabilitation hospitals and units. FRG was developed by Margaret Stineman and colleagues at the University of Pennsylvania and SUNY-Buffalo. This system is based on a rehabilitation coding system known as the *functional independence measure (FIM)*.

functional resumé Data sheet that highlights qualifications and skills.

functionally disabled Individual who has a physical or mental impairment that limits his or her capability for independent and self-sufficient living.

fund In a managed care capitation contract, the specific amount of dollars in reserve that is available to compensate the contracted provider of services.

fund account Accounting method that uses a formula for establishing insurance premium rates.

funding agency Entity that holds the assets of a retirement plan, which is often the insurance company.

funding deficiency See *accumulated funding deficiency.*

funding instrument See *funding vehicle.*

funding level Dollar amount of funds needed to finance a medical care program.

funding method System used by employers to pay for health insurance plans such as prospective premium payment, retrospective premium payment, shared risk, or self-funding.

funding standard account Bookkeeping account that is kept to determine if a defined benefit pension plan (DBPP) meets minimum funding standards set by law. Some of the entries to the account are derived actuarially. Failure to satisfy minimum funding standards can cause penalty taxes and enforcement actions. Also called *minimum funding standard account* and *minimum funding standards.*

funding vehicle Legal document (insurance contract) that states the policies and management of pension funds by a funding agency such as an insurance company. Also called *funding instrument.*

future increase option Insurance provision that allows an insured individual to buy additional stated amounts of life or disability income insurance at certain future dates without consideration of the insured's physical condition. Also called *guaranteed insurability option.*

future medical treatment In workers' compensation cases, potential medical care that may be necessary to maintain an injured worker's best possible condition or handle deterioration from the effects of an injury over time. Monetary awards for future medical treatment are established when a worker's condition is permanent and stationary (P & S).

future purchase option See *cost-of-living adjustment.*

future service Employee's projected service given to an employer from the date of the beginning of a pension plan or from the current date to the date of the employee's retirement. Pension benefits for this service are known as *future service benefits.*

FY See *fiscal year (FY).*

G

G-number See *group number.*

G1 HCPCS Level II modifier that may be used with CPT or HCPCS Level II codes indicating most recent urea reduction ratio (URR) reading of less than 60.

G2 HCPCS Level II modifier that may be used with CPT or HCPCS Level II codes indicating most recent urea reduction ratio (URR) reading of 60 to 64.9.

G3 HCPCS Level II modifier that may be used with CPT or HCPCS Level II codes indicating most recent urea reduction ratio (URR) reading of 65 to 69.9.

G4 HCPCS Level II modifier that may be used with CPT or HCPCS Level II codes indicating most recent urea reduction ratio (URR) reading of 70 to 74.9.

G5 HCPCS Level II modifier that may be used with CPT or HCPCS Level II codes indicating most recent urea reduction ratio (URR) reading of 75 or greater.

G6 HCPCS Level II modifier that may be used with CPT or HCPCS Level II codes indicating end-stage renal disease (ESRD) patient for whom less than six dialysis sessions have been provided in a month.

G7 HCPCS Level II modifier that may be used with CPT or HCPCS Level II codes indicating pregnancy resulted from rape or incest or pregnancy certified by physician as life threatening. Payment limits do not apply.

G8 HCPCS Level II modifier that may be used with CPT or HCPCS Level II codes indicating monitored anesthesia care (MAC) for deep complex, complicated, or markedly invasive surgical procedure.

G9 HCPCS Level II modifier that may be used with CPT or HCPCS Level II codes indicating monitored anesthesia care (MAC) for patient who has history of severe cardio-pulmonary condition.

GA 1. HCPCS Level II modifier that may be used with CPT or HCPCS Level II codes indicating a waiver of liability statement (advanced beneficiary notice) signed by the patient is on file. 2. Abbreviation for general agent. See *general agent (GA).*

GAAP See *generally accepted accounting principles (GAAP).*

GAAP reserves Insurance reserves that are calculated using generally accepted accounting principles. Also see *generally accepted accounting principles (GAAP).*

GAF See *geographic adjustment factor (GAF).*

gag clause Provision in a managed care contract that either limits the amount of information that a health care provider may share with a patient or limits the situations in which a provider may recommend a certain alternative treatment when the plan does not cover it. This may be experimental treatments or treatment that may be expensive even if this might be the best course of action for the patient.

gain from operations Amount of income that is in excess after benefit and administrative expenses have been accounted for.

gain-or-loss report Financial statement for insurance that shows underwriting and investment gains and losses for either an individual case, group of cases, or an entire category of group business.

gaming Illegal or unethical attempt to manipulate a system for financial gain such as billing to maximize income by listing a principal diagnosis that puts the patient in the highest-priced diagnosis-related group (DRG) in a prospective payment system (PPS) when a lower-priced diagnosis more precisely depicts the services given for a patient's medical problem.

gang visits 1. Significant number of daily evaluation and management (E&M) visits by the same physician to multiple patients at a facility within a 24-hour period. When insurance claims reach the insurance carrier in this type of situation, it may result in medical review to determine medical necessity for the visits. 2. In Medicare fraud, to bill based on gang visits (e.g., a provider who visits a nursing facility and bills for 20 visits without furnishing any specific service to, or on behalf of, individual patients).

GAO See *General Accounting Office (GAO).*

gap codes CPT codes that are not covered by the Medicare program; thus they do not have relative values under the resource-based relative value scale (RBRVS).

gap fill See *Medigap (MG) policy.*

gap, The See *The gap.*

gapfilling Term used when no comparable, existing test is available. Insurance carrier specific amounts are used to establish a national limitation amount for the following year.

gaps In the Medicare program, costs or services that are not covered under the Medicare plan; referred to as *Medicare gaps.*

garnishee 1. Debtor against whom a plaintiff has begun a process of garnishment. 2. Individual who has had his or her salary attached as payment toward a debt.

garnishment Court order attaching a debtor's property or wages to pay off a debt to the plaintiff.

gastroenterology (GE) Study and treatment of diseases affecting the gastrointestinal (GI) tract including the esophagus, stomach, intestines, gallbladder, and bile duct. It is a subspecialty of internal medicine.

gatekeeper In a managed care system, the primary care physician who is the first doctor the patient seeks for nonemergency care and determines whether referral to a specialist is medically appropriate. The gatekeeper also controls patient access to diagnostic testing services. In some managed care plans, a nurse practitioner or physician assistant is appointed to this role. Also called *primary care physician* and *referral provider.*

gatekeeping Process in which a managed care system's gatekeeper provides the initial patient care, schedules diagnostic testing services, and refers patients to specialists when necessary.

Gb See *gigabyte (Gb).*

GB HCPCS Level II modifier that may be used with CPT or HCPCS Level II codes indicating claim is being resubmitted for payment because it is no longer covered under a global payment demonstration.

GC HCPCS Level II modifier that may be used with CPT or HCPCS Level II codes indicating service has been performed by a resident under the direction of a teaching physician. The teaching physician submits the bill for the service.

GCM See *geriatric care manager (GCM).*

GDP See *gross domestic product (GDP).*

GE 1. HCPCS Level II modifier that may be used with CPT or HCPCS Level II codes indicating a service has been performed by a resident without the presence of a teaching physician under the primary care exception. 2. Abbreviation for gastroenterology. See *gastroenterology (GE).*

GEM system See *general equivalence mapping (GEM) system.*

gender rule System of establishing the insurance company that is the primary carrier for dependents when both parents have health insurance plans. Also see *birthday law.*

general account Type of undivided account that was formerly used by life and health insurance companies to handle all incoming funds. Beginning in the early 1960s, other types of accounts came into use such as separate accounts.

General Accounting Office (GAO) Investigative division of the United States Congress that reports to the Congress about studies assigned by Congressional committees or those mandated by legislative provisions.

general agency distribution system Part of the insurance agency system for selling individual life insurance. Each field office is independent and under contract to the insurance company. The office is directed by a general agent who employs a staff and pays the salaries and office expenses. Sales agents contract with the general agent and not the insurance company. Usually the insurance company pays all commissions to the general agent who retains a portion of each commission (overriding commission) and the remaining commission is paid to the sales agent. However, some offices use

a different procedure and pay commissions directly to the sales agents and overriding commissions directly to general agents.

general agent (GA) Insurance company representative licensed by the state that is under contract with an insurance company and sells insurance policies and services the policyholder for the insurer. Usually a general agent is in charge of a field office of the insurance company that uses a general agency distribution system and is compensated primarily by an overriding commission. Life insurance agents may also be called *life underwriters.* Also called *insurance agent* or *insurance broker.*

general anesthesia Absence of consciousness brought on by various anesthetic medications administered by inhalation or intravenous injection. General anesthesia can be administered only by an anesthesiologist, anesthesia assistant, or a certified registered nurse anesthetist.

general care floor Any all-purpose patient care unit in a hospital facility that is not designated as intensive care unit, critical care unit, or intermediate care unit.

general enrollment period (GEP) One of four periods during which an individual can enroll in Medicare Part A. This period is from January 1 through March 31 of each year. The Medicare Part A coverage is effective July 1 after the GEP in which he or she is enrolled.

general equivalence mapping (GEM) system Public domain reference crosswalk method developed as an aid to convert and test systems, link data in long-term clinical studies, develop application-specific mappings, and analyze data obtained during the transition from ICD-9-CM to ICD-10-CM and beyond. GEM is available at http://www.cdc.gov/nchs/about/otheract/icd9/icd10cm.htm.

general fund of the treasury Funds held by the treasury of the United States, other than revenue collected for a specific trust fund, such as supplemental medical insurance (SMI), and maintained in a separate account for that purpose. The majority of this fund is derived from individual and business income taxes.

general hospital Facility that receives all patients for inpatient care of acute illness or injury and obstetrics.

general journal Accounting books of original entry in which all financial transactions are first posted (recorded), except transactions recorded in specialized journals.

general liability insurance See *commercial general liability insurance (CGL)* and *commercial lines.*

general manager See *branch manager.*

general note When using the *International Classification of Diseases, Ninth Revision, Clinical Modification (ICD-9-CM)* code book, a note that is printed in italics or bold that helps clarify unique coding situations.

general office expenses (GOE) Necessary costs for a managed care plan's administrative activities and not claims administration costs.

G

general practitioner (GP) Family practice physician who gives comprehensive medical care regardless of age of the patient or presence of a condition that may need the services of a specialist. This term has been replaced by the term *family practitioner (FP)*.

general revenue Income to the supplemental medical insurance (SMI) trust fund from the general fund of the U.S. Department of the Treasury. Only a small percentage of total SMI trust fund income each year is attributable to general revenue.

general sessions See *small claims court*.

general supervision Direction and management of a medical procedure given by the physician, but the doctor's attendance is not necessary during the procedure (e.g., only available by telephone). Some medical procedures require general supervision to bill for a specific level of service. This level of supervision is never sufficient for meeting "incident-to" services. Also see *direct supervision* and *personal supervision*.

generalists Physicians who have received training that encompasses several branches of medicine including internal medicine, preventive medicine, pediatrics, surgery, psychiatry, and obstetrics and gynecology. These doctors provide comprehensive medical care, problem solve, and coordinate total health care delivery to all members of a family regardless of sex or age.

generally accepted accounting principles (GAAP) General guidelines and detailed procedures of customary accounting practice that are established and interpreted by the Financial Accounting Standards Board (FASB). FASB was formed in 1973. These accounting principles are used by business firms outside of the insurance industry, as well as by health and life insurance companies.

generic drugs Prescription drugs that have the same active ingredient formula as a brand name drug. Generic drugs usually cost less than brand name drugs and are rated by the Food and Drug Administration (FDA) to be as safe and effective as brand name drugs. Also called *generic equivalent*.

generic equivalent See *generic drugs*.

generic substitution Act of replacing a prescription brand drug for another drug that has the same active ingredient formula.

Genetically Handicapped Persons Program (GHPP) A state program for genetically disabled children.

geographic adjustment factor (GAF) Under the resource-based relative value scale (RBRVS) of the Medicare fee schedule, the weighted sum of the Geographic Practice Cost Indices (GPCI) for each geographic area. Also see *geographic practice cost indices (GPCIs)*.

geographic adjustment method In the Medicare program, this is a system used to convert the Medicare average United States fee-for-service per capita costs (USPCCs) to the local adjusted average per capita costs (AAPCCs). This is used to pay Medicare risk contracting health maintenance organizations (HMOs).

geographic practice cost indices (GPCIs) One of three components of the system in the Medicare program that is used in bringing fees for professional services in line for the region where each physician practices. It is pronounced "gypsies." Under the resource-based relative value scale (RBRVS) of the Medicare fee schedule, the indices are numbers used to adjust the Relative Value Units for each component of a service (physician's work, practice's overhead, and malpractice costs) to reflect geographic differences in cost to provide the services. Each component is multiplied by its own GPCI. The GPCI is a single measure that combines the three fixed shares, whereas the geographic adjustment factor (GAF) of the Medicare fee schedule allows for each service to reflect different shares, thus creating a GAF for each service.

geometric mean length of stay (GMLOS) Adjusted length of stay for all-patient allowances (diagnosis-related groups [DRGs]) for outliers, transfers, and negative outliers that would otherwise skew the data. The GMLOS is used to establish the per diem payment only for transfer cases.

GEP See *general enrollment period (GEP)*.

geriatric assessment Systematic collection and review of data (test results, signs, symptoms) pertaining to the elderly to identify problems, check functionality, and establish appropriate treatment.

geriatric care manager (GCM) Individual (usually social worker or nurse) who assists older people and their families in meeting the elderly person's health care needs (e.g., fill out insurance forms, perform a comprehensive needs assessment, identify available community resources, screen and arrange for in-home services, resolve disputes among family members). GCM services are typically not covered by insurance.

geriatric day care Ambulatory health care facility for the elderly that offers professional and community services for maximizing the patients' function and independence.

geriatrician Medical doctor (MD) who is licensed and certified, and who has specialized postgraduate education and experience in the medical care of older adults.

geriatrics Branch of medicine that specializes in handling the physiological characteristics of the elderly and the diagnosis and treatment of their medical problems.

gerontology Study of the biological, clinical, psychological, economical, and social processes of elderly adults and their problems as individuals, as well as society as a whole.

GF HCPCS Level II modifier that may be used with CPT or HCPCS Level II codes indicating nonphysician (nurse practitioner, certified registered nurse anesthetist, certified registered nurse, clinical nurse specialist, physician assistant) services performed in a critical access hospital.

GG HCPCS Level II modifier that may be used with CPT or HCPCS Level II codes indicating performance and payment of a screening mammogram and diagnostic mammogram on the same patient on the same day.

GH HCPCS Level II modifier that may be used with CPT or HCPCS Level II codes indicating a diagnostic mammogram converted from a screening mammogram on the same day.

GHAA Acronym for Group Health Association of America. See *American Association of Health Plans (AAHP)*.

ghost writing In medical legal reports, a medical report prepared in whole or in part by an individual other than the physician who did the actual examination. The law prohibits ghost writing.

GHPP See *Genetically Handicapped Persons Program (GHPP)*.

GI rider See *guaranteed insurability (GI) rider*.

GIC See *guaranteed investment contract (GIC)* and *separate account guaranteed investment contract (GIC)*.

gigabyte (Gb) Computer storage capacity that holds approximately 1 billion bytes or characters or 1000 megabytes. Gbs are used to represent large hard disk capacities.

GJ HCPCS Level II modifier that may be used with CPT or HCPCS Level II codes indicating an opt out physician or practitioner who has given emergency or urgent service to a Medicare patient.

GK HCPCS Level II modifier that may be used with CPT or HCPCS Level II codes indicating the actual item or service ordered by a physician. Item may be associated with GA or GZ modifier.

GL HCPCS Level II modifier that may be used with CPT or HCPCS Level II codes indicating a medically unnecessary upgrade provided instead of standard item, no charge, no Advance Beneficiary Notice (ABN).

glass insurance Insurance coverage for breakage of glass items caused by all risks but subject to exclusions of war and fire.

glaucoma screening Dilated eye examination with an intraocular pressure measurement and a direct ophthalmoscopic examination, or a slit-lamp biomicroscopic examination, to identify eye disorders or early signs of glaucoma.

global billing Act of increasing the fee for the purchased diagnostic service before billing.

global budget 1. Method of cost containment in which the government places a ceiling or cap on total public and private health care expenditures for a specific population within a specified time period. This type of cost containment applies to expenditures by insurers and individuals. 2. In the hospital setting, a limit of total budget as a cost containment method in which participating hospitals share one projected budget and give out each hospital facility's funds from that budget. Also called *total budget*.

global capitation Reimbursement method in which a managed care plan provides and pays for all health care services for an enrolled population of patients including physicians and hospitals. The plan accepts all risk for that population, which means it needs to keep costs for health care below the amount of premiums collected. A portion of the global cap may be withheld to pay for specialist care referred by primary care physicians. Each year excess funds may be either paid out or carried forward against future global capitation payments to the primary care physicians. Also called *full-risk capitation, full-risk contract*, or *fully capitated*.

global fee 1. All-inclusive payment for hospital and physician services (e.g., a surgery case with all preoperative and postoperative medical care in one fee). 2. Combined technical (equipment) and professional (physician) charges or payment.

global period Specific period of time during which all medical services pertaining to a condition or diagnosis are considered included in the payment for the initial surgery or treatment and may not be billed separately. Complications related to the procedure are considered outside of the global period and not included in payment for the initial surgery or treatment. Medicare global surgical policy (GSP) is from 0 to 90 days postoperatively.

global pricing Reimbursement method in which both the hospital and physician fees are packaged into one price (global fee) for a specific medical procedure such as coronary artery bypass graft (CABG) surgery. In addition, the global fee often includes diagnostic procedures, postsurgical recovery, rehabilitation, and follow-up office visits within a certain time period. Also called *package pricing* and *bundling*.

global service Medical service that has both a professional and technical component such as in some radiological procedures. CPT modifier -26 indicates the professional component and modifier -TC indicates the technical component. When billing if no modifier is present, it is assumed the physician provided the global service. Also see *professional component* and *technical component*.

global surgery package See *surgical package*.

global surgery policy (GSP) Medicare policy relating to surgical procedures in which preoperative and postoperative visits (24 hour prior [major] and day of [minor]), usual intraoperative services, and complications not requiring an additional trip to the operating room are included in one fee. See also *surgical package*.

GM HCPCS Level II modifier that may be used with CPT or HCPCS Level II codes indicating multiple patients were transported on one ambulance trip. List the total number of patients transported.

GME See *graduate medical education (GME)*.

GMLOS See *geometric mean length of stay (GMLOS)*.

GN HCPCS Level II modifier that may be used with CPT or HCPCS Level II codes indicating services delivered under an outpatient speech language pathology plan of care.

GNP See *gross national product (GNP)*.

GO HCPCS Level II modifier that may be used with CPT or HCPCS Level II codes indicating services delivered under an outpatient occupational therapy plan of care.

GOE See *general office expenses (GOE)*.

good health provision Rider in some group credit policies making a policy void if the insured was not in good health when the application was signed or delivered, whichever was mentioned in the contract.

government mandates Federal order or command for individuals to adhere to the legislation set down for the Medicare and Medicaid programs such as time limits in submitting insurance claims and correct use of diagnostic and procedural codes for billing.

government-sponsored health care program Health insurance plan such as Medicare, Medicaid, or TRICARE in which federal funds pay all or part of the fee for services for eligible individuals.

governmental assets Assets or liabilities that arise from transactions between a federal entity and a nonfederal entity. Also called *governmental liabilities*.

governmental liabilities See *governmental assets*.

GP 1. HCPCS Level II modifier that may be used with CPT or HCPCS Level II codes indicating services delivered under an outpatient physical therapy plan of care. 2. Abbreviation for general practitioner. See *general practitioner (GP)*.

GPCI See *Geographic Practice Cost Indices (GPCIs)*.

GPM See *group practice model (GPM)*.

GPPP See *group practice prepayment plan (GPPP)*.

GPWW See *group practice without walls (GPWW)*.

GQ HCPCS Level II modifier that may be used with CPT or HCPCS Level II codes indicating service provided using an asynchronous telecommunications system.

grace days 1. Inpatient hospitalized days that may be billed to the patient because they occurred after the hospital received a quality improvement organization (QIO) denial notice. 2. Number of days established by the QIO that are necessary for the physician or family to arrange for the patient's discharge from the hospital.

grace period Set number of days following the insurance policy's premium due date during which insurance remains in force, may not be canceled, and the policyholder may pay the premium without penalty or loss of benefits. Grace periods vary by contract from 30 to up to 120 days.

grace period liability Insurer's responsibility for insurance claims that are incurred during an insurance contract's grace period.

graded commission scale Payment schedule that lists the amount of money paid to an insurance agent for selling and servicing an insurance policy that is high for the first year and has a lower renewal commission for subsequent years.

graded level commissions Payment schedule that lists the amount of money paid to an insurance agent for selling and servicing an insurance policy that has the same commission percentages for premium increments of first and renewal years.

graded premium whole life insurance Type of whole life insurance in which premiums are increased once or at a certain time such as every 3 years until the premium reaches a specific level.

graduate medical education (GME) Period of formal medical training of a physician after he or she has obtained a Doctor of Medicine (MD) or Doctor of Osteopathy (DO) degree. It is referred to as *internship, residency,* and *fellowship training*.

Gramm-Rudman-Hollings Act Federal law known as the *Balanced Budget and Emergency Deficit Control Act of 1985*.

grandfather clause Section of a policy, law, or association's bylaws that allows continued eligibility or license for individuals who obtain benefits under the law without meeting all of the criteria regardless of a change in the law.

grantee See *trustee*.

greatest level of specificity In diagnostic coding, the code chosen with the highest level of detail and accuracy that corresponds with the patient's medical record.

grievance Written complaint by a dissatisfied patient submitted to a grievance committee of an insurance plan or program. It may be about availability, delivery, or quality of medical services, utilization review decisions, insurance claims payment, or the contract relationship between a plan member and an insurer. Also see *complaint*.

grievance committee Impartial panel of physicians who handle complaints by dissatisfied patients or their representatives against doctors.

grievance procedure Process or system in which a dissatisfied patient or participating provider of a managed care plan can express complaints to get a situation resolved. Such procedures include a due process provision and subject these procedures to a specific and standard adjudication method.

grievances and complaints Information from a discontented patient or dissatisfied provider transmitted to a managed care plan's grievance committee to seek remedies for resolution of the problem(s).

gross conversion factor Dollar amount that is obtained when converting a provider's fee schedule that is not based on the resource-based relative value scale (RBRVS) to one that is using only the current fee schedule. Because income is related to the fee for each service and to the frequency performed, this gives only a rough conversion factor. For a more accurate conversion factor formula, see *frequency-adjusted conversion factor (FACF)*.

gross charges per 1000 Statistic used to evaluate utilization management performance for inpatient, outpatient, partial hospitalization, and so on. Providers in a managed care environment need this information. The formula is to take the gross charges incurred by a specific group for a specific time period and divide it by the average number of members in that group during the same period and then multiply the result by 1000.

gross cost Total price of an insurance program for a certain time period such as 1 year before dividends and rate credits are considered.

gross costs per 1000 Statistic used to evaluate utilization management performance for inpatient, outpatient, partial hospitalization, and so on. The formula is to take the gross costs incurred for services received by a specific group for a certain time period and divide it by the average number of covered members in that group during the same period, and multiply the result by 1000. Providers in a managed care environment need this information because it is imperative to keep gross costs per 1000 below collections per 1000.

gross domestic product (GDP) Total current dollar value of all goods and services produced in the United States during a specific period, usually 1 year, regardless of who supplies the labor or property. GDP differs from the gross national product (GNP) by excluding net income that residents earn abroad. It is the primary indicator of the status of the economy. Formerly called *gross national product (GNP)*.

gross national product (GNP) See *gross domestic product (GDP)*.

gross premium Total price of an insurance policy to be paid by the policyholder before any discounts are applied such as subtracting costs for reinsurance or returning premium. The total price of the policy is the cost of a unit of insurance protection quoted from a rating manual plus the basic rate that covers expenses to the insurance company in maintaining the business.

group In insurance, insureds and their dependents who work for an employer or belong to an association through which they become entitled to insurance coverage.

group annuity Retirement plan that provides monthly (or quarterly, semiannual, or annual) income benefits at retirement to a group of individuals that are under a master contract usually issued to an employer. Each member of the annuity plan is given a verifying certificate.

group case Entire group insurance plan for a policyholder.

group contract Insurance agreement made with an employer or other entity that gives insurance coverage and benefits to employees and their dependents

under a single policy. It is issued for 12 months to the employer with individual certificates given to each insured individual or family and it may be renewed annually. Under the Health Insurance Portability and Accountability Act (HIPAA), insurance portability is tied to employer-group plans in which an employee changes jobs. Also called *group policy*.

group conversion Right of an individual covered by an employer's group insurance policy to convert to coverage under an individual insurance policy (different benefits and rates) and pay premiums directly to a health plan. Usually there is continuity of insurance, and it is not necessary for the individual to take a physical examination. This option may be made available when a person leaves the group, benefits are downgraded or terminated for a specific class, or when the group policy is terminated.

group coverage Insurance agreement between a health plan (contracting entity) and an employer (certificate holder) that gives coverage to all employees (group members) of the plan. The group members receive an identification card to show they have health insurance coverage. Under the Health Insurance Portability and Accountability Act (HIPAA), insurance portability is tied to employer-group plans in which an employee changes jobs.

group creditor life insurance Type of life insurance in which a master contract covers the lives of current and future debtors of the policy owner who is the beneficiary of the policy.

group deferred annuity Type of annuity that sometimes funds a retirement plan. The employer contributes under a group deferred annuity contract, and these funds are used to purchase deferred annuities for the retirement benefits of participants of the plan.

group enrollment agreement Contract between a health insurance plan and a group sponsor who acts as the intermediary for an insured group.

group enrollment period See *open enrollment period*.

Group Health Association of America (GHAA) See *American Association of Health Plans (AAHP)*.

group health coverage See *group health plan*.

group health plan 1. Any insurance plan by which a number of employees of an employer (and their dependents), or members of a similar homogeneous group, are insured under a single policy (master contract), issued to their employer or the group with individual certificates of insurance given to each insured individual or family. Usually, group insurance has lower monthly premiums compared with individual insurance. Group insurance is usually experience rated. Also called *group insurance* or *blanket insurance*. 2. Under the Health Insurance Portability and Accountability Act (HIPAA), an employee welfare benefit plan (as defined by ERISA) including any insured or self-insured plan that provides medical care including items and services paid for as medical care to employees or dependents either directly or through insurance, reimbursement, or otherwise if (a) the plan has 50 or more participants or (b) is administered by an entity other than the employer that established and maintains the plan. Also called *group health coverage*.

group HMO   Managed care organization that contracts with two or more groups of practices to provide health services.

group home   See *adult care home*.

group insurance   See *group health plan*.

group insurance number   See *group number*.

group leader   Member of a group insurance plan that is responsible for administration of the group's contract.

group life insurance   Type of life insurance on a group of individuals under a master policy that is issued without requiring a medical examination. It is issued to an employer, and each employee is given a certificate as verification of his or her insurance.

group medical plan   See *group health plan*.

group medicine   See *group practice*.

group model   Type of managed care organization (MCO) that contracts with a group of providers to give medical care to its members. The providers work out of their own office facilities. A group model may or may not give medical services exclusively for the MCO's members. Also called *network model*.

group model health maintenance organization (HMO)   Type of managed care plan (HMO) that contracts with one or more medical groups to give medical services to members. Usually all services, except hospital care, are provided under one roof and physicians share equipment, records, and personnel. Physicians are paid a predetermined per member, per month amount called *capitation*. From the capitation fund, the physicians' group pays its own physician members according to a prearranged schedule such as salary plus incentives. Also known as a *prepaid group practice plan*. Also see *staff model*.

group monthly premium in force   Total amount of monthly premiums billed at a specific time to cover all outstanding group insurance.

group name   Designated title under which a group is enrolled in an insurance plan.

group number   Number assigned to a group insurance plan that identifies the employer or specific insured group. It appears on each member's identification card and is used when submitting an insurance claim to the insurance company for payment. Also called *group insurance number, employer number, G-number, case number, file number, account number*, and *company code number*.

group ordinary life insurance   Type of group permanent life insurance that has premiums based on issue age. It accumulates and builds reserves and cash surrender values.

group paid-up life insurance   Type of group permanent life insurance in which the employee's contributions are used to purchase paid-up insurance. The employer's contributions are used to purchase term insurance. The employees' insurance coverage remains level each year. As the amount of paid-up insurance increases over time, the amount of term insurance that the employer purchases to make up the difference decreases. This type of life insurance has a cash surrender value.

group permanent life insurance   Type of life insurance that builds cash value and is composed of a group. It may be used to fund a group pension plan or to provide life insurance coverage that will continue after retirement.

group policy   See *group contract*.

group policy owner   See *group policyholder*.

group policyholder   Individual or company in whose name a group insurance policy is written. Also called *group policy owner*.

group practice   Three or more providers that share facilities, office personnel, expenses, equipment, financial and medical records, and income in a medical practice. A group practice may represent a partnership, but not necessarily, a single specialty, or a range of specialties (i.e., multispecialty group practice). Also called *group medicine* or *medical group practice*.

group practice model (GPM)   Type of health maintenance organization (HMO) in which the physicians in the plan share a central facility.

group practice prepayment plan (GPPP)   Managed care plan in which members pay a monthly premium and the plan offers medical services without additional fees. For some patients, Medicare Part B pays the GPPP directly for services given to beneficiaries.

group practice without walls (GPWW)   See *group without walls (GWW)*.

group provider number   A number assigned to a group of physicians submitting claims under the group name and reporting income under one name; used instead of the individual's physician's number (PIN) for the performing provider.

group representative   Salaried employee of the insurance company who assists insurance agents and brokers in acquiring, soliciting, and negotiating with potential buyers for group insurance and to service group contracts. The representative also renegotiates renewal policies.

group rider   Provision that adds group benefits to a basic insurance plan that is chosen by an employer for all employees who take out the insurance coverage.

group sponsor   Individual or professional association that acts as an agent for the group and its members. It pays the dues and service charges to a health insurance plan and agrees to receive the plan's certificate and information.

group universal life (GUL) insurance   Type of group life insurance policy that has flexible premiums, adjustable protection, not fixed, and it has investment earnings that allows for some tax benefits. The death benefit is established by the amount of the premium. In this type of policy, the insured can vary the premium and death benefit amounts during the life of the policy. A group member that leaves the group can continue coverage under the group plan. Also called *group universal life program (GULP)*.

group universal life program (GULP) See *group universal life (GUL) insurance*.

group without walls (GWW) Business composed of physicians or medical practices into one management arrangement. Physicians see patients in their own offices but share administrative, billing, and purchasing expenditures. GWW contracts with managed care plans as a sole entity. Also called *group practice without walls (GPWW)*.

grouper Automated computer coding software program that classifies numeric diagnostic codes and assigns DRGs of discharged patients using the following information: patient's age, sex, principal diagnosis, complications/comorbid conditions, principal procedure, and discharge status. A grouper is essential to reimbursement because it determines which type of complicated diagnosis and/or additional procedures affect a principal diagnosis and place the case into the appropriate DRG.

GSP See *global surgery policy (GSP)*.

GT HCPCS Level II modifier that may be used with CPT or HCPCS Level II codes indicating services provided by using interactive audio and video telecommunication systems.

guaranteed cash value Guaranteed amount available to the insured on surrender of a life insurance policy based on a table of guaranteed values scaled to the number of years in which the policy is in force.

guaranteed eligibility Specific period (3 to 6 months) in which patients who are insured in prepaid health plans are eligible for Medicaid regardless of their actual eligibility for Medicaid. A state may apply to the Centers for Medicare and Medicaid Services (CMS) for a waiver to have this put into its contracts.

guaranteed income contract See *guaranteed investment contract (GIC)*.

guaranteed insurability option See *future increase option*.

guaranteed insurability (GI) rider Life insurance policy amendment that allows the policyholder to buy additional insurance of the same type as that provided in the original policy. The amount is specified in the policy and may be purchased at specific premium rates and at certain times without new evidence of insurability. Also called *policy purchase rider*.

guaranteed interest contract See *guaranteed investment contract (GIC)*.

guaranteed investment contract (GIC) Mechanism of funding for a retirement plan in which an insurance company accepts a single deposit from a sponsor of the plan for a certain time period and retains the deposit

at a specific interest rate. At the end of the time period the deposited funds, with interest, are returned to the plan sponsor who may reinvest the plan assets with the insurance company or another party. Also called *guaranteed income contract* or *guaranteed interest contract*.

guaranteed issue 1. Provision in an employer's health plan that acceptance and coverage be offered to any employee of the company. 2. Legal requirement that an insurance company accept all individuals who apply for coverage. 3. Insurance coverage offered on a one-time basis that does not require that the individual give evidence of insurability. In some plans, it guarantees renewal of the coverage as long as the applicant pays the premium.

guaranteed-issue insurance Health insurance policy in which all eligible members of a certain group who apply and meet certain conditions are offered coverage.

guaranteed issue limit See *no-evidence limit*.

guaranteed issue rights Rights an individual has in certain situations when insurance companies are required by law to sell or offer a Medigap policy. In such situations, an insurance company cannot deny insurance coverage or place conditions on a policy but must cover the individual for all preexisting conditions and cannot charge more for a policy because of past or present health problems. Also called *Medigap protections*.

guaranteed renewable Clause in an insurance policy that means the insurance company must renew the policy as long as premium payments are made by the insured. However, the premium may be increased when it is renewed if it raises premiums for a particular class such as everyone in a geographic area with the same type of policy. These policies may have age limits of 60, 65, or 70 years or may be renewable for life.

guaranteed renewable contract Insurance policy that means the insured has the right to have the policy in force as long as he or she pays the premiums. However, the insurance company may increase the premium rate when the policy is renewed. These policies may have age limits of 60, 65, or 70 years or may be renewable for life. Also called *guaranteed renewable policy*.

guaranteed renewable policy See *guaranteed renewable contract*.

guaranteed replacement cost insurance Insurance policy that pays the full costs of replacing damaged property without any deduction for depreciation and without a dollar limit.

guarantor Individual who promises to pay the medical bill by signing a form agreeing to pay or who accepts treatment, which constitutes an expressed promise.

guaranty association In the insurance business, an organization that protects policy owners from losses when an insurance company becomes insolvent.

guardian Person appointed by the court who is designated to act on behalf of a minor or an incompetent

G

adult such as parent, trustee, committee, conservator, or other person or agency. Also called *legal guardian*.

guardianship Court-appointed authority given to an individual to act on behalf of a minor or incompetent adult.

guardianship of the estate Situation in which a person appointed by the court has the authority over property only for a minor or incompetent adult.

guardianship of the person Court-appointed authority given to a person with the right to carry out tasks only concerning personal matters such as medical decisions and residential questions.

guidelines 1. Information and instructions at the beginning of each of the six major sections of the *Current Procedural Terminology (CPT)* code book when coding medical services and procedures. Additional guidelines are provided at the beginning of each subsection and for code ranges. Guidelines present definitions and explanations of terms and phrases, applicable modifiers, explanation of notes, unlisted services, special reports information, and clinical examples. These are all factors to appropriately interpret and report the procedures and services contained in a particular section. 2. Written general rules and procedures to assist physicians in making a diagnosis and giving treatment. These are set down to change practice styles, lessen unnecessary care, and reduce costs. Depending on the region of the United States, may also be referred to as *medical practice parameters, clinical practice guidelines*, or *clinical protocols*.

GUL insurance See *group universal life (GUL) insurance*.

GULP See *group universal life program (GULP)*.

GV HCPCS Level II modifier that may be used with CPT or HCPCS Level II codes indicating attending physician was not employed or paid under arrangement by the patient's hospice provider.

GW HCPCS Level II modifier that may be used with CPT or HCPCS Level II codes indicating service was unrelated to the hospice patient's terminal condition. Append this modifier when medically necessary services are not part of the patient's hospice care.

GWW See *group without walls (GWW)*.

GY HCPCS Level II modifier that may be used with CPT or HCPCS Level II codes indicating item or service was statutorily excluded or does not meet the definition of any Medicare benefit.

gynecology Diagnosis, treatment (surgical and nonsurgical), and study of diseases of the female reproductive organs including the breasts. Usually it is studied and practiced with obstetrics.

GZ HCPCS Level II modifier that may be used with CPT or HCPCS Level II codes indicating item or service is expected to be denied as not reasonable and necessary.

H Abbreviation for history.

H & P See *history and physical (H & P)*.

H9 HCPCS Level II modifier that may be used with CPT or HCPCS Level II codes indicating a court-ordered service.

HA HCPCS Level II modifier that may be used with CPT or HCPCS Level II codes indicating a child/adolescent program. This modifier may be required for state Medicaid programs, so check with your state guidelines.

HAC See *Health Administration Center (HAC)*.

handicapped As defined by Section 504 of the Rehabilitation Act of 1973, any person who has a physical or mental impairment that substantially limits one or more major life activities, has a record of such impairment, or is regarded as having such an impairment.

handicapped dependent Unmarried dependent child who is not able to be self-supportive because of physical or mental disability.

HAP Abbreviation for hospital admission plan and hospital admission program. See *hospital admission plan (HAP)* and *hospital admissions program (HAP)*.

harass To irritate or persistently annoy.

harassment To aggressively bother an individual such as for payment of a debt.

hard copy A printout from a printer via computer.

hardware The physical components of a computer system (e.g., display screen, hard disk).

hazard Situation that exposes an individual to risk of injury or can be dangerous and increase the severity and/or probability of a loss, state or condition such as accident, illness, fire, flood, burglary, wet floor, and unsanitary location.

HB HCPCS Level II modifier that may be used with CPT or HCPCS Level II codes indicating a nongeriatric adult program. This modifier may be required for state Medicaid programs, so check with your state guidelines.

HBA See *health benefits advisor (HBA)*.

HC 1. HCPCS Level II modifier that may be used with CPT or HCPCS Level II codes indicating a geriatric adult program. This modifier may be required for state Medicaid programs, so check with your state guidelines. 2. Abbreviation for high complexity. See *high complexity (HC)*.

HCC model See *hierarchical condition categories (HCC) model*.

HCF See *health care finder (HCF)*.

HCFA See *Health Care Financing Administration*; also known as *Centers for Medicare and Medicaid Services (CMS)*.

HCFA-1450 See *CMS-1450* and *Uniform Bill (UB-04) claim form*.

HCFA-1500 See *health insurance claim form (CMS-1500)* and *CMS-1500*.

HCO See *Health Care Organization (HCO)*.

HCPCS See *Healthcare Common Procedure Coding System (HCPCS)* (pronounced "hick-picks").

HCPCS Level I See *Healthcare Common Procedure Coding System (HCPCS)*.

HCPCS Level II See *Healthcare Common Procedure Coding System (HCPCS)*.

HCPCS modifier See *Healthcare Common Procedure Coding System (HCPCS) modifiers*.

HCPP See *health care prepayment plan (HCPP)*.

HCQIA See *Health Care Quality Improvement Act (HCQIA) of 1996*.

HCQIP See *Health Care Quality Improvement Program (HCQIP)*.

HD 1. HCPCS Level II modifier that may be used with CPT or HCPCS Level II codes indicating a pregnant/parenting women's program. This modifier may be required for state Medicaid programs, so check with your state guidelines. 2. Abbreviation for hemodialysis. See *hemodialysis (HD)*.

HDE See *humanitarian device exemption (HDE)*.

HDHP See *high-deductible health plan (HDHP)*.

HE HCPCS Level II modifier that may be used with CPT or HCPCS Level II codes indicating a mental health program. This modifier may be required for state Medicaid programs, so check with your state guidelines.

headings In the *Current Procedural Terminology (CPT)* code book, the subdivisions of the six major sections that identify a group of CPT codes.

health State of physical, mental, and social well-being and the absence of disease or infirmity or other abnormal condition. It is not a static condition; constant change and adaptation to stress result in homeostasis.

Health Administration Center (HAC) Federal agency of the Department of Veterans Affairs that administers federal health benefit programs for veterans and their family members. These benefit programs include the Civilian Health and Medical Program of the Department of Veterans Affairs (CHAMPVA) including the CHAMPVA In House Treatment Initiative (CITI) and the CHAMPVA Meds by Mail program.

HAC also administers the Spina Bifida Health Care Program, the Children of Women Vietnam Veterans Health Care Program, and the Persian Gulf Examination Program for Dependents. HAC also runs two programs specifically designed to cater to veterans: (1) the Foreign Medical Program, which provides service to veterans living or traveling throughout the world, and (2) the Fee program, which provides services to veterans who need care outside a Veterans Affairs medical center. HAC's responsibilities are benefits management, eligibility determination, customer service, outreach and education, claims processing, appeals and grievances and fraud, and waste and abuse prevention.

health alliances See *consumer health alliances.*

Health and Human Services (HHS) See *Department of Health and Human Services (DHHS).*

health benefits advisor (HBA) Government employee (primary care coordinator) responsible for helping all military health system beneficiaries in the TRICARE program obtain medical care.

health benefits package See *benefit package.*

health care 1. Attention given to individuals or communities by representatives of the health services for the purpose of promoting, maintaining, monitoring, or restoring health. The phrase *health care* has the intent of a broader scope of meaning when compared with the phrase *medical care.* When one hears *medical care,* it infers treatment by or under the supervision of a physician. 2. Under the Health Insurance Portability and Accountability Act (HIPAA), care, services, or supplies related to the health of an individual. This includes preventive, diagnostic, therapeutic, rehabilitative, maintenance, or palliative care, and counseling, service, assessment, or procedure involving physical or mental conditions, or functional status. It also involves the sale or dispensing of a drug, device, equipment, or other item relating to a prescription.

health care advance directive See *advance directive.*

health care center Central location in which medical services are provided to group model health maintenance organization (HMO) members.

Health Care Claim Payment/Advice (835) See *electronic remittance advice (ERA).*

health care clearinghouse Under the Health Insurance Portability and Accountability Act (HIPAA), a third-party administrator (TPA) who receives insurance claims from the physician's office in a nonstandard format or with nonstandard data and puts it into standard data elements or a standard transaction, or that receives a standard transaction and processes or assists processing the data into nonstandard format for a receiving entity. The TPA performs software edits and redistributes the claims electronically to various insurance carriers.

health care coalition Unified body of health care providers, purchasers of care, industry, labor, and insurance companies to try to solve medical costs and problems.

Health Care Code Maintenance Committee Working group of individuals administered by the Blue Cross and Blue Shield Association. It is responsible for maintaining specific coding schemes used in the X12 transaction set such as claim adjustment reason codes, claim status category codes, and claim status codes.

health care consumer See *consumer.*

health care delivery Provide health care services to those in a community.

health care delivery system Method of structure and coordination encompassing medical facilities, health care services, and reimbursement methods to provide health care.

Health Care Financing Administration (HCFA) Former name of the federal agency within the Department of Health and Human Services (DHHS) established to administer and oversee Medicare, Medicaid, and State Children's Health Insurance Programs, as well as other governmental health programs. This agency is now called *Centers for Medicare and Medicaid Services (CMS).* See *Centers for Medicare and Medicaid Services (CMS).*

health care finder (HCF) Health care professionals, generally registered nurses, who are located at TRICARE Service Centers to act as liaison between military and civilian providers, verify eligibility, determine availability of services, coordinate care, facilitate the transfer of records, and perform first level medical review. This health care specialist helps TRICARE beneficiaries and providers with preauthorizations of medical services.

health care flexible spending account (HFSA) Employer-sponsored benefit that allows a fixed amount of pretax wages to be set aside for qualified expenses such as child care or uncovered medical expenses. Money in these accounts cannot be rolled over from year to year.

health care fraud See *fraud.*

health care ID See *national patient identifier.*

health care identification See *national patient identifier.*

Health Care Organization (HCO) Kind of association certified by the Department of Workers' Compensation to provide managed medical care within the workers' compensation system.

health care prepayment plan (HCPP) Type of managed care organization that contracts with Centers for Medicare and Medicaid Services (CMS) to provide Medicare-eligible Part B medical services to enrollees. In return for a monthly premium, plus any applicable deductible or copayment, all or most of an individual's physician services are provided by the HCPP. The HCPP pays for all services it has arranged for (and any emergency services) whether provided by its own physicians or its contracted network of physicians. If a member enrolled in an HCPP chooses to receive services that have not been arranged for by the HCPP, he or she is liable for any applicable Medicare deductible and/or coinsurance amounts, and any balance would be paid by the regional Medicare carrier.

health care professional Individual who has been trained in a health-related field, clinical or administrative. The professional may be licensed, certified, or registered by a state or government agency or professional organization or may be an employee of a health care facility.

health care provider 1. Under the Health Insurance Portability and Accountability Act of 1996 (HIPAA), a person or entity who is trained and licensed to provide care to a patient; also a place that is licensed to give health care such as a hospital, skilled nursing facility, inpatient/outpatient rehabilitation facility, home health agency, hospice program, physician, diagnostic department, outpatient physical or occupational therapy, rural clinics, or home dialysis supplier. Do not confuse this term with insurance companies that provide insurance. 2. Individual who provides medical services, which can include physician, nurse, physician assistant, pharmacist, physical therapist, occupational therapist, speech therapist, and other licensed medical professional persons.

health care provider taxonomy codes Administrative code set that classifies health care providers by type and area of specialization. The code set will be used in certain adopted transactions. Note: A given provider may have more than one health care provider taxonomy code.

health care provider taxonomy committee Organization administered by the National Uniform Claim Committee (NUCC) that is responsible for maintaining the provider taxonomy coding scheme used in the X12 transactions. The detailed code maintenance is done in coordination with X12N/TG2/WG15.

health care proxy See *power of attorney* and *durable power of attorney for health care.*

Health Care Quality Improvement Act (HCQIA) of 1996 Federal legislation that provides liability protection for physicians and hospital facilities who participate in peer review. This act established a national clearinghouse that collects information on physicians who have been sued for malpractice and types of disciplinary actions taken.

Health Care Quality Improvement Program (HCQIP) Program that supports the mission of the Centers for Medicare and Medicaid Services (CMS) to assure health care security for beneficiaries. HCQIP's mission is to promote the quality, effectiveness, and efficiency of services to Medicare beneficiaries by strengthening the community of those committed to improving quality; monitoring and improving quality of care; communicating with beneficiaries and health care providers, practitioners, and plans to promote informed health choices; protecting beneficiaries from poor care; and strengthening the infrastructure.

health care reform See *health system reform.*

health care services plan Any health insurance or managed care organization that contracts with physicians to provide hospital and medical services to enrollees on a prepaid basis.

health coach Individual, usually a registered nurse, who counsels patients on follow-up doctor visits, teaches a patient how to read prescription drugs, takes care of other medical needs, makes appointments with doctors, and helps discharged patients with their transition to home care. He or she makes regular house visits or talks to patients on the telephone and may be employed by an insurance company.

Health Employer Data and Information Set (HEDIS) Set of standard evaluation measures that gives information about the quality and performance of a health plan such as the quality of care, access, cost, patient satisfaction, membership and use, financial information, management, and other measures to compare managed care plans. Employers, health maintenance organizations, and the National Committee for Quality Assurance developed HEDIS. The Centers for Medicare and Medicaid Services (CMS) collects HEDIS data for Medicare plans.

health fair Community-based gathering of people with a festival atmosphere that offers vendors with health-related services, educational lectures, diagnostic screening, and counseling services for prevention of disease and to promote health.

Health Informatics Standards Planning Panel (HISPP) Organization accredited and staffed by the American National Standards Institute in 1991. It was replaced by the Healthcare Informatics Standards Board (HISB) in 1995. See *Healthcare Informatics Standards Board (HISB).*

health information Under the Health Insurance Portability and Accountability Act (HIPAA), any data, oral or recorded in any medium that is created or received by a health care provider, health plan, public health authority, employer, life insurer, school or university, or health care clearinghouse. The data relate to the past, present, or future physical or mental health or condition of an individual or future payment for the provision of health care to an individual.

health information exchange (HIE) Electronic transmission of health-related data among health care organizations that conforms to nationally recognized standards.

health information management (HIM) Department in a hospital facility that organizes, maintains, produces, stores, retains, disseminates, and keeps secure patient health information. Also referred to as *medical records.*

health information management (HIM) professional Trained specialist who may be certified and/or licensed and is responsible for designing and maintaining a method that assists with the collection, use, and dissemination of health and medical information.

health information organization (HIO) Association that oversees and governs the exchange of health-related data between organizations that conforms to nationally recognized standards.

health information system Computer system created for coding and billing data for hospital services provided to patients.

health insurance 1. Contract between the policyholder and/or member and insurance carrier or government program to reimburse the policyholder and/or member for all or a portion of the cost of medically necessary medical care rendered by health care professionals. 2. General category generic term that includes many types of insurance coverage such as insurance that applies to lost income arising from illness or injury—disability income insurance, accident and health insurance, hospital confinement insurance, hospital expense insurance, surgical expense insurance, major medical insurance, dental expense insurance, accidental death and dismemberment insurance, and medical expense insurance. Insurance may be obtained on either an individual or a group basis. Also referred to as *medical insurance*.

health insurance adjuster See *adjuster*.

Health Insurance Association of America (HIAA) In 2003, HIAA, Group Health Association of America (GHAA), and the American Managed Care and Review Association (AMCRA) merged with American Association of Health Plans (AAHP) and created what is now known as *America's Health Insurance Plans (AHIP)*. See *America's Health Insurance Plans (AHIP)*.

health insurance card See *identification card (ID card)*.

health insurance claim (HIC) Request for payment on behalf of the insured (patient) to an insurance company for professional services rendered by a provider.

health insurance claim form (CMS-1500) 1. Professional uniform insurance claim form developed and approved by the American Medical Association Council on Medical Service and the Centers for Medicare and Medicaid Services. The version in current use is the CMS-1500 (08-05). It is also known as the *UCF-1500*. It is used by physicians and other professionals to bill outpatient services and supplies to Medicare, TRICARE, and some Medicaid programs, as well as some private insurance carriers and managed care plans. Formerly known as *HCFA-1500*. 2. For electronically transmitted professional claims, the 837P replaces the paper CMS-1500 form and the electronic national standard format (NSF). 3. In Medicare fraud, altering insurance claim forms to obtain a higher payment amount.

health insurance claim number (HIC/HICN) Unique nine-digit Medicare entitlement number assigned to an individual by the Social Security Administration. It appears on the Medicare beneficiary's identification card and is used when submitting an insurance claim to the fiscal intermediary for payment. The HICN is used with a one- or two-letter or one-letter and one-number suffix. A letter prefix may indicate that the beneficiary is entitled to railroad retirement benefits.

health insurance issuer Under the Health Insurance Portability and Accountability Act (HIPAA), an insurance company, insurance service, or insurance organization that is licensed in the state to do business involving insurance and is subject to the state's laws regulating insurance. This phrase does not include a group health insurance plan.

health insurance networks (HINs) Groups of businesses that join together to lobby for better insurance policies or lower premiums from insurance companies.

health insurance portability Allows an individual to keep an employer-group medical insurance plan when changing jobs. See *Consolidated Omnibus Budget Reconciliation Act of 1985 (COBRA)*.

Health Insurance Portability and Accountability Act of 1996 (HIPAA) Federal law designed to limit exclusions for preexisting conditions, prohibit discrimination against employees and dependents based on their health status, guarantee that health insurance is available to small employers, and guarantee renewability of insurance to all employers regardless of size. However, people must go through the Consolidated Omnibus Budget Reconciliation Act program before using HIPAA. HIPAA allows portability in that it provides continuing insurance coverage when a person changes employment. It also simplifies administrative aspects of electronic health care transactions; mandates standard transaction code sets used by providers, plans, payers, and employers; and orders security, privacy, and confidentiality of patients' health information via electronic transmission. HIPAA requires use of national identification systems for health care patients, providers, payers or plans, and employers. This act is also known as *K2, Kennedy-Kasselbaum Bill, Kennedy-Kassenbaum Bill*, and *Public law 104-191*.

Health Insurance Portability and Accountability Act data dictionary See *HIPAA data dictionary (HIPAA DD)*.

health insurance prospective payment system (HIPPS) Code system for procedures that is used when billing Medicare patients in skilled nursing facilities, home health agencies, inpatient rehabilitation facilities, and swing bed facilities in rural hospitals. HIPPS codes are alphanumerical codes of five digits: The first three are derived from the resource utilization group (RUG), and the last two represent a modifier code for the specific assessment. This code is put in Form Locator 44 on the UB-04 Medicare claim form. Any patient coded in one of the top 26 RUGs is a skilled patient.

health insurance purchasing cooperatives (HIPCs) See *consumer health alliances.*

health insurance purchasing corporations See *consumer health alliances.*

health insuring organization (HIO) Entity that provides for or arranges for the provision of care and contracts on a prepaid capitated risk basis to provide a comprehensive set of services. This may involve state or federal programs such as Medicaid or Medicare beneficiaries. HIOs contract with providers on a discounted fee-for-service or a capitated basis to provide medical services.

Health IT Certification Provides professional training and certification for those responsible for planning, selecting, implementing, and managing electronic health records (EHRs) and other health information technology (HIT). See *Certified Professional in Electronic Health Records (CPEHR)* and *Certified Professional in Health Information Technology (CPHIT).* Website: www.HealthITCertification.com

Health Level Seven (HL7) Standard protocols and encoding rules published for developers to apply in the health industry. These were created by the Accredited Standards Committee X12 (ASC X12), a committee formed by American National Standards Institute (ANSI). HL7 sets some of the electronic standards for exchange of clinical and administrative information in health care applications (see Box H-1).

Health Level Seven, Inc. (HL7) Founded in 1987, a nonprofit, American National Standards Institute (ANSI)-accredited standards developing organization dedicated to providing a comprehensive framework and related standards for the exchange, integration, sharing, and retrieval of electronic health information that supports clinical practice and the management, delivery, and evaluation of health services.

Box H-1   HEALTH LEVEL SEVEN FORMAT OF DATE AND TIME OF BIRTH

To determine the date and time of a patient's birth date (e.g., for a neonate, for whom the age in hours might be relevant), the time of the birth, using military time, can be recorded with the birth date. From this, the age can be generated from the date of birth (DOB). Baby Jane was born on March 24, 2007, at 8:26 AM.

When the required HL7 format is YYYY MMDDHHMM, Baby Jane's date and time of birth will be entered for transmission as: 200703240826

YYYY	MM	DD	HH	MM
2007	03	24	08	26
Year	Month	Day	Hour	Minute

---

health literacy Ability to obtain, interpret, and understand basic medical information and health services and the capability to use the data and services to improve health.

Health Maintenance Act of 1990 Act developed by the National Association of Insurance Commissioners (NAIC) and used by most states as a model for legislation of health maintenance organizations (HMOs). This act mandates that HMOs have a certificate of authority to carry out their business in the state and they must provide the state with detailed financial and qualifying data.

health maintenance organization (HMO) Oldest of all prepaid health plans. A comprehensive health care financing and delivery organization that provides a wide range of health care services with an emphasis on preventive medicine to enrollees within a geographical area through a panel of contracted providers and hospital facilities. Members are required to use those participating in the plan. Primary care physicians called "gatekeepers" are usually reimbursed via capitation. One method is when enrollees pay a monthly premium and a small copayment for using medical services. Another method is when capitated rates are paid by payers for each member based on a projection of patients' costs. Payers may include employers, insurance companies, or government programs. There are four types of HMOs: group, staff, independent practice association, and network. HMOs can either be for profit or nonprofit. There are also specialized HMOs that provide vision, dental, or mental health care.

Health Maintenance Organization (HMO) Act of 1973 Public Law 93-222 created authority for the federal government to assist HMO development by providing grants, loans, and loan guarantees to offset the initial operating deficits of new HMOs that meet federal standards (e.g., are federally qualified) and to require most employers to offer an HMO to their employees as an alternative to traditional health insurance.

health maintenance organization (HMO) plan Type of Medicare Advantage Plan that is available in some areas of the United States. Plans cover all Medicare Part A and Part B health care. Some HMOs cover extra benefits (e.g., extra days in the hospital). In most HMOs the patient can only go to doctors, specialists, or hospitals on the plan's list except in an emergency.

Health Maintenance Organization Regulatory Agency State agency that administers, licenses, and regulates health maintenance organizations (HMOs). In most states, this agency is the state insurance department. Also called *HMO regulatory agency.*

health management See *preventive care.*

Health Manpower Shortage Area (HMSA) See *health professional shortage area (HPSA).*

health plan Entity that assumes the risk of paying for medical treatments and acts as an insurer for enrolled members under a fee-for-service or capitation system (i.e., insurance company, self-insured employer, group health plan, or managed care plan).

health plan document See *plan document.*

Health Plan Employer Data and Information Set (HEDIS) Set of standard performance measurements developed in 1989, 1993, and 1995 by the National Committee for Quality Assurance. It helps consumers, corporations, employers, and public purchasers of health care compare and determine the quality and value of managed care plans. HEDIS standardizes how health plans examine and report data including: quality of access to care, patient satisfaction, preventive medicine, membership and utilization, finance, and descriptive data on health plan management.

health plan ID See *national payer identifier.*

health plan purchasing cooperatives (HPPC) See *consumer health alliances.*

health professional shortage area (HPSA) Region based on a population per physician ratio. Three types of HPSAs are primary medical care, dental, and mental health. Physicians who perform services in HPSA areas receive incentive payments (also known as a *bonus payment program*). When billing, they must indicate their services were provided in an incentive-eligible HPSA by using a modifier. HPSAs replaced health manpower shortage areas (HMSAs).

health promotion Types of medical advertisements to help change behaviors that improve health and prevent disease such as those that influence self-care and lifestyle modifications. Promotions can appear as health information, education, diagnostic screening, and health care interventions.

health purchasing alliance (HPA) See *accountable health plan (AHP).*

health reimbursement account (HRA) Type of account to which only the employer can contribute and in which workers do not put their own funds. It is used to pay medical expenses for employees. An employer may keep the money in the account if a worker quits. Also see *consumer-directed health plan (CDHP).*

health savings account (HSA) Type of tax-favored savings plan in which a working person can deposit money in an HSA and deduct the amount of the deposits from taxable income. Withdrawal from an HSA is tax free when used for qualifying medical expenses. Money left unspent in an HSA may be rolled over year after year. HSAs are open to anyone younger than 65 years of age who enrolls in a high-deductible (e.g., more than $1000/individual or $2000/family) health plan (HDHP). Employers pay the monthly premiums. Also see *consumer-directed health plan (CDHP).*

health service agreement (HSA) Detailed contract describing enrollment, eligibility limitations, and benefits that an insurance plan will pay and services and procedures that are covered under the managed care plan. It is given to each enrolled group.

health services Medical services, given to individuals, that provide health care that may contribute either directly or indirectly to the physical or mental health and well-being of patients. These may be physicians' services, hospital services, acupuncture, alternative therapies, assisted living care, chiropractic care, dental care, drugs, home nursing care, skilled nursing care, and vision care.

health services area See *Health Systems Agency (HSA).*

health statement Form or section of a form that an insurance applicant completes to verify his or her own and dependents' health so that they can obtain membership in a managed care plan or become insured by an insurance company.

health status Statistical measurement of a certain individual's or population's health based on the individual's or population's own assessment; the incidence or prevalence of illness; or mortality and morbidity tables.

health system All medical services, functions, and resources within a geographical region that exist to affect the state of the health of that given population.

health system reform Attempts by the U.S. government to enact legislation to assist in reducing medical costs, increase access of health care, and establish a national health insurance program. Formerly known as *health care reform.*

Health Systems Agency (HSA) Agency funded by the federal government and states to provide services that include health planning, resource development, monitoring, education, and information for the population of a certain region within a state.

Healthcare Common Procedure Coding System (HCPCS) Three-tier coding system developed by the Centers for Medicare and Medicaid Services (CMS), formerly the Health Care Financing Administration (HCFA), used for reporting physician/supplier services and procedures. Providers must use HCPCS to receive payment by Medicare and Medicaid programs. Level I consists of national codes to code ambulatory, laboratory, radiology, and other diagnostic services for Medicare billing. This level contains only the American Medical Association's CPT codes. Level II consists of HCPCS national codes used to report ambulance services, durable medical equipment, and orthotic and prosthetic devices. Level III HCPCS regional/local codes have been discontinued. Pronounced "hick-picks" and formerly referred to as *Health Care Financing Administration Common Procedure Coding System (HCPCS).* Also known as *national codes.*

Healthcare Common Procedure Coding System (HCPCS) Level I See *Healthcare Common Procedure Coding System (HCPCS).*

Healthcare Common Procedure Coding System (HCPCS) Level II See *Healthcare Common Procedure Coding System (HCPCS).*

Healthcare Common Procedure Coding System (HCPCS) modifiers In HCPCS Level II coding, two alpha digits, two alphanumerical characters, or a single alpha digit placed after the usual five-digit CPT procedure code number. These modifiers are used to identify situations that change the description of service or supply. They are accepted by insurance carriers nationally and are updated annually by the Centers for Medicare and Medicaid Services (CMS) (see Box H-2 and Figure H-1).

Healthcare Financial Management Association (HFMA) Professional alliance of individuals who are organized to improve financial management of health care institutions and related health care organizations and do the following: (1) Foster and increase knowledge of and proficiency in financial management; (2) Conduct and participate in educational programs and activities concerning financial management; (3) Provide media for the interchange of ideas and dissemination of material relative to financial manage-

ment; (4) Strengthen cooperation among individuals of varying disciplines in financial management; (5) Develop curricula and financial management supporting material for use by educational institutions; (6) Cooperate with health care institutions and related health care organizations and agencies, as well as other interested groups in matters pertaining to financial management; (7) Establish and promulgate principles relative to financial management; (8) Promote and encourage financial management standards of performance for individuals and institutions in the various areas of financial management; and (9) Undertake research in financial management related to these objectives.

Healthcare Informatics Standards Board (HISB) Created by the American National Standards Institute's Executive Standards Council in December 1995 to replace the Health Informatics Standards Planning Panel (HISPP). Their basic objective is to achieve a high level of support of the health care users, providers, and business partners for development and use of health care information standards in a cooperative environment. HISB developed an inventory of candidate standards for consideration as possible Health Insurance Portability and Accountability Act (HIPAA) standards. In this forum, American health care providers, information systems vendors, organized users, and interested parties work together with Standards Development Organizations (e.g., Health Level 7, American Society for Testing and Materials, and Institute of Electrical and Electronics Engineers,

---

Box H-2   HCPCS MODIFIERS

When taking x-ray films of both feet, the billing portion of the insurance claim appears as follows:

05/06/XX	73620	**RT**	Radiologic examination, foot—right
05/06/XX	73620	**LT**	Radiologic examination, foot—left

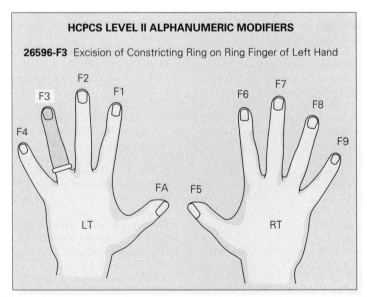

HCPCS LEVEL II ALPHANUMERIC MODIFIERS

26596-F3 Excision of Constricting Ring on Ring Finger of Left Hand

Figure H-1 HCPCS Level II alpha modifiers (LT and RT used to identify left and right hands) and alphanumerical modifiers (FA through F9) used to identify digits (fingers) of left and right hands.

Inc.) to resolve the many issues around harmonizing and coordinating standards evolution.

Healthcare Information Management Systems Society (HIMSS) Association focused on providing leadership for the optimal use of health care information technology and management systems for the betterment of human health. Founded in 1961 with offices in Chicago, Washington, D.C., and other locations across the country.

Healthcare Integrity and Protection Data Bank (HIPDB) National health care fraud and abuse data bank created by the Health Insurance Portability and Accountability Act (HIPAA) of 1996. Its information includes actions reported against health care providers, suppliers, and practitioners for fraud and abuse. The HIPDB is used with the national practitioner data bank (NPDB).

heaped commission schedule See *levelized commission schedule*.

hearing Second level of the appeal process for an individual applying for SSDI or SSI. This is a hearing before an administrative law judge who had no part in the initial or reconsideration disability determination.

hearing officer hearing In the Medicare program, this is Level 2, an independent determination related to insurance claims in which a party has appealed a review decision within 6 months of the date of notice of the decision; the hearing is rendered by a hearing officer assigned by the contractor. For Level 2, there is no requirement regarding the amount of money in controversy.

heart rate Frequency with which the heart beats, calculated by counting the number of QRS complexes or ventricular beats in one minute.

HEDIS See *Health Plan Employer Data and Information Set (HEDIS)*.

HEDIS measures from encounter data Measures from encounter data as opposed to having the plans generate Health Plan Employer Data and Information Set (HEDIS) measures. HEDIS is a collection of performance measures and their definitions produced by the National Committee for Quality Assurance (NCQA). Also see *Health Plan Employer Data and Information Set (HEDIS)*.

heir Person who inherits or is legally entitled to inherit under state law after the death of an individual who has created a will.

hematocrit Measure of red blood cell volume in an individual's blood.

hematology Branch of internal medicine concerned with the scientific study of blood and blood-forming tissues and with the treatment of diseases and disorders of the blood.

hemilaminectomy Surgical removal of one side (right or left) of the vertebral lamina. This is the posterior bony covering of the nerves.

hemodiafiltration Simultaneous hemodialysis and hemofiltration, which involves the removal of large volumes of fluid and fluid replacement to maintain hemodynamic stability. It requires the use of ultra pure dialysate or intravenous fluid for volume replacement. Also called *high-flux hemodiafiltration* and *double high-flux hemodiafiltration*.

hemodialysis (HD) 1. Method of dialysis in which blood from a patient's body is circulated through an external device or machine and then returned to the patient's bloodstream. Such an artificial kidney machine is usually designed to remove fluids and metabolic end products from the bloodstream by placing the blood in contact with a semipermeable membrane, which is bathed on one side by an appropriate chemical solution, referred to as *dialysate*. 2. Treatment usually done in a dialysis facility but can be done at home with the proper training and supplies. HD uses a special filter called a *dialyzer* or *artificial kidney* to clean the blood. The filter connects to a machine. During treatment, the blood flows through tubes into the filter to clean out wastes and extra fluids. Then the newly cleaned blood flows through another set of tubes and back into the body.

hemofiltration Fluid removal.

hepatitis B vaccine Preparation of killed microorganisms, living attenuated organisms, or living fully virulent organisms that is administered to produce or artificially increase immunity to hepatitis B.

hesitation payment See *token payment*.

HF HCPCS Level II modifier that may be used with CPT or HCPCS Level II codes indicating a substance abuse program. This modifier may be required for state Medicaid programs, so check with your state guidelines.

HFMA See *Healthcare Financial Management Association (HFMA)*.

HFSA See *health care flexible spending account (HFSA)*.

HG HCPCS Level II modifier that may be used with CPT or HCPCS Level II codes indicating an opioid addiction treatment program. This modifier may be required for state Medicaid programs, so check with your state guidelines.

HH HCPCS Level II modifier that may be used with CPT or HCPCS Level II codes indicating a mental health/substance abuse program. This modifier may be required for state Medicaid programs, so check with your state guidelines.

HHA See *home health agency (HHA)*.

HHABN See *Advance Beneficiary Notice (ABN)*.

HHC See *home health care (HHC)*.

HHS Also referred to as *DHHS*. See *Department of Health and Human Services (DHHS)*.

HI 1. HCPCS Level II modifier that may be used with CPT or HCPCS Level II codes indicating an integrated mental health and mental retardation/developmentally disabled program. This modifier may be required for state Medicaid programs, so check with your state guidelines. 2. Medicare Part A; see *hospital insurance.*

HIAA Abbreviation for Health Insurance Association of America, which is now known as *America's Health Insurance Plans (AHIP).* See *America's Health Insurance Plans (AHIP).*

HIC See *health insurance claim (HIC).*

HICN See *health insurance claim number (HICN).*

HIE See *health information exchange (HIE).*

hierarchical condition categories (HCC) model Risk adjustment prospective payment system used by Centers for Medicare and Medicaid Services (CMS) for managed care organizations (MCOs). It uses a hierarchical diagnosis classification system and other demographic adjusters to foretell costs and establish payment amounts for managed care services to Medicare beneficiaries.

hierarchy Numerical order of diagnostic codes in which each digit beyond three digits adds information. See Box H-3.

high complexity (HC) Phrase used to describe a type of medical decision making when a patient is seen for an E/M service.

high-cost alternative See *assumptions.*

high-deductible health plan (HDHP) Health plan that, when combined with a health savings account (HAS) or a health reimbursement arrangement (HRA), provides insurance coverage and a tax-advantage means to help consumers save for future medical expenses. This is a part of the Medicare Advantage Law of 2003.

Box H-3   ALPHANUMERICAL CODES FOR ICD-10-CM

FRACTURE OF UPPER LIMB (810-819)

810   Fracture of clavicle
Includes: collar bone
   interligamentous part of clavicle
The following fifth-digit subclassification is for use with category 810:
   0 unspecified part
   Clavicle NOS
   1 sternal end of clavicle
   2 shaft of clavicle
   3 acromial end of clavicle
✓5ᵗʰ   **810.0**
ICD-10-CM
   S42.00 Closed fracture of clavicle
   S42.001 Closed fracture of right clavicle
   S42.002 Closed fracture of left clavicle
   **S42.009 Closed fracture of clavicle,
      unspecified side**

---

high-flux hemodiafiltration See *hemodiafiltration.*

high-low commission scale Insurance payment schedule that gives individuals who sell insurance information that shows the amount of a high first-year commission and the reduced amounts for renewal commissions.

high risk A high chance of loss.

high-risk area Potential flaw in management controls requiring management attention and possible corrective action.

high-risk insurance pool State program that helps high-risk individuals who have health problems to join together to purchase health insurance. However, because the pool members are high risk, the insurance premium rates are high even with state subsidies.

high-severity presenting problem In CPT coding of a service or procedure, this is a problem where the risk of morbidity without treatment is high to extreme. There is a moderate to high risk of mortality without treatment or high probability of severe, prolonged functional impairment.

Hill-Burton Act Legislation and the programs operated under that legislation for federal support of constructing new and modernizing existing hospitals and other health facilities, beginning with Public Law 79-725, the Hospital Survey and Construction Act of 1946. The original law, which has been amended, provided for surveying state needs, developing plans for construction of hospitals and public health centers, and assisting in construction and equipping them in exchange for the hospitals' commitment to give free or discounted fees for services to individuals who cannot afford treatment. The Department of Health and Human Services (HHS) issued regulations that established standards for uncompensated care. It stated that care given to Medicare and Medicaid patients was not considered uncompensated care. Until the late 1960s, most of the amendments expanded the program in dollar amounts and scope. The administration has attempted to terminate the program, while Congress has tried to restructure it toward support of outpatient facilities, facilities to serve areas deficient in health services, and training facilities for health and allied health professions. The purpose of the existing Hill-Burton program was modified by Public Law 93-641 to allow assistance in the form of grants, loans, or loan guarantees for the following purposes: modernization of health facilities; construction of outpatient health facilities; construction of inpatient facilities in areas that have experienced rapid population growth; and conversion of existing medical facilities for the provision of new health services.

HIM See *health information management (HIM).*

HIM professional See *health information management (HIM) professional.*

HIMSS See *Healthcare Information Management Systems Society (HIMSS).*

H

HINN See *hospital-issued notice of noncoverage (HINN)*.

HINs See *health insurance networks (HINs)*.

HIO See *health insuring organization (HIO)* and *health information organization (HIO)*.

HIPAA See *Health Insurance Portability and Accountability Act of 1996 (HIPAA)*.

HIPAA data dictionary (HIPAA DD) Data dictionary that defines and cross-references the contents of all X12 transactions included in the Health Insurance Portability and Accountability Act (HIPAA) mandate. It is maintained by X12N/TG3.

HIPAA DD See *HIPAA data dictionary (HIPAA DD)*.

HIPCs Acronym that means health insurance purchasing cooperatives. See *consumer health alliances*.

HIPDB See *Healthcare Integrity and Protection Data Bank (HIPDB)*.

HIPPS See *health insurance prospective payment system (HIPPS)*.

HISB See *Healthcare Informatics Standards Board (HISB)*.

HISPP See *Health Informatics Standards Planning Panel (HISPP)* and *Healthcare Informatics Standards Board (HISB)*.

histologic Pertaining to the study of the microscopical, anatomical, and physiological characteristics of tissues and the cells found therein.

historical hospital cost data Cost information submitted by providers when submitting Medicare claims that is used to determine the future cost of medical professional services (referred to as *rate setting*).

history (Hx or H) 1. Record of past events. 2. Systematic account of the medical, emotional, and psychosocial occurrences in a patient's life and of factors in the family, ancestors, and environment that may contribute to a patient's condition.

history and physical (H & P) Detailed account obtained during an interview with the patient of the onset, duration, and character of the present illness and any acts or factors that aggravate or ameliorate the symptoms, as well as the findings on physical examination. Then the physician makes a medical decision based on the number of diagnoses or management options, amount of data or complexity of data reviewed, and complications and/or morbidity or mortality. An H & P may be performed before or on the day of admission as an inpatient to the hospital.

history of present illness (HPI) Chronological description of the development of the patient's present illness from the first sign or symptom or from the previous encounter to the present.

history statement Attending physician's statement that is usually part of an insurance application that contains specific health history of the proposed insured.

HIV See *human immunodeficiency virus (HIV)*.

HJ HCPCS Level II modifier that may be used with CPT or HCPCS Level II codes indicating an employee assistance program. This modifier may be required for state Medicaid programs, so check with your state guidelines.

HK HCPCS Level II modifier that may be used with CPT or HCPCS Level II codes indicating a specialized mental health program for high-risk populations. This modifier may be required for state Medicaid programs, so check with your state guidelines.

HL HCPCS Level II modifier that may be used with CPT or HCPCS Level II codes indicating services provided by an intern. This modifier may be required for state Medicaid programs, so check with your state guidelines.

HL7 See *Health Level Seven (HL7)* and *Health Level Seven, Inc. (HL7)*.

HM HCPCS Level II modifier that may be used with CPT or HCPCS Level II codes indicating a service provided by an individual without a bachelor's degree. This modifier may be required for state Medicaid programs, so check with your state guidelines.

HMO See *health maintenance organization (HMO)*.

HMO Act of 1973 See *Health Maintenance Organization (HMO) Act of 1973*.

HMO regulatory agency See *Health Maintenance Organization Regulatory Agency*.

HMSA See *health manpower shortage area (HMSA)*.

HN HCPCS Level II modifier that may be used with CPT or HCPCS Level II codes indicating a service provided by an individual with a bachelor's degree. This modifier may be required for state Medicaid programs, so check with your state guidelines.

HO HCPCS Level II modifier that may be used with CPT or HCPCS Level II codes indicating a service provided by an individual with a master's degree. This modifier may be required for state Medicaid programs, so check with your state guidelines.

hold harmless agreement 1. Liability of one entity is assumed by a second entity (insurance company). 2. Clause in an insurance contract that relieves the insurance payer of liability that may arise from the delivery of health care. 3. Provision that offers the insured protection in disputes between the insurer and the provider of a covered service. Also called *hold harmless provision*.

hold harmless clause 1. Provision in an insurance contract in which the liability of one party is assumed by a second party, usually the insurance company. 2. Legal section often used in managed care contracts that states if either the managed care plan or participating provider is held liable for corporate malfeasance or malpractice, the provider agrees not to sue or make any claims against a plan member. 3. Legal paragraph in a managed care contract that prohibits a provider from billing members (patients) if the managed care plan becomes insolvent or fails to meet its financial obligations. This is required by some state regulations. Also called *no balance billing clause*. 4. In cancer hospitals, the financial protection that ensures the hospitals recover all losses because of differences in their ambulatory payment classification (APC) payments and the pre-APC payments for Medicare outpatient services.

hold harmless provision See *hold harmless agreement*.

hold harmless release Clause that states a payee will pay an insurance company if a subsequent claimant successfully challenges the disbursement of the policy's proceeds.

holistic health Concept that concern for health requires a perspective of the individual as an integrated system rather than one or more separate parts including physical, mental, spiritual, and emotional.

holistic health care See *holistic medicine*.

holistic medicine System of comprehensive or total patient care that considers the physical, emotional, social, economic, and spiritual needs of the person; his or her response to illness; and the effect of the illness on the ability to meet self-care needs. Also called *holistic health care*.

home 1. Location, other than a hospital or other facility, where the patient receives care in a private residence. 2. When the physician's office or an outpatient hospital is billing, the "Place of Service" two-digit numerical code for home (12) is inserted in Block 24B of the CMS-1500 insurance claim form.

home and community-based service (HCBS) waiver programs Established under Section 2176 of the Omnibus Reconciliation Act; permit states to offer, under a waiver, a wide array of home and community-based services that an individual may need to avoid institutionalization. These programs offer different choices to some people with Medicaid such as case management, homemaker, home health aide, personal care, adult day health care, rehabilitation, respite care, and other services. Those that qualify may obtain care in their home and community so that they can stay independent and close to family and friends. HCBS programs help the elderly and disabled, mentally retarded, developmentally disabled, and certain other disabled adults. These programs give quality and low-cost services.

home and community care for the functionally disabled Home and community health care established under Section 1929 of the Social Security Act. It allowed states to provide a large range of services to the functionally disabled as an optional state plan benefit. In every state, except Texas, the option can serve only people older than 65. In Texas, people of any age are eligible if they meet the state's functional disability test and financial criteria. Also known as *frail elderly provision*.

home care See *home health care (HHC)*.

home care program Type of program with health and social services given to individuals and families where they reside for promoting, maintaining, or restoring health and minimizing effects of illness and disability.

home health agency (HHA) Public or private licensed, certified, or authorized state agency or organization that gives home care services that have been prescribed by a patient's physician such as skilled nursing care, physical therapy, occupational therapy, speech therapy, and personal care by home health aides. To be certified under the Medicare program, a provider or agency must meet certain health and safety standards and provide skilled nursing services and at least one additional therapeutic service (physical, speech, or occupational therapy; medical social services; or home health aide services) in the home. Some outpatient services may be covered if equipment is necessary and cannot be used in the patient's home. Also called *home health care agency*.

home health aide Person who, under the supervision of a home health or social service agency, assists elderly, ill, or disabled person with household chores, bathing, personal care, and other daily living needs. Social service agency personnel are sometimes called *personal care aides*.

home health care (HHC) 1. Limited part-time or intermittent skilled nursing care and home health aide services, as well as other health-related services given to the patient in his or her home. Examples of palliative and therapeutic care are assistance with medications, wound care, intravenous (IV) therapy, help with basic needs (e.g., bathing, dressing, mobility), physical and rehabilitation therapy, nursing, counseling, and social services. Usually this care is given to elderly, disabled, sick, or convalescent patients who do not need care in a facility. These services are provided by home health agencies (HHAs), hospitals, and other community organizations. Medicare pays for home care only if the type of care needed is skilled and required on an intermittent basis and is intended to help people recover or improve from an illness, not to provide unskilled services over a long period of time. There is no beneficiary cost sharing for home health care services. Also known as *home care*. 2. In Medicare fraud, certification or recertification by a provider of the need for home health care services, knowing that all of the requirements relating to being homebound and medical necessity have not been met.

home health care agency See *home health agency (HHA)*.

home health plan certification Physician receives, reviews, adjusts treatment, documents the plan in coordination with the care of the home health agency, and then bills for this service. For subsequent plan adjustment, see *home health plan recertification*.

home health plan recertification Physician receives, reviews, adjusts treatment, documents the plan in coordination with the care of the home health agency, and then bills for this subsequent plan adjustment. For initial certification, see *home health plan certification*.

home health services Supplies and services provided to patients by health care professionals in a patient's home. These individuals suffer from an injury, illness, or disabling condition or are terminally ill and require short- or long-term care. For Medicare to pay for the benefits, the services must be prescribed by a physician. Services consist of audiology, dental, medical supplies, part-time or intermittent skilled nursing care, nutrition counseling, occupational therapy, pediatric therapy, physical therapy, some rehabilitation equipment, social services, and speech-language pathology.

home health visit Service provided at the place of residence of a patient by a professional health worker.

home medical equipment See *durable medical equipment (DME)*.

home office administration System in which the insurance company maintains all clients' basic insurance agreement records at the home office.

home-office-to-home-office arrangement Understanding of a manufacturer and a distributor in which an insurance company selects not to offer a certain product or product line but acts as a brokerage general agent for specific product lines manufactured by another insurer.

home oxygen therapy requirements (HOTR) Physician's clinical documentation indicating that a patient's residential use of oxygen is medically necessary.

home patients Medically able individuals who have their own dialysis equipment at home and, after proper training, perform their own dialysis treatment alone or with the assistance of a helper.

home service agent Exclusive insurance agent who works for a home service company and who collects premiums and gives service at the policy-owner's residence. He or she offers monthly debit life, health, and fire insurance products and products for which premiums are billed by and remitted directly to the insurance company. Some of the business may also be in industrial insurance.

home service distribution system Method used for individual insurance that hires agents to collect premiums and give service at the policy owner's residence. The agent works in a defined geographical territory. See also *home service agent*.

homebound 1. Situation in which an individual is normally unable to leave home unassisted and to try to leave home takes considerable and taxing effort. Such a person may leave home for medical appointments; medical treatment; or short, infrequent absences for nonmedical reasons such as a trip to the barber or to attend a religious service. 2. In Medicare, one of the requirements to qualify for home health care.

homemaker services In-home health with meal preparation, shopping, light housekeeping, money management, personal hygiene, grooming, and laundry.

homeopath Practitioner of homeopathy.

Homeopathic Pharmacopoeia of the United States One of the official compendia in the United States. Also see *compendium*, *National Formulary*, and *United States Pharmacopoeia (USP)*.

homeopathy System of therapeutics based on the theory that was advanced in the late eighteenth century by Dr. Samuel Hahnemann, who believed that a large amount of a particular drug may cause symptoms of a disease and moderate dosage may reduce or relieve those symptoms; thus some disease symptoms could be treated by small doses of medicine.

homeowner's insurance Package policy that provides both property and personal liability insurance. It may cover the house, garage, other structures on the property, personal property inside the house and offer protection against fire, windstorm, riot or civil commotion, theft, vandalism, and accidental water damage from plumbing, a heating or air conditioning system, or a domestic appliance depending on the extent of the policy. Also called *homeowner's multiperil insurance*.

homeowner's multiperil insurance See *homeowner's insurance*.

homeowner's policy rates Cost of homeowner's insurance, which may depend on its location, age, construction, and replacement costs.

horizontal integration Merger between health care facilities that provides the same level of services (e.g., hospital with outpatient clinic).

hospice 1. Public agency or private organization primarily engaged in providing pain relief, symptom management, counseling, and supportive services to terminally ill patients and their families in their own homes, in a homelike center, or inpatient or outpatient hospital facility. The whole family is considered the unit of care and care extends through their period of mourning. 2. In the Medicare program, when a beneficiary chooses hospice benefits, all other Medicare benefits are discontinued except physician services and treatment of conditions not related to the terminal illness. Hospice care is covered under Medicare Part A (hospital insurance). The eligible beneficiary must have a life expectancy of 6 months or less. 3. Facility, other than a patient's home, in which palliative and supportive care for terminally ill patients and their families are provided.

hospice care Special manner of caring for people who are terminally ill and their families. This care includes home health services, volunteer support, physical care, pain management, and grief counseling. Hospice care is covered under Medicare Part A (hospital insurance). Also called *hospice services*.

hospice provider Hospital or home health care agency that may legally offer hospice care.

hospice services See *hospice care.*

hospital Licensed and accredited institution with organized medical staff, permanent facilities that include inpatient beds, and medical services including physician services and continuous nursing services for the diagnosis and treatment of patients with a variety of medical conditions, both surgical and nonsurgical, and preventive medical services.

hospital, accredited Official approval by The Joint Commission (TJC) that the hospital facility has met the quality and high standards after their scrutiny. TJC accredits clinics, hospitals, and other federal and military facilities. See *Joint Commission, The.*

hospital acquired conditions (HACs) High cost, high volume, complicating conditions or major complicating conditions that, when present as secondary diagnoses on insurance claims, result in a higher-paying diagnosis-related group category and are reasonably preventable through the application of evidence-based guidelines. Also see *never events.*

hospital admission plan (HAP) Proposal of action or method used to speed admitting a patient to a hospital and to assist with quick reimbursement to the hospital. Also called *hospital admissions program (HAP).*

hospital admissions program (HAP) See *hospital admission plan (HAP).*

hospital affiliation 1. Facility that has established a contractual arrangement to provide inpatient care for members of a managed care plan. 2. Inpatient facility where a physician has admitting privileges. 3. Facility that has an established relationship with a medical school.

hospital alliances Groups of hospitals that join together to share services and make purchases to reduce their costs. See also *integrated delivery system.*

hospital assumptions These include differentials between hospital labor and nonlabor indices compared with general economy labor and nonlabor indices; rates of admission incidence; the trend toward treating less complicated cases in outpatient settings; and continued improvement in diagnosis-related group (DRG) coding.

hospital audit companies Businesses that do retrospective audits for hospital facilities to try to obtain some percentage of savings from billed insurance claims.

hospital-based physician Doctor of medicine or osteopathy, salaried or unsalaried, under contract or arrangement who renders that service and treatment in a hospital setting rather than in an office environment.

hospital billing audit Independent evaluation of hospital bills by an external auditor (third party) to investigate if medical services and supplies billed to the patient were those actually given and if the fees were for the correct amounts.

hospital care Inpatient and outpatient care, procedures, supplies, and medical services provided and billed by a hospital facility.

hospital coinsurance Cost sharing in which a Medicare Part A beneficiary must pay a daily amount for the 61st through 90th day of hospitalization. It is equal to one fourth of the inpatient hospital deductible. For lifetime reserve days, a Medicare beneficiary must pay a daily amount that is equal to one half of the inpatient hospital deductible. See *lifetime reserve.*

hospital confinement Continuous stay in an acute hospital, skilled nursing facility, or other inpatient facility for a specific time period. This phrase is commonly seen in insurance contracts where benefits are listed.

hospital confinement insurance Type of health insurance that gives a predetermined benefit amount for each day an insured is in the hospital. Some policies provide higher benefit amounts if the insured is in an intensive or cardiac care unit. Also called *hospital indemnity insurance.*

hospital contract Formal legal agreement between a managed care plan or insurance company with a hospital facility to provide inpatient and outpatient medical services to members of the plan with payment for the care by the plan.

hospital day Twenty-four-hour period when a patient is admitted to the hospital as an inpatient. The day of admission is considered a hospital day, but the day of discharge from the hospital is not. The time a patient spends receiving medical services as an outpatient is not considered as a hospital day.

hospital days per 1000 Utilization measurement of the number of days per year of inpatient hospital care by members in a managed care plan. The formula is calculated by taking the total number of days spent in the hospital by the members and dividing it by the total number of members.

hospital expense insurance Type of insurance that has certain benefits for hospital services and associated medical expenses for treatment of a illness or injury. Most policies cover hospital charges for room and board and hospital services, surgeon's and physician's fees during a hospital stay, specific outpatient expenses, and extended care services such as convalescent or nursing home costs. Also called *hospital-surgical expense insurance.*

hospital extras allowance Group insurance benefit that covers hospital supplies and services other than room and board daily charges (e.g., x-rays, laboratory tests, medications, surgical dressings, anesthetics, use of an operating room). Also called *miscellaneous hospital expense benefit.*

hospital indemnity insurance Type of insurance that pays a certain cash amount for each day that the patient is in the hospital up to a specific number of days without taking into account the actual expense of the confinement. Some policies may provide higher benefit amounts if the insured is in an intensive or cardiac care unit. Indemnity insurance does not fill gaps in the Medicare coverage. Also called *hospital confinement insurance.*

hospital inpatient See *inpatient.*

hospital input price index Another name for "hospital market basket." See *hospital market basket.*

hospital insurance (HI) 1. See *hospital indemnity insurance.* 2. Medicare Part A under Title XVIII of the Social Security Act, in which coverage is generally provided automatically, and free of premiums, to (a) persons age 65 or older who are eligible for Social Security or Railroad Retirement benefits, whether they have claimed the monthly cash benefits or not, and (b) certain government employees and certain disabled individuals. This program provides basic protection against the costs of inpatient hospital services, posthospital skilled nursing care, home health services, and hospice care.

hospital insurance trust fund Trust fund that has as its primary source of income payroll taxes paid by employees and employers. This fund finances hospital and medical services covered under Medicare Part A.

hospital-issued notice of noncoverage (HINN) Printed document sent by a hospital to a Medicare beneficiary when the hospital determines the medical service the patient is receiving or is about to receive is not covered due to either medical necessity, not being delivered in the appropriate setting, or being considered custodial. An HINN may be given before admission, at admission, or any time during the inpatient stay.

hospital market basket Cost of the mix of goods and services (including personnel costs but excluding nonoperating costs) comprising routine, ancillary, and special care unit inpatient hospital services. Also referred to as *market basket.*

hospital miscellaneous services Inpatient services besides daily room and board charges and general nursing services that are given during a hospital stay (e.g., laboratory tests, drugs, x-ray studies).

hospital number Number given to each member hospital facility by the managed care plan or insurance company for identification purposes.

hospital outpatient See *outpatient.*

Hospital Payment Monitoring Program (HPMP) and the Comprehensive Error Rate Testing (CERT) Program Established by Centers for Medicare and Medicaid Services (CMS) to monitor and report the accuracy of Medicare fee-for-service (FFS) payments. The national error rate is calculated using a combination of data from the CERT contractor and HPMP with each component representing about 60% and 40% of the total Medicare FFS dollars paid. The CERT program measures the error rate for claims submitted

to carriers, durable medical equipment regional carriers (DMERCs), and fiscal intermediaries (FIs). The HPMP measures the error rate for the quality improvement organizations (QIOs). Beginning in 2003, CMS elected to calculate a provider compliance error rate in addition to the paid claims error rate. The provider compliance error rate measures how well providers prepare Medicare FFS claims for submission. CMS calculates the Medicare FFS error rate and estimate of improper claim payments using a methodology the Office of the Inspector General approved. The CERT methodology includes randomly selecting a sample of approximately 120,000 submitted claims, requesting medical records from providers who submitted the claims, and reviewing the claims and medical records for compliance with Medicare coverage, coding, and billing rules.

hospital reimbursement Payment to a facility for the health services given to treat an inpatient.

hospital services Inpatient and outpatient care, procedures, supplies, and medical services provided and billed by a hospital facility.

hospital staff State-licensed physicians with privileges to admit patients for treatment and medical services. May sometimes be referred to as *organized staff* or *medical staff.*

Hospital Standardization Program In 1913, the year of its founding, the American College of Surgeons appointed Codman to chair a committee on hospital standardization and to establish the College's standardization program. This endeavor represents an integral part of the College's history because it evolved into the Joint Commission on Accreditation of Hospitals in 1951 and the Joint Commission on Accreditation of Healthcare Organizations in 1987.

hospital-surgical expense insurance See *hospital expense insurance.*

hospitalist Physician who primarily takes care of patients when they are in the hospital. This doctor takes over the patient's care from the primary doctor when the patient is in the hospital and keeps the primary doctor informed about the patient's progress. The hospitalist returns the patient to the care of the primary doctor when the patient leaves the hospital.

hotline Special telephone number (1-800-HHS-TIPS) of the national Department of Health and Human Services and Office of the Inspector General for providers and the public who are encouraged to ask questions or to report suspected fraudulent or abusive activities of anyone associated with the Medicare or Medicaid programs.

HOTR See *home oxygen therapy requirements (HOTR).*

hour of service Phrase used in relation to the Employee Retirement Income Security Act (ERISA) that means an hour for which an employee is entitled to be paid or is paid. An hour of service can be earned while the employee is working for the employer or during the time of a vacation, holiday, illness, or other paid leave of absence.

HP HCPCS Level II modifier that may be used with CPT or HCPCS Level II codes indicating a service provided by an individual with a doctor's degree. This modifier may be required for state Medicaid programs, so check with your state guidelines.

HPA See *health purchasing alliance (HPA)*.

HPI Abbreviation for history of present illness. See *history of present illness (HPI)*. Also see *brief history of present illness (HPI)* and *extended history of present illness (HPI) 1997 guidelines*.

HPMP See *Hospital Payment Monitoring Program (HPMP)*.

HPPC See *health plan purchasing cooperatives (HPPC)*.

HPSA See *health professional shortage area (HPSA)*.

HQ HCPCS Level II modifier that may be used with CPT or HCPCS Level II codes indicating a service provided in a group setting. This modifier may be required for state Medicaid programs, so check with your state guidelines.

HR HCPCS Level II modifier that may be used with CPT or HCPCS Level II codes indicating a service provided with a family/couple with the client present. This modifier may be required for state Medicaid programs, so check with your state guidelines.

HRA See *health reimbursement account (HRA)*.

H.R. 10 plan See *Keogh Act*.

HS HCPCS Level II modifier that may be used with CPT or HCPCS Level II codes indicating a service provided for a family/couple without the client present. This modifier may be required for state Medicaid programs, so check with your state guidelines.

HSA Abbreviation for health service agreement, health systems agency, and health savings account. See *health service agreement (HSA)*, *health systems agency (HSA)*, and *health savings account (HSA)*.

HT HCPCS Level II modifier that may be used with CPT or HCPCS Level II codes indicating a service provided by a multidisciplinary team. This modifier may be required for state Medicaid programs, so check with your state guidelines.

HTA Acronym for health care technology assessment. See *technology assessment (TA)*.

https See *hypertext transport protocol secure (https)*.

HU HCPCS Level II modifier that may be used with CPT or HCPCS Level II codes indicating services or supplies that are funded by a child welfare agency. This modifier may be required for state Medicaid programs, so check with your state guidelines.

human immunodeficiency virus (HIV) Retrovirus that causes acquired immunodeficiency syndrome (AIDS), which attacks the human immune system, provoking the system to fail in containing diseases.

humanitarian device exemption (HDE) Exemption given by the Federal Drug Administration (FDA) for devices that treat rare medical conditions.

hurricane See *catastrophe insurance policy*.

HV HCPCS Level II modifier that may be used with CPT or HCPCS Level II codes indicating services or supplies funded by a state addictions agency. This modifier may be required for state Medicaid programs, so check with your state guidelines.

HW HCPCS Level II modifier that may be used with CPT or HCPCS Level II codes indicating services or supplies funded by a state mental health agency. This modifier may be required for state Medicaid programs, so check with your state guidelines.

Hx Abbreviation for history.

HX HCPCS Level II modifier that may be used with CPT or HCPCS Level II codes indicating services or supplies funded by a county/local agency. This modifier may be required for state Medicaid programs, so check with your state guidelines.

HY HCPCS Level II modifier that may be used with CPT or HCPCS Level II codes indicating services or supplies funded by a juvenile justice agency. This modifier may be required for state Medicaid programs, so check with your state guidelines.

hybrid entity Covered entity whose covered functions are not its primary functions.

hybrid medical record Transition from a paper-based medical record to an electronic record.

hydration Level of fluid in the body. Loss of fluid, or dehydration, occurs when the patient loses more water or fluid than he or she takes in. The body cannot keep adequate blood pressure, get enough oxygen and nutrients to the cells, or get rid of wastes if it has too little fluid.

hypertensive table Table that appears in the *International Classification of Diseases, Ninth Revision, Clinical Modification (ICD-9-CM)* code book Volume 1, Alphabetical Index, that provides the diagnostic codes for hypertension, a common disorder that is a known cardiovascular disease risk factor.

hypertext transport protocol secure (https) Language using a secure code at an Internet website that may be passed back and forth between servers and clients. Web addresses that begin with http and not https mean that it is possible for someone to eavesdrop on your computer's conversation with the website.

HZ HCPCS Level II modifier that may be used with CPT or HCPCS Level II codes indicating services or supplies funded by a criminal justice agency. This modifier may be required for state Medicaid programs, so check with your state guidelines.

H

I

I & D See *incision and drainage (I & D)*.

IADLs See *instrumental activities of daily living (IADLs)*.

IANC See *interest-adjusted net cost (IANC) method*.

IBNR See *incurred but not reported (IBNR)*.

IC See *independent contractor (IC)*.

ICA See *International Claim Association (ICA)*.

ICD See *International Classification of Diseases (ICD)*.

ICD-9-CM See *International Classification of Diseases, Ninth Revision, Clinical Modification (ICD-9-CM)*.

ICD-9-CM diagnostic code See *diagnostic code*.

ICD-9-CM Official Guidelines for Coding and Reporting Rules for coding diagnostic codes (ICD-9-CM) published in *Coding Clinic for ICD-9-CM* by the American Hospital Association.

ICD-10-CM See *International Classification of Diseases, Tenth Revision, Clinical Modification (ICD-10-CM)*.

ICD-10-CM diagnostic code See *diagnostic code*.

ICD-10-PCS See *International Classification of Diseases, Tenth Revision, Procedural Coding System (ICD-10-PCS)*.

ICD-O See *International Classification of Diseases, Oncology (ICD-O)*.

ICF See *International Classification of Functioning, Disability, and Health (ICF)*. Also see *intermediate care facility (ICF)*.

ICF MR See *intermediate care facility for mentally retarded (ICF MR)*.

ICHI See *International Classification of Health Interventions (ICHI)*.

ICN See *internal control number (ICN)*.

ICR See *intelligent character recognition (ICR)* and *image copy recognition (ICR)*.

ICU See *intensive care unit (ICU)*.

ID card See *identification card (ID card)*.

ID qualifier Alpha characters or numbers that relate to either the medical provider's state license number or national provider identifier. These data must be inserted on the CMS-1500 (08-05) claim form in Block 24I (see Figure I-2).

ID # See *identification number (ID #)*.

identification card (ID card) Health insurance card issued to the insured (member or subscriber) as proof of membership from a private insurance plan, managed care plan, or government program (see Figure I-1). ID cards do not guarantee eligibility for medical benefits but verify the patient has health coverage. It includes the insured's name, member number, group number, type of coverage, effective date, deductible, copayment, and other information. This card is produced when a patient wishes to receive medical services, and usually the provider's staff photocopies the front and back sides for reference when submitting an insurance claim. Also called *membership card* and *health insurance card*.

identification number (ID #) See *certificate number*.

identity theft See *medical identity theft*.

IDS See *integrated delivery system (IDS)*.

IDTF See *independent diagnostic testing facility (IDTF)*.

IEEE See *Institute of Electrical and Electronics Engineers, Inc. (IEEE)*.

IEP See *initial enrollment period (IEP)*.

IEQ See *initial enrollment questionnaire (IEQ)*.

IG See *implementation guide (IG)*.

IGI See *intergovernmental initiative (IGI)*.

IHDS Acronym for integrated health delivery system. See *accountable health plan (AHP)*.

IHN See *integrated health care network (IHN)*.

IHO Acronym for integrated health care organization. See *integrated delivery system (IDS)*.

IHS Acronym for integrated health system. See *accountable health plan (AHP)*.

IHS Acronym for integrated health care system (IHS). See *integrated delivery system (IDS)*.

illness perils Insurance category used by health insurance underwriters to review the type and degree of peril of particular jobs such as exposure to dust, poisons, and extreme temperatures.

IM See *internal medicine (IM)*.

image copy recognition (ICR) Same as *optical character recognition (OCR)*.

IME Abbreviation for independent medical evaluation, independent medical examiner, and independent medical evaluator. See *independent medical evaluation (IME)*, *independent medical examiner (IME)*, and *independent medical evaluator (IME)*.

immediate annuity Contract that begins making periodic payments to the annuitant within 1 year from the purchased date.

immediate maternity Insurance coverage for a pregnancy that begins before the date the individual becomes insured.

immediate nonemergency care Instant treatment for a medical, surgical, or dental condition or symptom that is not an emergent situation but is given for the health and well-being of the individual.

immediate participation guarantee (IPG) contract Agreement that does not completely protect the plan sponsor against investment loss or minimum investment returns.

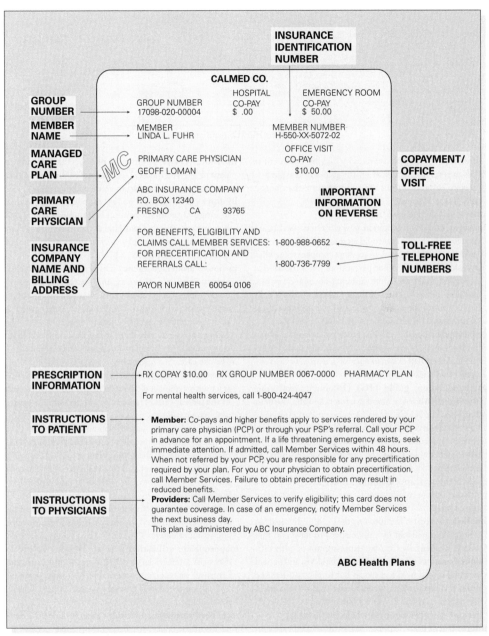

Figure I-1 Front *(top)* and back *(bottom)* sides of an insurance card.

immigrant See *alien*.

immunosuppressive drugs Transplant drugs used to reduce the risk of rejecting the new kidney after transplant. Transplant patients need to take these drugs for the rest of their lives.

immunosuppressive therapy Treatment by administering an agent that significantly interferes with the ability of the body's immune system to respond to antigenic stimulation by inhibiting cellular and humoral immunity such as preparing someone for a bone marrow transplant or to prevent rejection of donor tissue.

IMO See *independent marketing organization (IMO)*.

impact program Plan of managing and controlling expensive inpatient hospital costs that supports wise

Qualifier   Identifier

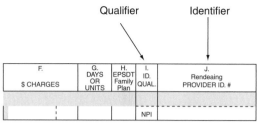

F. $ CHARGES	G. DAYS OR UNITS	H. EPSDT Family Plan	I. ID. QUAL.	J. Rendeaing PROVIDER ID. #
			NPI	

Figure I-2 ID qualifier.

utilization of medical services by moving treatment to less expensive settings when suitable and checking to be sure patients do not spend more time than necessary in the hospital.

impaired risk See *modified risk.*

impairment 1. Any condition of the insured's health, job, activities, or lifestyle that could increase his or her expected mortality or morbidity. 2. In workers' compensation when an injured worker cannot perform all job activities that he or she could do before suffering an injury but may perform some job duties. If the impairment substantially limits a major life activity, then a worker may qualify as disabled under the Americans with Disabilities Act.

impairment rider Health insurance policy provision that limits or denies coverage for a specific physical impairment. Also called *exclusion rider* or *impairment waiver.*

impairment waiver See *impairment rider.*

implementation guide (IG) Document explaining the proper use of a standard for a specific business purpose. The X12N Health Insurance Portability and Accountability Act (HIPAA) IGs are the primary reference documents used by those implementing the associated transactions and are incorporated into the HIPAA regulations by reference.

implementation specification Under HIPAA, precise instructions or requirements for putting a standard into operation.

implied authority Permission that an individual or company intends an insurance agent to have and that occurs incidentally from an express grant of authority.

implied contract Contract between physician and patient not manifested by direct words but implied or deduced from the circumstance, general language, or conduct of the patient. Insurance contracts are not implied contracts because every condition is included in the policy.

improvement plan Proposal for measurable process or outcome improvement. The plan is usually developed cooperatively by a provider and the managed care network. The plan must address how and when its results will be measured.

IMS Acronym for integrated medical system. See *integrated delivery system (IDS).*

in-area Within the geographical boundaries defined by a health maintenance organization as the area in which it will provide medical services to its members.

in-before-service Insurance phrase that means a patient is given medical services earlier than the effective date of membership in an insurance plan.

in force 1. Insurance policy that has not expired. 2. Original premium paid on an insurance policy that has not expired. 3. Total quantity of insurance at any specific time as far as cases, lives, amount (volume) of insurance, or premiums.

in-house brokerage agency Division in an exclusive-agency insurance company and staffed by company-employed brokerage sales agents. They solicit distribution agreements with other companies offering products that the exclusive-agent company does not have. The company's agents can then broker business with those companies through the in-house brokerage agency.

in-house care See *direct care.*

in network Group of physicians and hospitals who contract with a managed care plan to give care to members of the plan at certain rates and to do the administrative plan paperwork.

in plan Health care services obtained or chosen by a managed care plan member from a network or participating provider of the health plan.

in situ Description applied to a malignant growth confined to the site of origin without invasion of neighboring tissues.

inactive Term that refers to the health insurance status of a group or insured indicating it has been canceled and is not effective.

inappropriate utilization Use of services that are in excess of a beneficiary's medical needs and condition (overuse) or receiving a capitated Medicare payment and failing to provide services to meet a beneficiary's medical needs and condition (under use).

incentive coinsurance provision Rider included in a dental insurance policy that encourages regular dental care by stating that the insurance company will pay a higher percentage of dental expenses if the insured obtains regular dental examinations for preventive maintenance.

incentives Financial motivators offered to providers to help encourage efficiency and quality of health services and its delivery such as managed care contract agreements that offer profit-sharing, pooling, withhold pool, bonus pool, or risk pool. Arrangements are used to persuade physicians to decrease patients' hospital days, increase preventive health services, and consider alternative treatment.

incidence Frequency of new occurrences of a medical condition within a defined time interval. The incidence rate is the number of new cases of specific disease divided by the number of people in a population over a specified period of time, usually 1 year.

incidence rate Rate of new cases of a disease or health condition in a specified population over a defined period. To calculate an incidence rate, look at the number of new cases occurring in a population that is at risk for getting the disease over a specific time period.

incident of ownership Right to exercise any insurance policy privilege such as right to change the beneficiary, cancel or surrender a policy, assign the policy, obtain a policy loan, or use the policy as collateral for a loan.

incident-to billing 1. In the Medicare program, billing for medical services provided by an employee of a provider who is a nurse, physician's assistant, anesthetist, psychologist, technician, occupational therapist, or physical therapist. The services and supplies must be furnished under the direct supervision of the physician or other practitioner. The physician or other practitioner directly supervising the auxiliary personnel need not be the same physician or other practitioner on whose professional service the incident-to service is based. The physician does not need to be physically in the room with the ancillary provider, but he or she must be available in the immediate office suite. 2. Incident-to billing excludes inpatient hospital billing. Many hospital outpatient services need the presence and monitoring of a physician and contain incident-to language. Physicians must be in the same building when incident-to services are given by qualified providers, so physicians may need to sign in and out of a log book to document when they are on and off site. 3. Third-party payers may or may not recognize incident-to billing, and each insurance carrier has its own policies about it.

incident-to service 1. Benefit paid by Medicare for a service provided by an employee who is a nurse, physician's assistant, anesthetist, psychologist, technician, occupational therapist, or physical therapist. A physician bills Medicare for the service. When the services provided are integral, though incidental, to the physician's professional service and are performed under direct supervision of the physician, Medicare classifies this care as "incident to a physician's professional services" (e.g., a diabetic patient who reports to a clinic for checkups. 2. In the hospital setting, this term is used for revenue codes for pharmacy, supplies, and anesthesia with radiological procedures and other diagnostic services.

incision and drainage (I & D) To cut body tissue (e.g., wound or cavity) and remove fluid or infected material.

includes notes Phrase used in ICD-9-CM numeric code system to identify conditions that are included for coding diagnoses.

inclusion note Phrase used in ICD-9-CM numeric code system that identifies lists of conditions that are similar and may be coded or classified by the same medical code.

income limit 1. Maximum amount of income that a person can earn and still qualify for health insurance. 2. Maximum amount of income protection an insurance company will issue.

income protection insurance policy Type of disability income policy that states that an insured is disabled if he or she suffers an income loss due to a disability.

income rate Ratio of income tax revenues on an incurred basis (payroll tax contributions and income from the taxation of Old Age, Survivors, Health and Disability Insurance [OASDI] benefits) to the health insurance taxable payroll for the year.

income replacement ratio Percentage of pension income that a retiree would require after retirement to retain a standard of living that is equal to his or her preretirement standards. Because a retired individual's expenses are less when retired, this ratio is usually less than 100%.

incomplete claim Any Medicare claim missing required information; such claims are identified to the provider so that they may be resubmitted.

incontestable clause Provision in a health insurance contract or life insurance policy that states that the insurer is prohibited from disputing the coverage stated in the policy for certain conditions after it has been in force for 2 (or sometimes 3) years. Sometimes this clause is used in noncancelable guaranteed renewable insurance policies.

increase in coverage Additional health insurance benefits for an individual or group because of a change in class, wage or salary increase, occupational promotion, or negotiated benefits.

increasing term insurance Type of term insurance in which the death benefit increases during the coverage either at specific intervals, by a certain amount or percentage, or according to the cost of living.

incremental nursing charge In the hospital setting, a nursing service fee that is assessed in addition to the room and board charge.

incurred but not reported (IBNR) Dollar amount the insured payer's plan builds up to anticipate unknown medical expenses.

incur To suffer or become liable for a financial loss, medical claim, or health expense such as when a health insurance plan is legally responsible and must pay on a claim for an insured.

incurred basis Costs based on when the medical service was performed rather than when the payment was made.

incurred but not reported (IBNR) Cash reserve established by an insurance company or managed care plan to pay for medical services that have been provided to members but for which claims have not yet been received by the payer. These cash reserves are created by using an estimate based on prior insurance claims submissions. Also called *unreported claims.*

incurred but unpaid claims Reported and unreported insurance claims that have not been paid for a specific date.

incurred claim reserve Estimate of insurance claims that actually are incurred in a policy year plus the change of the claim reserves as of the end of the year. The change in reserves stands for the difference between the end-of-the-year and beginning-of-the-year claim reserves.

incurred claims Total dollar amount of insurance claims within a specific period of time regardless of when those claims are reimbursed.

incurred claims loss ratio Proportion of the claims incurred to the premiums earned to establish the loss. This ratio is based on a formula by taking incurred claims added to expenses and divided by premiums.

incurred-to-paid ratios Proportion of the annually incurred claims to the annually paid claims.

indefinite delivery/indefinite quantity (ID/IQ) Type of contract that provides for an indefinite quantity of supplies or services during a fixed period of time. Under the Federal Acquisition Regulations (FAR) in 16.501(a), when a government program manager is unsure of the exact quantity of products or services needed to fulfill his or her agency's needs, or the exact time at which these products or services will be necessary, an Indefinite Delivery/Indefinite Quantity (ID/IQ) contract provides the solution. Supplies or services are acquired through the issuance of individual delivery orders or individual task orders (i.e., Job Order Contracts). An ID/IQ contract is ideal for many government contracting officers because the tasks can be aligned in accordance with the agency's available funding. Also known as *job order contracting (JOC)* to public entities.

indemnification 1. Act of compensating for loss or damage sustained. 2. Compensation.

indemnification by corporation Corporation agrees to hold the doctor and his or her agents and employees harmless from any and all liability, loss, damage, claim, or expense of any kind including costs and attorneys' fees that result from negligent or willful acts or omissions by the corporation and its officers, agents, or employees in connection with the duties and obligations of the corporation under an agreement.

indemnification by physician Doctor agrees to hold corporation and payer and their officers, agents, and employees harmless from any and all liability, loss, damage, claim, or expense of any kind including costs and attorneys' fees that result from negligent or willful acts or omissions by the doctor or his or her agents or employees in connection with the duties and obligations of the physician under an agreement.

indemnify To compensate for a loss.

indemnity 1. Obligation to make good any loss, damage, or liability incurred by another. 2. Right of an injured individual to claim reimbursement for its loss, damage, or liability from a person who has such a duty. 3. Benefits paid to insured by an insurance policy for a loss; also known as *reimbursement.*

indemnity benefits plan Type of health insurance policy in which benefits in the form of cash payments are sent to the insured instead of service benefit payments to the service provider. The contract usually lists the maximum amounts paid for each covered service. Usually, after the service provider has billed the patient, the insured individual submits proof of payment to the insurance company and is reimbursed by the company for the covered costs and makes up the balance himself.

indemnity carrier See *insurance carrier.*

indemnity insurance Traditional health insurance plan, also known as *fee-for-service.* See *fee-for-service (FFS) reimbursement.*

indemnity limit See *maximum benefit period.*

indemnity plan Health insurance plan in which the insured pays 100% of all medical bills until he or she reaches the annual deductible and then the insurance company pays a percentage of covered benefits up to a maximum amount. Most indemnity plans pay 80% of total charges, leaving policyholders with a 20% coinsurance. The insured may obtain care from any health care provider and the provider is paid each time a service is rendered on a fee-for-service basis. The insured pays a fixed monthly premium, but these plans are more expensive than a managed care plan. These plans often provide coverage only for medically necessary doctor visits and not preventive care. A "pure" indemnity plan has no controls on utilization or price; a "managed" indemnity plan incorporates some utilization review and case management. Schedule of allowances, table of allowances, and usual, customary, and reasonable (UCR) are examples of indemnity plan fee schedules. Also known as *indemnity insurance, conventional group insurance,* and *traditional insurance.*

indemnity schedule See *schedule of allowances, fee schedule,* and *usual, customary, and reasonable (UCR).*

indented codes In ICD-9-CM, codes listed after stand-alone codes whose descriptions have a dependent status. To read the description, you must first read the description of the stand-alone code that comes before the semicolon (;) and then continue with the indented description listed by the subsequent code (indented code).

independent agent Self-employed insurance company representative who may represent two or more insurance companies and is paid on a commission basis.

independent contractor (IC) Individual who agrees to work under a negotiated contract (written or verbal) but is not under the control or an employee of the person or company with which the contract is made.

independent diagnostic testing facility (IDTF) Medicare provider or supplier that furnishes diagnostic tests such as a physician, group of physicians, or laboratory. Also called *testing facility*.

independent laboratory Freestanding clinical laboratory that meets conditions for participation in the Medicare program and bills through a carrier. It is not connected with a hospital, clinic, or physician's office. It is certified to perform diagnostic and/or clinical tests independent of an institution or a physician's office.

independent life broker Licensed insurance broker who operates independently and sells certain types of insurance products or handles estate planning.

independent living facility Living quarters composed of rental units in which services are not included as part of the rent. However, services may be available at the site and purchased by the residents for additional fees.

independent marketing organization (IMO) Association that contracts with an insurance company to distribute and carry out other marketing for the company's products.

independent medical evaluation (IME) In workers' compensation cases or disability cases, an impartial examination by a physician to settle a dispute about the nature and extent of an illness or injury.

independent medical evaluator (IME) Physician who is certified by the Industrial Medical Council (IMC) and conducts medicolegal evaluations of injured workers in workers' compensation cases for insurance companies or workers' compensation appeals board. IMEs render an unbiased opinion about the degree of disability of an injured worker. In addition to workers' compensation cases, sometimes an IME is required for disability insurance, liability lawsuit, or other legal proceedings. May be referred to as *agreed medical evaluator (AME)* or *qualified medical evaluator (QME)*.

independent medical examiner (IME) Physicians who make examinations of individuals, independent of the attending physician, and render an unbiased opinion regarding the degree of disability of a worker. IMEs are appointed by the referee or appeals board at state expense when a judge thinks additional medical evidence is necessary to provide a basis for a decision on an issue presented by the involved parties.

independent practice association (IPA) Type of managed care organization (MCO) in which a program administrator contracts with a number of physicians who agree to provide treatment to members (subscribers) in their own offices. This is a group association that has no common facilities and is open-panel because a physician's practice is not limited to IPA patients. Physicians are not employees of the MCO and are not paid salaries. They receive reimbursement on a capitation or fee-for-service basis; also referred to as a *medical capitation plan*. Also known as *individual practice organization (IPO)*.

independent property/casualty (P/C) brokers Independent insurance agents or agencies that distribute many property/casualty insurance industry products from what is commonly known as *independent agency system* or *American Agency System*.

indeterminate premium life insurance Type of non-participating whole life insurance that specifies both a maximum possible premium rate and a lower premium rate. The policy owner pays the lower rate for a certain period from when the policy is purchased and later the rate changes depending on the investment earnings of the insurance company. The premium rate will never be greater than the maximum premium rate. Also called *flexible premium life insurance, nonguaranteed premium life insurance*, and *variable premium life insurance*.

index case First infected person who started the outbreak of a disease (e.g., state department of health will investigate students attending a school to locate the index case of an outbreak of meningitis).

index convention Space-saving rule used in the Index, which is the last section of the annually published *Current Procedural Terminology* code book. For example:

Knee
Incision (of)

In this example, the word in parentheses (of) does not appear in the Index, but it is inferred. As another example:

Pancreas
Anesthesia (for procedures on)

In this example, because there is no such entity as *pancreas anesthesia*, the words in parentheses are inferred (i.e., anesthesia for procedures on the pancreas).

indexation Adjustment of postretirement benefits to compensate for the effects of inflation such as increasing pension benefits to the Consumer Price Index (CPI) to make up for a change in the cost of living.

indexed life insurance Whole life plan of insurance that provides for a premium rate increase automatically every year to correspond with any increase in the Consumer Price Index (CPI) to make up for a change in the cost of living.

indicator 1. Key clinical value or quality characteristic used to measure, over time, the performance, processes, and outcomes of an organization or some component of health care delivery. 2. Correct coding initiative (CCI) indicators designate which procedure codes can be pulled out of a bundle and which cannot.

indigent Individual who is not able to pay for medical services or treatments and is not eligible for benefits under the Medicaid or other public assistance program.

indigent care See *charity care.*

indigent medical care See *charity care.*

indirect costs 1. Medical practice business overhead costs that are not associated with the physician's medical service directly provided to the patient (e.g., rent, office supplies, utilities). 2. In managed care programs, cost that cannot be associated directly with a certain activity, service, or product. Indirect costs are usually distributed among the plan's services in proportion to each service's share of direct costs.

indirect medical education adjustment Change or modification applied to payments under the prospective payment system (PPS) for hospitals that operate approved graduate medical education programs. For operating costs, the adjustment is based on the hospital's ratio of interns and residents to the number of beds. For capital costs, the adjustment is based on the hospital's ratio of interns and residents to average daily occupancy.

indirect payer See *third-party payer, insurance company, insurer,* or *payer.*

indirect treatment relationship Association or connection between an individual and a health care provider in which the provider delivers care to the patient based on orders from another physician and the provider either gives services and supplies, reports diagnoses, or provides results directly to another provider who interacts with the patient. For example, a radiologist or a pathologist would be considered to have indirect treatment relationships with patients because they provide diagnostic services requested by other providers and furnish results to the patient through the direct treating physician.

individual Under the Health Insurance Portability and Accountability Act (HIPAA), the person who is the subject of protected health information.

individual account plan Retirement plan that is funded in accordance with a formula based on a certain percentage of the participant's compensation.

individual consideration Insurance claim that must be reviewed because of an unusual, unique, or variation from standard medical service to determine the benefit or payment allowance.

individual contract See *individual health plan.*

individual deductible See *deductible.*

individual employer groups Name of a segment of the insurance market of single employers that provide insurance coverage for their employees through a master contract that is issued to the employer.

individual fraud Type of medical insurance fraud that is committed by individuals on their insurance claims so that they can obtain benefits in excess of their medical expenses. Also see *provider fraud* and *fraud.*

individual funding method Retirement plan funding system that is determined by first separately calculating the contributions for each of the plan's participants and then adding those amounts to obtain the total required contribution.

individual health insurance See *individual health plan.*

individual health plan Insurance health plan in which one person and his or her dependents are insured under a policy. Also called *individual health insurance, individual contract, individual medical plan,* or *personal insurance.*

individual insurance Life insurance issued to an individual person. Also called *ordinary life insurance* and *whole life insurance.*

individual market Individual and his or her dependents who do not have group health insurance and may be insured under an individual plan.

individual medical plan See *individual health plan.*

individual membership Single type of membership in a managed care plan or insurance program in which one person is insured. Other types are family membership and group membership.

individual policy Health insurance policy purchased by an individual or family.

individual policy pension trust Type of retirement plan used for small groups and administered by trustees who are authorized to buy individual level premium policies or annuity contracts for each member of the plan. Usually the policies offer life insurance and retirement benefits.

individual practice association (IPA) See *independent practice association (IPA).*

individual practice organization (IPO) See *independent practice association (IPA).*

individual responsibility program (IRP) Infrequently seen state program in which physicians accept all patients but refuse to accept reimbursement from any third party, private or government. The provider directly bills the patient and the patient applies to the insurance company for reimbursement.

individual retirement account (IRA) Tax-deferred monies set aside for retirement in an approved account that allows individuals to make pretax contributions. Contributions and investment earnings are taxable as income when paid out of the account. IRAs can be established through financial institutions such as insurance companies and stock brokerages. Also see *Section 408(k) of the Internal Revenue Code.*

individual specific stop loss Situation when a member of a group of a managed care plan incurs insurance claims in excess of a certain dollar limit during the contract period and this excess it not charged against the group's experience. Also see *stop loss.*

individually identifiable health information Under the Health Insurance Portability and Accountability Act (HIPAA), data that comprises a subset of health information including demographic information collected from an individual and created or received by a health care provider, health plan, employer, or health care clearinghouse. It relates to past, present, or future physical or mental health or condition of an individual and it identifies the individual.

industrial accident Unforeseen, unintended event that takes place at the worker's job site. Also known as *workers' compensation injury.*

Industrial Accident Commission Office that administers and governs workers' compensation regulations in each state.

industrial insurance See *workers' compensation (WC) insurance.*

industry-wide liability See *enterprise liability.*

infectious disease Any communicable disease or one that can be transmitted from one human to another or from animal to human by direct or indirect contact.

infectious material Human body fluids that are considered potentially contagious are amniotic fluid, cerebrospinal fluid, pericardial fluid, peritoneal fluid, pleural fluid, saliva, semen, synovial fluid, vaginal secretions, any body fluid that is contaminated with blood, and all body fluids where it is difficult to differentiate among body fluids. Infectious material also refers to unfixed tissue or organ from a human (living or dead), cell or tissue cultures containing human immunodeficiency virus (HIV) and blood, and organs or tissues from animals infected with HIV or hepatitis B virus (HBV).

infertility Condition of being unable to produce offspring.

inflation guard clause Additional provision to a homeowner's insurance policy that automatically adjusts the dwelling limit on renewal of the policy because of current construction costs. Also called *inflation guard endorsement.*

inflation guard endorsement See *inflation guard clause.*

influenza vaccine Preparation of killed microorganisms, living attenuated organisms, or living fully virulent organisms that is administered to produce or artificially increase immunity to influenza.

informal review In the Medicare program, this was formerly referred to as the *first level of appeal process.* See *redetermination process.*

information model Conceptual example of the information needed to support a business function or process.

information services (IS) Administrators of the computer systems used by third-party payers and health care providers.

information technology (IT) System that is a merging of the computer (software and hardware) with high-speed telecommunication links carrying data, sound, and video. It is often used interchangeably with information system (IS). Physicians use IT to help run their practices such as obtaining treatment guidelines, exchanging clinical data with other physicians, accessing patient notes, generating reminders, and writing prescriptions.

informed consent The patient must acknowledge that he or she understands what choices are available, what the risks associated with each option are, and the information relayed. Informed consent is required before performing most invasive procedures and before admitting a patient to a research study. A signed permission document is obtained from a patient to perform a specific test or procedure.

informed consent form Signed permission obtained from a patient to perform a specific test or procedure. See *informed consent.*

infusion pump Device used for giving fluid or medication into a patient's vein at a specific rate or over a set amount of time.

initial claim determination First adjudication made by an insurance carrier or fiscal intermediary (FI) following a request for Medicare payment or the first determination made by a peer review organization either in a prepayment or postpayment context.

initial coverage Under a Medicare Part D plan, this phrase means the plan covers the first $2250 of total drug costs (the amount the insured and plan pays).

initial coverage election period For Medicare beneficiaries, this is a time 3 months immediately before a person is entitled to Medicare Part A and enrolled in Part B. If he or she chooses to join a Medicare health plan during the initial coverage election period, the plan must accept him or her. The only time a plan can deny enrollment during this period is when it has reached its member limit. This limit is approved by the Centers for Medicare and Medicaid Services (CMS). The initial coverage election period is different from the initial enrollment period (IEP). See *election period.*

initial enrollment period (IEP) One of four periods during which an individual can enroll in Medicare Part A. The IEP is the first chance the person has to enroll in Medicare Part A. This period starts 3 months before he or she first meets all the eligibility requirements for Medicare and continues for 7 months. Also see *annual enrollment period (AEP), general enrollment period (GEP), open enrollment period (OEP), special enrollment period (SEP),* and *transfer enrollment period (TEP).*

initial enrollment questionnaire (IEQ) Feedback form sent to the Medicare beneficiary when he or she becomes eligible for Medicare to learn if he or she has other insurance that should pay the medical bills before Medicare.

initial premium Amount to be paid at the beginning of insurance coverage but subject to change after additional experience or information has been obtained.

initial preventive physical examination (IPPE) First time an individual goes to see a physician for objective inspection and/or testing of organ systems or body areas to prevent the occurrence of illness, injury, and disease.

initial rate Premium amount paid on or before the effective date of a new insurance policy.

initial rehabilitation evaluation First procedures by a rehabilitation specialist after a case has been referred (i.e., contact the insured, employer, and physician). Factors investigated relate to medical, psychological, social, vocational, education, and economics to determine what action to take for rehabilitation of the insured.

initial reserve Funds set aside by an insurance company at the beginning of the insurance policy year. An initial reserve includes the net annual premium that is due on the policy.

injury 1. In a workers' compensation policy, this term signifies any injury or disease sustained, arising out of, and in the course of employment including injury to artificial members and medical braces of all types. 2. Bodily damage of an insured by an accident while the policy is in force.

injury, cumulative Industrial injury that occurs because of repetitive mentally or physically traumatic activities extending over a period of time, the combined effect of which causes a disability or need for medical treatment.

injury, specific Industrial injury that occurs as the result of one incident or exposure that causes disability or need for medical treatment.

inlier Hospital inpatient whose length of stay or cost of treatment is like those of most other patients in the same diagnosis-related group (DRG).

inpatient (IP) 1. Term used when a patient is admitted to the hospital or other health facility for overnight stay for the purpose of receiving a diagnosis, treatment, or other health service. 2. Relating to the care and treatment of a patient admitted as a bed patient to a facility or to a hospital for 24-hour care.

inpatient admission Registration of a patient as a bed patient who is provided with room, board, and continuous nursing service in a hospital or facility for overnight stay.

inpatient ancillary services Supplementary hospital inpatient services for which there are no additional charges (e.g., routine nursing care).

inpatient bed day See *bed day, inpatient.*

inpatient benefits Hospital inpatient benefits covered for an insured under an insurance plan such as daily room and board charges and other necessary services and supply charges.

inpatient care Medical services that the patient receives when he or she is admitted to a hospital, nursing home, postacute care institution, or psychiatric institution for overnight stay.

inpatient census Number of inpatients in a hospital facility during a specific time.

inpatient days of stay See *length of stay (LOS).*

inpatient hospital Medical facility, other than psychiatric, which primarily provides diagnostic, therapeutic (surgical and nonsurgical), and rehabilitation services by or under the supervision of physicians to patients admitted for a variety of medical conditions.

inpatient hospital claim Formal request for payment (bill) sent to the insurance company listing inpatient services with dollar amounts incurred by an insured.

inpatient hospital deductible Amount of money that is subtracted from the amount payable by Medicare Part A for inpatient hospital services furnished to a beneficiary during a spell of illness.

inpatient hospital services See *inpatient services.*

inpatient hospital stay See *inpatient hospitalization.*

inpatient hospitalization Period of time from the day of admission to the day of discharge from the hospital of a bed patient usually without interruption. This period includes the day of admission but not the day of discharge in the length-of-stay calculation.

inpatient prospective payment system (IPPS) Mandated system by the Tax Equity and Fiscal Responsibility Act (TEFRA) in 1983. It provides a predetermined rate of payment for each discharge for all acute hospital inpatient services and is known as the *diagnosis-related groups (DRGs).* See *diagnosis-related groups (DRGs).*

inpatient psychiatric facility Medical facility that provides care for an individual admitted for an overnight or longer stay for the diagnosis and treatment of mental illness on a 24-hour basis by or under the supervision of a physician.

inpatient reimbursement Insurance payment or payment by the patient to the hospital facility for the costs sustained to treat an individual admitted as a bed patient.

inpatient services Hospitalized benefits and items that are provided to an inpatient such as room and board, nursing care, diagnostic and therapeutic services, and medical and surgical services. Also called *inpatient hospital services.*

input That which goes into a computer memory bank.

inquiry See *tracer.*

inside build-up See *cash value.*

inside limit Maximum amount payable for a particular benefit under an insurance or managed care contract (e.g., $150 limit on daily hospital room and board). Inside limits may apply to procedures, services, confinement, disability, or calendar year.

insolvency Situation when a health plan has no money or other means to stay open, meet contract obligations, or give health care to patients.

insolvency clause Provision in many reinsurance contracts that specifies if the ceding company becomes insolvent, the reinsurer must pay the ceding company or its liquidator all reinsurance that comes payable even if the ceding company has failed to pay all or a portion of any claim. This provision is required by most state regulations.

insolvent 1. Unable to meet debts or discharge liabilities. 2. Bankrupt.

insolvent debtor Insolvent individual, partnership, corporation, or business association involved in a liquidation proceeding.

inspection Report that describes the evaluation of risk by an insurance company.

inspection company Professional independent agency that investigates individuals who apply for insurance.

inspection receipt Proof of payment slip that is given to an insurance applicant when he or she receives a policy for review. The receipt informs the applicant that the insurance is not effective until acceptance and legal delivery by the insurance company.

inspection report 1. Investigative report by a consumer reporting agency about a proposed insured's lifestyle, job, and financial background. 2. Document prepared by an inspection agency summarizing data about an applicant for a life or health insurance policy (i.e., financial, habits, morals, and physical condition).

installation 1. Procedure of helping a group policyholder in setting up initial and continuing administrative practices of the group's insurance plan. 2. Activities from the time an applicant decides to purchase a group insurance policy to the time the contract and its certificates are issued.

installment certificate Official document issued to the beneficiary of a life insurance policy that states the amount of each benefit payment and/or the period during which benefit payments are to be made under a settlement option. It also states if a beneficiary is allowed to withdraw all or part of the funds during the payment period.

installment disability income benefits Provision in a group term life insurance policy that equal installments are paid by the insurer over a specified time period in the event of an insured's total and permanent disability.

installment refund option Life income option with a refund that specifies that proceeds remaining on the death of the beneficiary will be paid in installments to the contingent payee.

installment settlement Payment of an insurance policy's proceeds in a series of payments at regular intervals instead of a lump sum.

Institute of Electrical and Electronics Engineers, Inc. (IEEE) Nonprofit professional association for the advancement of technology referred to by the letters I-E-E-E (pronounced "eye-triple-E"). IEEE is a leading authority on areas ranging from aerospace systems, computers, and telecommunications to biomedical engineering, electric power, and consumer electronics.

institution Under the Medicare program, a facility that meets Medicare's definition of a long-term care facility such as a nursing home or skilled nursing facility. This does not include assisted or adult living facilities or residential homes.

institutional health services Medical services provided on an inpatient basis in hospitals, nursing homes, or other inpatient facilities. Some institutions and departments within organized units use this phrase to refer to services delivered on an outpatient basis.

institutional providers Hospitals, ambulatory surgical centers, nursing homes, day care centers, and alcohol and substance abuse centers that have a contractual agreement with an insurance plan to provide health care services to members of managed care plans and eligible Medicare beneficiaries. Institutional providers bill the insurance carrier or fiscal intermediary directly.

institutional review boards (IRBs) Advisory boards composed of physicians, scientific professors, ethicists, and concerned nonscientists that have been created by federal legislation to oversee research on human subjects and to protect those subjects from research abuses.

instructional notes Detailed descriptions about diagnostic code selection for the insurance biller that appear at the beginning of a heading, in parentheses before or after a code, or in parentheses as part of the code's description. Also see *inclusion note.*

instrumental activities of daily living (IADLs) Physical activities that are necessary for living independently in the community such as cooking meals, shopping for groceries, managing money, taking medications, using the telephone, doing laundry, and housekeeping. Compare with *activities of daily living (ADLs).*

insurability Physical, moral, occupational, and financial characteristics of a risk that are evaluated by an insurance company to determine whether to insure the entity.

insurability provision Insurance rider that says for a policy to become effective, the insured must be insurable at the time of delivery of the policy according to the underwriting rules and practices of the insurance company.

insurability statement Evaluation form that an insurance agent may present to an applicant to fill out when a considerable amount of time has passed between the time the original application is received by the insurance company and the time the policy is issued. It is used to determine if any insurability factors have changed since the original application was completed.

insurability type temporary insurance agreement Contract issued together with a conditional premium receipt that gives temporary life insurance coverage from the date stated in the agreement on the condition that the proposed insured is insurable.

insurable interest Concern of an insured or beneficiary in property or the life of an individual in which there would be financial loss if the insured died or if the property is damaged or destroyed. For example, if an individual sells an automobile and is paid in installments, he or she has an insurable interest in the automobile in proportion to how much money remains unpaid. The buyer also has an insurable interest.

insurable risk Potential of a foreseen loss to the insured that has the following conditions: loss not under the control of the insured, others are subject to the same loss, chance of loss is calculable, cost is economically feasible, would not affect all insureds at the same time, and has the potential to be a serious financial hardship if not insured.

insurance Contractual relationship between a first party (insurer) and a second party (insured) in which the insurer agrees to protect against risk and reimburse the insured for financial loss caused by certain contingencies or hazards (fire, accident, illness, death) in return for payment of a monthly or annual premium.

insurance adjuster Individual at the workers' compensation insurance carrier overseeing an industrial case, authorizing diagnostic testing and medical treatment, and communicating with the provider of medical care.

insurance agency See *agency.*

insurance agent See *agent.*

insurance balance billing Billing statement that is sent to the patient after his or her insurance company has paid its portion of the claim.

insurance billing specialist Professional practitioner who carries out claims completion, coding, and billing responsibilities in accordance with legal state and federal regulations and third-party payer guidelines. He or she may or may not perform managerial and supervisory functions; also known as an *insurance claims processor, medical biller,* or *reimbursement specialist.* Also see *medical insurance billing specialist.*

insurance broker See *agent.*

insurance carrier Insurance company that underwrites, administers, and sells health insurance benefit plans. Sometimes called *contractor, insurer,* or *administrative agent.* See also *fiscal agent* or *fiscal intermediary.*

insurance claim See *claim.*

insurance claim form Document that is completed detailing the medical services rendered to a patient by the provider or facility and submitted to the insurance company for payment.

insurance claim number Social Security number of the wage earner, which appears on the Medicare identification card.

insurance claims processor See *insurance billing specialist.*

insurance clause See *provision.*

insurance clerk See *insurance billing specialist.*

insurance collection specialist 1. Individual who works with an insurance company to resolve billing and reimbursement problems. 2. Someone who works for a medical practice to bill and collect payments, solve billing problems, and help increase cash flow.

Insurance Commissioner See *Commissioner of Insurance.*

insurance company Agency chartered under state laws that underwrites, administers, and sells many types of insurance plans (e.g., fire and marine, life, casualty,

health, liability). For those it insures, it agrees to pay all legitimate claims that may arise under the policy in exchange for a monthly or annual premium. Also called *agency* or *insurance agency, indirect payer, insurer,* or *payer.* See also *insurance carrier, fiscal agent, fiscal intermediary (FI),* or *agency.*

insurance contract See *insurance policy.*

insurance counselor Person who assists the patient by obtaining information and identifying the amount that health insurance pays for a specific medical service and determines the amount the patient is responsible for paying. Also known as *patient account representative* or *patient service representative.*

insurance department Division or section within each state government that oversees, administers, and enforces state insurance laws and regulations. It is a valuable source of information about all types of insurance and handles consumer inquiries and complaints. It licenses insurance companies and agents.

insurance examiner Representative of a state department of insurance who performs official audits and investigates the compliance of insurance companies to regulations.

insurance fraud See *fraud.*

insurance information Data about the managed care plan or government program of which the patient is a member or beneficiary such as the program or plan's name and address, insured's name, insured's identification number, and group number and name.

insurance month Period beginning on a specific date (e.g., June 15) of any calendar month and ending on a day (July 14) of the next succeeding calendar month.

insurance policy Printed document that is a legally enforceable agreement stating the conditions and terms of the insurance contract between an individual or organization and the insurance company that is issued to the policyholder by the company; also referred to as *insurance contract* and *policy.*

insurance pool Group of insurance companies that combine some assets to provide an amount of insurance that is greater than that which can be provided by an individual company.

insurance provision See *provision.*

insurance register See *register.*

Insurance Regulatory Information System (IRIS) Information method developed by the National Association of Insurance Commissioners (NAIC) to help state regulatory agencies evaluate the financial stability of insurance companies by using a series of ratios from the companies' statutory annual statements.

insurance-to-value policy Insurance policy that is written in an amount that is close to the value of the property insured.

insurance trust Written agreement created during the lifetime of the individual who creates the trust. It is funded by insurance policies on the life of the trust's creator or by the proceeds from the policies.

insurance verification See *eligibility verification.*

insurance year of birth Insured individual's year of birth under a group insurance plan that represents the insurance age of the person on the policy anniversary.

insured Individual or organization protected in case of loss under the terms of an insurance policy. Also called *enrollee, beneficiary, enrolled patient, member, policyholder,* or *subscriber.*

insured funding To put monies into a retirement plan in which the sponsor of the plan buys annuity or life insurance contracts on behalf of each participant. The insurance company guarantees a specific benefit to each retiree.

insured plan Type of employer's funding instrument in which assets are held by a life insurance company under a group annuity contract guaranteeing payment of benefits.

insurer 1. See *insurance carrier.* 2. See *fiscal agent.* 3. See *fiscal intermediary.* Also known as *carrier, contractor, indirect payer, insurance company,* or *payer.*

insurer-administered group insurance plan Group insurance plan in which the insurance company does the administrative work such as computing premium amounts due and mailing monthly notices to the insureds.

insuring clause Section of an insurance policy that states the agreement and type of loss or damage that the insurer is protecting the insured against.

integrated carve-out plan System of combining two or more insurance benefit plans to prevent duplication of benefits or overinsurance. Also referred to as *integration.*

integrated deductible High preset amount (e.g., $2000) or the total benefits paid under a basic medical care plan, whichever is greater, that must be exceeded before supplemental major medical benefits are payable.

integrated delivery network See *integrated delivery system (IDS).*

integrated delivery system (IDS) Arrangement of several health care organizations rendering a network of medical services (facilities, physicians, ancillary service providers) to a specific population or geographical area. An advanced IDS form combines an insurance or third-party administrator so that there is no division between provider and payer. Also known as *integrated delivery network, integrated medical system (IMS), integrated healthcare system (IHS), integrated healthcare organization (IHO), integrated service network (ISN), integrated health delivery network,* or *organized care system.*

integrated dental plan Dental insurance plan that is part of a major medical insurance policy.

integrated health care network (IHN) Health care financing and delivery organizations established to give a continuum of care so that patients get the right care at the right time by the right provider. This continuum of care from primary care provider to specialist and ancillary provider under one corporate umbrella guarantees that patients get cared for appropriately, thus saving money and increasing the quality of care.

integrated health delivery network See *integrated delivery system (IDS).*

integrated health delivery system (IHDS) See *accountable health plan (AHP).*

integrated health system (IHS) See *accountable health plan (AHP).*

integrated healthcare organization (IHO) See *integrated delivery system (IDS).*

integrated healthcare system (IHS) See *integrated delivery system (IDS).*

integrated medical system (IMS) See *integrated delivery system (IDS).*

integrated pension plan Retirement plan in which benefits are coordinated with benefits of a government-sponsored pension plan.

integrated provider network (IPN) Arrangement of primary and secondary hospitals and physicians within a specific geographical area rendering a network of medical services.

integrated service network (ISN) See *accountable health plan (AHP).*

integration 1. Process used by hospital facilities and physicians in which they combine business operations to reduce expenses and increase health care services. There are different types of integration such as simple coordination (combine purchasing) to full integration (centralized administration and coordination of care). 2. Combination of two or more insurance benefit plans to prevent duplication of benefit payments. Also referred to as *integrated carve-out plan.*

integrative health care Medical care that incorporates the best approaches from conventional medicine and from complementary and alternative medicine. It includes the following specialty areas: acupuncturist, body work, chiropractic, conventional nursing, indigenous medicine, mental health care, minority health care, Oriental medicine, physical medicine, spiritual and prayer-based healing, Ayurvedic medicine, botanical medicine, clinical nutrition, holistic dentists and physicians, homeopathy, massage therapy, midwifery, naturopathic medicine, osteopathic medicine, and somatic educational. Alternative billing codes (ABCs) are used to bill for these services. Also called *integrative medicine.* See also *alternative medicine* and *alternative billing codes (ABCs).* Website: www.alternativelink.com

integrative medicine See *integrative health care.*

intelligent character recognition (ICR) Same as optical character recognition.

itemized billing statement Detailed invoice that lists charges, payments, adjustments, and total balance due. Also referred to as *billing statement* or *summary of charges.*

intensive care Constant complex health care as provided in various acute life-threatening conditions such as multiple trauma, severe burns, or myocardial infarction or after certain kinds of surgery. Life support systems are used such as respirators, monitors, and hypothermia equipment. Some insurance policies may increase the daily room and board benefit when an intensive care unit is necessary.

intensive care unit (ICU) Section in a hospital in which patients who require close monitoring and intensive care are kept. An ICU contains highly technical and sophisticated monitoring devices and equipment and is staffed by personnel to deliver critical care for various life-threatening conditions. A hospital may have several ICUs such as medical intensive care unit (MICU), surgical intensive care unit (SICU), pediatric intensive care unit (PICU), neonatal intensive care unit (NICU), and coronary care unit (CCU). Sometimes referred to as *special care unit.*

intensivist Physician who specializes in treating patients who need critical care.

inter vivo trust Trust created between living individuals that is usually revocable (it can be changed or revoked by the person who created it). Also known as *living trust.*

interactive telecommunication systems See *video conferencing.*

interactive transaction Back and forth communication between user and computer.

interagency agreement Written contract in which a federal agency agrees to provide to, purchase from, or exchange with another federal agency, services (including data), supplies, or equipment. Interagency agreements are between at least one component with the Department of Health and Human Services (DHHS) and another federal agency or component thereof.

interest Payment for the use of money during a specified period of time.

interest-adjusted cost Represents the average annual cost of a life insurance policy. This amount is obtained by calculating the premiums, dividends, and cash values. This cost amount is one figure calculated under the interest-adjusted net cost (IANC) method for comparing the costs of life insurance policies. Also called *surrender cost index (SCI).*

interest-adjusted net cost (IANC) method System of comparison of the costs of life insurance policies that weighs the dividends and cash values based on how much into the future the various amounts are payable. Three amounts are calculated: interest-adjusted cost, interest-adjusted payment, and the equivalent level annual dividend. Also known as *surrender cost index (SCI) method.*

interest-adjusted payment Represents the average annual payment of a life insurance policy. This amount is obtained by calculating premiums and dividends. This cost amount is one figure calculated under the interest-adjusted net cost (IANC) method for comparing the costs of life insurance policies. Also called *net payment cost index.*

interest option Provision in a life insurance policy in which the proceeds of the policy are temporarily left on deposit with the insurance company and the money earned on those proceeds is paid either annually, semiannually, quarterly, or monthly to the beneficiary.

interest-sensitive insurance See *investment-sensitive insurance.*

interest-sensitive whole life insurance See *current assumption whole life insurance.*

interface The point at which two different systems are linked (e.g., computer to printer or modem).

interfund borrowing Borrowing of assets by a trust fund (Old Age, Survivors, Health and Disability Insurance [OASHDI], health insurance [HI], or supplementary medical insurance [SMI]) from another of the trust funds when one of the funds is in danger of exhaustion. Interfund borrowing was authorized only during 1982-1987.

intergovernmental initiative (IGI) Cooperative relationship between governments or between agencies within a level of government together with federal, state, and local governments to provide integrated services and manage the delivery system (e.g., local dollars for indigent care are matched with federal Medicaid dollars).

interim bill Itemized statement that shows only the beginning stay at a hospital or skilled nursing facility. It is generated when the hospital expects to submit a series of inpatient insurance claims after a minimum confinement of 30 days. Interim bills may be submitted by a hospital that is under a prospective payment system every 60 days during the patient's confinement or course of treatment.

interim coverage Immediate initial insurance coverage of an individual who applies for insurance between the date of a prepaid premium and the date the insurance company notifies the applicant of its underwriting decision.

interim insurance agreement See *temporary insurance agreement (TIA).*

interim report Workers' compensation report submitted so that money can be paid to the physician during ongoing treatment of an industrial case.

intermediary See *fiscal intermediary (FI).*

intermediate care 1. Level of medical care for certain chronically ill or disabled individuals in which room and board are provided but skilled nursing care is not. Intermediate care is provided in a step-down unit that is also called an *intermediate care unit.*

2. Short-term care provided by many long-term facilities that may include rehabilitation services and care for certain conditions (stroke and diabetes) or postsurgical care. The goal is to discharge the patient to his or her home or to a lower level of care. Sometimes called *postacute care, subacute care,* or *transitional care.*

intermediate care facility (ICF) Institution furnishing health-related care and services to individuals who do not require the amount of care provided by hospitals or skilled nursing facilities.

intermediate care facility for mentally retarded (ICF MR) 1. Medical facility that primarily provides health-related care and services above the level of custodial care to mentally retarded and developmentally disabled individuals but does not provide the level of care available in a hospital or skilled nursing facility. 2. Optional Medicaid service. Each state defines its level of ICF MR care.

intermediate entities Entities that contract between a managed care organization (MCO) or one of its subcontractors and a physician or physician group, other than physician groups themselves. An independent practice association (IPA) is considered to be an intermediate entity if it contracts with one or more physician groups in addition to contracting with individual physicians.

intermediate repair Physical restoration of damaged tissue when the wound requires layered closure of one or more of the deeper layers of subcutaneous tissue and superficial (nonmuscle) fascia, in addition to the skin (epidermal and dermal) closure. Single-layer closure of heavily contaminated wounds that have required extensive cleaning or removal of particulate matter also constitutes intermediate repair and can be coded as such.

intermediate unit Hospital unit where patients are kept who do not require intensive care but who are not yet ready to be kept in a regular medical-surgical unit or are not ready to be released to independent care at home. Also called *step-down unit.*

intermittent peritoneal dialysis Periodic supine regimen that uses intermittent flow technique, automated assisted manual, or manual method in dialysis sessions two to four times weekly.

intermittent pain In a workers' compensation case, pain approximately 50% of the time.

intermittent symptoms Subjective indications of a disease or illness that occur about 50% of the time.

internal benchmarking See *benchmarking.*

internal control number (ICN) Number assigned by Medicare carriers to each insurance claim for control and inventory purposes. This number is composed of 15 digits, which indicate the claim type, region, year, Julian date, batch number, and sequence. This number should be referenced when communicating with the insurance carrier about a specific claim problem.

internal controls Business management systems and policies for reasonably documenting, monitoring, and correcting operational processes to prevent and detect waste and to ensure proper payment.

internal entrepreneur See *intrapreneur.*

internal limits Highest insurance plan amounts paid for each benefit or illness. The insured pays the remainder of the costs incurred. The insurance policy may state the limits in dollar amounts or in number of days payable.

internal medicine (IM) Branch of medicine concerned with the study of the physiologic and pathologic characteristics of the internal organs and the medical diagnosis and nonsurgical treatment of disorders of these organs. IM encompasses many subspecialties.

internal replacement To give up a life insurance policy because the insured wants to purchase another insurance policy issued by the same insurance company.

Internal Revenue Service (IRS)/Social Security Administration (SSA)/Centers for Medicare and Medicaid Services Data Match Process by which information on employers and employees is provided by the IRS and SSA and analyzed by the Centers for Medicare and Medicaid Services for use in contacting employers concerning a possible period of Medicare Secondary Payer (MSP). This information is used to update the Medicare Common Working File (CWF).

internal review Process of going over financial documents in the medical office before and after billing insurance carriers to determine documentation deficiencies or errors.

International Claim Association (ICA) ICA was founded in 1909 to promote efficiency, effectiveness, and high standards of performance in claim administration by member companies; provide a forum for research, education, and the exchange of ideas relating to various aspects of claim administration; and devise and effect measures for the benefit of policyholders and beneficiaries in matters relating to claims. ICA has been at the forefront of addressing a broad range of life, health, and disability claim issues including those relevant in the day-to-day operation of claim departments. The ICA provides a forum for information exchange and a program of education tailored to the needs of its member life and health insurance companies, reinsurers, managed care companies, TPAs, and Blue Cross and Blue Shield organizations worldwide.

International Classification of Diseases (ICD) Medical code set developed and maintained by the World Health Organization (WHO) primarily to classify causes of death. Eventually this code set became the standardized system of codes for diagnoses used to submit insurance claims for reimbursement to insurance carriers and for use in Health Insurance Portability and Accountability Act transactions.

International Classification of Diseases, Ninth Revision, Clinical Modification (ICD-9-CM) Diagnostic code book that uses primarily a numeric code system for classifying diseases and operations to assist collection of uniform and comparable health information. These codes are used by physicians and inpatient and outpatient facilities to effectively document the medical condition, symptom, or complaint of each patient when submitting insurance claims to insurance companies for payment. Its conventions include special terms, punctuation marks, abbreviations, or symbols to communicate special instructions to the coder. If the conventions are overlooked, the code number chosen may be incorrect. A code system to replace this is ICD-10, which has an implementation date set for October 1, 2013.

International Classification of Diseases, Oncology (ICD-O) Diagnostic code book first published in 1976 for classifying morphology of neoplasms. Of the five digits, the first four identify the histology of the neoplasm and the fifth identifies the neoplasm as either benign, uncertain, carcinoma in situ, primary malignant, secondary malignant, or unknown whether primary or secondary. Cancer registry centers in hospitals and ambulatory care centers use this code system for classification of tumors. Also known as *morphology of neoplasms*.

International Classification of Diseases, Tenth Revision, Clinical Modification (ICD-10-CM) Diagnostic code book that uses a system for classifying diseases and operations to assist collection of uniform and comparable health information. It has been modified, will be implemented on October 1, 2013, and will replace ICD-9-CM Volumes 1 and 2 when submitting insurance claims for billing hospital and physician office medical services. Presently it is used for mortality reporting in the United States.

International Classification of Diseases, Tenth Revision, Procedural Coding System (ICD-10-PCS) Procedural code system developed by 3M Health Information Systems (HIS) under contract with the Centers for Medicare and Medicaid Services (CMS). When implemented on October 1, 2013, it will replace ICD-9-CM Volume 3 for hospital inpatient procedure reporting in the United States.

International Classification of Functioning, Disability, and Health (ICF) Classification coding system developed by the World Health Organization (WHO) that is used to report an individual's functional capabilities or limits in situations that are the result of disease. The disease is not identified. This reporting system is not used in the United States but is being investigated at the National Center for Health Statistics for possible future use.

International Classification of Health Interventions (ICHI) Code system developed in Australia and distributed by the World Health Organization (WHO) to other countries. It is used to report interventions and procedures for the purpose of collecting data.

International Organization for Standardization Organization that coordinates the development and adoption of numerous international standards. ISO is not an acronym but rather the Greek word for "equal."

Internet-only manuals (IOMs) Medicare regulations online that replaced guidelines previously printed as paper-based manuals.

internist Doctor who finds and treats health problems in adults.

interoperable For e-prescriptions, able to communicate and exchange data accurately, effectively, securely, and consistently with different information technology systems, software applications, and networks in various settings and exchange data such that the clinical or operational purpose and meaning of the data are preserved and unaltered.

interoperability Ability of different information technology systems and software applications to communicate; exchange data accurately, effectively, and consistently; and use the information that has been exchanged. This is a definition created by member organizations of the National Alliance for Health Information Technology available online at www.nahit.org.

interplan Agreement between Blue Cross Plans through which a local plan may provide benefits for any out-of-area Blue Cross subscriber.

interpleader System of settling an insurance claim in which the insurance company pays the policy proceeds to a court because the insurer is not able to determine to whom the proceeds should be paid and asks the court to decide.

interpretation 1. Act or process of translating or explaining. 2. Health care provider's review of the patient's data expressing a verbal opinion or written documentation in a chart note or report. Interpretation of a test is a billable service.

intervention strategy Policy created to prevent harming of a patient or to improve the mental, emotional, or physical function of a patient. For example, a physiological process may be monitored or enhanced or a pathological process may be arrested or controlled.

interview Meeting an individual face to face for evaluating and questioning a job applicant.

intoxication Diagnostic coding term that relates to an adverse effect rather than a poisoning when drugs such as digitalis, steroid agents, and so on are involved.

intraagency agreement Written contract in which a federal agency agrees to provide to, purchase from, or exchange with another federal agency, services (including data), supplies, or equipment. Intraagency agreements are between at least two or more agencies within the Department of Health and Human Services (DHHS).

intragovernmental assets, liabilities Assets or liabilities that arise from transactions among federal entities.

intrapreneur Individual who works as an employee in an organization but focuses on creative and innovative products, services, and work methods. He or she often works independently or in loosely organized teams and is involved in rethinking current products, services, and organizational structures. Also referred to as *internal entrepreneur.*

intraservice time Documented face-to-face time or floor/unit time that may be used to calculate the level of Evaluation and Management code when time is the determining factor for the encounter with a patient.

invalid claim Any Medicare claim that contains complete, necessary information but is illogical or incorrect (e.g., listing an incorrect provider number for a referring physician). Invalid claims are identified to the provider and may be resubmitted.

invalid code Diagnostic code that is not as specific as it should be and has some missing digits. Insurance claims may be rejected by third-party payers.

inventory Detailed description of quantities and locations of kinds of facilities, equipment, and personnel that are available in a geographical area with the amount, type, and distribution of services these resources can support.

investigational medical procedure Clinical observation of an approved practice or procedure as to its immediate and long-term effectiveness, complications, and consequences.

investigative See *experimental.*

investigative care See *experimental care.*

investigative consumer report Investigative consumer report by a consumer reporting agency that interviews individuals who have knowledge about a specific consumer's character, living style, or reputation.

investment-sensitive insurance Category of insurance products that have death benefits and cash values that vary depending on the insurer's investment earnings such as variable annuities, variable life insurance, and variable universal life insurance. Also called *interest-sensitive insurance.*

investment year method (IYM) Accounting system in which an insurance company keeps records of the interest rates it annually earns on funds that relate to accounts in the general account. Also called *new money method.*

investor-owned hospital See *propriety hospital.*

involuntary plan termination Termination of a retirement plan initiated by a government organization rather than by a plan sponsor.

IP Abbreviation for inpatient. See *inpatient (IP).*

IPA See *independent practice association (IPA)* or *individual practice association (IPA).*

IPG contract See *immediate participation guarantee (IPG) contract.*

IPN See *integrated provider network (IPN).*

IPO See *independent practice association (IPA)* or *individual practice association (IPA).*

IPPE See *initial preventive physical examination (IPPE).*

IPPS See *inpatient prospective payment system (IPPS).*

IRA See *individual retirement account (IRA).* Also see *Section 408(k) of the Internal Revenue Code.*

IRB See *institutional review boards (IRBs).*

IRIS See *Insurance Regulatory Information System (IRIS).*

IRP See *individual responsibility program (IRP).*

irrevocable assignment Permanent legal transfer of an individual's interest in an insurance policy to another person.

irrevocable beneficiary See *beneficiary.*

IS See *information services (IS).*

ISN Acronym for integrated service network. See *accountable health plan (AHP).*

issuing bank Financial institution that sells and issues life insurance policies in its own name. It also issues its contracts, administers its records, and invests the assets of its insurance department.

IT See *information technology (IT).*

italicized code Diagnostic code in ICD-9-CM, Volume 1, Tabular List that may never be sequenced as the principal diagnosis.

itemized bill See *itemized statement.*

itemized statement Detailed summary of all transactions of a patient's account (i.e., dates of service, description of services, number of services provided, noncovered services, amount charged, payments [copayments and deductibles], date the insurance claim was submitted, adjustments, and account balance). Itemized statements are generated by physicians and hospital facilities after services have been provided to patients. Also called *itemized bill.*

IYM See *investment year method (IYM).*

J

J codes Subset of the HCPCS Level II alphanumeric codes used to identify certain drugs when administered by a provider and other items. The final Health Insurance Portability and Accountability Act (HIPAA) transactions and code sets rule states that the J codes will be deleted from the HCPCS and that national drug codes (NDCs) will be used to identify the associated pharmaceuticals and supplies.

JCAH See *Joint Commission on Accreditation of Hospitals (JCAH)*.

JCAHO See *Joint Commission on Accreditation of Healthcare Organizations (JCAHO)*.

JD Abbreviation for Doctor of Jurisprudence; lawyer; attorney.

jet screening Procedure used for quickly reviewing simple insurance applications using strictly defined underwriting standards.

job description Detailed explanation of the skills, duties, and physical and mental qualifications required for performing and carrying out tasks by an employee. This document is referred to in a disability case that will undergo rehabilitation and is used to evaluate work potential.

job-lock Situational phrase meaning a person's inability to change his or her employment because it would result in losing vital health insurance benefits.

job order contracting (JOC) See *indefinite delivery/indefinite quantity (ID/IQ)*.

joint and last survivorship annuity See *joint and survivor annuity*.

joint and several liability Legality that holds a defendant responsible for the full award in a medical liability case if the other defendants are not able to pay their share apportioned by fault.

joint and survivor annuity Annuity in which a series of payments is given to two or more annuitants until their deaths. Also called *joint and last survivorship annuity*.

joint and survivorship option Life insurance settlement choice in which payments are made to two or more payees until their deaths.

joint beneficiary Individual legally entitled to share in the proceeds of an insurance policy.

Joint Commision, The Formerly Joint Commission on Accreditation of Healthcare Organizations (JCAHO). Established in 1951 as Joint Commission on Accreditation of Hospitals (JCAH). It is a not-for-profit accrediting body for clinics, hospitals, and other federal and military facilities. The Joint Commission reviews the policies, patient records, credentialing

procedures, and quality assurance programs of the facility. When the Joint Commission awards official approval, it means the quality and high standards of the facility have been met after their scrutiny. This is the goal of every facility that goes through the process about every 3 years.

Joint Commission on Accreditation of Healthcare Organizations (JCAHO) See *Joint Commission, The*.

Joint Commission on Accreditation of Hospitals (JCAH) In 1913, the year of its founding, the American College of Surgeons appointed Codman to chair a committee on hospital standardization and to establish the College's standardization program. This endeavor represents an integral part of the College's history because it ultimately evolved into the Joint Commission on Accreditation of Hospitals in 1951 and the Joint Commission on Accreditation of Healthcare Organizations in 1987. See *Joint Commission, The*.

joint consent Written agreement by a covered entity giving sanction to use the approval of another covered affiliated entity.

joint credit life insurance Type of credit life insurance that pays a full benefit amount to a lender on the death of any of the cosigners of a loan.

joint venture Short-term business partnership of two or more entities.

joint whole life insurance policy Type of life insurance agreement that gives coverage to two lives and provides for payment of the proceeds at the time of the first insured's death.

judgment 1. Knowledge sufficient to understand the nature of a transaction. 2. Official and authentic decision of a court of justice on the respective rights of the parties to an action submitted to it for determination.

judicial Pertaining to the action in a court of law.

judicial review In the Medicare program, after payment or denial of an insurance claim and four levels of appeal, this is the fifth level in which the provider may file a civil action to be heard in a U.S. District Court. The amount in controversy must be $1000 or more.

Julian date 1. Date in the Julian calendar, or actual number of the day within the year (i.e., July 17, 2006, is Julian date 2453934.1471). Astronomers and calendricists use the term in this sense, according to which a Julian date is a number, denoting a point in time, which consists of an integer part and a fractional part (e.g., 2439291.301), where the integer part is a Julian day number and the fractional part specifies the time elapsed since the start of the day denoted by that Julian day number. 2. In the commercial world the term "Julian date" has been used for a quite different concept, that of the number of the chronological date of the year 001 through 365 preceded by a two-digit year designation, so that January 1st = day 001 and February 28th = day 059; thus 06121 would be Monday, May 1, 2006. For the number of the day in the year, the proper term for this concept is "ordinal date."

jumbo claim See *large claim.*

jurisdiction Legal territory over which a court has authority to hear and decide an issue and to enforce its decision.

jurisprudence Philosophy of law and the system of applied justice through the law and the courts.

justice courts See *small claims court.*

juvenile insurance policy Type of life insurance policy purchased by an adult to give coverage for a child.

JW HCPCS Level II modifier that may be used with CPT or HCPCS Level II codes indicating a drug amount discarded or not administered to any patient.

K

K See *kilobyte (K)*.

K0 HCPCS Level II modifier that may be used with CPT or HCPCS Level II codes indicating lower extremity prosthesis functional level 0—does not have the ability or potential to ambulate or transfer safely with or without assistance and a prosthesis does not enhance the patient's quality of life or mobility.

K1 HCPCS Level II modifier that may be used with CPT or HCPCS Level II codes indicating lower extremity prosthesis functional level 1—has the ability or potential to use a prosthesis for transfers or ambulation on level surfaces at fixed cadence. Typical of the limited and unlimited household ambulator.

K2 HCPCS Level II modifier that may be used with CPT or HCPCS Level II codes indicating lower extremity prosthesis functional level 2—has the ability or potential for ambulation with the ability to traverse low-level environmental barriers such as curbs, stairs, or uneven surfaces. Typical of the limited community ambulator.

K3 HCPCS Level II modifier that may be used with CPT or HCPCS Level II codes indicating lower extremity prosthesis functional level 3—has the ability or potential for ambulation with variable cadence. Typical of the community ambulator who has the ability to transverse most environmental barriers and may have vocational, therapeutic, or exercise activity that demands prosthetic utilization beyond simple locomotion.

K4 HCPCS Level II modifier that may be used with CPT or HCPCS Level II codes indicating lower extremity prosthesis functional level 4—has the ability or potential for prosthetic ambulation that exceeds the basic ambulation skills, exhibiting high impact, stress, or energy levels, typical of the prosthetic demands of the child, active adult, or athlete.

KA HCPCS Level II modifier that may be used with CPT or HCPCS Level II codes indicating an add-on option/accessory for a wheelchair.

Katie Beckett option See *TEFRA 134*.

KB HCPCS Level II modifier that may be used with CPT or HCPCS Level II codes indicating the Medicare beneficiary requested upgrade for Advance Beneficiary Notice (ABN) and that more than four modifiers are identified on the claim.

KC HCPCS Level II modifier that may be used with CPT or HCPCS Level II codes indicating replacement of special power wheelchair interface.

KD HCPCS Level II modifier that may be used with CPT or HCPCS Level II codes indicating that a drug or biological was infused through durable medical equipment (DME).

Keogh Act Federal legislation enacted in 1962 titled *Self-Employed Individuals Tax Retirement Act* to allow self-employed persons to set aside money for retirement. Eligible individuals deposit money in a government-approved account that is managed by a financial institution such as an insurance company or a bank. Also called an *H.R. 10 plan*.

key components Elements of documentation describing the amount of work performed that are used to determine code choice for many evaluation and management services (history, physical examination, and medical decision making). Two or three of these components must be verified (met or exceeded) by the documentation in the patient's medical record depending on the level of service (CPT code) by the provider.

key employee In retirement plans, an employee who makes a large salary and meets any one of four conditions that relates to compensation and company ownership. These criteria are stated in legislation for qualified pension plans and 401(k) tax regulations. Also see *Tax Reform Act of 1986*.

key groups See *anchor group*.

key-person insurance Type of life insurance created to protect a company against the loss of income resulting from the disability or death of an employee who is in a vital business position for the firm's success.

keypad A device, separate or part of the keyboard, that contains keys to control mathematical functions.

KF HCPCS Level II modifier that may be used with CPT or HCPCS Level II codes indicating the item billed has been designated by the Federal Drug Agency (FDA) as a Class III device.

KH HCPCS Level II modifier that may be used with CPT or HCPCS Level II codes indicating a durable medical equipment prosthestics, orthotics, and other supplies (DMEPOS) item—initial claim, purchase, or first month rental.

KI HCPCS Level II modifier that may be used with CPT or HCPCS Level II codes indicating a durable medical equipment prosthestics, orthotics, and other supplies (DMEPOS) item indicating a durable medical equipment prosthestics second or third month rental.

kickback To offer, solicit, pay, or receive payment, bribe, or rebate for referral of Medicare or Medicaid patients, for referrals for services, for ordering diagnostic tests, or items paid for, in whole or in part, by Medicare or Medicaid. This is considered fraudulent behavior and illegal by anti-kickback statutes. See *Stark I Regulations* and *Stark II Regulations*.

kidnap/ransom insurance Type of insurance that gives coverage up to a certain limit for payment of money demanded by kidnappers for the release of an individual who is held against his or her will.

kilobyte (K) An expression for standard quantity measurement of disk or computer storage capacity.

KJ HCPCS Level II modifier that may be used with CPT or HCPCS Level II codes indicating a durable medical equipment prosthetics, orthotics, and other supplies (DMEPOS) item, parenteral enteral nutrition (PEN) pump, or capped rental, months 4 to 15.

KM HCPCS Level II modifier that may be used with CPT or HCPCS Level II codes indicating replacement of facial prosthesis including new impressing/moulage.

KN HCPCS Level II modifier that may be used with CPT or HCPCS Level II codes indicating replacement of facial prosthesis using previous master model.

knowledge-based system Electronic database that uses stored expert knowledge to assist health care providers in making clinical decisions and solving medical and treatment problems.

Knox-Keene Act California legislation effective in 1975 that amended the Health and Safety Code that licenses health maintenance organizations separately from insurance companies. It provides for regulation by the Commissioner of Corporations.

KO HCPCS Level II modifier that may be used with CPT or HCPCS Level II codes indicating a single drug unit dose formulation.

KP HCPCS Level II modifier that may be used with CPT or HCPCS Level II codes indicating the first drug of a multiple drug unit dose formation.

KQ HCPCS Level II modifier that may be used with CPT or HCPCS Level II codes indicating the second or subsequent drug of a multiple drug unit dose formulation.

KR HCPCS Level II modifier that may be used with CPT or HCPCS Level II codes indicating a billing for partial month of a rental item.

KS HCPCS Level II modifier that may be used with CPT or HCPCS Level II codes indicating glucose monitor supply for diabetic beneficiary not treated with insulin.

KSOP Acronym that refers to Section 401(k) of the Internal Revenue Code, a stock ownership plan. See *Section 401(k) plan switchback*.

KX HCPCS Level II modifier that may be used with CPT or HCPCS Level II codes indicating specific required documentation is on file at the DMERC supplier.

Kyle provision Federal legislation in the Balanced Budget Act of 1997 that allows providers who choose to opt out of the Medicare program to enter into private agreements with Medicare recipients for services that would usually be covered by the Medicare program. The minimum time period that a provider may opt out is 2 years.

KZ HCPCS Level II modifier that may be used with CPT or HCPCS Level II codes indicating new coverage not implemented by managed care plan.

L

laboratory report Clinical record that indicates the findings after physical and chemical analysis of specimens.

lag study Report assembled by managed care plan managers to show how long insurance claims are pending and how much money is paid or expended each month.

LAN See *local area network (LAN)*.

lapse Expiration of an insurance policy because of nonpayment of the premium when it is due. Also referred to as *lapsed policy*.

lapsed policy See *lapse*.

large case management See *catastrophic case management*.

large claim Total of covered medical expenses of an insured that goes over a specified insurance claim limit. Also referred to as *jumbo claim* or *shock claim*.

large claim management See *case management*.

large claim pooling Financial system that identifies insurance claims above a certain dollar amount and charges them to a pool that is funded by the charges of all groups who share the pool. This system is established to assist in stabilizing premium fluctuations.

large group Dependent on each state's regulations, but generally defined as a group with 100 or more employees eligible for a group insurance plan.

large group health plan (LGHP) 1. Under Medicare Secondary Payer guidelines, this is a group health plan that covers (a) employees of either a single employer or employee organization that employed at least 100 full-time or part-time employees on 50% or more of its regular business days during the previous calendar year or (b) two or more employers or employee organizations, at least one of which employed at least 100 full-time or part-time employees on 50% or more of its regular business days during the previous calendar year. It includes individual policies (including Medigap policies) purchased by or through an employer or former employer of the individual or family member. 2. Employer-sponsored group health plan that gives insurance coverage for 20 or more employees and is primary to Medicare. This number of employees varies depending on each state's regulations.

last menstrual period (LMP) Last date of the patient's monthly discharge of blood and cellular debris from the uterus through the vagina. This date is expressed as eight digits and placed in Block 14 of the CMS-1500 claim form.

late applicant Eligible individual who applies for group health insurance after the 31-day open enrollment period.

late effect Inactive residual effect or condition produced after the acute phase of an illness or injury has ended. There is no time limit on when late effects can appear. For example, an individual could suffer an injury and then years later develop arthritis at that site. When listing the diagnostic code, sequence the condition code first and then the late effect code, unless the late effect code is combined with the manifestation in one code or the late effect is followed by the manifestation. Also known as *sequelae*.

late enrollment fee Dollar amount an individual must pay if there is a time limit for enrollment into a health plan and the patient delays enrollment beyond the deadline.

late-payment offer See *late-remittance offer*.

late penalty Under a Medicare Part D plan, this phrase means it is the extra dollar amount added to the monthly insurance premium if the Medicare beneficiary does not enroll when first eligible unless he or she is covered by creditable coverage from another plan. The penalty is 1% for every month past the end of the initial enrollment period that was May 15, 2006.

late-remittance offer Proposal to encourage reinstatement of a lapsed insurance policy by accepting an overdue premium after the grace period. Usually such offers do not require submission of evidence of insurability or completion of a reinstatement application. Also called *late-payment offer*.

late retirement age After the normal retirement age of 65. Qualified pension plans cannot force a plan participant to retire at a specific age and cannot stop accruing pension benefits if he or she wants to work beyond the normal retirement age.

laundering of monetary instruments To deposit into a general account illegally obtained funds (fraudulent claim payments) with legally obtained funds (legitimate claim payments). Also called *money laundering*.

law See *act*.

law enforcement official Under the Health Insurance Portability and Accountability Act (HIPAA), an officer or employee of any agency of the United States, a state, a territory, a political subdivision of a state or territory, or an Indian tribe, who has legal authority to investigate an official inquiry into a potential violation of the law or prosecute a criminal, civil, or administrative proceeding because of an alleged violation of the law.

law of large numbers Theory of probability that states the greater the number of observations of a certain event, the more likely the observed results will be the results anticipated by the mathematics of probability.

lawsuit Legal claim or dispute brought into a court of law. Also called *suit.*

LC 1. HCPCS Level II modifier that may be used with CPT or HCPCS Level II codes indicating a specific vessel (left circumflex coronary artery) in a stent placement, balloon angioplasty, and/or atherectomy. 2. Abbreviation for low complexity. See *low complexity (LC).*

LCAH See *life care at home (LCAH).*

LCD See *local coverage determination (LCD).*

LCD articles Local coverage determination articles and frequently asked questions (FAQs) that appear on Medicare contractor websites that address local coverage, coding, and medical review–related billing issues.

LCSW See *licensed clinical social worker (LCSW).*

LD HCPCS Level II modifier that may be used with CPT or HCPCS Level II codes indicating a specific vessel (left anterior descending coronary artery) in a stent placement, balloon angioplasty, and/or atherectomy.

leave of absence (LOA) days Period of time (number of days) during which a patient is discharged temporarily from the hospital. This situation can occur when surgery cannot be scheduled right away, a surgical team is not available, or treatment is necessary after diagnostic tests but cannot begin immediately. LOA days also refers to readmission after surgery for follow-up care, when a patient does not need hospital care during the interim period. LOA requires only one bill, and one diagnosis-related group payment is made.

ledger See *account, financial accounting record, financial record, ledger card,* or *patient account ledger.*

ledger card Individual financial account indicating charges, payments, adjustments, and balances owed for services rendered. Also called *financial accounting record, financial record,* or *patient account ledger.*

left employment To cease working at a company. The employee may be eligible for continuation of health insurance coverage with the group or may take out an individual policy.

legacy numbers Prenational provider identifiers such as provider identification numbers (PINs), unique physician identification numbers (UPINs), online survey certification and reporting system numbers (OSCARs), and national supplier clearinghouse numbers (NCSs) for DMERC claims. These were carrier-assigned numbers that every facility, physician, clinic, or organization that rendered services to patients when submitting insurance claims used. These have been replaced with the National Provider Identifiers (NPIs).

legal actions provision Individual health insurance clause that limits the period during which a claimant may file suit against the insurer to collect a disputed claim amount. It also specifies that no lawsuit can be brought against an insurance company until a specific time period after a claim is filed.

legal business name Name reported to the Internal Revenue Service (IRS) that is legally the business title.

legal father Male who is considered under the law to be the father of a child but may not necessarily be the biological father. Definitions vary by state, but most common is "the man married to the birth mother at the time of birth." In adoption cases, the legal father is called the *father of the adoptee* and his rights must be terminated for an adoption to be carried out.

legal guardian See *guardian.*

legal health record Patient medical record that complies with federal, state, and local laws and a definition developed by each organization based on its needs and what it requires to fulfill its mission. Each organization has its own custom legal health record definition.

legal majority See *age of majority* and *emancipated minor.*

legal red flag Special warning to specific legal danger that could happen with compliance and other health care issues and the possible problems that might result.

legal reserve See *statutory reserve.*

legal reserve life insurance company Life insurance company that operates under state insurance regulations that specify the minimum basis for the reserves the company must maintain on its policies.

legal residence Legal address where a person lives and also related to the region where he or she votes.

legal rule of comity Clause of the U.S. Constitution that gives citizens of one state the right to all privileges, immunities, and judicial decisions enjoyed by citizens of the other states.

legend drug Medication that can only be obtained with a written prescription.

length-of-service schedule Type of group insurance in which an employee is insured for an amount dependent on the length of time he or she has been employed for the employer.

length of stay (LOS) Number of calendar days a patient remains in a health care facility or is an inpatient in the hospital during an episode of illness or due to an injury. LOS statistics report the average number of days spent in a health care facility per admission and discharge. Also referred to as *average length of stay, days of stay, discharge days, duration of inpatient hospitalization,* and *inpatient days of stay.*

length-of-stay outliers Type of cases that fall outside, either longer or shorter than typical, from the average for a specific diagnosis, procedure, or diagnostic-related group.

lenses Curved transparent pieces of plastic or glass that are shaped, molded, or ground to refract light in a specific way, as in eyeglasses, microscopes, or cameras. Corrective lenses may be prescribed by an ophthalmologist or optometrist to improve vision.

LESOP See *leveraged employee stock ownership plan (LESOP).* Also see *employee stock ownership plan (ESOP).*

L

letter of request On organizational letterhead, a formal document detailing needs and purposes by a requestor for a federally funded project. In addition, a letter of support is required from the federal project officer on his or her organizational letterhead.

letter of support On organizational letterhead, a document from the federal project officer justifying the need for Centers for Medicare and Medicaid Services (CMS) data and supporting the requestor's use of such data.

Level I codes See *Current Procedural Terminology (CPT)*.

Level II codes See *Healthcare Common Procedure Coding System (HCPCS)*.

Level III codes See *Healthcare Common Procedure Coding System (HCPCS)*.

Level I emergency service Medical services provided to patients for conditions arising, often unexpectedly, that need at least one physician experienced in emergency care on duty in the emergency care area. There must be in-hospital physician coverage by members of the medical staff or by senior-level residents for at least medical, surgical, orthopedic, obstetric, gynecologic, pediatric, and anesthesiology services. When coverage can be demonstrated to meet suitably through another mechanism, an equivalent will be considered to exist for purposes of compliance with the requirement. Other specialty consultation must be available within approximately 30 minutes. Initial consultation through two-way voice communication is acceptable. The hospital's scope of services must include in-house capabilities for managing physical and related emotional problems on a definitive basis. Also see *emergency services*.

Level II emergency service Medical services provided to patients for conditions arising, often unexpectedly, that need at least one physician experienced in emergency care on duty in the emergency care area. Specialty consultation must be available within approximately 30 minutes by members of the medical staff or by senior-level residents. Initial consultation through two-way voice communication is acceptable. The hospital's scope of services must include in-house capabilities for managing physical and related emotional problems, with provision for patient transfer to another facility when required. Also see *emergency services*.

Level III emergency service Medical services provided to patients for conditions arising, often unexpectedly, that need at least one physician available to the emergency care area from within the hospital who is available immediately through two-way voice communication. Specialty consultation must be available by request of the attending medical staff member or by transfer to a designated hospital where definitive care can be rendered. Also see *emergency services*.

level commission scale System of applying the same insurance commission payment rate to the premium for each year that a policy is in force.

level of care (LOC) Type of assistance needed by a consumer that may establish his or her eligibility for a program or health care service such as protective, intermediate, or skilled. See also *level of service*.

level of service (LOS) 1. Intensity of medical services given to a patient when a physician provides one-on-one service (i.e., minimal, brief, limited, intermediate, comprehensive). 2. Other levels of service given by a health care organization (i.e., ambulatory surgery). Sometimes referred to as *level of care (LOC)*.

level of specificity Phrase used when assigning a diagnostic code to the highest degree. It means to assign (1) three-digit codes (category codes) if there are no four-digit codes within the code category or (2) four-digit codes (subcategory codes) if there are no five-digit codes for that category or (3) five-digit codes (fifth-digit subclassification codes) for those categories where they are available.

level premium annuity Type of deferred annuity in which the annuitant pays equal premium amounts, monthly or annually, until the date that benefit payments begin.

level premium billing Allows the insured to pay a specific amount of premium on each due date during the policy year that is based on an estimated annual premium. An adjustment is made at the end of the policy year for coverage changes that occurred during that year.

level premium insurance Life insurance for which the cost is evenly distributed over the period during which premiums are paid. Premiums are the same from year to year. Protection in the earlier years is more than the actual cost, building up a reserve, and in the later years, less than the actual cost.

level premium whole life insurance Type of whole life insurance policy in which equal premiums are paid throughout the premium payment period.

level premiums Annual premium payments that are the same each year that the life insurance policy is in force.

level schedule Group insurance plan in which all policyholders are insured for the same amount of benefits without regard to wages or job position.

level term insurance Type of term insurance that gives a death benefit that remains the same during a specified period. Premiums usually remain the same throughout each term of coverage.

levelized commission schedule Insurance commission table that provides different percentages for the first and renewal years of a policy. Also known as *heaped commission schedule*.

leveraged business See *minimum deposit business*.

leveraged employee stock ownership plan (LESOP) Plan that borrows money and uses the funds to purchase stock of the employer. In turn the employer makes contributions to the plan on behalf of the participating employees.

These are tax deductible for the employer and tax deferred for the employee. The ESOP uses the contributed money to pay the loan back and slowly gives the stock to the employees. Also see *employee stock ownership plan (ESOP)*.

LGHP See *large group health plan (LGHP)*.

LHWCA See *Longshoremen's and Harbor Workers' Compensation Act (LHWCA)*.

liability 1. Something one is bound to do, or an obligation one is bound to fulfill, by law and justice. A liability may be enforced in court. Liabilities are usually financial or can be expressed in financial terms. Also, the probable cost of meeting such an obligation. 2. Under Medicare Secondary Payer guidelines, responsibility or fault for damages arising out of a specified incident. 3. In insurance, any claim not yet paid.

liability determination In a Medicare case, to find out whether the beneficiary and the provider did not and could not have been reasonably expected to know that payment would not be made for services.

liability insurance 1. Form of insurance coverage that protects the insured against injury, illness, inappropriate action or inaction, or property damage claims from other parties. It includes automobile liability, uninsured and underinsured motorist, homeowner's liability, malpractice, product liability, and general casualty insurance. It includes payments under state "wrongful death" statutes that provide payment for medical damages. 2. Related to a physician, this is insurance against loss due to claims for damages alleging malpractice by a physician while exercising his or her profession. Also known as *professional liability insurance (PLI)* or *malpractice insurance*.

liability insurance payment Under Medicare Secondary Payer guidelines, payment by a liability insurer including a payment to cover a deductible required by a liability insurer by any individual or other entity that possesses liability insurance or is covered by a self-insured plan.

license 1. In insurance, a formal certification issued by a state department of insurance that an insurance agent is qualified to solicit insurance applications during a specified time period. 2. Approval granted by a state or government agency to engage lawfully in a practice, occupation, or specific activity of health care.

licensed 1. Formal permission obtained from legal authorities to execute specific professional activities that conform to state regulations or federal regulations and compliance standards. This certification is applicable to individuals and health care facilities. 2. In reference to a long-term facility, this means the facility has met certain standards set by a state or local government agency. 3. For a health maintenance organization (HMO), that it has met all regulatory requirements before it started to operate in a locale and that the state authority reviewed and approved its fiscal soundness, network capacity, and quality assurance. Also referred to as *licensure*.

licensed beds See *beds, licensed*.

licensed broker See *broker*.

licensed by the state as a risk-bearing entity Entity that is licensed or otherwise authorized by the state to assume risk for offering health insurance or health benefits coverage. The entity is authorized to accept prepaid capitation for providing, arranging, or paying for comprehensive health services under a Medicare+Choice (M+C) contract. Designation that an M+C organization has been reviewed and determined "fully accredited" by a Centers for Medicare and Medicaid Services (CMS)-approved accrediting organization for those standards within the deeming categories that the accrediting organization has the authority to deem.

licensed clinical social worker (LCSW) See *clinical social worker (CSW)*.

licensed health care professional Individual who is licensed by the state to render medical care to patients such as physician, registered nurse, and licensed practical nurse.

licensed physician Doctor who is authorized to perform services within limitations imposed by the state on the scope of practice; issuance by a state of a license to practice medicine constitutes legal authorization.

licensed practical nurse (LPN) Individual educated in basic nursing techniques and direct patient care who passes a state board of nursing and has legal authorization (license) to practice. LPNs practice under the supervision of a licensed physician or registered nurse (RN). Also called *licensed vocational nurse (LVN)* or *practical nurse*. In California and Texas, licensing is as a licensed vocational nurse (LVN). In Canada, an LPN is called a *certified nursing assistant*.

licensed vocational nurse/licensed visiting nurse (LVN) See *licensed practical nurse (LPN)*.

licensing To give license or permit formally.

licensure See *licensed*.

lien 1. Claim on the property of another as security for a debt. 2. In litigation cases, it is a legal promise to satisfy a debt owed by the patient to the physician out of any proceeds received on the case.

life annuity See *annuity*.

life annuity with period certain A policy in which if the annuitant dies before the end of the specific time period, the insurer will continue to pay to a contingent beneficiary until the end of the designated period. Also called *life income with period certain annuity*.

life care at home (LCAH) Type of health care program in which the elderly live at home instead of at a centralized location. It resembles a continuing care retirement community (CCRC).

life expectancy In insurance, the average number of years of life remaining for individuals of a given age according to a particular mortality table. Also called *expectation of life*.

L

life income option Life insurance settlement option in which the insurance company uses the policy proceeds and interest to pay the beneficiary as long as the beneficiary lives.

life income option with period certain Life insurance settlement in which the insurance company guarantees to pay the beneficiary for a specific time to continue as long as the original beneficiary lives. If the original beneficiary dies during the guaranteed period, payments are made to a recipient specified by the original beneficiary until the end of the guaranteed period and then all payments cease.

life income option with refund Type of life insurance settlement in which the insurance company guarantees that if the beneficiary dies before the total amount paid under the option equals the proceeds of the policy, then the insurer pays the difference to a contingent payee. Also called *refund life income option*.

life income with period certain annuity See *life annuity with period certain*.

life insurance Type of insurance that provides protection against financial loss resulting from death of the insured individual.

life insurance trust, funded Trust established to distribute life insurance proceeds. Because insurance companies cannot act as trustees or guardians, the policy proceeds are paid to a trust company and distributed under the terms of a trust agreement creating greater flexibility in distribution of the proceeds. The trustee has control over both the policy proceeds and also securities or other property to provide funds out of which to pay the premiums. This type of arrangement is a funded life insurance trust.

life insurance trust, unfunded Trust established to distribute life insurance proceeds. Because insurance companies cannot act as trustees or guardians, the policy proceeds are paid to a trust company and distributed under the terms of a trust agreement creating greater flexibility in distribution of the proceeds. This type of arrangement is an unfunded life insurance trust.

life underwriters See *agent*.

lifetime disability benefit Insurance contract terms that provide for payment of disability income for an insured's lifetime as long as he or she is totally disabled.

lifetime limit Maximum amount of insurance benefits payable under an insurance policy.

lifetime maximum See *lifetime maximum benefit*.

lifetime maximum benefit Largest dollar amount that an insurance company will pay for an insured's claims in a lifetime and/or the greatest dollar amount paid for all illnesses and injuries for each insured as long as the certificate is in effect. Also called *total certificate membership benefit maximum* and *lifetime maximum*.

lifetime reserve See *lifetime reserve days (LRDs)*.

lifetime reserve days (LRDs) Medicare Part A coverage that means a reserve of 60 days of inpatient hospital care available over an individual's lifetime that the individual may use after he or she has used the maximum 90 days allowed in a single benefit period. For each lifetime reserve day, Medicare pays all covered costs except for a daily coinsurance ($534 in 2009). Also referred to as *lifetime reserve* or *reserve days*.

light duty Refers to assignment of job duties that are less physically or mentally stressful than those that an individual previously performed before a work injury. This inexact phrase should not be used in workers' compensation reports.

lighting up Phrase used in workers' compensation cases that describes an aggravation of a preexisting or underlying condition. This occurrence causes a temporary or permanent increase in disability that may require new medical treatment or a change in the existing treatment.

limit 1. Maximum amount of insurance benefits payable under an insurance or managed care contract. 2. Restriction or denial of insurance coverage to certain age groups.

limitation of liability 1. Statement in an insurance contract that the maximum amount an insurance company agrees to pay in case of loss. 2. In the Medicare program, agreement given to the patient to read and sign before rendering a service if the participating physician thinks that it may be denied for payment because of medical necessity or legal responsibility. The patient agrees to pay for the service; also known as *Advance Beneficiary Notice (ABN), waiver of liability,* or *responsibility statement*.

limitations Situations or conditions under which the insurance company will not pay or will limit payments. Such exclusions are found in a document called *certificate of insurance*. If it is a group policy, the employer receives a detailed contract and each employee receives a booklet summarizing and explaining the insurance plan.

limited coverage policy Type of medical insurance policy that covers only medical expenses caused by a specific disease that is named in the policy. Also called *dread disease policy*.

limited liability company (LLC) Hybrid form of business that combines the elements of partnerships and corporations. The owners are called *members* and receive protection from individual liability for company debts. For tax purposes, it is considered a partnership. Gains and losses are claimed by members on their own income tax returns.

limited license Kind of state license in which the type and number of services are less than for a full license to practice medicine. It is often limited to certain services within a specialty.

limited license practitioner (LLP) Professional individual state licensed to provide specific health care services in private practice dependent on his or her specific scope of training such as chiropractors, dentists, optometrists, podiatrists, psychologists, and social workers. Also called *limited practitioner*.

limited payment life insurance See *limited payment whole life insurance*.

limited payment whole life insurance Type of whole life insurance that may specify the number of years that premium payments are payable or the specific age when premiums are no longer paid. The policy may also state that premiums are payable until death if death occurs before the end of the specified period. Also referred to as *limited payment life insurance*.

limited policy Insurance contract that gives coverage only to specific accidents or illnesses.

limited practitioner See *limited license practitioner (LLP)*.

limiting charge Maximum amount a nonparticipating physician may legally charge a Medicare patient for services billed on nonassigned insurance claims. In the original Medicare plan, it is usually the highest amount of money a beneficiary can be charged for a covered service by doctors and other health care suppliers who do not accept assignment. The limiting charge is 15% over Medicare's approved amount. The limiting charge only applies to certain services and does not apply to supplies or equipment. This was previously called a *maximum allowable actual charge (MAAC)*. Also referred to as *billing limit* or *limiting fee charge*.

limiting fee charge See *limiting charge*.

line item Medical service or other item listed as a line entry on an insurance claim form or other computer-generated document. Usual data are date of the service, procedural code, service fee amount, and so on.

line item denial Insurance carrier or fiscal intermediary's refusal to pay one or more of the line items on an insurance claim due to a technical error or because of insurance policy benefit issues. Denied line items must be appealed by the provider except for emergency department visits in which the patient died during a procedure categorized as an inpatient procedure. In that situation, the claim is resubmitted as an inpatient claim.

line item posting Financial accounting procedure in which each payment is posted to the exact transaction for which the payment is received.

line item rejection Insurance carrier or fiscal intermediary's elimination of one or more of the line items on an insurance claim due to a technical error such as omission or erroneous information, or because it does not follow Medicare guidelines. In these situations the claim may be corrected and resubmitted by the provider, but they cannot be appealed.

line of business (LOB) 1. Private indemnity insurance plan or managed care plan that is set up as a separate business unit within another larger organization (e.g., life insurance company, fidelity line, HMO, PPO). The LOB makes a distinction between the managed care plans from the free-standing company or one set up as a subsidiary. 2. Refers to a distinctive type of program within a health plan such as Medicaid. 3. Different types of health plans offered by a large insurance company or insurance broker as a product line.

linking codes For establishing medical necessity, software computer edits check procedure and HCPCS Level II codes that are connected (linked) to ICD-9-CM diagnostic codes submitted on insurance claims for payment. These must be supported by the documentation in the patient's medical record.

Linton yield method See *rate of return method*.

liquidated damages Amount stipulated in a contract that estimates a value to be recovered by an individual if the other party breaches. The sum is a measure of damages for a breach, whether it exceeds or falls short of the actual damages.

liquidation See *liquidation proceeding*.

liquidation proceeding Course of action of converting all assets into cash and paying all outside creditors according to the order of their preference and distributing what is left over to the owners in proportion and in the order of preference of ownership. Also called *liquidation*.

liquidator Individual who is administering assets in any liquidation proceeding.

list service (listserv) An online computer service run from a website where questions may be posted by subscribers. It is a single e-mail address that resends to many others and allows a discussion to continue among a group of participants. Also called *distribution list* or *e-mailing list*.

litigation A lawsuit.

lives Unit of measurement used by managed care plans or insurance companies to find out the number of people covered in the contract or policy. The formula for determining this number is to multiply the number of plan members by 2.5.

living benefit rider Insurance policy provision that allows the insured to receive all or part of the policy's death benefit before the insured's death dependent on specific conditions. This type of rider may be used to help an insured individual pay medical expenses if he or she develops a terminal illness.

living benefits See *accelerated benefits*.

living donor kidney transplant Surgical procedure of excising a kidney from a living donor and implanting it into a suitable recipient.

living trust See *inter vivo trust*.

living will Legal document that states the wishes of an individual concerning life support or other medical treatment in certain circumstances, usually when death is imminent or if the person is unconscious and unable to make a decision. Also known as a *medical directive, advance directive,* or *health care advance directive.*

LL HCPCS Level II modifier that may be used with CPT or HCPCS Level II codes indicating when a durable medical equipment (DME) lease or rental fee is to be applied against the purchase price.

LLC See *limited liability company (LLC).*

LLP See *limited license practitioner (LLP).*

LMP See *last menstrual period (LMP).*

LMRP See *local medical review policy (LMRP).*

LMRP articles See *LCD articles.*

LOA See *leave of absence (LOA) days.*

loading Dollar amount or percentage added to the insurance policy's basic rate or premium that is used to cover the expense to the insurance company of maintaining the business (e.g., in life insurance to provide for expenses, contingencies, or profits or to adjust the premium rate for special situations such as older average age, hazardous industry, many unskilled employees, and adverse experience).

loan value In life insurance, this is a specific amount that can be borrowed from the issuing company by the policy owner, using the cash value of the policy as collateral. If the policy owner dies and the debt is not completely paid, then the amount borrowed plus any interest is deducted from the face amount of the loan.

LOB See *line of business (LOB).*

LOC See *level of care (LOC).*

local anesthesia Absence of sensation in a small area of the body that is time limited. It may be brought on by various anesthetic medications administered through local tissue infiltration, topical application, or subcutaneous or intradermal field block or nerve block injection. Benefits include reduced cost, ease of administration of medication, low toxicity, and quick recovery.

local area network (LAN) Interlink of multiple computers contained within a room or building that allows sharing of files and devices such as printers.

local code(s) Generic term for code values that are defined for a state or other political subdivision, or for a specific payer. This term applies to state-assigned institutional (hospital facility) revenue codes, condition codes, occurrence codes, value codes, and so on. Previously this term was most commonly used to describe Level III HCPCS regional/local codes, but these have been discontinued.

local coverage determination (LCD) Decision by a Medicare fiscal intermediary whether to cover a particular service on an intermediary-wide or carrier-wide basis in accordance with the Social Security Act. This determination is based on whether the service is considered reasonable and necessary. The difference between local medical review policies (LMRPs) is that LCDs consist of only "reasonable and necessary"

information, whereas LMRPs may also contain category or statutory provisions. Formerly known as *local medical review policy (LMRP).*

local medical review policy (LMRP) Regional guideline or rule used to make local Medicare medical coverage decisions because a national coverage regulation is absent. Such policies were developed after review of medical literature, local practice, and comments from the medical community and Carrier Advisory Committee. Beginning December 7, 2003, all LMRPs were converted to local coverage determinations (LCDs). See *local coverage determination (LCD).*

local medical review policy articles See *LCD articles.*

local public health clinic See *state public health clinic.*

locality Certain geographical region (state, county, aggregation of counties, parts of counties, population density, metropolitan size, or townships) within which Medicare carriers or fiscal intermediaries establish prevailing charges. Also called *area.*

locality code Three-digit number that represents a group of zip codes.

location 1. Place of service (POS) where a medical service is performed such as a hospital (inpatient or outpatient), doctor's office, or skilled nursing facility. When the physician's office or an outpatient hospital is billing, the two-digit POS code is inserted in Block 24B of the CMS-1500 insurance claim form (e.g., 11 is doctor's office and 12 is patient's home). 2. Anatomical location of a medical problem.

location code See *place of service (POS) code.*

location-selling distribution system Distribution of insurance products by finding insurance offices and agents in locations where consumers commonly shop for groceries or take care of other personal or business matters. Also known as *retail outlet distribution system.*

lock-in In managed care plans and health maintenance organizations, a provision in which members must receive their medical care from the network providers unless it is an emergency.

logical observation identifiers names and codes (LOINC) Code system that consists of universal names and identification codes that identify and are used to report laboratory and clinical observations. It is maintained by the Regenstrief Institute. These codes are expected to be used in the HIPAA claim attachments standard. Also see *Regenstrief Institute.*

LOINC See *logical observation identifiers names and codes (LOINC).*

long-form reinstatement application Insurance reinstatement application form for a policy that is no longer in force. The applicant must complete a long-term health history.

long range The next 75 years.

long-stay hospital Facility with patients who have an average length of stay of at least 30 days.

long-term acute care (LTAC) Medical facilities that provide patients with acute care for extended inpatient stays (defined by federal statute as an average of 25 days or more). The health care objective is stabilization of physical condition, medical recovery, and return to home.

long-term acute care hospital See *long-term care hospital (LTCH)*.

Long Term Acute Care Hospital Association of America (LTACHAA) See *Acute Long Term Hospital Association (ALTHA)*.

long-term care (LTC) Medical and personal care services rendered to patients who are not in an acute phase of illness but chronically ill, aged, or disabled and generally residing in a nursing home or assisted living facility. Sometimes home health care is provided on a long-term basis, and this may be referred to as *LTC*. Patients require help with activities of daily living (ADLs) such as bathing, continence, dressing, eating, mobility, transferring in and out of bed or a chair, using the toilet, and walking. Most long-term care is custodial care, and Medicare does not pay for this type of care if this is the only kind of care the patient needs.

long-term care facility Health care facility that offers extended nursing care and subacute care services to resident patients whose illness does not require acute care. To participate in the Medicare or Medicaid programs, such a facility must be certified as a skilled nursing facility (SNF) or other nursing facility (NF).

long-term care hospital (LTCH) 1. Facility that treats patients not in an acute phase of illness but who need medical and nursing services not available in nursing homes (e.g., rehabilitation hospital). 2. In the Medicare program, this type of facility is called a *short-term acute care hospital*. Average inpatient stay is greater than 25 days. Also called *long-term hospital* and *long-term acute care hospital*.

long-term care insurance Type of private insurance policy to help pay for some skilled, intermediate, custodial, and long-term medical and nonmedical care such as help with activities of daily living. Because Medicare and Medigap policies generally do not pay for long-term care, this type of insurance policy may help provide coverage for long-term care that the individual may need in the future. Some long-term care insurance policies offer tax benefits called *tax-qualified policies*. This type of insurance may be expensive, and coverage may be denied on health status or age.

long-term care ombudsman Advocate (supporter) for nursing home and assisted living facility residents who investigate and work to resolve problems between residents and nursing homes or assisted living facilities. This individual monitors federal and state regulations that pertain to long-term care facilities, provide information to the public about the elderly in facilities, and train volunteers to help with this program. Also called *ombudsman*. See *ombudsman*.

long-term care ombudsman program Program that is federally authorized by Title III of the Older Americans Act. See *long-term care ombudsman*.

long-term disability Condition in which an insured employee suffers a nonoccupational accident or illness and is not able to perform the duties of his or her occupation for an extended period of time.

long-term disability income insurance See *long-term disability insurance*.

long-term disability insurance Type of disability income insurance that has a provision to pay benefits to a covered disabled person as long as he or she remains disabled, up to a specified period exceeding 2 years. This kind of insurance may be purchased by an employer or an individual. Also called *long-term disability income insurance*.

long-term hospital See *long-term care hospital (LTCH)*.

longer term care minimum data set Core set of screening and assessment elements of the Resident Assessment Instrument (RAI). This assessment system provides a comprehensive, accurate, standardized, reproducible assessment of each long-term care facility resident's functional capabilities and helps staff to identify health problems. This assessment is performed on every resident in a Medicare and/or Medicaid-certified long-term care facility including private pay.

longitudinal patient record Medical record, electronic or paper, that contains the patient's lifetime health care history, diagnoses, treatments, medications, and tests.

Longshoremen's and Harbor Workers' Compensation Act (LHWCA) Federal act that provides benefits for private and public employees who perform maritime work nationwide.

loop Repeating structure or process.

looping The automated diagnosis-related group (DRG) grouper process (computer software program that assigns DRGs) that searches all listed diagnoses for the presence of any comorbid condition or complication or searching all procedures for operating room procedures or other specific procedures.

LOS See *length of stay (LOS)* and *level of service (LOS)*.

loss 1. Reason for an insurance claim for recovery of indemnity or payment for damages. 2. Any reduction of the quantity, quality, or value of a property.

loss of preinjury capacity Change in a person's ability to perform physical or other activities as compared with his or her condition before the injury after the condition has become stable.

loss-of-time insurance See *disability income insurance*.

loss ratio 1. The proportion between the cost to deliver health care and the amount of money taken in by the managed care plan. 2. The relative amount of insurance claims incurred to insurance premium monies received. An indicator used by insurance companies to measure the amount of benefits returned to policyholders. The formula for obtaining the ratio is incurred claims plus expenses divided by premiums. Low loss ratio indicates that the premiums collected were more than necessary to fund the actual claims. High loss ratio shows that claims exceeded the premiums for the given time period. Also known as *incurred claims loss ratio, medical loss ratio (MLR), medical cost ratio*, or *paid claims loss ratio*.

lost claim Insurance claim that cannot be located after sending it to an insurer.

lost-time claim In workers' compensation cases, this is a claim filed for the time lost from work as a result of an industrial injury or occupational illness.

low complexity (LC) Phrase used to describe a type of medical decision-making when a patient is seen for an evaluation and management (E/M) service. Medical record documentation must consist of a limited number of diagnoses or management options, a limited amount of data or complexity of data reviewed, and a low risk of complications and/or morbidity or mortality.

low severity presenting problem Medical problem in which the risk of morbidity without treatment is low and there is little or no risk of mortality without treatment. Usually full recovery without functional impairment is expected.

low utilization payment adjustment (LUPA) In the home health prospective payment system, an episode of four or fewer visits is paid using the national standardized per visit rates instead of the home health resource group (HHRG).

LPN See *licensed practical nurse (LPN)*.

LR HCPCS Level II modifier that may be used with CPT or HCPCS Level II codes indicating laboratory round-trip service.

LS HCPCS Level II modifier that may be used with CPT or HCPCS Level II codes indicating a U.S. Food and Drug Administration–monitored intraocular lens implant.

LT HCPCS Level II modifier that may be used with CPT or HCPCS Level II codes indicating procedures performed on the left side of the body.

LTAC See *long-term acute care (LTAC)*.

LTACHAA See *Long Term Acute Care Hospital Association of America (LTACHAA)*.

LTC See *long-term care (LTC)*.

LTCH See *long-term care hospital (LTCH)*.

lump sum commutation settlement Under Medicare Secondary Payer guidelines, the injured party accepts a lump sum payment that compensates for all future medical expenses and disability benefits related to the work injury or disease.

lump sum compromise settlement Under Medicare Secondary Payer guidelines, a settlement that provides less in total compensation than the individual would have received if he or she had received full reimbursement for lost wages and lifelong medical treatment for the injury or illness. This situation may occur when compensability is contested.

LUPA See *low utilization payment adjustment (LUPA)*.

LVN Abbreviation that means licensed vocational nurse/licensed visiting nurse. See *licensed practical nurse (LPN)*.

lysis 1. Breakdown, decomposition, destruction, or dissolution of a cell or molecule through the action of a specific agent such as lysin. 2. Slow and steady lessening of the symptoms of a disease.

lysis of adhesions Operation performed to free an organ from adjoining restrictive scar tissue.

M

M codes Tissue-type codes for morphology of neoplasms that appear in the ICD-9-CM system. These codes are used to gather statistical data on the occurrences of specific tumors in the general population.

M+C Abbreviation for Medicare+Choice. See *Medicare Plus (+) Choice (M+C) program, Medicare Plus (+) Choice (M+C) plan*, and *Medicare Part C.*

MA See *medical assistant (MA)*.

MAAC See *maximum allowable actual charge (MAAC)*.

MAC See *maximum allowable charge (MAC), maximum allowable*, and *Medicare administrative contractor (MAC)*.

magnetic resonance imaging (MRI) Medical imaging diagnostic test based on the resonance of atomic nuclei in a strong magnetic field. MRI is the method of choice for a growing number of disease processes. Advantages are its superior soft-tissue contrast resolution, ability to image in multiple planes, and lack of ionizing radiation hazards.

main term 1. When coding a diagnostic statement, identifies the condition, disease, or injury word(s) to look up in the alphabetical index of the *International Classification of Diseases, Ninth Revision, Clinical Modification (ICD-9-CM)* code book. 2. Alphabetical major headings printed in boldface that appear in the "Index," which is the last section of the annually published *Current Procedural Terminology* code book. These main terms relate to procedures, services, organs, other anatomical sites, conditions, synonyms, eponyms, and abbreviations.

maintenance expenses Costs of keeping an insurance policy in force such as processing premium payments, making policy dividend payments, and servicing time of agents and help by customer service personnel to clients.

major diagnosis Patient's condition that uses the most resources during hospitalization. This may differ from the admitting and principal diagnoses.

major diagnostic categories (MDCs) Broad classifications of diagnoses grouped by organ system that are medically related by diagnosis, treatment, or similarity, or that are statistically similar by length of stay in a hospital. There are 83 coding system–oriented MDCs in the original diagnosis-related groups (DRGs) and 23 body system–oriented MDCs in the revised set of DRGs. MDCs are used in DRG payment.

major medical Health insurance policy designed to offset heavy medical expenses resulting from catastrophic or prolonged illness or injury. Usually there is a deductible, coinsurance, and large benefit maximums.

Also called *catastrophic coverage, catastrophic insurance, catastrophic health insurance*, or *major medical expense insurance.*

major medical expense insurance Type of health insurance that has benefits for medical expenses up to a high maximum benefit. Generally these policies have internal limits and the insured must pay a deductible and coinsurance. Sometimes referred to as *major medical.*

major procedure 1. Commonly used phrase in describing a surgical intervention that may have 30 to 90 follow-up days. A major primary operative procedure may be considered by insurance third-party payers to be part of a surgical package or Medicare global package. 2. Medical procedures greater than 5 minutes that involve the operating room setting and there is risk and complexity of decision-making throughout the procedure.

major services In dental insurance, dental benefits including inlays, crowns, prosthodontics, and orthodontics that are covered at 50% of their reasonable and customary fees.

major teaching hospital Medical facility that is associated with a university, has an accredited program in various specialties of medical practice, has an approved graduate medical education program, and has a ratio of interns and residents to beds of 25% or greater. It gives clinical experience to medical students while they deliver supervised medical care to patients.

majority Age, generally either 18 or 22, when a minor becomes of adult age as per state law and can assume civil duties and rights such as serving on a jury or voting.

maldistribution Surplus or lack of health care providers based on a population per physician ratio either geographically or by specialty. Also see *health professional shortage area (HPSA)*.

malfeasance Performance of an unlawful, wrongful act.

malignant tumor Abnormal growth that has the properties of invasion and metastasis (i.e., transfer of diseases from one organ to another). The word "carcinoma" (CA) refers to a cancerous or malignant tumor.

malingering To deliberately pretend or fake symptoms of a disease or injury to intentionally profit in some way to reach a desired end (collect insurance benefits) or to feign symptoms as the result of mental illness.

malnutrition Health problem caused by the lack of, or too much, needed nutrients.

179

malpractice Professional misconduct or lack of ordinary skill in the performance of a professional act that results in damage to another person. A physician is liable for damages or injuries caused by malpractice. Also see *malpractice insurance.*

malpractice costs One of three components used in determining the relative value units under the resource-based relative value scale. Malpractice costs stand for the cost of professional liability insurance for each procedure.

malpractice expense Cost of professional liability insurance coverage incurred by a physician.

malpractice insurance Professional liability insurance coverage for a physician against the risk of suffering financial damage because of professional negligence, misconduct, or lack of standard skills. Sometimes referred to as *medical malpractice insurance, professional liability insurance (PLI),* or *liability insurance.*

malpractice reform Effort to lower costs in health care by reducing the number of lawsuits against physicians and other health care providers and/or the amounts awarded in such lawsuits.

mammogram Special x-ray of the breasts. Medicare covers the cost of a mammogram once a year for women older than age 40.

mammography screening X-ray examination of the breasts for early detection of cancer.

managed behavioral health program (MBHP) Program in a managed care organization (MCO) under a carve-out arrangement that provides services to the members such as behavioral services, utilization management services, or organizing an employee assistance program (EAP).

managed care 1. System of health care delivery designed to reduce unnecessary utilization of medical services, control costs, and measure performance while managing access and giving quality, cost-effective health care. Emphasis is placed on prevention, early intervention, and outpatient care. A variety of arrangements for health care delivery and financing includes health maintenance organizations (HMOs), preferred provider organizations (PPOs), point-of-service (POS) plans, and competitive medical plans (CMPs). The plans provide health services on prepayment terms that are based on either cost or risk. 2. Reimbursement method by third-party payers who implement some requirements to control costs of health care while retaining quality care. 3. Under Medicare, includes HMOs, CMPs, and other plans that provide health services on prepayment terms, which are based on either cost or risk, depending on the type of contract they have with Medicare. The term *managed care* has been replaced with *Senior Advantage plans.* See also *Medicare Plus (+) Choice (M+C) program* and *Senior Advantage plans.* Also called *managed health care.*

managed care committee See *managed care coordinator.*

managed care coordinator Individual or committee that receives managed care plan referral authorization requests and depending on precise rules can either approve or deny the request. Also may be known as *managed care committee.*

managed care organization/prepaid health plan (MCO/PHP) standards Principles that states set for plan structure, operations, and the internal quality improvement/assurance system that each MCO/PHP must have in order to participate in the Medicaid program.

managed care organizations (MCOs) 1. Generic term applied to managed care plans such as exclusive provider organizations (EPOs), health maintenance organizations (HMOs), preferred provider organizations (PPOs), and point-of-service (POS) plans. MCOs are usually prepaid group plans and physicians are typically paid by the capitation method. Also referred to as *managed health care plan.* 2. MCOs are entities that serve Medicare or Medicaid beneficiaries on a risk basis through a network of employed or affiliated providers. In the Medicaid program, other organizations may set up managed care programs to respond to Medicaid managed care. These organizations include federally qualified health centers, integrated delivery systems, and public health clinics.

managed care payment suspension See *suspension of payments.*

managed care plan 1. Prepayment health care program in which a specified set of health benefits is provided in exchange for a yearly fee or fixed periodic payments to the provider by the plan. This category of third-party payers includes health maintenance organizations (HMOs), preferred provider organizations (PPOs), and independent or individual practice associations (IPAs). 2. Under the Medicare program, type of prepaid medical plan that must cover all Medicare Part A and Part B health care. Some managed care plans cover extra benefits such as extra days in the hospital. In most cases, a type of Medicare Advantage Plan that is available in some areas of the country. Cost to the patient may be lower than in the Original Medicare Plan.

managed care plan with a point-of-service option (POS) Prepaid health plan that lets the patient use doctors and hospitals outside the plan for an additional cost.

managed care plans See *coordinated care (CC) plans.*

managed care system Health delivery method that integrates the financing and provision of appropriate health care services to covered individuals by means of arrangements with contracted providers to furnish a comprehensive set of health care services to members, explicit criteria for the selection of health care providers, and significant financial incentives for members to use providers and procedures associated with the plan. Managed care plans typically are either health maintenance organizations (HMOs), preferred provider organizations (PPOs), or point-of-service (POS) plans. Managed care services are paid by a variety of methods including capitation, fee-for-service, or a combination of the two.

managed competition Health care reform system wherein health plans offer their most competitive rates to provide health insurance coverage. This system changes competition in the health insurance market from risk (insuring healthy persons instead of those with preexisting conditions) to price. Employers form large purchasing networks to obtain insurance coverage at reduced rates. The employers pay for the employees and the employees choose a health plan they want during open enrollment and pay the difference between the employer's contribution and the cost of the plan. The insurance coverage is transferable if the employee changes jobs. Also known as *managed cooperation*. See also *consumer health alliances*.

managed cooperation See *managed competition*.

managed fee-for-service System composed of a combination of fee-for-service (FFS) and managed care components to control inappropriate use such as precertification, second surgical opinion, and utilization review. The costs of covered services given to members are paid by the plan after the services have been used. Also referred to as *managed fee-for-service product*.

managed fee-for-service product See *managed fee-for-service*.

managed health care See *managed care*.

managed health care plan See *managed care organization (MCO)*.

managed indemnity plan Standard fee-for-service (FFS) health insurance plan that uses some managed care components such as concurrent utilization review and precertification for hospital and outpatient services. This type of plan allows members freedom of choice among providers.

Management and Administrative Reporting Subsystem (MARS) One of the systems approved by the Centers for Medicare and Medicaid Services (CMS) that supports the operation of the Medicaid program. MARS is a federally mandated comprehensive reporting module of the Medicaid Management Information System (MMIS) that includes data and reports as specified by federal requirements.

management services organization (MSO) Type of publicly or privately held administrative group that gives strategic, financial, and operational plans needed by physicians, clinics, and ancillary service providers for a successful managed care business enterprise. The MSO contracts with payers, hospitals, and physicians to provide services such as negotiating fee schedules, handling administrative functions, billing, and collections. An MSO may own the facilities and employ nonphysician staff to deliver care or may be a direct subsidiary of a hospital or owned by investors. Sometimes referred to as *medical services organization (MSO)* or *physician management corporation (PMC)*.

managing general agent (MGA) Independent contractor authorized to appoint personal producing general agents (PPGAs) on behalf of an insurance company and who may represent more than one company.

mandated benefits 1. Medical services required by state or federal statutes but not necessarily covered as an insurance benefit (e.g., medical services for child abuse or rape or mandated 48-hour maternity stays following delivery of a baby). Also referred to as *mandated services*. 2. Minimum insurance benefits specified under federal or state regulations (e.g., specific smallest amount of benefits that must be paid for alcoholism under all insurance contracts sold in the state). Also called *state legislated benefits*.

mandated providers 1. Health care professionals who must be state or federal licensed providers to render services under a managed care plan (e.g., chiropractors, optometrists, podiatrists, psychologists). 2. Health care suppliers whose medical services must be included in insurance coverage offered by a health plan as required by state or federal regulations.

mandated services Under Medicaid programs, medical services required by state statutes for needy individuals such as inpatient and outpatient hospital services, laboratory tests, x-rays, home health care, family planning, nurse midwives, nursing facility care, dental services, renal dialysis services, and medical transportation. Also referred to as *mandated benefits*.

mandatory enrollment Required membership in a program (e.g., Medicaid managed care, Medicare Part D).

mandatory outpatient surgery List of surgical procedures that should be performed as an outpatient to reduce unnecessary inpatient hospital admission.

mandatory securities valuation reserve (MSVR) Liability account designed to absorb, within specified limits, realized and unrealized gains and losses that result from an insurance company's investments.

mandatory spending Outlay of funds for entitlement programs such as Medicare and Medicaid that are not subject to the federal appropriations process.

mandatory supplemental benefits Medical services not covered by Medicare that enrollees must purchase as a condition of enrollment in a Medicare Advantage Plan. Usually those services are paid for by premiums and/or cost sharing. Mandatory supplemental benefits can be different for each Medicare Advantage Plan. Medicare Advantage Plans must ensure that any particular group of Medicare beneficiaries does not use mandatory supplemental benefits to discourage enrollment.

M

manifestation Characteristic signs or symptoms associated with an illness.

manipulation Reduction or correction of a fracture or joint dislocation by applying manual force to move it into its normal anatomical position or alignment.

manual Book published by an insurance company or rating bureau that is used as a guide. It contains rates, classifications, specifications, and rules pertaining to various types of insurance policies.

manual billing Processing statements by hand; may involve typing statements or photocopying the patient's ledger and placing it in a window envelope, which then becomes the statement.

manual claim review Physical analysis of an insurance claim, prepayment or postpayment, that requires the intervention of program safeguard contractor (PSC) personnel.

manual premium rate See *manual rate*.

manual rate Cost of a unit of insurance protection (premium) obtained from the insurance company's standard rating table that appears in the underwriting manual. Also referred to as *manual premium rate* or *manual rating*.

manual rating See *manual rate* .

manual transmittal Online instruction manual that the Centers for Medicare and Medicaid Services (CMS) transmits to Medicare carriers. It includes guidelines for processing and paying Medicare claims, preparing reimbursement forms, billing procedures, and Medicare regulations. The manual system has been replaced by online, Internet-only manuals (IOMs)—the, *National Coverage Determinations Manual, Medicare Benefit Policy Manual, Publication 100*, one-time notifications, and manual revision and update notices. This information is helpful to providers when dealing with Medicare contractors for issues such as researching information, claims processing, and appealing denials. Formerly known as *Medicare Coverage Manual (MCM)*. See *Medicare Coverage Manual (MCM)*.

mapping See *data mapping, crosswalk*, and *crosswalking*.

MAR See *medication administration record (MAR)*.

margin Insurance provision to allow for an error when estimating premium rates and reserve requirements.

marine insurance Type of insurance coverage for protection of cargo (goods) in transit and the vessels and vehicles of transportation (i.e., ocean transit, over land, and by air). Also called *ocean marine insurance*.

market area Specific geographical region where an insurance plan's chief market potential is located. It may not be the same as its service area, but many times it can overlap.

market basket See *hospital market basket*.

market basket index Table used by the Centers for Medicare and Medicaid Services (CMS) to compute and update the indexes for most facilities. It takes into consideration three elements: a set of input categories (labor, supplies, purchased services); a set of price proxies that represent price levels for the input categories; and a fixed set of weights (proportions) that represent the importance of each input category for providers' input expenditures for the base year. The formula is to take the actual or projected values of the price proxies for a year, multiply them by the category weights, and total them to get the overall market basket index value for the year. For physicians' office practices, see *Medicare Economic Index (MEI)*.

market pressure Situation that affects primary decision-making by providers or health plans that is related to competitive levels of insurance benefits or types of medical services.

market price Amount paid or value considered in the open market at which a security or stock can be bought or sold.

market segment Phrase that refers to the section, part, or portion of a specific class or type of potentially enrolled consumer for selling an insurance contract (e.g., groups under 100 employees or self-funded groups).

market share Section or portion of a potential market, usually expressed as a percentage, that a managed care plan has captured.

market value Current assets worth that is based on the daily stock market such as stocks, bonds, and real estate.

market value clause Provision in an insurance policy that provides that the insurance company, in the event of loss, will pay the selling price of the completed merchandise instead of cost replacement or its actual value.

marketing 1. All activities pertaining to the selling of insurance and its products to the consumer such as advertising and packaging. 2. Under the Health Insurance Portability and Accountability Act (HIPAA), make a communication about a product or service that encourages recipients of the communication to purchase or use the product or service. Marketing may also include an agreement between a covered entity and any other entity when the covered entity releases protected health information to the other entity in exchange for direct or indirect payment so that the other entity can market its product or service. Covered entities are not engaged in marketing when it exchanges information to persons about (a) participating providers and health plans in a network, the services offered by a provider, or the benefits covered by a medical plan; (b) the individual's treatment; or (c) case management or care coordination for that individual, or directions or recommendations for alternative treatments, health care providers, or settings of care to that individual.

married In a managed care contract, a hospital facility and a managed care plan that agree to work exclusively with each other. Also see *unmarried*.

MARS See *Management and Administrative Reporting Subsystem (MARS)*.

mass immunization center Location where providers administer pneumococcal pneumonia and influenza virus vaccination and submit these services as electronic media claims or paper claims or use the roster billing method. This generally takes place in a mass immunization setting such as a public health center, pharmacy, or mall but may include a physician's office setting.

mass marketing Sales technique employed by insurance companies to immediately reach a vast number of potentially interested individuals.

master charge list See *charge description master (CDM)*.

master contract Insurance policy issued to a group insurance policyholder that lists the provisions (terms and conditions) of the group insurance plan. Also called *master policy*.

master patient index (MPI) File for a facility's patients that contains demographic information such as gender, date of birth, Social Security number, medical record number, address, race and ethnicity, admission and discharge dates, encounter types, and disposition (i.e., intended care setting following discharge). Optional additional elements might be emergency contacts, allergies, and problem lists. This file lists a unique identification number for each patient and is a cross-reference used to obtain a patient's health record. Also referred to as *member index*.

master plan Employee-benefit retirement plan created by a financial institution or insurer that can be adopted only by plan sponsors who use the financial institution to fund the plan.

master policy See *master contract*.

matching contributions Contributions made by an employer on behalf of an employee's pension plan that are equal to the employee's contributions up to a specific amount or percentage of compensation.

material fact Statement of a situation that is of such importance that disclosure would alter an underwriting decision regarding issuance or rating of an insurance policy or loss settlement.

material misrepresentation See *misrepresentation*.

Material Safety Data Sheet (MSDS) Document that informs industrial purchasers and users of hazardous chemicals of the reasonably foreseeable physical and chemical hazards that may arise from the use of those chemicals. Most materials packaged for consumer use are exempt from the requirements of the Hazard Communication Standard (HCS). The MSDS should include precautions for normal use, handling, storage, disposal, and spill cleanup. The HCS requires that accurate information be provided on the MSDSs. This applies as much to "overwarning" on the MSDS and label, as well as the absence of information ("underwarning").

material weakness Serious flaw in management controls that requires high-priority corrective action.

Maternal and Child Health Program (MCHP) A state service organization to assist children younger than 21 years of age who have conditions leading to health problems. It operates with federal grant support under Title V of the Social Security Act. In some states this program may be known as *Children's Special Health Care Services (CSHCS)* or *State Children's Health Insurance Program (SCHIP)*.

maternity benefit Provision that may appear in a hospital or medical insurance policy; allows payment for normal pregnancy.

maternity care In an obstetrical case, inpatient hospital care that includes use of the delivery room, postpartum care, and care of the newborn infant.

mature minor Individual (mid- to late-teen) considered mature enough to understand a physician's recommendations for treatment and give his or her informed consent. Also see *minor* and *emancipated minor*.

matured endowment Endowment insurance policy that has reached the end of its term during the lifetime of the insured and is due for payment.

maturity date Date on which an endowment policy matures and begins to pay out benefits to the policyholder.

maturity factor Dollar amount sum (factor) to annualize insurance claims where less than 1 year's experience is obtainable. For example, if only 10 months of claims exist, the total dollar amount is multiplied by a maturity factor of 1.2 to obtain a 1-year claim amount (10 × 1.2 = 12).

maximum allowable Sum set by an insurance company as the greatest amount that it will pay for a specific medical benefit or procedure. Third-party actual payment may be less than the maximum allowable because of the insured's deductible and coinsurance. Also called *maximum allowable charge, maximum allowable amount, allowed amount*, or *approved amount*.

maximum allowable actual charge (MAAC) Formerly a provision of the Medicare program that affected nonparticipating (nonpar) physicians before January 1, 1991. It set a limit on fees billed by a nonpar provider for professional and incident to professional services. This system was replaced with the resource-based relative value scale (RBRVS). See *limiting charge*.

maximum allowable amount See *maximum allowable* and *maximum allowable charge (MAC)*.

maximum allowable charge (MAC) Highest amount a health care provider or pharmacy vendor who participates in an insurance plan may be paid for a specific service to members of the plan under a certain contract. Also called *fee maximum, maximum allowable, maximum allowable amount, allowed amount*, or *approved amount*.

maximum allowable cost (MAC) list Pharmacy benefit manager (PBM) or insurance health plan's schedule or table that shows the greatest price they will pay for a generic drug. It is usually a dollar amount that is near the low end of the price scale. Participating pharmacies receive this list, and it may be reviewed from time to time by the PBM or health plan. If a member of the plan orders a brand name, he or she must pay the difference between the MAC price and the brand. See *drug price review (DPR)*.

maximum allowable cost (MAC) program 1. Federal regulation that limits payment for prescription drugs under the Medicaid program. 2. Administration of a pharmacy benefit manager's (PBM's) or insurance health plan's maximum allowable cost (MAC) list. See *maximum allowable cost (MAC) list*.

maximum allowable fee Largest dollar amount established by a managed care plan that a physician may charge for a medical service or procedure.

maximum benefit Largest dollar amount that an insured may receive under an insurance policy. This insurance provision may be set annually or for the lifetime of the policy. It is generally indexed to inflation so that it increases as price levels increase.

maximum benefit period Greatest length of time that benefits are payable in any one period of disability. Also called *indemnity limit*.

maximum benefits for related confinements provision Insurance rider that may be seen in basic hospital and surgical policies. It limits the maximum benefits for hospital confinements and for surgery done during one episode of illness or for any single injury.

maximum claim liability Greatest dollar amount of insurance claims payment for which an insurance company is responsible.

maximum daily hospital benefit Health insurance policy provision that states the greatest dollar amount paid for the daily inpatient hospital room rate.

maximum defined data set Under HIPAA, necessary data elements for a particular standard based on a certain implementation specification. The sender who creates the transaction may include whatever data the receiver might require. The receiver of the data may ignore any part of the data that is not necessary to carry on its portion of the business transaction unless some unnecessary data are necessary for coordination of benefits with another insurance company.

maximum enrollee out-of-pocket costs Medicare beneficiary's highest dollar liability amount (copayments, deductibles, and coinsurance) for a specified time period.

maximum fee schedule Third-party reimbursement arrangement in which a participating provider agrees to accept the contract's schedule of allowances as the total fee for each covered health care service rendered.

maximum lifetime benefits Total amount a health insurance plan will pay for medical care for any individual insured.

maximum medical improvement (MMI) In workers' compensation, the point of greatest recovery after all treatment has been used within a reasonable time period to allow for optimal recovery and other physiological adjustments to occur. Also see *permanent and stationary (P & S)*.

maximum medical improvement and impairment (MMI) In workers' compensation disability rating, it is a measurement of long-term impairment often expressed as a percentage of total body function.

maximum out-of-pocket costs Limit on the total medical expenses (number of copayments, deductibles, and coinsurance) that an insured must pay that are not covered under a managed care contract.

maximum plan benefit coverage Highest dollar amount per time period that a plan will insure. This is only applicable for service categories where there are enhanced benefits being offered by the plan because Medicare coverage does not allow a maximum plan benefit coverage expenditure limit.

maximum tax base Annual dollar amount above which earnings in employment covered under the health insurance (HI) program are not taxable. Beginning in 1994, the maximum tax base was eliminated under HI. Also called *contribution base*.

maximum taxable amount of annual earnings See *maximum tax base*.

maximums Greatest amount an insurance carrier will pay for a specific benefit or policy during a specified time period.

MBHP See *managed behavioral health program (MBHP)*.

MC See *moderate complexity (MC)*.

MCCA See *Medicare Catastrophic Coverage Act (MCCA)*.

McCarran-Ferguson Act Federal legislation (Public Law 15) enacted in 1945 providing that even though the insuring or provision of health care may be national in scope, the regulation of insurance is left to the states. Under the Act, insurance is exempt from some federal antitrust statutes to the extent that it is regulated by the states. The exemption primarily applies to gathering data in concert for the purpose of ratemaking. Otherwise, antitrust laws prohibit insurers from boycotting, acting coercively, restraining trade, or violating the Sherman or Clayton Acts.

MCCR See *Medical Care Cost Recovery (MCCR) program*.

MCD See *Medicaid (MCD)*.

MCE See *Medicare code editor (MCE)* or *medical care evaluation (MCE)*.

MCM See *Medicare Carriers Manual (MCM)*.

MCO/PHP standards See *managed care organization/ prepaid health plan (MCO/PHP) standards*.

MCOs See *managed care organizations (MCOs)*.

MCR See *modified community rating (MCR)* and *Medicare Contracting Reform (MCR)*.

MD 1. Acronym that means a Doctor of Medicine degree. See *medical doctor (MD)*. 2. See *Doctor of Osteopathy (DO)*.

MDCs See *major diagnostic categories (MDCs)*.

MDM See *medical decision-making (MDM)*.

MDO See *monthly debit ordinary (MDO) insurance*.

MDS See *minimum data set (MDS)*.

ME See *medical examiner (ME)* and *medical examination (ME)*.

measurement Systematic process of data collection, repeated over time or at a single point in time.

med-surg Abbreviation for medical-surgical. See *medical-surgical nursing* and *medical-surgical procedures*.

medblogging See *medical blogging*.

MedCHAMP See *Medicare and CHAMPUS (MedCHAMP)*.

MEDCIN® Reference medical terminology classification system created by the National Committee on Vital Health and Statistics that is used to code text data after they are captured by an electronic health record (EHR) system. It assists in the standardization of clinical point of care terminology used in EHRs.

mediate To settle differences between two parties.

Medicaid (MCD) Medical assistance program established in 1965 by Title XIX of the Social Security Act that is jointly funded by the federal government and the states. It provides medical benefits for certain low-income persons in need of health and medical care. Recipients' benefits, data for claims processing, and payments vary from state to state. Medicaid is jointly funded by the federal and state governments to assist states in providing long-term care assistance to people who meet certain eligibility criteria. California's Medicaid program is known as *Medi-Cal*.

Medicaid eligibility verification system (MEVS) Lets providers electronically access the state's eligibility file using a point-of-sale device, computer software, and automated voice response system. Also called *recipient eligibility verification system (REVS)*.

Medicaid expansion program Any federal or state health insurance program that receives funds via the Medicaid legislation with the intent to provide additional health services to Medicaid recipients.

Medicaid fiscal agent Organization under contract to the state to process claims for a state Medicaid program.

Medicaid Integrity Program (MIP) Federal program created by the Deficit Reduction Act of 2005 to track and prevent Medicaid fraud. Government contractors will review the actions of those seeking payment from Medicaid, conduct audits, identify overpayments, and educate providers and others on program integrity and quality of care.

Medicaid managed care organization (MCO) Prepaid health plan that provides comprehensive services to Medicaid beneficiaries but not to commercial or Medicare enrollees. Also called *Medicaid-only managed care organization (MCO)*.

Medicaid Management Information System (MMIS) System approved by the Centers for Medicare and Medicaid Services (CMS) that supports the operation of the Medicaid program. It includes the following types of subsystems or files: recipient eligibility, Medicaid provider, claims processing, pricing, Surveillance and Utilization Review System (SURS), Management and Administrative Reporting Subsystem (MARS), and potentially encounter processing. The objectives of this system and its enhancements include the Title XIX program control and administrative costs, service to recipients and providers, answers to inquiries, operations of claims control and computer capabilities, and management reporting for planning and control.

Medicaid-only managed care organization (MCO) See *Medicaid managed care organization (MCO)*.

Medicaid state agency State division that is responsible for administering federal and state policies and overseeing the state's Medicaid program.

Medi-Cal California's version of the nationwide program known as *Medicaid*. See *Medicaid (MCD)*.

medical application See *application form*.

medical assistant (MA) Person who, under the direction of a physician, performs various routine administrative and nontechnical clinical tasks in a hospital, clinic, or other medical facility. See *administrative medical assistant* and *clinical medical assistant*.

medical biller See *insurance billing specialist*.

medical blogging Online publications by physicians or health care workers over the Internet. Content ranges from medical studies and opinions of interpretations of medical studies to hot topics in the news related to health care such as tort reform and Medicare reimbursement, with links to interesting news items. Often called *medblogging*.

medical capitation plan See *independent practice association (IPA)*.

medical care When one hears *medical care*, it infers treatment of illness or injury, maintenance of health, and prevention of disease by or under the supervision of a physician. The phrase *health care* has the intent of a broader scope of meaning when compared with the phrase *medical care*. See also *health care*.

Medical Care Cost Recovery (MCCR) program Program developed by the Department of Veterans Affairs (VA) to allow the VA to bill third-party payers for non-service-connected care rendered by the VA to veterans and to collect copayments from veterans with less than a 50% service-connected disability rating for non-service-connected care given, based on ability to pay.

medical care evaluation (MCE) 1. Form of health care review in which a component of the quality assurance program audits and monitors the quality of both the delivery and organization of medical services. The purpose is to ensure that health care services are appropriate to the patients' needs and of the highest quality and that the managed care plan in

M

place supports and provides the care. 2. The Medicare Conditions of Participation require an audit with the use of screening criteria for evaluation by diagnosis and/or procedure. Utilization review requirements under Medicare and Medicaid require utilization review committees in hospitals and skilled nursing facilities to have at least one such study in progress at all times. Such studies are required by the Quality Improvement Organization (QIO) program. This is called *medical care evaluation studies (MCE studies)*.

medical care evaluation studies (MCE studies) See *medical care evaluation (MCE)*.

medical case management See *case management*.

medical code sets Codes that characterize a medical condition or treatment. These code sets are usually maintained by professional societies and public health organizations. Compare with administrative code sets.

medical coder See *coder*.

medical coding See *coding*.

medical condition Any physical or mental state that results from illness, disease, injury, pregnancy, or congenital malformation.

medical consultation See *consultation*.

medical cost ratio (MCR) See *loss ratio*.

medical decision making (MDM) Health care management process done after performing a history and physical examination on a patient that results in a plan of treatment. It is based on establishing one or more diagnoses and/or selecting a management or treatment option, amount of data or complexity of data reviewed, and complications and/or morbidity or mortality. Four types of MDM are straightforward, low complexity (LC), moderate complexity (MC), and high complexity (HC).

medical direction Defined by Medicare, an anesthesiologist's involvement with a certified registered nurse anesthetist (CRNA) or anesthesiology assistant (AA) in one, two, three, or four concurrent procedures where the anesthesiologist is physically present and where all the seven requirements are met and documented. Medicare does not recognize medical direction by the anesthesiologist if he or she is involved in more than four concurrent procedures. When the anesthesiologist takes on five or more cases, he or she is supervising or has failed to meet the medical direction requirements, with a few exceptions [Medicare Carriers Manual, Section 4830].

medical directive See *living will*.

medical director Usually a physician who is employed by a hospital or managed care organization (MCO) in an administrative capacity as head of the organized medical staff. He or she acts as a liaison for the staff with the administration and governing body.

medical doctor (MD) See *physician*.

medical documentation See *documentation*.

medical editor (ME) Individual who reviews onscreen notes or a computer-generated hard copy document while listening to the physician's voice on tape. The correctionist makes changes related to voice recognition errors such as corrections, changes, additions, and deletions. The final product is given to the physician for review before becoming part of the patient's medical record. Also referred to as a *correctionist*. See also *medical proofreader*.

medical emergency See *emergency (EMG)*.

medical examination (ME) Physical examination performed by a physician to determine if an insurance applicant has any physical, moral, occupational, or financial characteristics of risk. These qualities are evaluated by the insurance company to determine whether to insure the entity. An ME may also be performed when an insured claims to have disability and to determine whether he or she is actually disabled.

medical examiner (ME) 1. Physician approved by the insurance company to perform a medical examination on an individual who is applying for health or life insurance. 2. Member of a national or state board of medical examiners. 3. Physician authorized by a government agency to determine cause of death for a situation that does not occur under natural circumstance. See also *coroner*.

medical expense coverage See *no-fault insurance*.

medical expense insurance Type of health insurance that provides benefits for health care costs incurred for medical care such as hospital room and board, surgeon's fees, office visits to doctors, prescription drugs, medical treatments, and nursing care. Some managed care plans offer benefits for preventive care.

medical foundation See *foundation for medical care (FMC)*.

medical group 1. Group of physicians and/or providers structured as a sole professional business that is recognized under state law as an entity to practice a medical profession. 2. In a managed care plan, a professional organization of physicians that contracts with a health plan to deliver both primary or basic and special medical care to plan members.

Medical Group Management Association (MGMA) National membership organization that provides information, networking, and professional development for the individuals who manage and lead medical group practices. Its purpose is to improve the effectiveness of medical group practices and the knowledge and skills of the individuals who manage and lead them. It provides its members data on physician compensation, performance efficiency, and medical practice comparisons.

medical group practice See *group practice*.

medical identity theft When an individual uses a person's name and sometimes other parts of the identity such as insurance information without the person's knowledge or consent to obtain medical services or goods or uses the person's identity information to make false claims for medical services or goods. Also called *identity theft.*

medical informatics Study of storage, retrieval, analysis, and communication of biomedical and clinical information to improve medical decision-making by physicians and managers of health care organizations. Also referred to as *medical information science* and *informatics.*

medical information Data needed about the onset and history of a specific illness so that a managed care plan may establish if benefits are available for treatment.

Medical Information Bureau (MIB), Inc. Nonstock, nonprofit membership association of life insurance companies of the United States and Canada that provides information and database management services to the financial services industry. Organized in 1902, MIB's core fraud protection services protect insurers, policyholders, and applicants from attempts to conceal or omit information material to the sound and equitable underwriting of life, health, disability, and long-term care insurance. Fair pricing of insurance products is dependent on accurate "risk assessment," "risk classification," and "risk selection." A determination of these factors begins with the assurance of accurate health information supplied on the insurance application concerning the proposed insured.

medical insurance See *health insurance.*

medical insurance billing specialist Employee who works for a physician or in a health care facility and handles source documents, codes procedures and diagnoses, processes insurance claims, and follows up on delayed reimbursement and delinquent accounts. Also known as an *insurance claims processor, medical biller,* or *reimbursement specialist.* Also see *insurance billing specialist.*

medical-legal (ML) evaluation In workers' compensation, the independent assessment of an employee that results in the preparation of a narrative medical report prepared and attested to in accordance with the state labor code. It must be performed by either a qualified medical evaluator, agreed medical evaluator, or the primary treating physician for the purpose of proving or disproving a contested workers' compensation claim.

medical-legal expense Any costs and expenses incurred by or on behalf of any party, the administrative director, the board, or a referee for x-rays, laboratory fees, other diagnostic tests, medical reports, medical records, medical testimony, or interpreter's fees, for the purpose of proving or disproving a contested workers' compensation claim.

medical-legal testimony In workers' compensation cases, expert testimony given by a physician at a deposition or appeals board hearing about the medical opinion submitted by the physician.

medical licensing board See *physician licensing board.*

medical loss ratio (MLR) See *loss ratio.*

medical malpractice insurance See *professional liability insurance (PLI)* and *malpractice insurance.*

medical management System employed by health insurance and managed care plans that uses administration and policy and the individuals who make the decisions and supervise to achieve business objectives and reduce costs and use of health care services.

medical meaningfulness Phrase used in statistics that explains patients in the same diagnosis-related groups (DRGs) that are anticipated to have a set of clinical responses that result in a comparable pattern of use of medical services and supplies.

medical model of health care delivery Medical care given only when an individual is ill with emphasis on the diagnosis and treatment of disease instead of health promotion and prevention of disease.

medical necessity 1. Performance of services and procedures required by the patient, indispensable, and consistent with the diagnosis in accordance with standards of good medical practice, performed at the proper level, and provided in the most appropriate setting. Medical necessity must be established (via diagnostic and/or other information presented on the individual claim under consideration) before the carrier may make payment. 2. Cal. Wel. & Inst. Code 14059.5 defines medical necessity when it is reasonable and necessary to protect life, to prevent significant illness or significant disability, or to alleviate severe pain. Also see *medically necessary care.*

medical nutrition therapy (MNT) Specific nutritional procedures including assessment, counseling sessions, and interventions in the treatment of an acute or chronic illness, injury, or disease condition. MNT is provided by registered dietitians (RDs) and state-licensed dietitians.

medical-only claim In workers' compensation cases, a claim in which time lost from work does not exceed 7 calendar work days.

medical payments coverage See *no-fault insurance.*

medical payments insurance Liability insurance coverage in which the insurance company agrees to pay the insured and others, subject to a limit, for medical, surgical, hospital, and funeral expenses sustained because of bodily injury or death by accident regardless of whether the insured is liable or not. Usually this type of coverage is included in automobile and other public liability policies.

medical practice parameters See *guidelines.*

medical practice plan See *faculty practice plan (FPP).*

medical proofreader Medical transcriptionist who checks medical reports that have blanks or questionable terminology and flags them for correction by the dictator. See also *medical editor (ME).*

medical protocols See *clinical protocols.*

medical provider network (MPN) In workers' compensation insurance, group of health care providers created by an insurer or self-insured employer to treat workers injured on the job.

medical provider number See *national provider identifier (NPI)*.

medical rationing Limiting health care because of the high cost or the patient's age or chance of recovery.

medical record Written and graphic information documenting facts and events during the rendering of patient care. Records must be comprehensive and data must be accurately documented.

medical record documentation See *documentation*.

medical records employee Individual who works in a facility in the health information management department and is responsible for handling and safeguarding patient medical records such as medical records file clerk, health information management (HIM) professional, registered health information administrator (RHIA), and registered health information technician (RHIT).

medical records See *health information management (HIM)*.

Medical Records Institute Organization that promotes the development and acceptance of electronic health care record systems.

medical report Permanent, legal document (letter or report format) that formally states the results of the patient's examination or treatment.

medical review (MR) 1. Evaluation of services by contractor medical personnel; includes analysis of claims data to identify potential billing problems resulting in inappropriate utilization situations; includes various plans of action to correct the problem. 2. In the Medicaid program, an analysis by a team composed of physicians and other appropriate health and social service personnel may be required to assess the patient's condition and need for care (e.g., medical evaluations of inpatients in a long-term care facility). Also called *continued stay review*. 3. In the Medicare program, an evaluation by a Medicare administrative contractor and/or quality improvement organization (QIO) of services rendered by health care providers. This assessment is done to determine if the services are reasonable and necessary; services meet Medicare guidelines; quality of service is in line with the standards of health care; services are medically appropriate in an inpatient, outpatient, or other setting; and services are supported by documentation. Also called *utilization review*.

medical savings account (MSA) Type of tax-free savings account that allows individuals and their employers to set aside money to pay for health care expenses. An employer can set up an MSA for his or her employees and make an annual contribution to the MSA, which is tax deductible for both employer and employee. MSA balances accumulate from year to year tax-free, but unused funds may not

be carried over in a flexible spending account (FSA) (another type of MSA). Earned interest is not taxed. MSAs are portable, allowing individuals to take their MSAs with them when they change jobs or relocate. Medicare beneficiaries are eligible to enroll in a similar tax-advantaged savings account, which may be referred to as a *Medicare medical savings account*. See *dependent-care spending account*.

medical scribe See *scribe*.

medical service order An authorization from the employer that is given to the physician, either written or verbal, to treat the injured or ill employee.

medical services contract Agreement between an insurer, physician, or provider and a managed care plan; between an insurer and a physician or provider; between a managed care plan and a provider or group of providers; between medical or mental health facilities; and between a medical or mental health clinic and a physician or provider to provide medical or mental health services.

medical services organization (MSO) See *management services organization (MSO)*.

medical staff See *hospital staff*.

medical staff-hospital organization (MeSH) Association that bonds hospital facilities and attending medical staff as a network. Also known as *physician hospital organization (PHO)*. See *physician hospital organization (PHO)*.

medical student Individual who participates in an accredited education program that is not an approved graduate medical education (GME) program. A medical student is never considered to be an intern or a resident. Medicare does not pay for medical services provided by a student.

medical-surgical nursing Nursing care of adult patients whose conditions or disorders are treated pharmacologically or surgically.

medical-surgical procedures Phrase that refers to the services provided by a physician. Sometimes abbreviated as med-surg.

medical terminology Technical vocabulary of the science of medicine used throughout the health care industry.

medical transcription Act of keying voice-recorded dictation into a final document (medical report).

medical treatment In workers' compensation cases, any medical, surgical, chiropractic, and hospital care including nursing, medicines, medical and surgical supplies, crutches, and artificial members that is reasonably necessary to cure or relieve from the effects of the injury.

medical underwriting Process that an insurance company uses to decide, based on the patient's medical history, whether or not to take his or her application for insurance, whether or not to add a waiting period for preexisting conditions (if the state law allows it), and how much to charge for the insurance plan. The insurance company sets higher premiums for those deemed to be higher medical risks.

medically dependent children's program (MDCP) Medicaid program that provides a variety of services (nursing and respite) to support families caring for medically dependent children in their homes to encourage deinstitutionalization of children in nursing homes.

medically driven In a workers' compensation case, issues that require medical information for decision-making.

medically indigent (MI) See *medically needy (MN)*.

medically necessary care 1. Health care services covered by insurance that are necessary to preserve and maintain the health of a member of a managed care plan. The medical service provided must be necessary, appropriate according to current standards of medical practice, provided in the most appropriate setting, and performed at the proper level of service. 2. Cal. Wel. & Inst. Code 14059.5 defines medical necessity when it is reasonable and necessary to protect life, to prevent significant illness or significant disability, or to alleviate severe pain. See also *medical necessity* and *medically (or psychologically) necessary services*.

medically (or psychological) necessary services Medical or psychological services that are considered appropriate care; that meet standards of good medical practice; that are generally accepted by qualified professionals to be reasonable and adequate for the diagnosis and treatment of illness, injury, pregnancy, and mental disorders; that are not provided mainly for the convenience of the patient or the physician; or that are reasonable and adequate for well-baby care.

medically necessary days (MUD) That portion of a patient's inpatient hospital stay during an episode of illness or injury that is called *excessive* when care may be given in a less expensive or more efficient setting. It may be considered too long a stay when considering current standards of good medical practice.

medically needy (MN) Persons in need of financial assistance and/or whose income and resources will not allow them to pay for the costs of medical care. Also called *medically indigent* in some states. See also *charity allowance* and *charity care*.

medically underserved areas (MUAs) County, group of counties, or neighborhood that is considered to have three shortage area categories: primary care, dental care, and mental health care. Designation of a particular service area is based on the percentage of population below poverty level, percentage of population age 65 and older, infant mortality rate, and ratio of primary care physicians per 1000 population.

medically unlikely edits (MUEs) Medicare frequency edits that limit the number of units of service (UOS) that a provider may bill for certain HCPCS/CPT codes on an insurance claim for the same beneficiary

on the same date of service. MUEs were developed to catch errors and prevent inappropriate payments and are applied to each line of the claim. Thus the entire claim is not denied, and the provider only appeals the denied codes.

Medicare (M) Nationwide federal government health insurance program for persons age 65 years and older, people with certain disabilities, and people of all ages with end-stage renal disease (permanent kidney failure requiring dialysis or kidney transplant). This program is administered by the Centers for Medicare and Medicaid Services, formerly known as the *Health Care Financing Administration (HCFA)*. Local Social Security offices take applications and supply information about the program. This fee-for-service health plan lets the patient go to any physician, hospital, or other health care supplier who accepts Medicare and is accepting new Medicare patients. The patient pays the deductible. Medicare pays its share of the Medicare-approved amount, and the patient pays his or her share (coinsurance). The Original Medicare Plan has two parts: Part A (hospital insurance) and Part B (medical insurance). Also called *Original Medicare Plan* or *Medicare fee-for-service plan*.

Medicare administrative contractor (MAC) 1. Organization under contract to the state to process claims for a state Medicaid program. Also see *A/B jurisdictions*. 2. Insurance carrier that enters into an agreement with the Centers for Medicare and Medicaid Services (CMS). It receives and processes claims from physicians, hospital facilities, other suppliers of service, and durable medical equipment (DME) for Parts A and B of Medicare. Medicare contractors must have the provider customer service program (PCSP) in place to assist physicians and their staff in understanding and complying with Medicare's operational processes, policies, and billing procedures. Formerly referred to as *fiscal intermediary*, *Medicare carrier, fiscal agent, Medicare Part B carrier*, or *contractor*. Also see *Medicare Contracting Reform (MCR)* and *A/B jurisdiction*.

Medicare Advantage Law of 2003 See *high-deductible health plan (HDHP)* and *Medicare Advantage (MA) plan*.

Medicare Advantage (MA) plan Plan offered by a private insurance company that contracts with Medicare to provide beneficiaries with Medicare Part A and Part B benefits. Depending on where the patient lives, plans may or may not offer Medicare Part D prescription drug coverage. A Medicare Advantage Plan can be a health maintenance organization (HMO) plan, preferred provider organization (PPO) plan, special needs plan, or a private fee-for-service plan. In 2006 MA replaced the Medicare Plus (+) Choice program. Also referred to as *Medicare Health Plans*.

M

Medicare and CHAMPUS (MedCHAMP) Program for CHAMPUS-eligible individuals younger than the age of 65 who qualify for both Medicare and CHAMPUS. Medicare is the primary payer and CHAMPUS is the secondary payer.

Medicare-approved amount Dollar amount a physician or supplier can be paid including what Medicare pays and any deductible, coinsurance, or copayment that the patient pays. It may be less than the actual amount charged by a doctor or supplier. Sometimes called *approved charge* or *allowed amount*.

Medicare beneficiary See *beneficiary*.

Medicare Benefit Policy Manual (BP) Online instruction handbook that the Centers for Medicare and Medicaid Services (CMS) makes available to Medicare carriers. It includes guidelines for processing and paying Medicare claims, preparing reimbursement forms, billing procedures, and Medicare regulations. This system has online, Internet-only manuals (IOM): National Coverage Determinations Manual, Publication 100, one-time notifications, and manual revision and update notices. This information is helpful to providers when dealing with Medicare contractors for issues such as researching information, claims processing, and appealing denials. Formerly found in Chapter II of the *Medicare Carriers Manual, the Medicare Intermediary Manual* and various provider manuals and program memorandums.

Medicare benefits Health insurance available under Medicare Part A and Part B through the traditional fee-for-service payment system.

Medicare Benefits Notice (MBN) Document that the patient receives after the physician files an insurance claim for Part A services in the Original Medicare Plan. It lists the services the provider billed, the Medicare-approved amount, the Medicare payment, and the amount the patient must pay. The patient may also receive a Medicare Summary Notice (MSN) (formerly known as an *Explanation of Medicare Benefits [EOMB]*). See also *Medicare Summary Notice (MSN), remittance advice (RA)*, and *Explanation of Medicare Benefits (EOMB)*.

Medicare carrier See *fiscal agent (FA)* and *Medicare administrative contractor (MAC)*.

Medicare Carriers Manual (MCM) See *Medicare Benefit Policy Manual (BP)*.

Medicare carve-out Medical benefits offered by employers to retired employees that lowers medical expense benefits so that those benefits are provided by the Medicare program.

Medicare carved out plans See *Medicare/employer supplemental insurance*.

Medicare Catastrophic Coverage Act (MCCA) Enacted July 1, 1988, this law provided the most significant expansion of the Medicare program since its inception. It also contained numerous technical amendments to the Medicare and Medicaid programs, as well as three new Medicaid provisions. However, in December 1989, the President signed into law Public Law 101-234, which repealed the major expansions of the Medicare program enacted the previous year.

Medicare-certified provider Physician, other individual, or entity meeting certain quality standards that provides outpatient self-management training services and other Medicare-covered items and services.

Medicare code editor (MCE) Computer software program used by Medicare fiscal intermediaries that identifies code inconsistencies in data on inpatient insurance claims. The MCE evaluates the coverage, codes, and clinical information and screens for accuracy and consistency such as the patient's age, sex, discharge status, DRG payment, principal and secondary diagnoses, and procedures.

Medicare Contracting Reform (MCR) Medicare Prescription Drug Improvement and Modernization Act (MMA) of 2003 was passed by Congress in which Section 911 required the Centers for Medicare and Medicaid Services (CMS) to replace the fiscal intermediary and carrier contracts for the administration of Medicare benefits with Medicare administrative contractors (MACs). Its intention is to improve Medicare's administrative services to beneficiaries and health care providers and to bring standard contracting principles to Medicare (i.e., competition and performance incentives). In this reform, the United States will be divided into 15 A/B jurisdictions and each A/B jurisdiction will be assigned to one MAC who administers both Part A and Part B claims. Also see *Medicare administrative contractor (MAC)* and *A/B jurisdictions*.

Medicare contractor See *Medicare administrative contractor (MAC)*.

Medicare coordination of benefits contractor Medicare contractor who collects and manages information on other types of insurance or coverage that pay before Medicare. Some examples of other types of insurance or coverage are group health coverage, retiree coverage, workers' compensation, no-fault or liability insurance, veterans' benefits, TRICARE, Federal Black Lung Program, and COBRA. Also see *coordination of benefits (COB)*.

Medicare cost plan Type of health maintenance organization (HMO). If the patient receives medical services outside of the plan's network without a referral, the Medicare-covered services will be paid for under the Original Medicare Plan, except the patient's plan pays for emergency services, or urgently needed services outside the service area.

Medicare coverage Medical benefits composed of two parts: hospital insurance (Part A) and medical insurance (Part B). See *Medicare Part A* and *Medicare Part B*.

Medicare Coverage Advisory Committee (MCAC) Committee that informs the Centers for Medicare and Medicaid Services (CMS) on whether specific medical items and services are reasonable and necessary under Medicare law. They perform this task via a careful review and discussion of specific clinical and scientific issues in an open and public forum. The MCAC is advisory in nature, with the final decision on all issues resting with CMS. The advice given by the MCAC is most useful when it results from a process of full scientific inquiry and thoughtful discussion, in an open forum, with careful framing of recommendations and clear identification of the basis of those suggestions. MCAC supplements CMS's internal expertise and ensures an unbiased and contemporary consideration of state-of-the-art technology and science. MCAC members are valued for their background, education, and expertise in a wide variety of scientific, clinical, and other related fields. In composing the MCAC, CMS was diligent in pursuing ethnic, gender, geographical, and other diverse views and in carefully screening each member to determine potential conflicts of interest.

Medicare durable medical equipment regional carrier (DMERC) Regional insurance carrier that has entered into an agreement with the Centers for Medicare and Medicaid Services (CMS) to administer durable medical equipment for a region.

Medicare economic index (MEI) Table used by the Centers for Medicare and Medicaid Services (CMS) to update the annual physician fee schedule to set limits for payment. This index considers annual changes in the economy taking into account inflation, productivity, and changes in health care expense factors such as malpractice insurance, personnel salaries, rent, and other expenses.

Medicare/employer supplemental insurance Aged individuals who have supplemental insurance coverage with complementary benefits by employment plans after retirement. In some cases, coverage may be paid by a former employer after retirement. For working-aged individuals who have group health insurance through their employer or the employment of their spouse, usually Medicare is the secondary payer (MSP). Usually crossover insurance claims processing relationships exist with many insurance carriers who insure Medicare beneficiaries.

Medicare fee schedule (MFS) List of Medicare payment fees based on resource-based relative value scale

(RBRVS) factors. These factors are based on the physician's work, medical practice expense, and malpractice insurance costs. The fee schedule is based on relative value units (RVUs). A formula is used to obtain the RVU consisting of three components: relative value unit (RVU) for the service, a geographical adjustment factor (GAF), and a monetary conversion factor (CF). Synonymous with and also see *resource-based relative value scale (RBRVS)*. Also called *Medicare physician's fee schedule (MPFS)*.

Medicare Handbook Publication that is given to all Medicare beneficiaries when first enrolled in the program. It provides information about how to file an insurance claim and what type of care is covered under the program.

Medicare health plan Medicare advantage plan (e.g., HMO, PPO, or private fee-for-service plan) or other plan such as a Medicare cost plan. Everyone who has Medicare Part A and Part B is eligible for a plan in their area, except those who have end-stage renal disease (unless certain exceptions apply).

Medicare identification card Insurance card issued to the beneficiary of the Medicare government program (see Figure M-1). It includes the patient's name, insurance claim number, type of hospital and medical coverage (Part A and/or B), and effective date. The insurance claim number is the Social Security number of the wage earner with an alpha suffix.

Medicare Integrity Program (MIP) Plan that permits Medicare to contract with other entities to examine the activities of providers, audit cost reports, educate providers, and maintain a list of authorized durable medical equipment.

Medicare Intermediary Manual See *Medicare Benefit Policy Manual (BP)*.

Medicare managed care plan Type of Medicare Advantage Plan that is available in some areas of the United States. In most of these plans, the member can only go to doctors, specialists, or hospitals on the plan's list. Plans must cover all Medicare Part A and Part B health

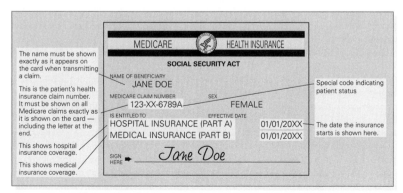

Figure M-1 Medicare health insurance identification card.

care. Costs to the member may be lower than in the Original Medicare Plan.

Medicare/Medicaid (Medi-Medi) Refers to an individual who receives medical and/or disability benefits from both Medicare and Medicaid programs. Sometimes referred to as a *Care/Caid* or *Medi-Medi case.* This term is no longer used and has been replaced by dual eligible. See *dual eligible.*

Medicare Medical Savings Account (MSA) Plan Type of Medicare health plan that is made up of two parts. One part is a Medicare MSA health insurance policy with a high deductible, and the other part is a special savings account where Medicare deposits money to help the insured pay the medical bills.

Medicare Modernization Act (MMA) See *Medicare Prescription Drug, Improvement, and Modernization Act (MMA).*

Medicare National Coverage Determinations Manual See *National Coverage Determinations Manual.*

Medicare Part A Hospital benefits of a nationwide health insurance program for persons age 65 years and older and certain disabled or blind individuals regardless of income, administered by Centers for Medicare and Medicaid Services (CMS), formerly HCFA. It was established by §1811 of Title XVIII of the Social Security Act of 1965. Local Social Security offices take applications and supply information about the program. Benefits include hospital, nursing home, hospice, home health, and other inpatient care. Insurance claims are transmitted to fiscal intermediaries for payment. Ten regional offices provide CMS with a decentralized administration and delivery of Medicare programs. Each regional office oversees private insurance companies that contract with the government to process and pay for Medicare Part A benefits. Medicare hospital insurance is also referred to as "HI."

Medicare Part A fiscal intermediary See *fiscal intermediary.*

Medicare Part B Medical insurance that is a nationwide health insurance program for persons age 65 years and older and certain disabled or blind individuals regardless of income, administered by the Centers for Medicare and Medicaid Services (CMS), formerly HCFA. It was established by §1831 of the Title XVIII of the Social Security Act of 1965. Local Social Security offices take applications and supply information about the program. Benefits include physicians' services, outpatient hospital care, durable medical equipment, and some medical services that are not covered by Part A. Physicians transmit their insurance claims to fiscal agents/intermediaries for payment. Ten regional offices provide CMS with a decentralized administration and delivery of Medicare programs. Each regional office oversees private insurance companies that contract with the government to process and pay for Medicare Part B benefits. Also referred to as *supplementary medical insurance (SMI).*

Medicare Part B carrier See *fiscal agent (FA).*

Medicare Part B premium (PBP) reduction amount Managed care organizations (MCOs) are able to use their adjusted excess to reduce the Medicare Part B premium for beneficiaries. When offering this benefit, a plan cannot reduce its payment by more than 125% of the Medicare Part B premium. In order to calculate the Part B premium reduction amount, the PBP system must multiply the number entered in the "indicate your MCO plan payment reduction amount, per member" field by 80%. The resulting number is the Part B premium reduction amount for each member in that particular plan rounded to the nearest multiple of 10 cents.

Medicare Part C Medicare Plus (+) Choice (M+C) plans offer a number of health care options in addition to those available under Medicare Part A and Part B. It was created under the Balanced Budget Act (BBA) in 1997. Plans may include health maintenance organizations (HMOs), fee-for-service plans, provider-sponsored organizations (PPOs), point-of-service (POS) plans, provider-sponsored organizations (PSOs), religious fraternal benefit society plans (RFPs), and Medicare medical savings accounts (MSAs). Also see *Medicare Plus (+) Choice (M+C) plan* and *zero premium plan.*

Medicare Part D Prescription Drug Plan Stand-alone drug plan, presented by insurance and other private companies that offer drug coverage that meets the standards established by Medicare. Other names for these plans are *Part D prescription drug plans, PDPs,* or *MA-PDs.*

Medicare Payment Advisory Commission (MedPAC or MedPac) Commission established by Congress in the Balanced Budget Act of 1997 to replace the Prospective Payment Assessment Commission (ProPAC) and the Physician Payment Review Commission (PPRC). MedPAC is directed to provide the Congress with annual advice and recommendations on payment policies affecting Medicare Parts A, B, and C. These recommendations are factored into CMS rates for Parts A and B and payments to Part C plans.

Medicare Plus (+) Choice organization Public or private entity organized and licensed by a state as a risk-bearing entity (with the exception of a provider-sponsored organization receiving waivers) that is certified by the Centers for Medicare and Medicaid Services (CMS) as meeting the M+C contract requirements. Also referred to as *Medicare Part C,* which was replaced in 2006 by the Medicare Advantage (MA) program. See *Medicare Part C.*

Medicare Plus (+) Choice (M+C) plan Health benefits coverage offered under a policy or contract by an M+C organization under which a specific set of health benefits are offered at a uniform premium and uniform level of cost-sharing to all Medicare beneficiaries residing in the service area of the M+C plan. An M+C plan may be a coordinated care plan (with or without point-of-service options), a combination of an M+C medical savings account (MSA) plan, and a contribution into an M+C MSA or an M+C private fee-for-service plan. Also referred to as *Medicare Part C*, which was replaced in 2006 by the Medicare Advantage (MA) program. See *Medicare Part C.*

Medicare Plus (+) Choice (M+C) program Medicare program created in 1997 and also referred to as *Medicare Part C*, which was replaced in 2006 by the Medicare Advantage (MA) program. See *Medicare Part C.*

Medicare Preferred Provider Organization (PPO) Plan Type of Medicare Advantage Plan in which the member uses doctors, hospitals, and providers that belong to the network but can also use physicians, hospitals, and providers outside of the network for an additional cost.

Medicare Premium Collection Center (MPCC) Contractor that handles all Medicare direct-billing payments for direct-billed beneficiaries. MPCC is located in Pittsburgh, Pennsylvania.

Medicare Prescription Drug, Improvement, and Modernization Act (MMA) Federal legislation enacted in 2003 that amended Title XVIII of the Social Security Act to provide for a voluntary program for prescription drug coverage under the Medicare program, to modernize the Medicare program, to amend the Internal Revenue Code of 1986 to allow a deduction to individuals for amounts contributed to health savings security accounts and health savings accounts, to provide for the disposition of unused health benefits in cafeteria plans and flexible spending arrangements, and for other purposes.

Medicare prescription drug plan See *Medicare Part D prescription drug plans.*

Medicare private fee-for-service plan Type of Medicare Advantage Plan in which the member may go to any Medicare-approved doctor or hospital that accepts the plan's payment. The insurance plan, rather than the Medicare program, decides how much it will pay and what the patient pays for the services. The patient may pay more or less for Medicare-covered benefits. The patient may have extra benefits the Original Medicare Plan does not cover.

Medicare Program Integrity Manual (PIM) Written guidelines that reflect the principles, values, and priorities for the Medicare Integrity Program. The primary principle of program integrity is to pay claims correctly.

Medicare program memorandums See *Medicare transmittals.*

Medicare remittance advice remark codes National administrative code set used in the X12 835 claim payment and remittance advice transaction. It provides either claim-level or service-level Medicare-related

messages that cannot be communicated with a claim adjustment reason code.

Medicare remittance notice (MRN) Paper-summarized statement for providers including payment information for one or more beneficiaries; equivalent to the *electronic remittance notice (ERN)*. See also *electronic remittance notice (ERN), remittance advice (RA)*, and *explanation of benefits (EOB).*

Medicare risk contract Agreement between Medicare and a federally qualified HMO or competitive medical plan that provides Medicare-covered services for enrollees, receives monthly capitated payments from Medicare, and assumes insurance risk for its enrollees.

Medicare risk HMO See *Medicare risk contract.*

Medicare savings program State Medicaid programs that help pay some or all Medicare premiums and deductibles if an individual meets certain income limits criteria.

Medicare Secondary Payer (MSP) Primary insurance plan of a Medicare beneficiary that must pay for any medical care or services first before Medicare is sent a claim. MSP may involve aged or disabled patients who are under group health plans and cases related to end-stage renal disease, black lung disease, workers' compensation, automobile accidents (e.g., medical no-fault and liability insurance), and individuals receiving benefits under the Department of Veterans Affairs and Medicare. For a Medicare patient suffering from end-stage renal disease (ESRD), MSP is the payer for the first 30 months that the beneficiary is entitled to benefits.

Medicare Secondary Payer alert (MSP alert) Medicare edit on inpatient, outpatient, and physician insurance claims that indicates Medicare is the secondary payer. The outpatient code editor (OCE) marks claims with specific trauma diagnosis codes to identify claims about accidents because patients may be covered under other liability insurance that would be a primary payer. The insurance carrier places these claims in suspense for additional review and determination.

Medicare Select Type of Medigap (supplemental) health insurance policy that may require a member to use hospitals and, in some cases, doctors within its network to be eligible for full benefits. Emergency care may be sought outside the preferred provider network.

Medicare Summary Notice (MSN) Document received by the patient explaining amount charged, Medicare approval, deductible, and coinsurance for medical services rendered. See also *remittance advice, Explanation of Medicare Benefits (EOMB)*, and *Medicare Benefits Notice (MBN).*

Medicare supplement (Medsupp) policy See *Medigap (MG) policy.*

Medicare transmittals Informative messages issued by the Centers for Medicare and Medicaid Services

M

(CMS) to update program policies and procedures; formerly called *Medicare program memorandums*.

Medicare trust funds Treasury accounts established by the Social Security Act for the receipt of revenues, maintenance of reserves, and disbursement of payments for the health insurance and supplemental medical insurance programs.

Medicare UPIN numbers See *national provider identifier (NPI)*.

Medicare Volume Performance Standard (MVPS) Percentage figure that represents an acceptable rate of increase in physicians' Medicare reimbursement for 1 year. MVPS is based on inflation, mix, and age of Medicare population, technological changes, improper utilization, and inadequate access to care. The Department of Health and Human Services uses a formula to establish the annual Medicare Part B increase in physicians' payments.

Medicare wrap See *Medigap (MG) policy*.

medication administration record (MAR) Drug history during the admission/encounter of the patient in the hospital.

medication aide See *Medication Assistant-Certified (MA-C)*.

medication assistant See *Medication Assistant-Certified (MA-C)*.

Medication Assistant-Certified (MA-C) Title received by a Certified Nursing Assistant (CNA) who takes additional education in preparing for a role in administering oral and topical medications, works under the supervision of a licensed nurse, and passes a state certification examination. Medication assistants primarily work in nursing homes.

medication therapy management Type of help that individuals with multiple prescriptions, chronic diseases, and high drug costs receive to help them manage all of their medications for the purpose of making sure all of the drugs work well together.

Medication Therapy Management Services (MTMS) CPT Category III code series that allows for billing by the pharmacist when he or she reviews pertinent patient history, reviews the medication profile (prescription and nonprescription), and makes recommendations for improving health outcomes and treatment compliance.

medicine section Division of the *Current Procedural Terminology (CPT)* code book that contains information about injections, psychiatric procedures, dialysis services, gastroenterology procedures, ophthalmology services, otorhinolaryngologic services, cardiovascular therapeutic services, noninvasive vascular diagnostic studies, allergy and immunology tests, neurology and neuromuscular procedures, chemotherapy administration, physical medicine, acupuncture, chiropractic treatment, and other special services and procedures.

Medifill See *Medigap (MG) policy*.

Medigap Compare Several websites have been created that help Medicare beneficiaries to find insurance companies that sell Medigap insurance plans and to compare coverage costs (e.g., http://www.medicare.gov/medigap/default.asp). A Google search using key words "Medigap Compare" can also be used to do this research.

Medigap (MG) policy Specialized Medicare supplemental insurance policy whose predefined minimum benefits are regulated by the federal government and devised for the Medicare beneficiary. It typically covers the deductible and copayment amounts not covered under the Medicare policy. This coverage is available only to individuals who are covered by Medicare and is purchased by individuals or by employers to cover retired employees. Except in Massachusetts, Minnesota, and Wisconsin, there are 12 standardized plans labeled Plan A through Plan L. Medigap policies only work with the Original Medicare Plan. Also known as *complementary program, gap fill, Medifill, Medicare supplement policy, Medsupp, Medicare wrap, supplemental health insurance*, or *wraparound plan*.

Medigap protections See *guaranteed issue rights*.

Medi-Medi case Sometimes referred to as a *Care/Caid case*. See *Medicare/Medicaid (Medi-Medi)*. Also see *crossover patient*.

MedPAC See *Medicare Payment Advisory Commission (MedPAC)*.

MEDPARD Directory State and county directory that contains names, addresses, and specialties of Medicare-participating physicians who have agreed to accept assignment on all Medicare claims and covered services.

Medsupp Acronym for Medicare supplement (Medsupp) policy. See *Medigap (MG) policy*.

meeting of the minds Situation in which both parties agree and understand their responsibilities and rights under an insurance contract.

megabyte Computer storage capacity in which one megabyte is equal to 1000 kilobytes (1024 characters).

MEI See *Medicare economic index (MEI)*.

member 1. Person covered under the Blue Cross/Blue Shield subscriber's contract including the subscriber or contract holder who is the person named on the membership identification card and in the case of (1) two-person coverage, (2) one adult–one child coverage, or (3) family coverage, eligible family dependents enrolled under the subscriber's contract. 2. Individual who purchases health insurance coverage. Also called *certificate holder, enrollee, insured, policyholder*, and *subscriber*.

member continuity Continuation of insurance coverage without lapse when making a change from one group to another or one health plan to another.

member contribution See *percentage contribution*.

member health index Health insurance plan's complex formula that measures and tracks the insured's overall health levels such as how often they are in emergency departments, how often they receive preventive care, and whether they take needed medications.

member index See *master patient index.*

member months Total managed care plan membership each month for a given time period (e.g., 200 members serviced each month for 6 months equals 1200 member months). Operating figures for managed care companies may be expressed in terms of member months (e.g., per member per month [PMPM] or per member per year [PMPY]).

member services department Payment section of the insurance carrier that acts as a patient advocate to resolve problems and take insurance claims appeals to a committee after all other processes have been used.

membership State of belonging to a managed care plan as a subscribing member and entitled to the benefits, right, privileges, and obligations. For family coverage, this may include enrollment of eligible dependents.

membership agreement Formal contract with a health plan that consists of enrollment application, health statements, and certificate of coverage including any amendments. Also referred to as *membership service agreement.*

membership application form Prospective applicant's enrollment form when applying to a health plan for health coverage. It must be signed and may serve as an agreement between the member and the health plan. Also see *application form.*

membership benefits See *benefit* and *benefit package.*

membership card See *identification card (ID card).*

membership file Insurance company's electronic master file of information on insured individuals such as names, certificate numbers, and contract data.

membership service agreement See *membership agreement.*

memorandum of understanding Document that provides a general description of the responsibilities that are to be assumed by two or more parties in their pursuit of some goals. It is used when agencies enter into a joint project in which (1) they each contribute their own resources and the scope of work is broad and not specific to any one project or (2) there is no exchange of goods or services between the participating agencies.

memory Storage in computer.

mental health parity Equality of health insurance coverage for the diagnosis and treatment of mental disorders and substance abuse services. National and state organizations have made efforts to obtain progress in this direction. See Mental Health Parity Act (MHPA).

Mental Health Parity Act (MHPA) Federal legislation enacted on September 26, 1996, that prohibits a lifetime dollar amount on mental health benefits by group health insurance plans and those that issue coverage under such plans.

mental health provider Psychiatrist, social worker, psychiatric nurse, psychiatric hospital, or other institution for mental disease that is licensed to render mental health services.

mental health/substance abuse Insurance payer phrase for health care services given to members of a managed care or private plan for emotional problems or chemical dependency.

mental illness Any type of illness in which psychological syndrome, intellectual, emotional, or behavioral dysfunction is the main feature.

mental retardation Disorder characterized by significantly below average general intellectual function with deficits or impairments in the ability to learn and to adapt socially. The cause may be genetic, biological, psychosocial, or traumatic.

mentor Guide or teacher who offers advice, criticism, wisdom, guidance, and perspective to an inexperienced but promising protégé to help reach a life goal.

MeSH See *medical staff-hospital organization (MeSH).*

messenger model Agent or third party that conveys to purchasers information obtained individually from providers in the network about the prices the network participants are willing to accept and conveying to providers any contract offers made by purchasers. Each provider then makes an independent, unilateral decision to accept or reject each contract offer.

MET See *multiple employer trust (MET).*

metadata See *supportive data.*

metastasis 1. Process by which tumor cells spread to distant parts of the body. 2. Tumor that develops away from the site of origin.

method I composite rate Alternative payment system for dialysis services. If a patient selects method I, the facility rendering the dialysis care assumes responsibility for giving home dialysis equipment, supplies, and home support services. The facility receives payment under the composite rate system. The patient pays the Medicare Part B deductible and coinsurance at the facility's composite rate.

method II dealing direct Alternative payment system for dialysis services. If the patient selects method II, the patient contacts the supplier of the home dialysis equipment and supplies and not a dialysis facility. The patient has only one supplier and pays the Medicare Part B deductible and coinsurance. The dialysis facility may not be paid for home dialysis equipment or supplies under this reimbursement system. The facility only receives method II payment for home dialysis support services.

metropolitan statistical areas (MSAs) Major urban population areas designated by the U.S. Department of Commerce that have aggregate populations in excess of 1 million individuals. MSA designations are used as a factor in the Medicare fee schedule calculations for

M

physician office costs and in the prospective payment system (PPS) calculation of hospital labor costs.

MEVS See *Medicaid eligibility verification system (MEVS)*.

MEWA See *Multiple-Employer Welfare Association (MEWA)*.

MFS See *Medicare fee schedule (MFS)*.

MGA See *managing general agent (MGA)*.

MGMA See *Medical Group Management Association (MGMA)*.

MHPA See *Mental Health Parity Act (MHPA)*.

microfiche Sheet of microfilm about 4 × 6 inches (10 × 15 cm) that has multiple microphotograph film images of pages of books and documents recorded. Special equipment is used to enlarge each image for viewing.

microfilm Photographic film for recording small film images of pages of a book or documents in files in a consecutive manner. Special equipment is used to enlarge each image for viewing.

midlevel practitioner (MLP) Medical professional who renders medical care under the direct supervision of a state-licensed physician (e.g., nurse midwife, nurse practitioner, physical therapist, physician assistant). Commonly referred to as *midlevel provider (MLP)*, *nonphysician practitioner (NPP)*, or *physician extenders (PEs)*.

midlevel provider (MLP) See *midlevel practitioner (MLP)*.

military identification card Card issued to active duty service members that may be used to present to providers when seeking medical care under the TRICARE Prime Remote program (see Figure M-2). Also known as a *sponsor identification card*.

military retiree (service retiree) Individual who is retired from a career in the armed forces; also known as *service retiree*.

military service wage credits Credits recognizing that military personnel receive other cash payments and wages in kind (such as food and shelter) in addition to their basic pay.

military suspension Interruption of insurance coverage during the time period in which an insured is in the military.

military treatment facility (MTF) Under the TRICARE program, all uniformed service hospitals. MTF also refers to certain former U.S. Public Health Services (USPHS) facilities now designated as Uniformed Service Treatment Facilities (USTF). Also known as *military hospitals* or *uniformed service hospitals*.

minimal care Medical care given to patients who can ambulate and are partially self-sufficient, requiring limited therapeutic and diagnostic services, and in the final stages of recovery. Services might include administration of medications and treatments that cannot be done by the patient and giving self-care instructions and posthospitalization health maintenance.

minimal care unit Hospital department for the treatment of inpatients who are ambulatory and able to meet many of their own daily living needs but require minimal nursing care.

minimal pain In a workers' compensation case, pain that would represent an annoyance but would cause no handicap in the performance of the particular activity and would be regarded as a nonratable permanent disability.

minimal presenting problem In CPT coding of a service or procedure, this is a problem that may not require the presence of the physician, but service is provided under the physician's supervision.

minimum age requirement For retirement plans, a condition that an employee must attain a specific age before being allowed to participate in an employer's pension plan. Usually pension plans cannot have a minimum age requirement older than age 21.

minimum data set (MDS) Core set of screening, clinical, and functional elements used for long-term care patient assessment. Resource utilization group (RUG-III) is a classification system based on MDS.

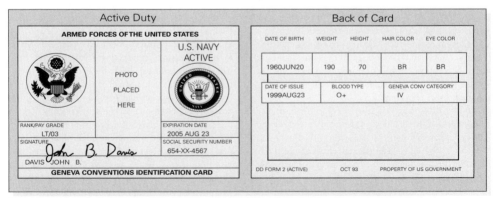

Figure M-2 Military identification card for an active duty individual in the armed forces. It is used as the identification card for the TRICARE Prime Remote Program and is considered a sponsor identification card.

Medicare prospective payment systems and skilled nursing facilities use MDS as the data for classifying patients for case mix. Beginning in June 1998, electronic collection and transmission of MDS data were required.

minimum deposit arrangement Agreement that a policy owner can apply the first-year cash value of an insurance policy to the initial premium amount.

minimum deposit business System to use policy loans to pay premiums in which the policy owner instructs the insurer to pay the premium out of the policy's cash value and to bill the policy owner for a premium only if the cash value is insufficient to pay the premium. Also called *leveraged business.*

minimum funding standards See *funding standard account.*

minimum funding standard account See *funding standard account.*

minimum premium plan (MPP) Group health insurance plan that is partially self-insured by the group policyholder but fully administered by an insurer. Premiums are low because the group policyholder pays most of the claims.

minimum premium rate Lowest premium amount that an insurance company will charge a policyholder for the first year or a specified period of a group insurance policy. Also referred to as *minimum premium.*

minimum scope of disclosure Principle that, to the extent practical, individually identifiable health information should only be disclosed to the extent needed to support the purpose of the disclosure.

minimum service requirement In retirement plans, a condition that an employee complete a specific period of employment before participating in the employer's pension plan.

Minimum Standards Model Regulation Policies declared official in 1974 by the National Association of Insurance Commissioners (NAIC) for setting insurance categories for basic forms of coverage with necessary minimum benefits.

minor Person not of legal age in the state in which he or she resides; a person younger than the age of majority. Also see *mature minor* and *emancipated minor.*

minor procedure 1. Surgical procedure with 0 to 10 follow-up days that may be considered by third-party payers to be part of the surgical package or Medicare global package for a primary surgical service. It cannot be billed separately from the primary operative procedure. 2. Medical procedure that takes 5 minutes or less and involves relatively little decision-making once the need for the operation is determined (e.g., simple sutures, chest tubes, débridements).

MIP See *Medicaid Integrity Program (MIP)* and *Medicare Integrity Program (MIP).*

MIS See *management information system (MIS).*

miscellaneous hospital expense benefit See *hospital extras allowance.*

miscoding Incorrect choice or transposition of diagnostic or procedural code numbers.

misfeasance Improper performance of a lawful act, especially in a way that may cause damage or injury.

misrepresentation 1. Pertaining to an insurance application or insurance claim, appearance of a written or verbal falsehood or misleading statement. Such deceptions will cause voiding or rescinding an insurance policy or denying payment of a claim. 2. In Medicare fraud, to give an inaccurate or deliberate false account of services rendered, amounts charged for services rendered, identity of the person receiving the service, or dates of service.

misstatement of age Insured that gives an age that is younger or older than his or her actual age. In life insurance policies, there is a provision specifying that either the policy's benefit amount or premium amount will be adjusted depending on whether it is an individual or group policy.

mixed model Managed care plan that mixes two or more types of medical care delivery systems (e.g., open-panel and closed-panel systems). It contracts directly with individual physicians. Also called *hybrid model.*

MLA See *multiple-line agency (MLA) system.*

MLP See *midlevel practitioner (MLP).*

MMA See *Medicare Prescription Drug, Improvement, and Modernization Act (MMA).*

MMI See *maximum medical improvement and impairment (MMI).*

MMIS See *Medicaid Management Information System (MMIS).*

MNT See *medical nutrition therapy (MNT).*

mobile facility Transportable independent diagnostic testing clinic with medical equipment provided in a vehicle for service to multiple locations (e.g, portable x-rays, portable mammograms). Also called *portable unit.*

modality 1. Method of application of a therapeutic agent to produce changes to biological tissue (i.e., thermal, acoustic, light, mechanical, cold packs, or electric appliances). 2. Homeopathic term for a condition that modifies drug action. 3. Specific sensory entity such as taste or vision. 4. Form of imaging such as x-ray, fluoroscopy, ultrasound, nuclear medicine, duplex Doppler, computed tomography (CT), and magnetic resonance imaging (MRI).

mode of premium payment Method and frequency insurance premiums are to be paid (i.e., annually, quarterly, or monthly).

model bill Sample legislation developed by the National Association of Insurance Commissioners (NAIC). States may adopt a model bill exactly as written or use it to develop their own laws.

Model Life Insurance Solicitation Regulation Official rule adopted by the National Association of Insurance Commissioners (NAIC) in 1976 requiring

M

insurers to give consumers information that will improve their ability to select the most appropriate life insurance plan to meet their needs, an understanding of the basic features of the policy that is purchased or is being considered, and the ability to evaluate the costs of similar plans of life insurance.

Model Rules Governing the Advertisement of Life Insurance National Association of Insurance Commissioners (NAIC) model law that provides a set of complete guidelines that covers almost all aspects of advertisements for life insurance policies and annuity contracts.

Model Unfair Trade Practices Act National Association of Insurance Commissioners (NAIC) model law that forbids unfair trade practices such as defamation, rebates, unfair discrimination, and unfair claim settlement. The law prohibits any form of advertising that is false, deceptive, or misleading.

modem MOdulator DEModulator unit, a device that converts data into signals for telephone transmission and then (at the receiving end) back again into data.

moderate complexity (MC) Phrase used to describe a type of medical decision-making when a patient is seen for an E/M service. Medical documentation must consist of multiple diagnoses or management options, a moderate amount of data or complexity of data to be reviewed, and a moderate risk of complications and/or morbidity or mortality.

moderate pain In a workers' compensation case, pain that would be endurable but would cause marked handicap in the performance of the activity precipitating the pain.

moderate sedation Also called *conscious sedation*.

moderate severity presenting problem In CPT coding of a service or procedure, this is a problem where the risk of morbidity without treatment is moderate. There is moderate risk of mortality without treatment and uncertain prognosis or increased probability of prolonged functional impairment.

modification Under the Health Insurance Portability and Accountability Act (HIPAA), this is a change adopted by the Secretary, through regulation, to a standard or an implementation specification.

modified average-cost method Under this system of calculating summary measures, the actuarial balance is defined as the difference between the arithmetic means of the annual cost rates and the annual income rates, with an adjustment included to account for the offsets to cost that are due to (1) the starting trust fund balance and (2) interest earned on the trust fund.

modified community rating (MCR) Rating method in which premiums are based on the average health care costs within a specific geographical region as modified by rating factors such as age and sex that have been filed with the state insurance department.

modified fee-for-service Third-party payer system in which physicians are paid for a unit of service provided with a set maximum fee for each service.

modified job See *modified work*.

modified life Ordinary life insurance that has premiums during the first few years (usually 5) that are slightly larger than the rate for term insurance. After that time period, the annual premium is higher.

modified net premiums Net premiums, other than level, that are lower for the first year and higher in subsequent years.

modified-premium whole life insurance Type of whole life insurance in which the policy owner pays a lower than normal premium for a certain initial period and then the premium increases to a specific amount that is higher than usual, which is then paid for the life of the policy.

modified risk In life and health insurance, individual whose physical condition is less than standard or who has a dangerous occupation or hobby (e.g., history of stroke or race driver). An additional premium is required because of the possibility of loss from an impairment. Also called *substandard risk* or *impaired risk*.

modified work In workers' compensation cases, job that has been changed to allow an injured worker to perform (e.g., to alter a workstation so that the job can be done seated instead of standing or to adjust the content of the work to exclude tasks the worker is not able to perform). Also called *modified job*.

modifier 1. In *Current Procedural Terminology (CPT)* coding, a two-character (numeric or alphanumeric) add-on indicator placed after the usual procedure code number to indicate circumstances in which a procedure as performed differs in some way from that described by its usual five-digit code (see Box M-1). Also called *code modifier*. 2. In HCPCS Level II coding, a one- or two-digit alpha or alphanumeric number placed after the usual Level I or II code that helps further describe a procedure or service. Also see *Healthcare Common Procedure Coding System (HCPCS) modifiers*.

modifier -22 CPT modifier used for unusual procedural services. When the services provided are greater than those usually required for the listed procedure, they may be identified by adding modifier -22 to the usual procedure number. A report may also be appropriate. This modifier may affect reimbursement, depending on the payer.

Box M-1   MODIFIER
27372-51 (typed on one line)

modifier -23 CPT modifier used for unusual anesthesia. Occasionally, a procedure that usually requires either no anesthesia or local anesthesia must be done under general anesthesia because of unusual circumstances. This circumstance may be reported by adding the modifier -23 to the procedure code of the basic service. This modifier may affect reimbursement, depending on the payer.

modifier -24 CPT modifier used for unrelated evaluation and management service by the same physician during a postoperative period. The physician may need to indicate that an evaluation and management service was performed during a postoperative period for a reason(s) unrelated to the original procedure. This circumstance may be reported by adding the modifier -24 to the appropriate level of E/M service. This modifier may affect reimbursement, depending on the payer.

modifier -25 CPT modifier used for significant, separately identifiable evaluation and management (E/M) service by the same physician on the day of a procedure or other service. The physician may need to indicate that on the day a procedure or service identified by a CPT code was performed, the patient's condition required a significant, separately identifiable E/M service above and beyond the other service provided or beyond the usual preoperative and postoperative care associated with the procedure that was performed. The E/M service may be prompted by the symptom or condition for which the procedure and/or service was provided. As such, different diagnoses are not required for reporting the E/M service on the same date.

modifier -26 CPT modifier used for the professional component. Certain procedures are a combination of a professional physician component and a technical component. When the professional (physician) component is reported separately, the service may be identified by adding the modifier -26 to the usual procedure number. Use of this modifier may affect reimbursement. The professional component comprises only the professional services performed by the physician during radiologic, laboratory, and other diagnostic procedures. These services include a portion of a test or procedure that the physician does such as interpretation of the results. The technical component includes personnel; materials including usual contrast media and drugs, film, or xerograph; space; equipment; and other facilities but excludes the cost of radioisotopes. When billing for the technical component, use the usual five-digit procedure number with modifier -TC.

modifier -27 CPT modifier used for multiple outpatient hospital E/M encounters on the same date. For hospital outpatient reporting purposes, utilization of hospital resources related to separate and distinct E/M encounters performed in multiple outpatient hospital settings on the same date may be reported by adding the modifier -27 to each appropriate level outpatient and/or emergency department E/M code(s). This modifier provides a means of reporting circumstances involving E/M services provided by physician(s) in more than one (multiple) outpatient hospital setting(s) (e.g., hospital emergency department, clinic). Do not use this modifier for physician reporting of multiple E/M services performed by the same physician on the same date. See *evaluation and management (E/M) codes, emergency department*, or *preventive medicine codes*.

modifier -32 CPT modifier used for mandated services. Services related to mandated consultation and/or related services (e.g., PRO, third-party payer, governmental, legislative or regulatory requirement) may be identified by adding the modifier -32 to the basic procedure. The modifier is informational in nature. Do not ask for an adjustment in reimbursement. Monitor reimbursement when using this modifier.

modifier -47 CPT modifier used for anesthesia by surgeon. Regional or general anesthesia provided by the surgeon may be reported by adding the modifier -47 to the basic service (this does not include local anesthesia). This modifier may affect reimbursement, depending on the payer. Modifier -47 would not be used for anesthesia procedures 00100 through 01999.

modifier -50 CPT modifier used for a bilateral procedure. Unless otherwise identified in the listings, bilateral procedures requiring a separate incision performed during the same operative session should be identified by the appropriate five-digit code describing the first procedure. The second (bilateral) procedure is identified by adding modifier -50 to the procedure number. It is important to read each surgical description carefully to look for the word "bilateral." A bilateral modifier on a unilateral procedure code indicates that the procedure was performed on both sides of a paired organ during the same operative session.

modifier -51 CPT modifier used for multiple procedures. When multiple procedures, other than E/M services, are performed at the same session by the same provider, the primary procedure or service may be reported as listed. The additional procedure(s) or service(s) may be identified by adding the modifier -51 to the additional procedure or service code(s). This modifier should not be appended to designated "add-on" codes (see Appendix E of CPT). Always list the procedure of highest dollar value first.

modifier -51 exempt (⊘) Symbol used in the procedure code book titled *Current Procedural Terminology (CPT)*

M

to indicate a procedure code listed is exempt from the use of modifier -51 but have *not* been designated as CPT add-on procedures/services. A summary of five-digit procedural codes exempt from modifier -51 are shown in Appendix E in CPT.

modifier -52 CPT modifier for reduced services. Under certain circumstances a service or procedure is partially reduced or eliminated at the physician's election. Under these circumstances the service provided can be identified by its usual procedure number and the addition of the modifier -52, signifying that the service is reduced. This provides a means of reporting reduced services without disturbing the identification of the basic service. This modifier affects reimbursement, but there will be no effect on the physician's fee profile in the computer data. It is not necessary to attach a report to the claim when using this modifier because it indicates a reduced fee. When a physician performs a procedure but does not charge for the service such as a postoperative follow-up visit that is included in a global service, remember to use code 99024. Some physicians prefer to bill the insurance carrier the full amount and accept what the carrier pays as payment in full. In such cases, a modifier would not be used. If only part of a procedure is performed and the physician feels a reduction in the service is warranted, to develop a reduced fee, try calculating the reduced service by time. Calculate the amount (cost) per minute of the complete procedure by dividing the amount (cost) by the usual time it takes to complete the procedure. To determine how long the reduced procedure took, multiply the amount (cost) per minute by the time it took to do the reduced procedure.

modifier -53 CPT modifier used for discontinued procedure. Under certain circumstances, the physician may elect to terminate a surgical or diagnostic procedure. Due to extenuating circumstances or those that threaten the well-being of the patient, it may be necessary to indicate that a surgical or diagnostic procedure was started but discontinued. This circumstance may be reported by adding the modifier -53 to the code for the discontinued procedure. This modifier is not used to report the elective cancellation of a procedure before the patient's anesthesia induction and/or surgical preparation in the operating suite. For outpatient hospital/ambulatory surgery center (ACS), see *modifier -73* and *modifier -74*.

modifier -54 CPT modifier used for surgical care only: When one physician performs a surgical procedure and another provides preoperative and/or postoperative management, surgical services may be identified by adding the modifier -54 to the usual procedure number. This modifier may affect reimbursement. Because many surgical procedures encompass a "package" concept that includes normal uncomplicated follow-up care, the surgeon will be paid a reduced fee when using this modifier.

modifier -55 CPT modifier used for postoperative management only. When one physician performs the postoperative management and another physician performs the surgical procedure, the postoperative component may be identified by adding the modifier -55 to the usual procedure number. The fee to list would be approximately 30% of the surgeon's fee.

modifier -56 CPT modifier used for preoperative management only. When one physician performs the preoperative care and evaluation and another physician performs the surgical procedure, the preoperative component may be identified by adding the modifier -56 to the usual procedure number. This modifier may affect reimbursement, depending on the payer.

modifier -57 CPT modifier used for decision for surgery. An evaluation and management service that resulted in the initial decision to perform the surgery may be identified by adding the modifier -57 to the appropriate level of E/M service. This modifier is informational in nature. Do not ask for an adjustment in reimbursement. Monitor reimbursement when using this modifier.

modifier -58 CPT modifier used for staged or related procedure or service by the same physician during the postoperative period. The physician may need to indicate that the performance of a procedure or service during the postoperative period was (1) planned prospectively at the time of the original procedure (staged); (2) more extensive than the original procedure; or (3) for therapy after a diagnostic surgical procedure. This circumstance may be reported by adding the modifier -58 to the staged or related procedure. This modifier is informational in nature. Do not ask for an adjustment in reimbursement. Monitor reimbursement when using this modifier. This modifier is not used to report the treatment of a problem that requires a return to the operating room. See *modifier -78*.

modifier -59 CPT modifier used for distinct procedural service. Under certain circumstances, the physician may need to indicate that a procedure or service was distinct or independent from other services performed on the same day. Modifier -59 is used to identify procedures/services that are not normally reported together but are appropriate under the circumstances. This may represent a different session or patient encounter, different procedure or surgery, different site or organ system, separate incision/excision, separate lesion, or separate injury (or area of injury in extensive injuries) not ordinarily encountered or performed on the same day by the same physician. However, when another already established modifier is appropriate, it should be used rather than modifier -59. Only if no more descriptive modifier is available, and the use of modifier -59 best explains the circumstances, should modifier -59 be used.

modifier -62 CPT modifier used for two surgeons. When two surgeons work together as primary surgeons performing distinct parts of a single reportable procedure, each surgeon should report his or her distinct operative work using the same procedure code and adding the modifier -62. If additional procedures (including add-on procedures) are performed during the same surgical session, separate codes may be reported without the modifier -62. If the cosurgeon assists in the performance of additional procedure(s) during the same surgical session, those services may be reported using separate procedure code(s) with modifier -80 or -81.

modifier -63 CPT modifier used for procedure performed on infants less than 4 kg. Procedures performed on neonates and infants up to a present body weight of 4 kg may involve significantly increased complexity and physician work commonly associated with these patients. This circumstance may be reported by adding the modifier -63 to the procedure number. Unless otherwise designated, this modifier may only be appended to procedures/services listed in the 20000-69999 code series. Modifier -63 should not be appended to any codes listed in the Evaluation and Management Services, Anesthesia, Radiology, Pathology/Laboratory, or Medicine sections.

modifier -66 CPT modifier used for surgical team. Under some circumstances, highly complex procedures (requiring the concomitant services of several physicians, often of different specialties, plus other highly skilled, specially trained personnel and various types of complex equipment) are carried out under the "surgical team" concept. Such circumstances may be identified by each participating physician with the addition of the modifier -66 to the basic procedure number used for reporting services. This modifier may affect reimbursement.

modifier -73 CPT modifier used for discontinued outpatient hospital/ambulatory surgery center (ASC) procedure before the administration of anesthesia. Because of extenuating circumstances or those that threaten the well-being of the patient, the physician may cancel a surgical or diagnostic procedure subsequent to the patient's surgical preparation (including sedation when provided, and being taken to the room where the procedure is to be performed), but before the administration of anesthesia (local, regional block[s], or general). Under these circumstances, the intended service that is prepared for but canceled can be reported by its usual procedure number and the addition of modifier -73. The elective cancellation of a service before the administration of anesthesia and/or surgical preparation of the patient should not be reported. For physician reporting of a discontinued procedure, see *modifier -53*.

modifier -74 CPT modifier used for discontinued outpatient hospital/ambulatory surgery center (ASC) procedure after administration of anesthesia. Because of extenuating circumstances or those that threaten the well-being of the patient, the physician may terminate a surgical or diagnostic procedure after the administration of anesthesia (local, regional block[s], or general) or after the procedure was started (incision made, intubation started, scope inserted). Under these circumstances, the procedure started but terminated can be reported by its usual procedure number and the addition of modifier -74. The elective cancellation of a service before the administration of anesthesia and/or surgical preparation of the patient should not be reported. For physician reporting of a discontinued procedure, see *modifier -53*.

modifier -76 CPT modifier used for repeat procedure by same physician. The physician may need to indicate that a procedure or service was repeated subsequent to the original service. This circumstance may be reported by adding modifier -76 to the repeated service. This modifier may affect reimbursement.

modifier -77 CPT modifier used for repeat procedure by another physician. The physician may need to indicate that a basic procedure performed by another physician had to be repeated. This situation may be reported by adding modifier -77 to the repeated service. This modifier may affect reimbursement, depending on the payer.

modifier -78 CPT modifier used for return to the operating room for a related procedure during the postoperative period. The physician may need to indicate that another procedure was performed during the postoperative period of the initial procedure. When this subsequent procedure is related to the first and requires the use of the operating room, it may be reported by adding the modifier -78 to the related procedure. (For repeat procedures on the same day, see *modifier -76*.) This modifier may affect reimbursement, depending on the payer.

modifier -79 CPT modifier used for unrelated procedure or service by the same physician during the postoperative period. The physician may need to indicate that the performance of a procedure or service during the postoperative period was unrelated to the original procedure. This circumstance may be reported by using the modifier -79. (For repeat procedures on the same day, see *modifier -76*.) This modifier may affect reimbursement, depending on the payer.

modifier -80 CPT modifier used for assistant surgeon. Surgical assistant services may be identified by adding the modifier -80 to the usual procedure number(s). This modifier may affect reimbursement. Some insurance policies do not include payment for assistant surgeons such as for 1-day surgery but do pay for major or complex surgical assistance. In some instances,

M

prior approval may be indicated due to the patient's physiologic condition. Medicare will not pay assistant surgeons for operations that are not life threatening. Therefore Medigap insurance will not pay on this service because the service is nonallowable. Assisting surgeons usually charge 16% to 30% of the primary surgeon's fee.

modifier -81 CPT modifier used for minimum assistant surgeon. Minimum surgical assistant services are identified by adding the modifier -81 to the usual procedure number. Payment is made to physicians but not registered nurses or technicians who assist during surgery. This modifier may affect reimbursement.

modifier -82 CPT modifier used for assistant surgeon (when qualified resident surgeon is not available). The unavailability of a qualified resident surgeon is a prerequisite for use of modifier -82 appended to the usual procedure code number(s). This modifier may affect reimbursement. This modifier is usually used for services rendered at a teaching hospital.

modifier -90 CPT modifier used for reference (outside) laboratory. When laboratory procedures are performed by a party other than the treating or reporting physician, the procedure may be identified by adding the modifier -90 to the usual procedure number. This modifier may affect reimbursement, depending on the payer. Use this modifier when the physician bills the patient for the laboratory work and the laboratory is not doing its own billing.

modifier -91 CPT modifier used for repeat clinical diagnostic laboratory test. In the course of treatment of the patient, it may be necessary to repeat the same laboratory test on the same day to obtain subsequent (multiple) test results. Under these circumstances, the laboratory test performed can be identified by its usual procedure number and the addition of modifier -91. This modifier may not be used when tests are rerun to confirm initial results; due to testing problems with specimens or equipment; or for any other reason when a normal, one-time, reportable result is all that is required. This modifier may not be used when other code(s) describe a series of test results (e.g., glucose tolerance tests, evocative/suppression testing). This modifier may only be used for laboratory test(s) performed more than once on the same day on the same patient.

modifier -99 CPT modifier used for multiple modifiers. Under certain circumstances, two or more modifiers may be necessary to delineate a service completely. In such situations modifier -99 should be added to the basic procedure, and other applicable modifiers may be listed as part of the description of the service. This modifier is informational in nature. Do not ask for an adjustment in reimbursement. Monitor reimbursement when using this modifier.

modify See *modification*.

modifying factors Details that change the definition or extent of a medical problem.

modifying terms Main term that may be followed by a series of up to three indented terms (subterms) that modify the main term shown in the annually published *Current Procedural Terminology* code book. These subterms have an effect on the selection of the appropriate CPT code for a procedure or service.

money laundering See *laundering of monetary instruments*.

money-purchase pension plan Type of retirement plan that states a rate of contribution to each participant's account by the employer that results in benefits equal to the amount in the account (investment gains and losses) at retirement. At retirement, the contributions plus investment earnings are often used to purchase an annuity to provide a regular pension benefit.

monitored anesthesia care State of depressed consciousness, with or without analgesia, that is medically controlled with maintenance of the patient's airway, protective reflexes, and responsiveness to stimulation and verbal commands.

monitoring Planned, systematic, and ongoing process to gather and organize data and aggregate results in order to evaluate performance.

monitoring of managed care organization/prepaid health plan standards Activities related to the monitoring of standards that have been set for plan structure, operations, and quality improvement/assurance to determine that standards have been established, implemented, adhered to, and so on.

monthly adjustment billing To bill the insured for the premium on the due date for insurance coverage for the actual number of individuals covered by the group insurance contract.

monthly debit ordinary (MDO) insurance Type of hybrid life insurance policy that has the face value of industrial policies and is handled as ordinary insurance. Monthly premiums are usually paid to an agent.

monthly increment process System of payment of one or two months' dues when receivables have been created for quarterly or annual dues.

monthly indemnity Benefit paid monthly under a health insurance policy.

monthly outstanding balance method Arrangement for contributory plans in group creditor insurance in which the lender adds to the outstanding balance of the loan an amount to insure that balance for 1 month.

moral hazard Refers to risk that results from an insured's personal habits that increases the possibility of loss or intensifies the severity of a loss because of carelessness or dishonesty. For example, this phenomenon may be connected to someone who may have had a series of fires.

morbidity In clinical usage, any diseased condition or state including diagnosis and complications. It is often used in the context of a "morbidity rate" (i.e., the rate of disease or proportion of diseased people in a population).

morbidity rate Phrase seen in health care contracts that refers to an actuarial statistic of the number of cases of a disease or illness in a population divided by the total population at risk for that illness during a specific period of time categorized by age. Insurance premiums are based in part on the morbidity rate for the person's age group. Also referred to as *incidence rate* or *prevalence rate*.

morbidity table List of actuarial statistics that shows the expected average frequency and duration of disability, illness, and accidents in a well-defined class of individuals categorized by age.

moribund In a dying state.

mortality Cause of death. Mortality rate is the number of deaths in a given time or place.

mortality charge Price of insurance coverage for a universal life policy that is based on the net amount of risk, insured's risk classification, and insured's age.

mortality curve Line graph that shows the mortality rates as they change from age to age.

mortality experience Actual number of deaths that occur within a defined group of people.

mortality rate Death rate often made explicit for a particular characteristic (e.g., gender, sex, specific cause of death). Mortality rate contains three essential elements: the number of people in a population exposed to the risk of death (denominator), a time factor, and the number of deaths occurring in the exposed population during a certain time period (the numerator). Insurance premiums are based in part on mortality rate for a person's age group.

mortality table Statistical chart that shows death rate for various age groups usually expressed per thousand.

mortgage Legal document that conveys property on condition as security for payment of a debt and becomes void on payment.

mortgage insurance Type of life insurance that pays off any mortgage balance outstanding at the time of death of the head of the family. A family beneficiary is named instead of the mortgagee. Also referred to as *principal mortgage insurance (PMI)*.

mortgage redemption insurance Type of decreasing term life insurance that gives coverage to the person who takes out a mortgage. If the individual dies during the term of the insurance, the policy proceeds pay the remaining amount of the mortgage loan.

most-favored-nation clauses Provision stated in health care contracts that requires the physician to bill the third-party payer the lowest fee charged to any other person.

most prevalent charge See *most prevalent rate*.

most prevalent rate Dollar amount that is applicable to the largest number of semiprivate or private beds in a hospital facility. Also called *most prevalent charge*.

mouse Device used to input computer data.

MPCC See *Medicare Premium Collection Center (MPCC)*.

MPFS Acronym for Medicare physician's fee schedule. See *Medicare fee schedule (MFS)*.

MPI See *master patient index (MPI)*.

MPN See *medical provider network (MPN)*.

MPP See *minimum premium plan (MPP)*.

MR See *medical review (MR)*.

MRI See *magnetic resonance imaging (MRI)*.

MRN See *Medicare remittance notice (MRN)*.

MS HCPCS Level II modifier that may be used with CPT or HCPCS Level II codes indicating a 6-month maintenance and servicing fee for reasonable and necessary parts and labor that are not covered under any manufacturer or supplier warranty.

MSA See *medical savings account (MSA)*.

MSAs See *metropolitan statistical areas (MSAs)*.

MSDS See *Material Safety Data Sheet (MSDS)*.

MSHP See *multiskilled health practitioner (MSHP)*.

MSN See *Medicare Summary Notice (MSN)*.

MSO See *management services organization (MSO)*.

MSP See *Medicare Secondary Payer (MSP)*.

MSP alert See *Medicare Secondary Payer alert (MSP alert)*.

MSVR See *mandatory securities valuation reserve (MSVR)*.

MTF See *military treatment facility (MTF)*.

MUAs See *medically underserved areas (MUAs)*.

MUD See *medically necessary days (MUD)*.

MUEs See *medically unlikely edits (MUEs)*.

multi-employer group health plan Group health plan that is sponsored jointly by two or more employers or by employers and employee organizations. If an employee leaves one employer who is a member of the group and goes to work for another member of the group, he or she may continue insurance coverage under the plan. Also called *multi-employer plan*.

multi-employer plan See *multi-employer group health plan*.

multiperil policy Type of insurance that packages several different perils into one form and provides coverage.

multiple birth Two or more newborns delivered without complications.

multiple coding Use of more than one diagnostic code to identify both etiology and manifestation of a disease.

multiple coverage See *duplication of coverage*.

multiple employee group Workers of two or more employers that are covered under one master insurance contract. This situation may occur in trade associations or employers in the same industry or union members who work for more than one employer.

multiple employer plan Group health plan that is sponsored jointly by two or more employers or by employers and unions.

multiple employer group health plan Group of employers (two or more) who contract together to a managed care plan. This is cost saving and broadens the risk pool. It is different from a multiple employer trust. Also referred to as *multi-employer group health plan*.

multiple employer plan Health plan sponsored by two or more employers. These are generally plans that are offered through membership in an association or a trade group.

multiple employer trust (MET) 1. Group of employers who procure group health insurance for their employees using self-funded monies. This helps to lower costs, promotes larger membership, and makes available the selection for greater benefits. 2. One master insurance policy that covers several employers with specific benefit packages and limitations.

Multiple-Employer Welfare Association (MEWA) Type of purchasing group that is defined in the Employee Retirement Income Security Act of 1974. It is composed of a group of employers who purchase health insurance using self-funded monies and offers benefits to employees of two or more employers. This helps to lower costs, promotes larger membership, and makes available the selection for greater benefits.

multiple indemnity Insurance contract provision in which the principal sum of the policy is multiplied by 100, 200, 300, or more percent in the event of death from specific accidents.

multiple-life case Group insurance situation in which several applicants apply for coverage at the same time such as owners, employees, association members, or members of another group.

multiple-line agency (MLA) system Method in which full-time insurance career agents distribute life and health and property/casualty insurance products for groups that are financially interrelated. Also known as *multiple-line exclusive agency system* or *all-lines exclusive agency system*.

multiple-line exclusive agency system See *multiple-line agency (MLA) system*.

multiple option plan Group health plan offering employees a choice from a number of health plans such as health maintenance organization, preferred provider organization, point-of-service plan, or major medical indemnity plan.

multiple-participant billing To list all insured individuals on one statement as a convenience for premium payment.

multiple surgery Situation when more than one surgical procedure is performed at the time of the operation. A five-digit CPT code number is used with an attached modifier -51 to list the procedure. If listing more than one modifier, the appropriate sequence is to list -51 first and any one of these modifiers in the next position (-54, -55, -62, -66, -80). For two surgeons and surgical care, only list -62 and -54 after -51 modifier. For team surgery and surgical care, list only -66 and -54 after -51 modifier. Also called *multiple surgical procedure*.

multiple surgical procedure See *multiple surgery*.

multipurpose billing form All-encompassing billing form personalized to the practice of the physician or hospital outpatient facility that reflects the services performed and any associated charges (i.e., supplies and anesthesia). This form acts as a historical record used in case a charge must be researched to identify any discrepancy or billing errors. It may be used if a patient submits his or her own insurance billing. Also called *charge document, charge slip, communicator, encounter form, fee ticket, patient service slip, routing form, superbill*, and *transaction slip*.

multiskilled health practitioner (MSHP) Individual cross-trained to provide more than one function, often in more than one discipline. These combined functions can be found in a broad spectrum of health-related jobs, ranging in complexity and including both clinical and administrative functions. The terms *multiskilled, multicompetent*, and *cross-trained* can be used interchangeably.

multispecialty group practice Several physicians who work together in a group practice and are from different clinical and specialty practices.

multisystem examination 1997 guidelines Examination must include at least six organ systems or body areas. For each system or area selected, performance and documentation of at least two elements identified in a table by a bullet (•) are expected. Alternatively, a detailed examination may include performance and documentation of at least 12 elements identified in a table by a bullet (•) in two or more organ systems or body areas.

musculoskeletal system All of the muscles, bones, joints, and related structures such as the tendons and connective tissue that function in the movement of body parts and organs.

mutual company See *mutual insurance company*.

mutual insurance company Life insurance company that has no capital stock or stockholders, is owned by its policy owners, and is managed by a board of directors chosen by the policy owners. It issues participating insurance. Earnings left over after operating expenses of the company are given to the policy owners in the form of dividends. Also called *mutual company* or *mutual life insurance company*.

mutual life insurance company See *mutual insurance company*.

mutualization Process of conversion of a stock insurance company to a mutual insurance company.

mutually exclusive code pairs Medical service or procedure combinations that would not or could not reasonably be performed at the same session, by the same provider, on the same patient.

mutually exclusive edit One of two main types of Correct Coding Initiative (CCI) edits. This type of edit is applied to code combinations in which one of the codes is considered either impossible to perform or improbable to be performed with the other code. See also comprehensive/component edit.

MVPS See *Medicare volume performance standard (MVPS)*.

M

N

NA See *nursing assistant (NA)*.

N/A Abbreviation for not applicable.

NACHC See *National Association of Community Health Centers (NACHC)*.

NADP See *National Association of Dental Plans (NADP)*.

NAHDO See *National Association of Health Data Organizations (NAHDO)*.

NAHMOR Formerly National Association of HMO Regulators. See *National Association of Managed Care Regulators (NAMCR)*.

NAIC See *National Association of Insurance Commissioners (NAIC)*.

NAIC Model Privacy Act Model bill written by the National Association of Insurance Commissioners and designed to set standards for the use of information collected from insurance applications. State law forbids any insurer or agent from impersonating someone else to gain information about an applicant, unless there is reasonable cause to suspect criminal activity. It provides that an insurer must give timely notice of renewal and other company policies. It governs the method in which an insurer can collect, use, and disclose information about a policyholder. Applicants are allowed access to information that the insurer has collected about them, the right to correct it if wrong, and to learn the reason they were turned down for insurance.

named perils Specified perils in an insurance policy against which the policyholder is insured.

NAPDP See *National Association of Dental Plans (NADP)*.

NAS See *Nonavailability Statement (NAS)*.

NASMD See *National Association of State Medicaid Directors (NASMD)*.

national alphanumeric codes Alphanumeric codes developed by Health Care Financing Administration (HCFA), now known as *Centers for Medicare and Medicaid Services (CMS)*. See *Healthcare Common Procedure Coding System (HCPCS)*.

National Association of Blue Shield Plans (NABSP) Former name of the national coordinating organization for all Blue Shield plans, which is now known as *Blue Cross and Blue Shield Association (BCBSA)*.

National Association of Community Health Centers (NACHC) Nonprofit organization founded in 1970 to enhance and expand access to quality, community-responsive health care for America's medically underserved and uninsured. In serving its mission, NACHC represents the nation's network of more than 1000 federally qualified health centers (FQHCs) that serve 16 million people through 5000 sites located in all of the 50 states, Puerto Rico, the District of Columbia, the U.S. Virgin Islands, and Guam.

National Association of Dental Plans (NADP) Nonprofit trade association whose mission is "to promote and advance the dental benefits industry to improve consumer access to affordable, quality dental care." Formerly called *National Association of Prepaid Dental Plans (NAPDP)*.

National Association of Health Data Organizations (NAHDO) Group that promotes the development and improvement of state and national health information systems.

National Association of Insurance Commissioners (NAIC) Organization of insurance regulators from the 50 states, the District of Columbia, and the four U.S. territories created in 1871. NAIC provides a forum for the development of uniform policy when uniformity is appropriate. Its mission is to assist state insurance regulators, individually and collectively, in serving the public interest and achieving the following fundamental insurance regulatory goals in a responsive, efficient, and cost-effective manner, consistent with the wishes of its members; protect the public interest; promote competitive markets; facilitate the fair and equitable treatment of insurance consumers; promote the reliability, solvency, and financial solidity of insurance institutions; and support and improve state regulation of insurance.

National Association of Managed Care Regulators (NAMCR) Organization composed of both regulator members and associate industry members. Originally known as the *National Association of HMO Regulators (NAHMOR)*. NAMCR provides expertise and a forum for discussion to state regulators and managed care companies about current issues facing managed care. NAMCR also provides expertise to the National Association of Insurance Commissioners (NAIC) in preparation of NAIC Model Acts used by many states. Regulator members come from state insurance or health departments. Associate (nonvoting) membership is available on the NAMCR website, and an NAMCR newsletter will again be published.

National Association of Prepaid Dental Plans (NAPDP) See *National Association of Dental Plans (NADP)*.

National Association of State Medicaid Directors (NASMD) Bipartisan, professional, nonprofit organization of representatives of state Medicaid agencies (including the District of Columbia and the territories).

Since 1979, NASMD has been affiliated with the American Public Human Services Association (APHSA). The primary purposes of NASMD are to serve as a focal point of communication between the states and the federal government and to provide an information network among the states on issues pertinent to the Medicaid program. NASMD is composed of the officials who administer the Medicaid program in the states, the District of Columbia, and the territories. Generally these officials are the state Medicaid director and his or her senior staff. For the purpose of carrying out association business, each entity is limited to one voting member.

National Cancer Registrars Association (NCRA) Not-for-profit association representing cancer registry professionals and Certified Tumor Registrars (CTR). NCRA's primary focus is education and certification with the goal to ensure all Cancer Registry professionals have the required knowledge to be superior in their field.

National Center for Complementary and Alternative Medicine (NCCAM) Federal government's lead agency since 1991 for scientific research on complementary and alternative medicine (CAM) that sponsors and conducts research using scientific methods and advanced technologies to study CAM. Also see *complementary and alternative medicine (CAM)*.

National Center for Health Statistics (NCHS) One of the Centers for Disease Control and Prevention (CDC), which is part of the U.S. Department of Health and Human Services. NCHS is the United States' principal health statistics agency. It designs, develops, and maintains a number of systems that produce data related to demographic and health concerns. These include data on registered births and deaths, the National Health Interview Survey (NHIS), the National Health and Nutrition Examination Survey (NHANES), the National Health Care Survey, and the National Survey of Family Growth (NSFG). NCHS maintains the ICD-9-CM code system and developed the Clinical Modification for the ICD-10.

National Center for Vital and Health Statistics (NCVHS) Health statistics agency that compiles statistical information to guide actions and policies to improve the health of the American people. NCVHS data systems include data on vital events, as well as information on health status, lifestyle, and exposure to unhealthy influences. This is a governmental agency within the Department of Health and Human Services that advises the secretary about possible changes to the Health Insurance Portability and Accountability Act (HIPAA) standards.

National Certified Insurance and Coding Specialist (NCICS) Insurance and coding certification that is awarded by an independent testing agency, the National Center for Competency Testing (NCCT).

national claims history (NCH) system Database that is an integral part of a single-site repository for all Medicare Part A and Part B claims and utilization data record per claim.

national codes Alphanumeric codes developed by Health Care Financing Administration (HCFA), which is now known as *Centers for Medicare and Medicaid Services (CMS)*. See *Healthcare Common Procedure Coding System (HCPCS)*.

National Committee for Quality Assurance (NCQA) Independent, 501(c)(3) nonprofit organization whose mission is to improve health care quality everywhere. NCQA accredits Medicare health plans, managed care plans, and health maintenance organizations (HMOs). It does this by maintaining and using the Health Employer Data and Information Set (HEDIS), a set of data reporting standards that compares performance between plans.

National Committee for Vital Health Statistics (NCVHS) Committee established by Congress to serve as an advisory body to the Department of Health and Human Services on health data, statistics, and national health information policy. It fulfills important review and advisory functions relative to health data and statistical problems of national and international interest, stimulates or conducts studies of such problems, and makes proposals for improvement of the nation's health statistics and information systems. In 1996 the Committee was restructured to meet expanded responsibilities under the Health Insurance Portability and Accountability Act of 1996 (HIPAA).

national conversion factor See *conversion factor (CF)*.

National Correct Coding Council (NCCC) Committee that reviews established coding patterns and develops code methodologies to control improper coding that has generated inappropriate and increased payment of Medicare Part B insurance claims.

National Correct Coding Initiative (NCCI) Federal legislation that attempts to eliminate unbundling or other inappropriate reporting of procedural codes for professional medical services rendered to patients. The NCCI is updated quarterly. Hospitals always use the prior quarter's edits and physicians use the current quarter's edits. An annual list of codes from the Centers for Medicare and Medicaid Services (CMS) is published for Part B Medicare fiscal intermediaries to identify services that are considered either part of a comprehensive code or exclusive of it. Also known as *Correct Coding Initiative (CCI)*.

National Council for Prescription Drug Programs (NCPDP) Not-for-profit ANSI-accredited standards development organization that maintains a number of standard formats for use by the retail pharmaceutical industry, some of which have been adopted as HIPAA standards. NCPDP creates and promotes standards for the transfer of data to and from the pharmacy services sector of the health care industry. The organization provides a forum and support wherein the membership can efficiently and effectively develop and maintain these standards through a consensus building process. Members consist of chain and independent pharmacies, consulting companies and pharmacists, database management organizations, federal and state agencies, health insurers, health maintenance organizations, mail service pharmacy companies, pharmaceutical manufacturers, pharmaceutical services administration organizations, prescription service organizations, pharmacy benefit management companies, professional and trade associations, telecommunication and systems vendors, wholesale drug distributors, and other parties interested in electronic standardization within the pharmacy services sector of the health care industry.

national coverage analyses (NCA) Numerous documents support the national coverage determination process. They include tracking sheets to inform the public of the issues under consideration and the status (e.g., pending, closed) of the review, information about and results of Medicare Coverage Advisory Committee (MCAC) meetings, technology assessments, and decision memoranda that announce the Centers for Medicare and Medicaid Services' (CMS's) intention to issue a national coverage determination (NCD). These documents, along with the compilation of medical and scientific information available, any Food and Drug Administration (FDA) safety and efficacy data, and clinical trial information, provide the rationale behind the evidence-based NCDs.

national coverage analyses (NCA) closed Date when the Medicare decision memorandum is issued and the NCA is considered closed; policy change is not effective until the manual transmittal is issued.

national coverage analyses (NCA) decision memorandum Document that provides the reasons that support a Medicare national coverage determination.

national coverage analyses (NCA) new Instance when the Centers for Medicare and Medicaid Services receives a coverage request or a current national coverage determination is being edited.

national coverage analyses (NCA) pending Situation in which a national coverage analyses is under review and the decision memorandum has not been issued.

national coverage analyses (NCA) reconsideration Formal reassessment of a Medicare policy can be requested if documentation is presented that meets one of the following criteria: additional medical material or scientific information that was not considered during the initial review or arguments that the NCA conclusion materially misrepresented the existing evidence at the time the national coverage determination was made.

national coverage determinations (NCDs) Government policies that grant, eliminate, or exclude Medicare coverage for specific services, items, and tests. The Centers for Medicare and Medicaid Services (CMS) guidelines state the circumstances when these services, items, and tests are considered reasonable and necessary or may not be considered a Medicare benefit. Medicare contractors are required to follow NCDs. If an NCD does not specifically exclude/limit an indication or circumstance, or if the item or service is not mentioned at all in an NCD or in a Medicare online manual, it is up to the Medicare contractor to make the coverage decision (see local medical review policy). Before an NCD takes effect, CMS must first issue a manual transmittal, CMS ruling, or *Federal Register* notice giving specific directions to the claims-processing contractors. That issuance, which includes an effective date and implementation date, is the NCD. If appropriate, the agency must also change billing and claims processing systems and issue related instructions to allow for payment. The NCD will be published in the *Medicare National Coverage Determinations Manual*. An NCD becomes effective as of the date listed in the transmittal that announces the manual revision.

National Coverage Determinations Manual (NCDM) The Centers for Medicare and Medicaid Services (CMS) manual that contains national coverage decisions and specific medical items, services, and treatment procedures or technologies. It is used by Part A Medicare fiscal intermediaries, Part B insurance carriers, and quality improvement organization (QIO) programs. Formerly known as *Coverage Issues Manual (CIM)*.

national coverage policy Government guidelines and mandates for the Medicare program that affect all states and regions. These rules are published daily online via the Internet by the Centers for Medicare and Medicaid Services (CMS) in the *Federal Register* as a final notice, contained in a CMS ruling, or issued as a program instruction. These guidelines explain under what circumstances services and supplies are benefits for Medicare and Medicaid beneficiaries.

national coverage request Request from any entity, Medicare administrative contractor, or Centers for Medicare and Medicaid Services (CMS) internal staff for the CMS to consider an issue for a national coverage decision.

national drug code (NDC) Medical code set maintained by the U.S. Food and Drug Administration (FDA) to identify codes for FDA-approved drugs. The 11-digit drug product identifier code identifies manufacturer, repackager or distributor, drug product (strength, dosage, and formulation), and package size. The codes are used to bill for drugs when transmitting insurance claims electronically. The Secretary of the Department of Health and Human Services (HHS) adopted this code set as the standard for reporting drugs and biologicals on standard transactions.

National Electronic Information Corporation (NEIC) Large clearinghouse that receives, processes, edits, and sorts health insurance claims that are transmitted to participating insurers for payment.

national employer identifier Identifying system used for recognizing sponsors of health care benefits.

National Flood Insurance Program (NFIP) Program that makes federally backed flood insurance available to homeowners, renters, and business owners in communities for events that are not covered by traditional homeowners' policies. Community participation in the NFIP is voluntary. Three components of the NFIP are flood insurance, floodplain management, and flood hazard mapping. Also see *Federal Emergency Management Agency (FEMA)* and *Federal Insurance Administration (FIA)*.

National Formulary One of the official compendia in the United States. Also see *compendium, United States Pharmacopoeia*, and *Homeopathic Pharmacopoeia of the United States*.

national health expenditures (NHE) Economic indicator that reports the amount the United States spends annually on health care (e.g., dental services, drugs, home nursing care, medical research, physician and hospital services). It is expressed as a percentage of the gross domestic product (GDP).

National Health Information Infrastructure (NHII) Health Insurance Portability and Accountability Act (HIPAA) Administrative Simplification (A/S) initiative that set forth to improve patient safety and the quality of health care, as well as to better inform individuals regarding their own health information and to help them understand health care costs. NHII is overseen by the Department of Health and Human Services (HHS) with the National Committee on Vital and Health Statistics (NCVHS) serving as a public advisory committee.

national health insurance Method of insurance protection for medical expenses that is provided by a federal government. Also called *socialized medicine, statutory health insurance*, and *universal coverage*.

national improvement projects Health Care Quality Improvement Program (HCQIP) projects developed by a group consisting of representatives of some or all of the following groups: Centers for Medicare and Medicaid Services (CMS), Public Health Service (PHS), networks, renal providers, and consumer communities. The object is to use statistical analysis to identify better patterns of care and outcomes and to feed the results of analysis back into the provider community to improve the quality of care provided to renal Medicare beneficiaries. Each project will have a particular clinical focus.

national individual identifier (NII) See *national patient identifier*.

National Institutes of Health (NIH) Predecessor agency, Marine Hospital Services, was established in 1798 to provide for the medical care of merchant seamen. NIH fosters medical research to improve health and expand knowledge base in medical and associated sciences to enhance the United States' economic well-being and ensure a continued high return on the public investment in research.

National Library of Medicine (NLM) World's largest medical library that collects materials and provides information and research services in all areas of biomedicine and health care.

national median charge Exact middle amount of the amounts charged for the same service. This means that half of the hospitals and community mental health centers charged more than this amount and the other half charged less than this amount for the same service.

National Oceanic and Atmospheric Administration (NOAA) Agency that enriches life through science with roots dating back to 1807 when the United States' first scientific agency, the Survey of the Coast, was established. Members of NOAA are eligible for TRICARE benefits.

National Organization of Life and Health Guaranty Associations (NOLHGA) Voluntary association founded in 1983 that is made up of the life and health insurance guaranty associations of all 50 states, the District of Columbia, and Puerto Rico. NOLHGA assists its member associations in quickly and cost-effectively providing coverage to policyholders in the event of a multistate life or health insurer insolvency. When an insurer licensed in multiple states is declared insolvent, NOLHGA, on behalf of affected member state guaranty associations, assembles a task force of guaranty association officials. This task force analyzes the company's commitments to policyholders; ensures that covered claims are paid; and, where appropriate, arranges for covered policies to be transferred to a healthy insurer. The task force may also support the efforts of the receiver to dispose of the company's assets in a way that maximizes their value. When there is a shortfall of estate assets needed to pay the claims of covered policyholders, guaranty associations assess the licensed insurers in their states a proportional share of the funds needed.

national patient identifier Identifying system used for recognizing all recipients of health care services. Also known as *health care identification, health care ID*, and *national individual identifier (NII)*.

national payer identifier Numbering system to identify organizations that provide reimbursement for medical services. Now known as *NPLANID*. Previously known as *health plan ID, payer ID*, or *plan ID*. See *NPLANID*.

national plan identifier (NPLANID) See *NPLANID*.

national practitioner data bank (NPDB) Data bank established through Title IV of Public Law 99-6660, the *Health Care Quality Improvement Act of 1986*. It is primarily an alert or flagging system intended to

N

facilitate a comprehensive review of health care practitioners' professional credentials. It helps improve the quality of health care by encouraging state licensing boards, hospitals, other health care entities, and professional societies to identify and discipline those individuals who engage in unprofessional behavior. These groups can also restrict the ability of incompetent physicians, dentists, and other health care practitioners to move from state to state without disclosure or discovery of previous medical malpractice payment and adverse action history such as those involving licensure, clinical privileges, professional society members, and exclusions from either the Medicare or Medicaid program.

national provider file Database envisioned for use in maintaining a national provider registry.

national provider identifier (NPI) Medicare lifetime 10-digit number that replaces the provider identification number (PIN), unique physician/practitioner identification number (UPIN), Online Survey Certification and Reporting (OSCAR) system number, and National Supplier Clearinghouse (NSC) number. It is the standard identifier for providers of health care services, supplies, and equipment. Providers who submit claims to government-sponsored insurance programs insert the NPI on their claims. See Figure N-1.

national provider registry Organization that assigns national provider identifier (NPI) numbers and has a compiled national list of professional providers' names. As of the publication of this dictionary, it is in the developmental stage.

national provider system Administrative system envisioned for supporting a national provider registry.

national standard format (NSF) 1. Generically, this applies to any nationally standardized data format, but it is often used in a more limited way to designate the electronic media claims NSF used to submit professional health insurance claims. 2. Name of the standardization of data to reduce paper and have more accurate information and efficient organization.

national standard per visit rates National rates for each six home health disciplines based on historical claims data. Used in payment of low utilization payment adjustments (LUPAs) and calculation of outliers.

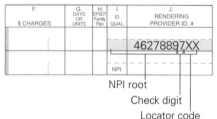

NPI root

Check digit

Locator code

Figure N-1 National provider identifier *(NPI).*

National Supplier Clearinghouse (NSC) number See *national provider identifier (NPI).*

National Uniform Billing Committee (NUBC) NUBC was brought together by the American Hospital Association (AHA) in 1975. It includes the participation of all the major national provider and payer organizations. The NUBC was formed to develop a single billing form and standard data set that could be used nationwide by institutional providers and payers for handling health care claims. In 1982 the NUBC voted to accept the UB-82 and its associated data manual for implementation as a national uniform bill. Improvement of the design led to the development of Uniform Bill (UB-92) and subsequently Uniform Bill (UB-04).

National Uniform Billing Committee, Electronic Data Interchange, Technical Advisory Group (NUBC EDI TAG) Coordinates issues that affect both the NUBC and the X12 standards.

National Uniform Claim Committee (NUCC) Voluntary organization presided over by the American Medical Association. It maintains the CMS-1500 insurance claim form and under HIPAA regulations a set of data element specifications for professional claims submission using the CMS-1500 claim form, the professional electronic media claims (EMC) national standard format (NSF), and the X12 837 health care claim. Under HIPAA, NUCC maintains the provider taxonomy codes and is consulted for transactions affecting nondental, noninstitutional professional health care services. NUCC replaced the Uniform Claim Form Task Force in 1995.

natural father See *biological father* and *birth father.*

natural mother See *birth mother* and *biological mother.* Adoptive parents do not prefer this term because it implies that the adoptive mother was unnatural.

naturopath Practitioner of naturopathy who uses natural healing and does not use medicine or surgery for treatment.

naturopathy System of health care that uses no drugs and has many varieties of therapies such as heat, massage, exercise, fresh food, hydrotherapy, and herbal medicine. Its aim is treating the entire person to stimulate his or her own healing power and to prevent illness.

NBICU See *newborn intensive care unit (NBICU).*

NC See *no charge (NC).*

NCA See *national coverage analyses (NCA).*

NCCAM See *National Center for Complementary and Alternative Medicine (NCCAM).*

NCCC Abbreviation for National Correct Coding Council. See *National Correct Coding Council (NCCC).*

NCCI See *National Correct Coding Initiative (NCCI).*

NCDM See *National Coverage Determinations Manual (NCDM).*

NCDs See *national coverage determinations (NCDs).*

NCHS See *National Center for Health Statistics (NCHS).*

NCICS See *National Certified Insurance and Coding Specialist (NCICS)*.

NCPDP See *National Council for Prescription Drug Programs (NCPDP)*.

NCPDP batch standard National Council for Prescription Drug Programs format for use by low-volume dispensers of pharmaceuticals such as nursing homes. The Secretary of the Department of Health and Human Services (HHS) adopted this format as a standard transaction under the Health Insurance Portability and Accountability Act (HIPAA).

NCPDP telecommunication standard National Council for Prescription Drug Programs format designed for use by high-volume dispensers of pharmaceuticals such as retail pharmacies. Use of this standard has been mandated under the Health Insurance Portability and Accountability Act (HIPAA).

NCQA See *National Committee for Quality Assurance (NCQA)*.

NCVHS See *National Center for Vital and Health Statistics (NCVHS)*.

ND See *nondisability (ND) claim* or *Doctor of Naturopathy (ND)*.

NDC See *national drug code (NDC)*.

nebulizers Equipment to give medicine in a mist form to the patient's lungs.

NEC See *not elsewhere classifiable (NEC)*.

needs analysis Phase during the process of creating a detailed personal and financial picture of a prospect to evaluate an individual's insurance requirements.

needs assessment Estimation of the requirements for health services by a community or population.

neglect When caretakers do not give a person they care for the goods or services needed to avoid harm or illness.

negligence Conduct that intentionally disregards others' rights and lacks the standard of care that an individual would carry out in the same situation.

negotiated discount System of payment to contracted providers as stated in the managed care plan agreement that allows a specific percentage by which a fee may be reduced.

negotiated trusteeship Agreement that results from collective bargaining (negotiation between a union and one or more employers) that provides group insurance for the members of the union. Also called a *Taft-Hartley Trust*.

NEIC See *National Electronic Information Corporation (NEIC)*.

neighborhood health center See *community health center (CHC)*.

NEMB See *notice of exclusions from Medicare benefits (NEMB)*.

neo ICU See *neonatal intensive care unit (neo ICU or NICU)*.

neonatal intensive care unit (neo ICU or NICU) Section or department within a hospital that uses special equipment for the care of premature, ill, newborn infants.

neonatal period Period of an infant's life from birth to the age of 27 days, 23 hours, and 59 minutes.

neonatology Art, science, and study of diagnosis and treatment of disorders of premature and/or high-risk newborn infants.

neoplasm Spontaneous new growth of tissue forming an abnormal mass; also known as a *tumor*; may be benign or malignant.

neoplasm table In Alphabetical Index, Volume 2 of ICD-9-CM diagnostic coding, table used to locate a code for a neoplasm.

nephrology Study of the kidney—anatomy, physiology, and treatment of diseases and disorders.

nervous system Organ system of the body that is composed of the central and peripheral nervous systems. The central nervous system is composed of the brain and spinal cord. The peripheral nervous system includes all of the other neural elements.

net amount at risk Life insurance policy's death benefit minus the policy's reserve at the end of the policy year.

net benefit premium Portion of the insurance premium that funds the benefit reserve. Generally accepted accounting principles (GAAP) are used to calculate the net benefit premium.

net cash value See *cash surrender value*.

net charge 1. For a CPT professional component service, the fee of the interpreting physician. 2. For a CPT technical component service, the fee of the supervising physician.

net cost 1. For group insurance, total sum that equals the insurance claims plus the reserves plus the expenses; or premiums less dividends. 2. In individual insurance, cost of an insurance policy obtained from any one of several different figures.

net level premium reserve Amount of liability for an insurance policy that is calculated using net level annual premiums.

net loss ratio Total insurance claims liability plus total expenses divided by the insurance premiums.

net payment cost index See *interest-adjusted payment*.

net premium 1. For insurance, the amount paid after any discount amount is applied. 2. Part of the gross premium that covers insurance policy benefits (e.g., the amount of the premium sent to the home office by an insurance agent after subtracting the commission). 3. Amount of money needed to provide life insurance benefits for a policy.

net premium rate Portion of the premium rate of a group that represents anticipated insurance claims.

net proceeds See *policy proceeds*.

net revenue Amount of money actually received by a hospital for billed services rendered. This is the amount after deductions for bad debts, charity, and contract adjustments.

net single premium Present value of expected benefits of an insurance policy, which is the amount of money that would have to be collected at the time an insurance policy is issued.

netback Evaluating a collection agency's performance by taking the amount of monies collected and subtracting the agency's fees.

network 1. Use of contacts to gain information or obtain some professional advantage. 2. Group of physicians, hospitals, and pharmacies that have health contracts with an insurance plan to provide medical care to the plan's members. 3. Process in which computer software and hardware interact in a multiuser system. 4. For electronic transmission of insurance claims, connection among clearinghouses, telephone companies, insurance plans, software vendors, and so on.

network HMO Managed care organization that contracts with two or more group practices to provide health services.

network model Managed care plan that contracts with several groups of providers or networks to give health care to the members of the plan. Also called *group model*.

networking Exchanging information or services among individuals, groups, or institutions and making use of professional contacts.

neurology Study of the nervous system including diagnosis and treatment of its diseases.

neurosurgery Diagnosis and surgery of the nervous system including the brain.

never events Occurrences related to surgical procedures that are performed on the wrong side, wrong site, wrong body part, or wrong person; retention of a foreign object in a patient following a procedure; patient death or disability associated with the use of contaminated drugs, devices, or biologics provided by the health care facility; patient death or serious disability associated with a medication error; stage 3 or 4 pressure ulcers acquired after admission to the health care facility; and patient death or disability associated with a fall while being cared for at the health care facility. This phrase was created because such happenings should never occur in medical practice and are usually preventable. Some insurance companies have stopped reimbursing hospitals for never events. Also see *hospital acquired conditions (HACs)*.

new business department See *underwriting department*.

new cost funding Type of conventional insurance contract that refunds cash surplus to its members but limits the amount that may be carried over to the next year.

new money method See *investment year method (IYM)*.

new patient (NP) 1. Current Procedural Terminology (CPT) defines new patient as an individual who has not received any professional services from the physician or another physician of the same specialty who belongs to the same group practice within the past 3 years. 2. Medicare interprets a new patient to mean a patient who has not received any professional services (i.e., evaluation and management [E & M] service or other face-to-face service [e.g., surgical procedure]) from the physician or physician group practice (same physician specialty) within the previous 3 years. For example, if a professional component of a previous procedure is billed in a 3-year time period (e.g., a laboratory interpretation is billed and no E & M service or other face-to-face service with the patient is performed), then this patient remains a new patient for the initial visit. An interpretation of a diagnostic test, reading an x-ray or electrocardiograph, in the absence of an E & M service or other face-to-face service with the patient does not affect the designation of a new patient.

newborn admission Infant born in the hospital facility. Newborns are reported separately from inpatient admissions and excluded from the admission data when registration of the mother is performed.

newborn intensive care unit (NBICU) Special hospital care unit for premature and very ill infants.

NF See *nursing facility (NF)*.

NFIP See *National Flood Insurance Program (NFIP)*.

NHE See *national health expenditures (NHE)*.

NICU See *neonatal intensive care unit (neo ICU or NICU)*.

NIH See *National Institutes of Health (NIH)*.

NLM See *National Library of Medicine (NLM)*.

no balance billing clause See *hold harmless clause*.

no charge (NC) Waiving of the entire fee owed for professional care.

no-evidence limit In group insurance, maximum amount that an insurance company will insure someone without securing evidence of insurability. Also known as *guaranteed issue limit*.

no-fault insurance Type of insurance that under state regulations permits automobile accident victims to collect directly from their own insurance company for medical and hospital expenses and loss of income regardless of who may have been responsible for causing the accident. Also called *medical payments coverage, personal injury protection*, or *medical expense coverage*. Automobile no-fault insurance is also called *personal injury protection (PIP)*. Homeowners and commercial medical payments insurance is also known as *Med-pay coverage*.

no loss/no gain Group insurance regulation that means no employee shall suffer a loss of benefits if a policyholder transfers the insurance plan from one company to another.

no man's land See *zone 2*.

no-payment bill or claim Insurance claim submitted to the third-party payer for which the physician does not anticipate reimbursement. Such claims are submitted to the insurance carrier to let them know of reimbursable periods of confinement or ending dates of care. Also called *nonpayment claim*.

no show Situation in which a patient does not appear for his or her scheduled appointment and did not call to cancel the appointment. Also referred to as *did not show (DNS)*.

NOI See *notice of intent (NOI)*.

NOLHGA See *National Organization of Life and Health Guaranty Associations (NOLHGA)*.

nomenclature Act of naming or describing a term or procedure (e. g., a CPT or HCPCS code description).

nominal payment See *token payment*.

non-face-to-face time Amount of time spent performing work before and after seeing the patient or family that is not a component of evaluation and management codes.

nonadmitted assets Items that cannot be included on the balance sheet of a life insurance company's annual statement.

nonadmitted reinsurer Insurance company that is not licensed to accept reinsurance in a given area.

nonallowed amount See *disallowance*.

nonassigned claim Type of insurance claim that may only be filed by a nonparticipating Medicare physician. When a claim is filed nonassigned, the beneficiary is reimbursed directly. Medicare pays 80% of the allowable amount to the beneficiary. The patient pays the provider the total amount of the charge for the service event if it is larger than the Medicare allowable amount.

Nonavailability Statement (NAS) In the TRICARE or CHAMPVA program, a statement issued on request and signed by the commanding officer before treatment when the military treatment facility cannot provide inpatient care and the patient lives in a certain ZIP code near a military hospital. INAS is an acronym for inpatient nonavailability statement.

noncancelable clause or policy Insurance policy clause that means the insurance company cannot increase premium rates and must renew the policy until the insured reaches the age stated in the contract. Some disability income policies have noncancelable terms.

noncomplying employer In workers' compensation, an employer who either allowed insurance coverage to lapse or failed to provide workers' compensation insurance that is required by law.

nonconfining sickness Illness that disables an insured individual but not enough that restricts him or her to home or hospital.

noncontributory group insurance plan See *noncontributory plan*.

noncontributory plan 1. Group insurance plan in which premiums are paid by the employer and the employees do not contribute to the cost. Usually enrollment of group members is automatic. 2. In a pension plan, contributions are made entirely by the plan sponsor.

noncontributory wage credits Wages and wages in kind that were not subject to the health insurance (HI) tax but are deemed as having been. Deemed wage credits exist for the purposes of (1) determining HI program eligibility for individuals who might not be eligible for I coverage without payment of a premium were it not for the deemed wage credits; and (2) calculating reimbursement due the HI trust fund from the general fund of the Treasury. The first purpose applies in the case of providing coverage to persons during the transitional periods when the HI program began and when it was expanded to cover federal employees; both purposes apply in the cases of military service wage credits and deemed wage credits granted for the internment of persons of Japanese ancestry during World War II. Also called *deemed wage credits*. See *military service wage credits* and *quinquennial military service determinations and adjustments*.

noncovered inpatient days Hospital inpatient days of medical care that are not covered by the insurance carrier. In the Medicare program, noncovered days may not be claimed as Medicare patient days for cost reporting by the hospital and the patient is not charged for using Part A hospital services.

noncovered procedure In the Medicare program, a medical service that is not a benefit and if billed to the fiscal intermediary, it will be denied for payment.

noncovered services 1. Medical services and supplies that are not covered and therefore not paid in keeping with the requirements of an insurance policy. 2. In the Medicare program, a service that does not meet the requirements of a benefit category, is statutorily excluded from coverage, and is not considered reasonable and necessary under federal guidelines. 3. In Medicare fraud, to bill for a service that has no coverage as if it were a covered service (e.g., to bill routine foot care as a more involved form of foot care to obtain payment).

noncustodial parent Divorced parent who generally is awarded visitation rights with the child and does not have legal custody.

nondisability (ND) claim An on-the-job injury that requires medical care but does not result in loss of working time or income.

nondisabling injury benefit In disability income policies, insurance provision that pays for medical expenses because of injury when the insured is not entirely disabled.

nonduplication clause Insurance policy provision that excludes expenses incurred by a policyholder that are covered by two or more policies. It is stricter than a coordination of benefits provision.

nonduplication of benefits Insurance provision that coordinates medical benefit payments between two or more insurance companies. The secondary payer reimburses if there is any difference between the amount paid by the primary plan and the total bill. However, some plans that have this clause may state that any services covered in whole or in part by another plan are excluded from coverage.

nonemergent condition In insurance coverage, there may be no payment for services such as routine physical examination, diagnostic workup for a chronic condition, routine eye examination, routine prenatal care, and elective surgery. These are considered nonemergent.

nonentity assets Resources that are held by an entity but are not available to the entity. These are also amounts that, when collected, cannot be spent by the reporting entity.

nonessential modifiers In ICD-9-CM diagnostic coding, additional descriptive words that do not affect the code assignment and are enclosed in parentheses after a main term.

nonexclusive territory Area in which more than one insurance agent may represent the same insurance company.

nonexclusivity Provision in an agreement that allows the physician or corporation to enter into similar agreements with other entities.

nonexempt assets One's total property (in bankruptcy cases) not falling in the exemption category including money, automobile equity, and property, over a specified amount, depending on the state in which the person lives.

nonexempt employees Employee classification that specifically states who is subject to overtime compensation and work time limits under the Federal Labor Standards Act (FLSA).

nonexempt trust See *Section 402(b) of the Internal Revenue Code.*

nonfacility practice expense Physician's direct and indirect medical practice costs with reference to each service provided in the office, patient's home, or residential care facility—not in a hospital setting.

nonfeasance In malpractice, the failure to act when a duty to act existed.

nonfederal agency State or local government agency that receives records contained in a system of records from a federal agency to be used in an electronic matching program.

nonforfeiture factors Certain amounts that some insurance companies use to calculate their policies' cash values.

nonforfeiture option Life insurance choice available to a policyholder if he or she discontinues the premium payments. The policy value, if any, may be taken in cash as extended term insurance or as reduced paid-up insurance.

nonforfeiture reduced paid-up benefit Life insurance policyholder with cash value may choose a smaller, fully paid-up policy with no further premium payments. The amount of the paid-up policy is established using the insured's age and cash surrender amount.

nonforfeiture values Insurance policy benefits that the insurance company guarantees to the policyholder if the insured ceases to pay premiums. These amounts may be used by choosing a value as stated in the nonforfeiture option clause of the policy.

nonformulary drugs Medications not on a government program or insurance plan approved list. Usually these drugs require a higher copayment by the patient.

nongroup Subscribers or members of an insurance plan that are not connected to a company-sponsored group. Nongroups are directly enrolled in plans.

nonguaranteed premium life insurance See *indeterminate premium life insurance.*

noninnovator, multiple-source drugs Classification of drugs used by the Centers for Medicare and Medicaid Services (CMS) when establishing the payment rate. These are generic drugs approved by the Food and Drug Administration (FDA).

noninvasive diagnostic test Diagnostic service or procedure that does not involve insertion of an instrument or device through the skin or body orifice.

nonmedical application Formal request for insurance coverage that does not require that the applicant undergo a medical examination. The document contains questions that the proposed insured must answer about his or her health.

nonmedical declaration See *nonmedical supplement.*

nonmedical supplement Report that describes the proposed insured's medical history. This document may be completed by the insurance agent from information from the proposed insured and may be a part of a nonmedical application. Also called *nonmedical declaration.*

nonmember hospital Hospital facility that has not contracted with a health insurance plan to render hospital services to its members. Also called *nonparticipating hospital.*

nonoccupational insurance See *disability income insurance.*

nonoccupational policy See *disability income insurance.*

nonpar See *nonparticipating physician (nonpar).*

nonpar policy See *nonparticipating policy.*

nonparticipating hospital See *nonmember hospital.*

nonparticipating insurance Life insurance in which the premium is calculated to cover the anticipated cost of the protection and no dividends are payable.

nonparticipating physician (nonpar) Provider who does not have a signed agreement with Medicare and has an option regarding assignment. Physician who does not agree to accept Medicare's allowed amount as payment in full and may charge the beneficiary, up to the limiting charge, for the services. The physician may not accept assignment for all services or has the option of accepting assignment for some services and collecting from the patient for other services performed at the same time and place. Also called *nonparticipating provider.*

nonparticipating policy Life insurance agreement in which the policyholder does not receive dividends. Also called *nonpar policy.*

nonparticipating provider (nonpar) Provider who decides not to accept the determined allowable charge from an insurance plan as the full fee for care. Payment goes directly to the patient in this case, and the patient is usually responsible for paying the bill in full. See *nonparticipating physician (nonpar).*

nonpatient service Service that is not given to a patient seen at the hospital such as laboratory test or pathology service performed on a sample sent to the hospital laboratory from an outside source to process. Thus the service is on the specimen and not a patient seen at the hospital or present when the service is performed.

nonpayment claim Insurance claim sent to a third-party payer for which the physician does not anticipate any reimbursement (e.g., to inform the insurance carrier of reimbursable periods of confinement, ending dates of medical care, Medicare benefits are exhausted, Medicare lifetime reserve days are exhausted, Medicare services are not covered, submission of additional information on a possible workers' compensation case). Also called *no-payment bill or claim.*

nonphysician practitioner (NPP) Health care provider who meets state licensing requirements to provide specific medical services. Medicare allows payment for services furnished by nonphysician practitioners including but not limited to advance registered nurse practitioners (ARNP), certified registered nurse practitioners, clinical nurse specialists (CNS), licensed clinical social workers (LCSW), physician assistants (PA), nurse midwives, physical therapists, speech therapists, and audiologists. Also referred to as *limited license practitioner (LLP), midlevel practitioner, midlevel provider (MLP),* or *physician extenders (PEs).*

nonplan provider Health care provider who does not have an agreement with an insurance company.

nonprivileged information Information consisting of ordinary facts unrelated to the treatment of the patient. The patient's authorization is not required to disclose the data unless the record is in a specialty hospital or in a special service unit of a general hospital such as the psychiatric unit.

nonreportable procedure Diagnostic services that should not be billed because they comprise supervision, interpretation, technical, or professional services only. For hospital billing, always list and report codes for the complete procedure. Coding tips under the hospital revenue codes mention exceptions to this rule.

nonparticipating policy Insurance that does not provide for payment of a dividend.

nonprofit/not-for-profit Organization that reinvests all profits back into that same organization.

nonprofit insurers Companies or corporations that give medical benefits on a not-for-profit basis. Formerly, Blue Cross and Blue Shield plans were structured under this system.

nonrenewable policy Insurance agreement that covers an insured during a period of short-term risk.

nonresident license State license that authorizes an insurance agent who lives in another state to sell insurance in the licensing state.

nonresidential treatment center Facility that gives medical services for treatment of alcohol and substance abuse and other psychiatric problems to individuals who do not need inpatient hospitalization.

nonretroactive disability benefits Disability benefit that is paid only for the period of disability that is after an elimination period.

nonroutine disclosure To reveal data that are not necessary for treatment, payment, or health care operations and that require the patient to sign an authorization for release of medical information.

nonscheduled dental plan Insurance plan with dental coverage that pays for procedures based on the dentist's actual charges (i.e., usual, customary, and reasonable charges).

nonservice-connected Medical condition that did not take place and was not caused during an individual's military service.

nonsmoker risk class Underwriting risk class of individuals who have never smoked or have not smoked for 12 months before applying for insurance and therefore pay lower than standard insurance premiums.

nonspecific code Diagnostic code that specifies the diagnosis as ill defined, other, or unspecified and if no other code closely describes the diagnosis, this may be considered a valid code. See *not otherwise specified (NOS).*

nonsystemic condition Physical problem that affects a specific area of the body (e.g., cataracts, bunion, ear disorder, kidney stone).

nonvested reserves Group insurance reserves owned by the policyholder that are considered voluntary allocations of earnings and may be used for his or her benefit to pay claims but are not returned if and when the contract is ended.

normal cost Amount designated to a specific year for the insurance plan's operation.

normal delivery Process of childbirth in which the birth of an infant is without medical complications.

normal/reasonable Applying normal collection processes to Medicare, as well as non-Medicare patients.

North Atlantic Treaty Organization (NATO) Alliance of 26 countries from North America and Europe committed to fulfilling the goals of the North Atlantic Treaty signed on April 4, 1949. Members of this branch of the uniformed services are eligible for TRICARE benefits.

North Carolina Healthcare Information and Communications Alliance Organization that promotes the advancement and integration of information technology into the health care industry.

NOS See *not otherwise specified (NOS).*

nosocomial Pertaining to or originating in a hospital (e.g., disease, other pathologic condition).

not elsewhere classifiable (NEC) This term is used in the ICD-9-CM diagnostic coding system when the code lacks the information necessary to code the term in a more specific category. It is used only in Volume 2.

not otherwise specified (NOS) Unspecified. Used in ICD-9-CM numeric code system for coding diagnoses. It refers to a lack of sufficient detail in the diagnosis statement to be able to assign it to a more specific subdivision within the code classification. It is used only in Volume 1. When coding an unspecified case, the fourth digit of the diagnostic code is always 9. Fourth digits 0 through 7 identify more specific information of the main condition (term). The fourth digit number 8 is used for identifying other information.

notice of admission Form sent to an insurance company by the hospital when an insured is admitted for inpatient services. It lists the patient's name, address, gender, age, date of admission, reason for admission, and certificate number.

notice of claim Formal written document to the insurance company by the insured who claims a loss that is covered under the insurance policy.

notice of exclusions from Medicare benefits (NEMB) Document (CMS 20007 form) that may be used by a medical practice informing a Medicare beneficiary that the service he or she is receiving is not a Medicare benefit. It is not a required document but increases the likelihood of collecting for the service from the patient.

notice of intent (NOI) Federal document describing a regulation that is being considered and inviting comments from interested parties. Comments are used to develop a notice of proposed rule making (NPRM) or a final regulation.

notice of noncoverage See *Advance Beneficiary Notice (ABN)*.

Notice of Privacy Practices (NPP) Under the Health Insurance Portability and Accountability Act (HIPAA), a document given to the patient at the first visit or at enrollment explaining the individual's rights and the physician's legal duties in regard to protected health information (PHI). Also called *privacy notice*.

notice of proposed rule making (NPRM) Federal document explaining a new regulation or revision of an old rule being considered and inviting comments from interested parties. Comments are used to develop a final regulation.

notification of claim Official information, written or electronic, to a third-party payer on behalf of an insured relaying the facts relevant to an insurance claim.

NP See *nurse practitioner (NP)* and *new patient (NP)*.

NPDB See *national practitioner data bank (NPDB)*.

NPI See *national provider identifier (NPI)*.

NPLANID Acronym used by the Centers for Medicare and Medicaid Services (CMS) that means national plan identifier. It is a numbering system used to identify organizations that provide reimbursement for medical services. Previously known as *health plan ID, national payer identifier, payerID*, or *plan ID*. Also see *national payer identifier*.

NPP See *notice of privacy practices (NPP)* and *nonphysician practitioner (NPP)*.

NPRM See *notice of proposed rule making (NPRM)*.

NR HCPCS Level II modifier that may be used with CPT or HCPCS Level II codes indicating when durable medical equipment (DME) is new when rented and is subsequently purchased.

NSF See *national standard format (NSF)*.

NU HCPCS Level II modifier that may be used with CPT or HCPCS Level II codes indicating new equipment.

NUBC See *National Uniform Billing Committee (NUBC)*.

NUBC EDI TAG See *National Uniform Billing Committee, Electronic Data Interchange, Technical Advisory Group (NUBC EDI TAG)*.

NUCC See *National Uniform Claim Committee (NUCC)*.

number holder See *wage earner*.

number of units 1. In outpatient or physicians' office billing, the total amount of days or units that apply to each line of service in Block 24G of the CMS-1500 insurance claim form (e.g, multiple office or hospital visits, anesthesia minutes, oxygen volume, number of miles, units of supplies including drugs). However, not all codes need the number of units reported. 2. In hospital inpatient billing, the quantitative measurement of the medical procedures, services, supplies, tests, accommodation days, treatments, and so on identified by a certain revenue code. However, not all revenue codes need the number of units reported. Revenue codes are inserted in Field 42 of the Uniform Bill (UB-04) inpatient hospital billing claim form.

numerical rating system Risks based on classifying each medical and nonmedical factor with a numerical value on its expected influence on mortality.

nurse 1. Individual specifically trained and graduated from a nursing program who performs certain standards of education and clinical competence and is licensed by the state to practice nursing. 2. To give services necessary to promote, maintain, and restore health.

nurse aide Individual who provides nursing or nurse-related services to patients and is not state licensed.

nurse midwife See *Certified Nurse-Midwife (CNM)*.

nurse practitioner (NP) Registered nurse qualified and specially trained to give basic primary health care in physicians' offices, patients' homes, ambulatory care facilities, long-term care facilities, and other health care institutions. NPs generally function under supervision of a physician but not necessarily in his or her presence, diagnosing and treating common acute illnesses and injuries. In many states, NPs may prescribe certain medications. Also referred to as *physician extender (PE)*.

nurse triage Method performed by a nurse of sorting patients by type of injury or disorder and its severity either during a telephone call or other emergency situation. Some managed care plans use this system to direct care and use resources effectively. Also referred to as *telephone triage system*.

nursing To give services necessary to promote, maintain, and restore physical or mental health to individuals who are not able to provide such services for themselves.

nursing assistant (NA) Individual trained in basic nursing techniques and direct patient care who practices under the supervision of a registered nurse.

nursing facility (NF) Specially qualified facility that has the staff and equipment to provide skilled nursing care and health-related services above the level of custodial care to other than mentally retarded individuals. These services are medically necessary for a patient's recovery. NFs must be licensed by each state for individuals receiving care under the Title XIX (Medicaid) long-term care program. NF was formerly known as a *skilled nursing facility*.

nursing home Residence that provides a room, meals, and help with activities of daily living and recreation. Generally, nursing home residents have physical or mental problems that keep them from living on their own. They usually require daily assistance such as bathing, dressing, eating, and using the toilet.

nursing home care Treatment and services to assist nursing home residents with activities of daily living such as bathing, dressing, eating, and using the toilet.

nursing notes Medical record entries by an attending nurse that detail the medical care given to a patient.

nutrition To get enough of the right foods with vitamins and minerals that a body needs to stay healthy. Malnutrition, or the lack of proper nutrition, can be a serious problem for elderly individuals.

nutrition therapy See *medical nutrition therapy (MNT)*.

N

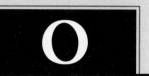

OA See *open access (OA)*.

OAA See *Older Americans Act (OAA)*.

OAS See *Office of Audit Services (OAS)*.

OASDI See *Old Age, Survivors, and Disability Insurance (OASDI) Program*.

OASHDI See *Old Age, Survivors, Health and Disability Insurance (OASHDI) Program*.

OASIS See *outcomes and assessment information set (OASIS)*.

OB See *obstetrician (OB)*.

objective 1. Viewing events or phenomena as they exist in the external world impersonally or in an unprejudiced way. 2. Open to observation by oneself and by others such as objective findings.

objective data Information that is factual, observed, and directly measurable.

objective factors See *objective findings*.

objective findings In workers' compensation, factors of impairment that can be determined by either seeing (visual), feeling (palpation), smelling; listened to (auscultation); or measured (i.e., size of a cyst, range of motion, strength, findings on x-ray, and results of laboratory or diagnostic tests). Also called *objective factors*.

obligation Budgeted funds committed to be spent.

obligatory actions Actions that are anticipated or demanded by ordinary moral standards (e.g., health information management professionals are expected to perform at a higher minimum standard of conduct than a layperson when it involves accuracy and privacy of medical information).

obliterate To eliminate completely such as illegally changing a medical record by erasing or covering an entry in a medical chart note with whiteout liquid or opaque adhesive tape. Also called *sanitizing*.

OBRA See *Omnibus Budget Reconciliation Act (OBRA) of 1980, 1981,* and *1987*.

observation patient Individual who presents with signs and symptoms of a significant degree of instability that warrants monitoring and needs to be evaluated and assessed to establish if he or she should be admitted for inpatient care or referred to another facility. Usually someone under observation is released within 24 hours.

observation services Under the orders of a physician or other licensed individual, outpatient hospital services given to a patient to evaluate the need for admission to the hospital as an inpatient. This may include the use of a bed and periodic monitoring by nurses or other hospital staff. Observation services are usually 23 hours or less.

observation status Patient not formally admitted to the hospital but instead admitted to "observation status" while his or her condition is being observed and a decision is made regarding admittance or discharge. The patient need not be in a separate observation area in the hospital to meet the observation criteria.

observation unit Department in the hospital in which patients are placed so that their disorders and/or complications can be watched for no longer than 23 hours and 59 minutes. The patient is then released or admitted to an inpatient unit. Such observation cases usually come from the emergency department.

obsolete care Medical care that from the insurance company's opinion is no longer accepted as standard care because of prevailing current standards of medical practice.

obstetrical services Medical and/or surgical care given by an obstetrician related to pregnancy (prenatal care) and/or delivery of a baby (postnatal care).

obstetrician (OB) Individual who specializes and practices in the branch of surgery that deals with the management of pregnancy, labor, and the puerperium.

obstetrics (OB) Pertaining to the specialty of medicine related to management of pregnancy and childbirth.

occasional pain In a workers' compensation case, pain approximately 25% of the time.

occasional symptoms In workers' compensation, a subjective indication of a disease or a change in condition as perceived by the patient that occurs approximately 25% of the time.

occupancy rate Measure of the average percentage of a hospital's occupied beds (entire facility or one specific department). This percentage is determined by dividing the number of available bed days by patient days.

occupational class See *occupational classification*.

occupational classification Group of job descriptions that have a similar risk to an insurance company and may have either a variable premium or the same insurance premium rate if all other factors are the same. Also called *occupational class*.

occupational disease See *occupational illness (or disease)*.

occupational exposure Experience of coming into contact with the skin, eye(s), mucous membranes, or parenteral contact with blood or other infectious materials during the course of employment.

occupational health services Medical services that deal with physical, mental, and social well-being of an individual relative to his or her work safety environment and with the adaptability of individuals to their work (i.e., job satisfaction).

occupational illness (or disease) Abnormal condition or disorder caused by environmental factors associated with employment. It may be caused by inhalation, absorption, ingestion, or direct contact and usually exists over a period of time.

occupational rate Insurance premium based on an occupation class.

Occupational Safety and Health Administration (OSHA) A federal agency that regulates and investigates safety and health standards in work locations.

occupational schedule Type of insurance table in which individuals are insured for an amount based on their job classifications.

occupational therapist (OT) Allied health professional who has graduated from a program in occupational therapy approved by the Committee on Allied Health Education and Accreditation of the American Medical Association, has obtained clinical experience before registration by the American Occupational Therapy Association, and practices occupational therapy.

occupational therapy (OT) Various services and treatment to an individual who is recovering from illness, injury, or physical or emotional problems by having him or her perform activities meant to improve joint range of motion and/or ability to cope with the demands of daily life (e.g., bathing, preparing meals, housekeeping). OT can be provided either on an inpatient or outpatient basis.

occupational therapy department Division or unit that provides various services and treatment in a medical community such as evaluation of patients' disabilities and performance capabilities and giving occupational therapy.

occupied by transient patient bed See *bed, occupied by transient patient.*

occurrence code Two-digit number and date for reporting services related to a specific type of accident, date beneficiary or spouse is retired, date the beneficiary was notified of the intent to bill for accommodations or procedures, and date physical, occupational, or speech-language pathology therapy treatments were begun. Occurrence codes are inserted in Fields 31 through 36 of the Uniform Bill (UB-04) inpatient hospital billing claim form. The electronic version requires an eight-character date listing year, month, and day: 20XX0328. A total of 12 occurrence codes and dates may be reported on a UB-04.

occurrence span code Two-digit number and the beginning and ending date for reporting circumstances related to the claim being submitted (e.g., benefit eligibility period, patient or provider liability period, residential level of care). Occurrence codes are inserted in Fields 35 and 36 of the Uniform Bill (UB-04) inpatient hospital billing claim form.

OCE See *outpatient code editor (OCE).*

ocean marine insurance See *marine insurance.*

OCFAA See *Office of Civil Fraud and Office of Administrative Adjudication (OCFAA).*

OCL See *other carrier liability (OCL).*

OCNA number Acronym that translates as Other Carrier Name and Address. Medicare patients who have a Medigap supplemental insurance plan must show the PAYERID number (often called the *OCNA key*) in Block 9d of the CMS-1500 insurance claim form. The Medicare fiscal intermediary transmits a Medigap claim electronically to the Medigap carrier after processing it for participating physicians. This is called a *crossover claim.*

OCR See *optical character recognition (OCR)* or *Office for Civic Rights (OCR).*

OD See *Doctor of Optometry (OD).*

OEP See *open enrollment period (OEP).*

OESS See *Office of E-Health Standards and Services (OESS).*

off-peak Periods of time, generally after business hours, when insurance claims can be electronically transmitted to insurance carriers quicker than during standard business hours.

off-site Location other than the provider's regular place of medical practice.

offer In property and casualty insurance, the application for a policy. In life insurance it must be accompanied by the first premium.

office 1. Location, other than a hospital, skilled nursing facility (SNF), military treatment facility, community health center, state or local public health clinic, or intermediate care facility (ICF), where the health professional routinely provides health examinations, diagnosis, and treatment of illness or injury on an ambulatory basis. 2. Position of authority.

Office for Civil Rights (OCR) Office that is part of the Department of Health and Human Services (HHS) promoting and ensuring that people have equal access to and opportunity to participate in and receive services in all HHS programs without facing unlawful discrimination. Through prevention and elimination of unlawful discrimination, OCR helps HHS carry out its overall mission of improving the health and well-being of all people affected by its many programs. OCR is responsible for enforcement of the Health Insurance Portability and Accountability Act of 1996 (HIPAA) privacy rules.

office manager Supervisor in a physician's medical practice who has administrative responsibilities.

Office of Audit Services (OAS) Organization of independent auditors for the Department of Health and Human Services (HHS). It identifies fraud, abuse, and waste in operations and programs and reports ways to improve, through a shared commitment with management, the economy, efficiency, and effectiveness of operations and services to beneficiaries of HHS programs.

O

Office of Civil Fraud and Office of Administrative Adjudication (OCFAA) Department responsible for coordinating activities that result in the negotiation and imposition of Civil Monetary Penalty Statutes (CMPS), assessments, and other program exclusions. It works with the Office of Investigations, Office of Audit Services (OAS), Centers for Medicare and Medicaid Services (CMS), and other organizations in the development of health care fraud and exclusion cases.

Office of E-Health Standards and Services (OESS) Department of Health and Human Services (HHS) that is responsible for enforcing HIPAA's transactions and code sets rule. Formerly known as *HHS' Office of HIPAA Standards (OHS)*.

Office of Inspector General (OIG) Agency established as an independent entity on March 29, 1989. The OIG provides independent and objective audits and investigations relating to agency programs and operations, provides leadership and coordination, recommends policies to prevent and detect fraud and abuse in Medicare and Medicaid and other government health care programs and operations, and provides a means for keeping the Chairman, Commissioners, and Congress fully informed about problems and deficiencies at the agency. The Inspector General (IG) reports to, and is under the general supervision of the, Federal Communications Commission (FCC) Chair and assists the Commission as it continues to improve its efficiency and effectiveness. The IG informs the Chairman and Congress of fraud or any serious problems with the administration of FCC programs and operations discovered during audits, investigations, and reviews. The IG recommends corrective action, where appropriate, and reports on progress made in the implementation of actions. The IG refers criminal matters to the Department of Justice for potential prosecution and coordinates referrals to managers for administrative action by the agency.

Office of Investigations (OI) Department within the Office of the Inspector General (OIG) that investigates allegations of crime, cyber-crime, Medicare fraud, waste, abuse, and misconduct affecting National Aeronautics and Space Administration (NASA) programs, projects, operations, and resources. OI refers its findings to either the Department of Justice for prosecution or NASA management for action. Through its investigations, OI identifies crime indicators and recommends effective measures for NASA management that are designed to reduce NASA's vulnerability to criminal activity.

Office of Management and Budget (OMB) Body within the Executive Office of the President of the United States (EOP) that helps with coordinating U.S. federal agencies. It is a senior management team of the White House. The OMB performs this coordination by gathering and filtering budget requests, issuing circulars dictating agency management practices, and reviewing proposed federal regulations. Six positions within the OMB—the Director, Deputy Director, Deputy Director for Management, and Administrators of the Office of Information and Regulatory Affairs, the Office of Federal Procurement Policy, and the Office of Federal Financial Management—are presidentially appointed and Senate-confirmed positions.

Office of Strategic Operations and Regulatory Affairs (OSORA) Federal agency that coordinates the preparation of manuals and other policy instructions to ensure accurate and consistent implementation of the Centers for Medicare and Medicaid Services (CMS) programs. It directs maintaining and amending of CMS-wide records for confidentiality and disclosure related to the Privacy Act and includes planning, organizing, initiating, and controlling privacy matching assignments.

office visit (OV) Formal face-to-face contact between a physician and a patient in an office, health facility, or hospital outpatient department.

Official Guidelines for Coding and Reporting See *ICD-9-CM Official Guidelines for Coding and Reporting*.

offset 1. Provision in tax law that lets an insurer use the amount paid for one type of tax reduce another part of the insurance company's tax liability. 2. Recovery by Medicare of a non-Medicare debt by reducing present or future Medicare payments and applying the amount withheld to the indebtedness (e.g., Public Health Service debts or Medicaid debts recovered by the Centers for Medicare and Medicaid Services [CMS]). This situation occurs if money is to be rebated to the fiscal intermediary (FI) and the provider is slow in doing so. When issuing the next payment check to the provider, the FI subtracts the rebate amount from the payment. This can lead to confusion when posting to accounts, so overpayments must be quickly refunded.

offset approach Method of putting together the benefits from a private defined benefit pension plan with the benefits from a government plan. This allows the benefits payable from the private plan to be reduced by a certain percentage of the benefits received from the government plan.

OHCA See *organized health care arrangement (OHCA)*.

OHI See *other health insurance (OHI)*.

OI See *Office of Investigations (OI)*.

OIB See *outpatient in a bed (OIB)*.

OIG See *Office of Inspector General (OIG)*.

OL See *outlier threshold (OT)*.

Old Age, Survivors, and Disability Insurance (OASDI) Program Federal program created by the Social Security Act in 1965. It taxes both employees and employers to pay benefits to retired and disabled individuals, their dependents, widows or widowers, and children of deceased workers. It also provides rehabilitation services to the disabled.

Old Age, Survivors, Health and Disability Insurance (OASHDI) Program Federal program administered by the Social Security Administration that provides monthly cash benefits to retired and disabled workers and their dependents and to survivors of insured workers; it also provides health insurance benefits for persons aged 65 and older and for the disabled younger than age 65. The health insurance component of OASHDI was initiated in 1965 and is generally known as *Medicare*. Commonly known as *Social Security*, the legislative authority for the program is found in the Social Security Act, originally enacted in 1935. The program is an example of social insurance. Medicaid legislation also falls under this program. Sometimes referred to as *disability insurance*.

Older Americans Act (OAA) Federal legislation that addresses the needs of elderly adults in the United States and provides funds for aging services (home-delivered meals, congregate meals, senior centers, employment programs) and creates the structure for federal, state, and local agencies that oversee these programs.

OMB See *Office of Management and Budget (OMB)*.

ombudsman 1. Individual who assists enrollees in resolving problems they may have with their managed care organization (MCO) or prepaid health plan (PHP). He or she acts as a neutral party who works with enrollees, the MCO/PHP, and the provider (as appropriate) to resolve individual enrollee problems. 2. Advocate or supporter who works to solve problems between residents and nursing homes, as well as assisted living facilities. Also called *long-term care ombudsman*. See *long-term care ombudsman*.

OME See *other medical expenses (OME)*.

Omnibus Budget Reconciliation Act (OBRA) of 1980 This Act made Medicare the secondary payer when an injured person has automobile medical, no-fault, or liability insurance.

Omnibus Budget Reconciliation Act (OBRA) of 1981 Provisions of this Act made Medicare the secondary payer for up to 12 months when a beneficiary entitled to Medicare solely on the basis of end-stage renal disease also has coverage under an employer group health plan.

Omnibus Budget Reconciliation Act (OBRA) of 1987 Federal legislation that required all nursing facilities and intermediate care facilities to meet skilled nursing facility certification requirements if handling Medicare patients.

OMRA See *other Medicare-required assessment (OMRA)*.

on-site Provider's regular office or clinic location for conducting his or her practice of medicine.

on-site review Evaluation performed at the managed care organization or prepaid health plan's health care delivery system location to assess the physical resources and operational practices in place to deliver health care.

oncology Branch of medicine concerned with the study of malignancy and with the diagnosis and treatment of cancerous growths.

Online Medical Evaluation CPT Category III code series that allows billing by a physician or qualified health care professional for services to a patient using Internet resources in response to the patient's online inquiry or problem (e.g., telephone call, prescription provision, laboratory orders).

online medical record See *electronic medical record (EMR)*.

Online Survey Certification and Reporting (OSCAR) system Centers for Medicare and Medicaid Services (CMS) system that came online in October 1991 to replace the Medicare/Medicaid Automated Certification System (MMACS) and the Rapid Data Retrieval System (RADARS). CMS uses OSCAR in its survey of Medicare and Medicaid providers to monitor state agency and provider performance. OSCAR contains data for current and previous surveys. Some data are overwritten as new information is entered (e.g., number of beds, address, employment information, scope and severity of deficiencies), but deficiency data remains and is tracked historically. Part of the OSCAR data is self-reported information by the nursing homes about the facility and its patients. Remaining data are generated by the surveyors based on deficiencies. Federal regulations detailing survey requirements are classified into 17 major categories. Specific survey requirements within these categories were consolidated from 325 individual items to 185 items effective July 1, 1995.

Online Survey Certification and Reporting (OSCAR) system number See *national provider identifier (NPI)*.

onset of condition Date a disease, illness, or injury first begins. This is usually when the patient seeks medical treatment.

OOA See *out of area (OOA)*.

OOPs See *out-of-pocket expenses (OOPs)*, *out-of-pocket limit*, and *out-of-pocket maximum*.

OP See *outpatient (OP)*.

OPD See *outpatient department (OPD)* and *outpatient diagnostic rider (OPD)*.

open access (OA) Phrase in a managed care plan's agreement that allows a member to self-refer for specialty medical care. Also called *open-ended* or *open panel*.

open access plan Members of a managed care plan may receive services outside the provider network without a referral authorization but may be required to pay an additional copayment and/or deductible amount. Also called *open panel* or *open-ended plan*.

open accounts Accounts from which charges are made from time to time and payment is expected within a specified period without a formal written contract.

open adoption Adoption of a child in which the individuals involved know each other and may maintain a relationship over time. This type of situation may or may not be legally sanctioned or legally binding.

open contract Insurance agreement used by fraternal benefit societies in which their charter, constitution, and bylaws become part of the contract.

open debit Insurance policy owners that have not been assigned to a service agent in a home service sales region.

open-ended plan See *open access plan.*

open enrollment See *federal open enrollment.*

open enrollment period (OEP) 1. Generally, time in the fall allowed by most managed care plans to encourage enrollment with an effective date of January 1. 2. Time when new subscribers may choose to enroll in, re-enroll in, or transfer between health insurance plans offered by federal health programs through his or her employer. Usually no physical examination or waiting period is required. Also called *open enrollment.* See also *election period, federal open enrollment, group enrollment period,* and *enrollment period.* 3. Opportunity each year when physicians may change participation status in the Medicare program for the following calendar year, usually in November.

open formulary List of drugs covered by a benefit plan in which the drugs on it are preferred but not required. See also *closed formulary* and *restricted formulary.*

open fracture Broken bone with an open skin wound; also referred to as a *compound fracture.*

open panel See *open access panel.*

open-panel HMO Type of managed care plan that contracts with physicians who operate out of their own offices and allows plan members to seek medical care from a participating provider without referral from another physician.

open panel 1. Phrase used to describe private physicians who agree to accept a managed care plan's terms to render care to members of the plan in his or her office. Also called *open access* or *open-ended.* 2. Type of managed care plan that contracts with physicians who operate out of their own offices and allows plan members to seek medical care from a participating provider without referral from another physician.

open system interconnection (OSI) Multilayer International Organization for Standardization (ISO) data communications standard. Health Level Seven (HL7) of this standard is industry specific, and HL7 is responsible for specifying the level seven OSI standards for the health industry.

open treatment Treatment of a fracture in which the site is surgically opened for visualization and possible internal fixation with a plate or pins.

operating bed See *bed, operating.*

Operation Restore Trust (ORT) Federal 2-year pilot program created in 1995 to fight fraud, waste, and abuse in Medicare and Medicaid programs. It targeted home health agencies, nursing homes, hospice, and medical equipment and supplies. It was concentrated in five states: California, Florida, Illinois, New York, and Texas.

operative notes Written or dictated information relating to a patient's surgical procedure that is prepared by the operating surgeon(s). It becomes part of the patient's health record.

operative report Surgical document describing a patient's surgical procedure that is written or dictated and signed by the operating surgeon(s).

ophthalmologist Individual who has a state license to practice medicine relating to the diagnosis and treatment of disorders and diseases of the eye.

ophthalmology Branch of medicine that deals with the study of the physiology, anatomy, and pathology of the eye and the diagnosis and treatment of disorders of the eye.

OPL See *other party liability (OPL).*

optical character recognition (OCR) Device that reads typed characters at high speed and converts them to digitized files that can be saved in memory. Data must appear within each item number so that the scanner can obtain the information. Some insurance contractors use OCR to scan insurance claims information directly into their claims processing system. Also known as *intelligent character recognition (ICR)* and *image copy recognition (ICR).*

optician Maker of or individual who dispenses eyeglasses with corrective lenses that have been prescribed by either an ophthalmologist or optometrist.

option Choice of an insured individual to decide how to apply settlements, dividends, or nonforfeiture values.

optional benefits 1. Additional insurance coverage that may be purchased when applying for insurance such as benefits for chemical dependency, drug addiction treatment, or mental illness treatment. 2. Lump sum payment for an injury, which may be available under a health insurance policy.

optional modes of settlement In a life insurance policy, proceeds received as periodic payments instead of receiving a lump sum.

optional provisions Additional benefits that an insurance company may include in the insurance contract.

optional renewable policy Insurance contract that has a renewal provision in which the insurer has the right to refuse to renew the policy on a premium renew date and may add coverage limitations or increase premium rates.

optional service or benefits In Medicaid, various medical benefits that a state plan may decide to offer individuals in the program such as diagnostic services, intermediate care facility for mentally retarded patients, personal care, prescription drugs, and rehabilitation therapies.

optional supplemental benefits Services not covered by Medicare that enrollees can choose to buy or reject. Enrollees who choose such benefits pay for them directly, usually in the form of premiums and/or cost sharing. Those services can be grouped or offered individually and can be different for each Medicare + Choice plan offered.

optionally renewable Insurance policy renewal provision in which the insurer has the right to refuse to renew the policy on a date and may add coverage limitations or increase premium rates.

optometrist See *Doctor of Optometry (OD)*.

order 1. Written or verbal communication from the treating physician that requests a diagnostic test or other medical service be performed on a patient. 2. In the Medicare program, communication (written, verbal, or electronic mail) from the treating physician/practitioner requesting that a diagnostic test be performed for a beneficiary. If the communication is via telephone, both the treating physician or his or her office and the testing facility must document the call in their respective copies of the patient's medical records.

ordering physician The physician ordering nonphysician services for a patient (e.g., diagnostic laboratory tests, pharmaceutical services, durable medical equipment) when an insurance claim is submitted by a nonphysician supplier of services.

ordinary agency system See *agency system*.

ordinary care See *due care*.

ordinary insurance See *individual insurance*.

ordinary life insurance See *whole life insurance* and *individual insurance*.

organ Structural part of a system of the body that is composed of tissues and cells that enable it to perform a particular function such as the digestive organs, heart, kidney, liver, pancreas, reproductive organs, spleen, and organs of special sense.

organ procurement Process of timely retrieval of vital tissues or an organ (heart or kidney) from a donor for transplant to another individual.

organ procurement organization Association that performs or coordinates the retrieval, preservation, and transportation of donor organs and maintains a system of locating prospective recipients for available organs.

organizational determination Health plan's decision on whether to pay all or part of a bill, or to give medical services after the patient files an appeal. If the decision is not in the patient's favor, the plan must give a written notice. This notice must give a reason for the denial and a description of steps in the appeals process.

organized care system An advanced integrated delivery system (IDS) that combines an insurance or third-party administrator so that there is no division between provider and payer. This results from mergers and affiliations between physicians and managed care organizations. See *integrated delivery system (IDS)*.

organized delivery systems See *accountable health plan (AHP)*.

organized health care arrangement (OHCA) Under the Health Insurance Portability and Accountability Act (HIPAA), an agreement that allows two or more covered entities (CEs) that participate in joint activities to share protected health information to manage and benefit their joint operations.

organized staff See *hospital staff*.

original age conversion Act of changing a term insurance policy to a whole life policy in which the premium rate is based on the age of the insured at the time the term policy was set up.

Original Medicare Plan See *Medicare (M)*.

orphan drugs Food and Drug Administration (FDA) phrase used for medications created to treat diseases or conditions that either affect fewer than 200,000 persons or more than 200,000 persons in the United States but for which there is no reasonable expectation that the cost of developing and marketing the drug would be recovered from U.S. sales. This classification is used by the Centers for Medicare and Medicaid Services if the drug has no use other than to treat the rare disease or condition and for establishing payment for the drug.

orthopedic (orthopaedic) Pertaining to the medical and surgical treatment and correction of deformities of the musculoskeletal system (i.e., bones, joints, ligaments, muscles, and tendons).

orthotics Field of knowledge that relates to orthopedic appliances or apparatus used to support a paralyzed muscle, align, prevent, or correct deformities or to improve the function of movable parts of the body (e.g., braces, splints, contour insoles).

OSCAR See *Online Survey Certification and Reporting (OSCAR) system*.

OSCAR system number See *Online Survey Certification and Reporting (OSCAR) system number*.

OSI See *open system interconnection (OSI)*.

OSORA See *Office of Strategic Operations and Regulatory Affairs (OSORA)*.

osteopath See *Doctor of Osteopathy (DO or MD)*.

osteopathy 1. Any disease of a bone. 2. A system of therapy founded by Andrew Taylor Still (1828-1917), based on the theory that the body makes its own remedies against disease and other toxic conditions when it is in normal structural relationship and has favorable environmental conditions and adequate nutrition. It uses physical, medicinal, and surgical methods of diagnosis and therapy, as well as manipulative methods of detecting and correcting any peculiar position of the joints or tissues.

osteoporosis Disorder characterized by abnormal loss of bone density and deterioration of bone tissue, with an increased risk of fracture. Often called the "silent disease" because bone loss occurs without symptoms. Medicare provides coverage of bone mass measurements once every 24 months (more often if medically necessary) for people at risk for osteoporosis.

OT See *occupational therapist (OT)* and *occupational therapy (OT)*.

OTC See *over-the-counter (OTC) drug*.

other carrier liability (OCL) See *other party liability (OPL)*.

other carrier name and address (OCNA) See *PAYERID number*.

"other" claims Medicare claims not considered "clean" claims that require investigation or development on a prepayment basis (developed for Medicare Secondary Payer information).

other diagnoses 1. All conditions that coexist at the time of admission, that develop subsequently, or that affect the treatment received and/or the length of stay as defined by the uniform hospital discharge data set (UHDDS). Diagnoses that relate to an earlier episode that have no bearing on the current hospital stay are excluded. UHDDS definitions apply to inpatients in an acute care, short-term, hospital setting. This definition also applies to outpatient encounters. 2. Additional conditions that affect patient care in terms of requiring clinical evaluation, therapeutic treatment, diagnostic procedures, extended length of hospital stay, or increased nursing care and/or monitoring. Also referred to as *secondary diagnoses* or *additional diagnoses*.

other health insurance (OHI) Health care coverage for TRICARE beneficiaries through an employer, an association, or a private insurer. A student in the family may have a health care plan through school.

other insurance clause Provision in an insurance contract that states the effect on the policy of other insurance coverage.

other managed care arrangement Another type of agreement used if the plan is not considered either a primary care case management (PCCM), prepaid health plan (PHP), comprehensive managed care organization (MCO), Medicaid-only MCO, or health insuring organization (HIO).

other medical expenses (OME) Medical expenses excluding hospital facility charges.

other Medicare-required assessment (OMRA) Additional assessment required within 8 to 10 days of discontinuance of treatment in a skilled nursing facility for medical care to be covered.

other party liability (OPL) Phrase used in the coordination of benefits (COB) clause of an insurance plan that states that the other insurance plan is the primary plan. This policy provision is used for workers' compensation and carve-out programs to clarify when another party is the primary payer. Sometimes called *other carrier liability (OCL)*.

other specified See *not otherwise specified (NOS)*.

other teaching hospital Medical center with an approved graduate medical education program and a ratio of interns and residents to beds of less than 25%.

other unlisted facility Other health service facility not previously identified.

otolaryngologist Medical doctor who specializes in the diagnosis and medical and surgical treatment of illnesses and injuries of the ears, nose, and throat (ENT).

otolaryngology Branch of medicine relating to the diagnosis and treatment of diseases and disorders of the ears, nose, throat, and adjacent structures of the head and neck.

out of area (OOA) 1. Services provided to enrollees by providers who have no contractual or other relationship with Medicare+Choice organizations. 2. Services obtained by an individual outside the area where the person is insured.

out-of-area benefits Coverage for members for services outside of the stated geographic area in the managed care plan contract such as emergency care and benefits for out-of-state students. Some plans require members to file claim forms for payment of these out-of-pocket expenses.

out-of-area services See *out-of-area benefits*.

out-of-hospital psychiatric care Mental health care, such as psychoanalysis, given in a physician's office.

out of network Phrase used to describe a facility or provider who does not participate in the managed care plan's contracted network but renders services to a member or subscriber. This situation can occur when an enrollee suffers an illness or injury while doing out-of-an area travel. Some plans may require that the member pay the fee for the service, whereas other plans allow for coverage but the member must meet a higher copayment amount. Also referred to as *out of plan, out-of-area emergency*, and *out-of-area transfer agreement*.

out-of-network benefit Type of service that allows a beneficiary with the option to access plan services outside the plan's contracted network of providers. In some cases a beneficiary's out-of-pocket costs may be higher for an out-of-network benefit.

out-of-panel physician or provider Doctor or provider who is not a part of a managed care plan's panel.

out of plan Phrase used to describe a provider who is not a member of a managed care plan.

out-of-plan referral Referral to a medical specialist who is not a participating provider in the managed care plan. Such referrals must have prior authorization by the managed care plan.

out-of-pocket cost Dollar amount a patient pays as his or her share of an insurance plan such as monthly premium, deductible, and coinsurance. In Medicare Part D drug plans, this is the coverage gap amount that is also known as the *doughnut hole*.

out-of-pocket expenses (OOPs) Medical costs that do not have insurance coverage and must be paid by the insured such as coinsurance, copayments, and deductibles. Also called *direct costs* or *out-of-pocket payment*.

out-of-pocket limit See *out-of-pocket maximum* and *coinsurance maximum*.

out-of-pocket maximum Largest amount of money the insured must pay in a calendar year for deductibles and coinsurance. Also called *out-of-pocket limit* and *coinsurance maximum*.

out-of-pocket payment See *out-of-pocket expenses (OOPs)*.

out-of-service area Phrase used in managed care plan contracts that refers to medical care services received out of the geographical area that is specified in the agreement. Such services may or may not be a benefit depending on the plan. In some plans, out-of-area coverage is limited to emergency services only. Also referred to as *out-of-area coverage*.

out-of-state corporation See *foreign corporation* and *foreign company*.

outcome Expected, desired, or actual result of performance or nonperformance of a function or process relating to patient care.

outcome data Information that measures the health status of people enrolled in managed care plans resulting from specific medical and health interventions (e.g., the incident of measles among plan enrollees during the calendar year).

outcome indicator Resulting statistic or conclusion that assesses what happens or does not happen to a patient following a process; agreed on desired patient characteristics to be achieved; and undesired patient condition to be avoided (e.g., mortality following coronary artery bypass surgery, neonatal death rate, nosocomial infection rate, readmission rate following discharge).

outcomes and assessment information set (OASIS) Standard core assessment data tool developed to measure the outcomes of adult patients receiving home health services under the Medicare and Medicaid programs. This assessment is performed on every patient receiving services of home health agencies that are approved to participate in the Medicare and/or Medicaid programs. OASIS is done for the purpose of outcome-based quality improvement (OBQI).

outcomes management See *disease management*.

outcomes measurement Formal process to measure the quality of medical care, the standard against which the end result (outcomes) of the intervention is assessed.

outcomes measures Assessments that estimate the results of treatment for a specific disease or condition such as objective data (health status, morbidity, and mortality) and subjective data (patient's perception of restored function, quality of life, and functional status).

outcomes research Study that assesses the effect of certain medical and health interventions (treatments) on health care costs and is measured in terms of a patient's ability to function, quality of life, and length of life.

outlawed claim In the legal sense, no further claim is legally permitted if the plaintiff does not take action within a specified period of time.

outlay Issuance of checks, disbursement of cash, or electronic transfer of funds made to liquidate an expense regardless of the fiscal year the service was provided or the expense was incurred. When used in the discussion of the Medicaid program, outlays refer to amounts advanced to the states for Medicaid benefits. Also called *expenditure*.

outlier Inpatient medical case whose course of treatment has unusually higher costs or a longer length of stay (LOS) when compared with other patients who were discharged in the same diagnosis-related group (DRG). The day outlier is no longer used. This term is used in utilization review. Also referred to as *stay outlier*.

outlier threshold (OT) Maximum hospital inpatient length of stay (admission date to discharge date), which is a component used in calculating the payment for a diagnosis-related group (DRG).

outpatient (OP) 1. Patient who receives services in a health care facility such as a physician's office, clinic, urgent care center, emergency department, or ambulatory surgical center but does not occupy a bed. 2. Refers to care given in organized programs such as outpatient clinics.

outpatient admission Registration of a patient for medical services who is provided with room, board, and continuous nursing service in a facility where patients generally do not stay overnight. Outpatient services are also known as *ambulatory services*.

outpatient care See *ambulatory care*.

outpatient code editor (OCE) Computer software program used by Medicare fiscal intermediaries that identifies code inconsistencies on outpatient insurance claims. The OCE detects incorrect billing and coding data, assigns an ambulatory payment classification for services that are a benefit, and determines the proper reimbursement. It tests validity of the codes and does compatibility edits of diagnostic codes and HCPCS codes and modifiers. It lists the errors and shows the action to take with the claim such as "suspended, denied." For inpatient insurance claims the computer software program is known as *Medicare code editor (MCE)*.

outpatient department (OPD) Section of a facility that is regularly maintained by a health care organization for patients who require medical services for less than 24 hours and do not require admission as inpatients. Medical services may include physical therapy, diagnostic x-rays, laboratory tests, dialysis for end-stage renal disease (ESRD), and so on. OPDs are subject to the outpatient prospective payment system (OPPS).

O

outpatient diagnostic facility State-licensed, free-standing facility that gives laboratory, radiology, and/or nuclear imaging testing on an outpatient basis to patients referred by physicians or contracted for by managed care plans.

outpatient diagnostic rider (OPD) Medical benefits that can be added to an insurance plan for diagnostic studies, tests, and treatment of illness or injury in the hospital's outpatient department.

outpatient facility See *ambulatory care facility* and *freestanding surgical center.*

outpatient hospital 1. Portion of a facility that provides diagnostic, therapeutic (surgical and nonsurgical), and rehabilitation services to sick or injured persons who do not require hospitalization or institutionalization. 2. Part of the hospital that provides services covered by supplementary medical insurance including services in an emergency department or outpatient clinic, ambulatory surgical procedures, medical supplies (such as splints), and laboratory tests billed by the hospital. 3. Under Medicare Part B, benefits do not include an overnight hospital stay but will pay for blood transfusions, certain drugs, hospital-billed laboratory tests, mental health care, medical supplies (splints and casts), emergency department, outpatient clinic, same-day surgery, x-rays, and other radiation services.

outpatient hospital claim Request to an insurance company for reimbursement of outpatient services given to a patient.

outpatient in a bed (OIB) Patient who is still in the hospital but does not meet inpatient or observation criteria. In this type of case, a hospital cannot bill an insurance claim as an inpatient but when billing can bill everything except for room and observation charges. Bill all ancillary and procedure charges as for an outpatient claim.

outpatient maintenance dialysis services Treatments and procedures given to patients who have end-stage renal disease in an outpatient facility. They are paid under a composite payment rate that includes all services, equipment, supplies, and certain laboratory tests and drugs for dialysis treatment.

outpatient physical therapy services 1. Treatments and procedures provided by a group of professional personnel to patients in an outpatient facility using physical agents and methods to assist in rehabilitating and restoring function after an illness or injury. Treatment may consist of massage, manipulation, therapeutic exercises, cold, heat, paraffin, shortwave and microwave diathermy, ultrasonic heat, hydrotherapy, or electric stimulation. Speech-language pathology services are also considered outpatient physical therapy services. 2. Physical therapy given by a physical therapist in an office setting or patient's home.

outpatient pricer Computer software program developed by the Centers for Medicare and Medicaid Services (CMS) that is used to establish the dollar amount for each service or supply, as well as the deductible and coinsurance amounts. It determines the ambulatory payment classification line-item price and calculates outlier payments for each claim.

outpatient prospective payment system (OPPS) Medicare prospective payment system used for hospital-based outpatient services and procedures that uses assignment of ambulatory payment classifications (APCs). OPPS was mandated by the Balanced Budget Act of 1997 (BBA). It changed Medicare payments from cost based to prospective based on national average capital costs per case. This complex payment system helps Medicare control its spending by encouraging providers to furnish care that is efficient, appropriate, and typical of practice expenses for providers. Patients and resource needs are statistically grouped, and the system is adjusted for patient characteristics that affect the cost of providing care. A unit of service is then established, with a fixed, predetermined amount for payment. The Centers for Medicare and Medicaid Services (CMS) administers the APC (ambulatory payment classification)-based OPPS. It is updated on a quarterly basis.

outpatient review Evaluation and assessment of outpatient services for appropriateness of treatment and observation of ongoing care.

outpatient services 1. Medical and other services provided by a facility to a patient who is not being admitted as a bed patient and is discharged within 24 hours (more hours would define the patient as an inpatient). These services may take place at a hospital outpatient department or community mental health center and include emergency department services, surgical procedures, rehabilitation therapy, physical therapy, occupational therapy, speech pathology services, diagnostic radiological procedures, laboratory tests, and dialysis in the facility. 2. Patient appointment system used in a physician's medical office practice.

outpatient surgery See *ambulatory surgery.*

outpatient surgery list List of operative procedures that can be performed without having the patient admitted as a bed patient.

outpatient treatment Medical therapy given in a hospital, clinic, or office setting in which the patient is admitted, treated, and released the same day.

outpatient visit Visit by a patient to an outpatient hospital or freestanding medical or dental treatment facility that provides medical care on an outpatient basis, without an overnight stay. The visit may include diagnostic, therapeutic, and rehabilitative services; preventive care; emergency medicine; and minor surgery to individuals. Also called *ambulatory visit.*

output Information transferred from internal memory storage to external storage.

outside laboratory Clinical laboratory that bills the physician for tests that the physician purchased on behalf of a patient. The physician bills the patient's medical plan by completing Block 32 on the CMS-1500 claim form or for an e-claim 837P Data Elements 19, 116, 156, 166, and 1035.

outstanding balance See *beginning balance.*

outstanding check Check issued by a payer that has not cleared the bank and has not appeared on the bank statement.

outstanding fee bill list In workers' compensation, a monthly list of all outstanding bills for each payee.

OV See *office visit (OV).*

over bill Type of hospital invoice (patient's financial accounting statement) assessed by someone auditing a hospital bill who has charged items that have not been documented in the hospital chart. Also see *clean bill* and *under bill.*

over line Insurance coverage that is more than the normal insurance capacity of an insurance company. Also called *over retained.*

over retained See *over line.*

over-the-counter (OTC) drug Medication that does not need a prescription under federal or state law and is sold directly to the consumer.

over-the-counter selling of insurance System of selling insurance wherein the insured buys directly from the insurance company and not through an agent.

overage To issue a credit to a group or an insured's billing.

overcoding See *upcoding.*

overhead expense disability income policy Type of disability income policy that provides funds for ongoing monthly business expenses such as employees salaries, equipment payments, rent, and utility fees if the insured (owner) becomes disabled.

overinsurance Condition in which the insurance benefit amount exceeds the real loss of the insured.

overinsurance provision 1. In an individual's health insurance policy, clause in which benefits are reduced if the insured has more insurance than necessary to cover medical expenses. 2. In disability insurance, if the insured's disability income exceeds his or her predisability earnings.

overlapping insurance Insurance by two or more insurance policies that give the same coverage for the same risk.

overlapping territory Geographical area in which some portion of the region is open to an insurance agent other than the general agent and the rest of the area is the exclusive domain of the general agent.

overpayment 1. Money paid over and above the amount due by the insurance carrier or the patient. 2. In Medicare, the funds a physician, supplier, or beneficiary has received in excess of the amount due and payable under Medicare statute and regulations. The amount of overpayment is a debt owed to the U.S. government.

overpayment assessment Decision that an incorrect amount of money has been paid for Medicare services and a determination of what that amount is.

override 1. Type of claims payment in which the adjudicator tells the computer the amount to pay and to whom; thus computer logic is not used—the claims adjuster overrides the system. 2. See *overriding commission.*

overriding commission Additional earned fee paid to a broker, general agent, or insurance agent on any type of insurance written by other agents in a specific geographical area. Some companies may base it on the overall production of the insurance field office. Also called *override.*

overutilization Health care services delivered to patients more frequently than medically necessary.

overvalued procedures Physicians' medical services for which prevailing charges have been reduced because they are considered financially overrated by historical comparative performance report (CPR).

O

P

P & T See *pharmacy and therapeutics committee (P & T)*.

P value See *probability*.

P1 Two-character alphanumeric modifier appended to five-digit CPT procedure codes and used for billing to indicate anesthesia was given to a normal, healthy patient.

P2 Two-character alphanumeric modifier appended to five-digit CPT procedure codes and used for billing to indicate anesthesia was given to a patient with mild systemic disease.

P3 Two-character alphanumeric modifier appended to five-digit CPT procedure codes and used for billing to indicate anesthesia was given to a patient with severe systemic disease.

P4 Two-character alphanumeric modifier appended to five-digit CPT procedure codes and used for billing to indicate anesthesia was given to a patient with severe systemic disease that is a constant threat to life.

P4P Abbreviation of a Medicare reimbursement model titled *pay-for-performance*.

P5 Two-character alphanumeric modifier appended to five-digit CPT procedure codes and used for billing to indicate anesthesia was given to a moribund patient who is not expected to survive without the operation.

P6 Two-character alphanumeric modifier appended to five-digit CPT procedure codes and used for billing to indicate anesthesia was given to a declared brain-dead patient whose organs are being removed for donor purposes.

PA See *physician advisor (PA), physician's assistant (PA), prior approval (PA),* and *prior authorization (PA)*.

PAC Acronym that translates as preadmission certification or preauthorized check system. See *precertification, automatic bill payment, electronic funds transfer (EFTS),* and *preauthorized payment*.

PACE See *Program of All-Inclusive Care for the Elderly (PACE)*.

package Several combined insurance contracts in one group wherein each agreement specifies a type of benefit (e.g., behavior health, dental, prescription drugs).

package policy One insurance contract that has all the coverage in a group plan.

package pricing See *global pricing*.

packaging 1. Professional service that is put together with a medical procedure. Packaged services may be coded and billed for payment. See *bundling*. 2. System of insurance in which several coverages are grouped together and offered in one plan. Eligible participants must either accept or reject the whole package. Also called *package plan*.

paid amount That part of a submitted insurance claim that has actually been paid by both the third-party payer and the insured including deductible, copayments, and balance bills.

paid claim Insurance claim that has been applied to an insurance plan, a check has been issued, and the check has cleared through the bank system.

paid claims loss ratio See *loss ratio*.

paid-up additions See *dividend additions*.

paid-up insurance 1. Insurance contract on which all required premiums have been paid. 2. Insurance contract that provides benefits in the future but does not require additional premium payments. Also called *paid-up policy*.

paid-up policy See *paid-up insurance*.

palliative care Treatment designed to relieve or reduce intensity of uncomfortable symptoms but not to produce a cure (e.g., narcotics to relieve pain in a cancer patient, creation of a colostomy to bypass an inoperable obstruction of the bowel, débridement of necrotic tissue in a patient with malignant metastasis).

palliative service Medical care given to a patient who is chronically ill to lessen symptoms of an illness or disability.

palliative treatment Therapy designed to relieve or reduce intensity of uncomfortable symptoms but not to produce a cure (e.g., use of narcotics to relieve pain in a patient with advanced cancer).

panel Managed care plan network of providers who render medical services to members of the plan.

panel physician See *panel provider*.

panel provider Physician, health care facility, or medical supplier who enters into an agreement with a managed care plan to provide specific service to the plan's members. Also called *panel physician*.

panel size Number of patients served by a physician or physician group. If the panel size is greater than 25,000 patients, then the physician group is not considered to be at substantial financial risk because the risk is spread over the large number of patients. Stop loss and beneficiary surveys would not be required.

Pap test See *Papanicolaou (Pap) test* and *screening Pap (Papanicolaou) smear*.

Papanicolaou (Pap) smear See *Papanicolaou (Pap) test* and *screening Pap (Papanicolaou) smear*.

Papanicolaou (Pap) test Simple smear method for precancerous cellular changes and early detection of cancer of the cervix, the opening to a woman's womb. It is done by removing cells from the cervix. The cells are then prepared so that they can be seen with the use of a microscope. Also called *Papanicolaou (Pap) smear, Pap test,* or *screening Pap (Papanicolaou) smear*.

paper claim An insurance claim submitted on paper including those optically scanned and converted to an electronic form by the insurance carrier.

paperless patient chart See *electronic medical record (EMR)*.

PAPs Acronym that translates as patient assistance programs. See *Partnership for Prescription Assistance (PPA)*.

par Abbreviation for participating provider. See *participating provider (par)*.

PAR Abbreviation for preadmission review. See *precertification*.

par policy See *participating policy*.

par provider Abbreviated phrase for a provider who is participating in an insurance plan. See *participating provider (par)*.

paramedical examination Physical examination performed by a medical practitioner other than a physician on someone who has applied for insurance.

paramedical report Medical document detailing a medical history and a physical examination performed by a medical technician, a physician's assistant, or a nurse. It describes the health of a proposed insured and may be used as part of an application for an insurance policy.

parent company Insurer in a group of insurance companies that has control over the other companies (subsidiaries). Generally, the parent company is the group policyholder.

parenteral contact Absorption of substances within the body by structures other than the digestive tract.

parenteral nutrition (PEN) Nourishment delivered to a patient by some means other than through the gastrointestinal tract (e.g., intravenously).

parentheses 1. In ICD-9-CM coding, symbols used to enclose nonessential modifiers because their presence or absence does not affect the code assigned and these data provide additional description. 2. In CPT coding, symbols used to enclose a note listed at the end of a code section.

Part A hospital insurance coverage See *Medicare Part A*.

Part A premium Monthly fee paid by or on behalf of individuals who are entitled to voluntary enrollment in the Medicare health insurance program.

Part B hospital insurance coverage Generally Medicare Part B is for medical insurance. However, Part B hospital insurance coverage applies under the following circumstances: (1) when a beneficiary receives inpatient hospital services and these cannot be reimbursed under Part A because the benefits are exhausted either before or after admission and before the stay reaches outlier status; (2) the outlier days are not covered or the waiver of liability payment is not made; (3) a noncovered level of care is received; or (4) the patient is not entitled to Part A or elects not to use lifetime reserve days. See *Medicare Part B*.

Part C Medicare Plus (+) Choice Program See *Medicare Part C*.

Part D Medicare Prescription Drug Program See *Medicare Part D Prescription Drug plan*.

part-time work In workers' compensation cases, employment of fewer than 30 hours per week for one employer.

partial capitation Managed care capitation contract that concerns a capitated payment plus a payment for the actual cost of providing care and medical services to enrollees. This combination of capitation and fee-for-service reimbursement is sometimes a method for developing toward the total capitation of providers in a medical group or market area.

partial disability 1. Disability from an illness (congenital or acquired) or injury that prevents an insured person from performing one or more of the functions of his or her regular job. Loss of function may be expressed as a percentage. 2. Individual who has permanently lost a specific percentage of earning capacity.

partial disability benefit Dollar amount stated in a disability income insurance policy that is paid when the insured has a partial disability (prevented from doing one or more of his or her daily job duties). See *residual disability benefit*.

partial hospitalization Structured therapeutic program that is less than 24-hour care (usually during the day) in a hospital facility or other institution (mental or substance abuse facility, rehabilitation hospital, intermediate care facility) for patients moving from full-time inpatient care to outpatient care. Cardiac and chronic pain patients could also use this service.

partial hospitalization psychiatric facility Program in which a patient attends for several hours during the day (e.g., 8:30 AM to 3:30 PM). The patient is not there on a 24-hour basis. When completing the CMS-1500 for billing this type of case, the place of service code 52 is inserted in Block 24B of the paper claim form.

partial payment Incomplete reimbursement by a third-party payer to the provider or patient for medical services listed on a patient's insurance claim.

partial plan termination Process of ending a pension or employee-benefit plan for a group of participants but not for another group. Sometimes this is done so that sponsors can reclaim some of the assets of an overfunded plan.

partial procedure Procedure that is a part of a larger surgical procedure and needs a separate code (e.g., partial cystectomy vs. complete cystectomy). See *separate procedure* to learn the difference between partial and separate procedure. See also *complete procedure* to learn the difference between partial versus complete.

partial surrender See *withdrawal provision*.

partially capitated Stipulated dollar amount established for certain health care services while other services are reimbursed on a cost or fee-for-service basis.

partially self-funded See *self-insurance*.

participant See *beneficiary*.

participating dentist State-licensed dentist who has signed a contract with an insurance plan to give dental services to the plan's members.

participating hospitals 1. State-licensed hospital that has signed a contract with an insurance plan to provide hospital services to the plan's members. 2. Inpatient facilities that participate in the Medicare program.

participating insurance Type of insurance provision in which the insured is entitled to receive policy dividends that reflect the difference between the premium charged and actual costs. Premiums are calculated to give some margin over the expected cost of the insurance protection. Also called *participating policy*.

participating pharmacy Pharmacy that has signed a contract with an insurance plan to give medical services to the plan's members.

participating physician 1. A physician who contracts with an HMO or other insurance company to provide services to the plan's members. 2. A physician who has agreed to accept a plan's payments for services to subscribers (e.g., some Blue plans). Eighty percent of practicing American physicians are participating physicians. 3. Doctor or supplier who agrees to accept assignment on all Medicare claims. These physicians or suppliers may bill the patient only for the Medicare deductible and coinsurance amounts. Also called *affiliated health care provider, participating provider, in-network provider, network provider*.

participating physician (par) agreement 1. Physician agrees to accept payment from Medicare (80% of the approved charges) plus payment from the patient (20% of approved charges) after the deductible ($131 in 2007) has been met. 2. Under the (TRICARE) program, the provider agrees to accept an assignment, agrees to accept the TRICARE-determined allowable charge as payment in full, and transmits claims to the regional contractor directly.

participating policy Annuity or life insurance policy in which dividends are paid to the policyholder. Also called a *par policy*. Also see *participating insurance*.

participating provider (par) Physician, health care facility, or medical supplier that has a contractual agreement with an insurance plan to render care to eligible beneficiaries and bills the insurance carrier directly. Also called *participating physician, in-network provider, network provider* and *affiliated health care provider*. Also see *participating physician, participating hospitals, participating dentist,* and *participating pharmacy*.

participating provider panel Association of physicians and/or medical facilities or suppliers that are a single entity and enter into an agreement to provide specific services to all of a managed care plan's members.

participating provider's fee See *base charge*.

participation 1. Total number of insured individuals covered under a group insurance plan versus the total number of individuals who are eligible to have coverage. This is expressed in a percent. 2. A physician participates in an insurance plan when agreeing to accept assignment for all services he or she will give to members of the plan. Also see *participating provider (par)* and *participation program*.

participation limit See *relation of earnings to insurance clause*.

participation program Medicare program in which a physician voluntarily enters into an agreement to accept assignment for all services provided to Medicare patients.

partnership Group of two or more providers who set up and share in the investment risk and profits of the medical practice.

partnership entity plan Buy-sell insurance agreement that provides on the death of a business partner that the partnership will purchase the share of the deceased partner and the deceased partner's estate will sell its share to the partnership. Premiums are paid by the partnership out of income and any cash value of the insurance.

Partnership for Prescription Assistance (PPA) Assistance programs used to fill gaps in Medicare Part D that are offered by pharmaceutical companies to help patients who are struggling to pay for their medications. Also referred to as *patient assistance programs (PAPs)*.

partnership life and health insurance Business insurance that provides funds so that the partners in a business may purchase the business interest of a disabled partner or one who has died. Also see *business-continuation insurance*.

partnership program A program that lets TRICARE-eligible individuals receive inpatient or outpatient treatment from civilian providers of care in a military hospital or from uniformed service providers of care in civilian facilities.

PAS norms See *professional activity study (PAS)*.

pass through See *first pass*.

password Combination of letters and/or numbers selected by individuals, reported to management, and assigned to access computer data and for security measures.

past, family, and social history (PFSH) Review and documentation of the patient's past history, family history, and social history for the patient's health record. When billing an evaluation and management service there must be documented review of two, or for comprehensive assessment all three areas (past, family, and/or social history) are required.

past history (PH) Patient's past experiences with allergies, illnesses, hospitalizations, operations, injuries, and treatments.

past service benefit Pension plan credit given for an employee's past service before the establishment of the plan.

past service cost Total value (single sum) of the past service benefits plan beginning with the effective date of the plan.

PATH See *physicians at teaching hospitals (PATH)*.

pathologist Physician specializing in the study of disease (i.e., autopsies, clinical pathology, surgical pathology, or research).

pathology Study of the characteristics, causes, and effects of disease, as observed in the structure and function of the body. Also see *clinical pathology*.

pathology and laboratory section Division of the CPT code book that contains information about pathology and laboratory tests.

patient (pt) Person under treatment or care by a physician or surgeon or in a hospital.

patient account ledger See *account, financial accounting statement, ledger,* or *ledger card*.

patient account number Number with or without an alpha given to each patient's health and financial records for internal identification by the provider of health care. See also *patient's account number*.

patient account representative See *insurance counselor*.

patient accounting system Software program for posting charges for medical services rendered to patients, sending bills, tracking amounts owed, and compiling accounts to show outstanding bills.

patient acuity Measurement of the intensity of care needed for a patient that is based on six categories from minimal care (I) to intensive care (VI).

patient advocate 1. Hospital employee whose job is to speak on a patient's behalf and help patients get any information or services they need. 2. Individual who assists patients with understanding the changes being made by the facility to protect their confidential information.

patient control number Alphabetic and/or numeric identifier that is used in an internal medical office system or hospital facility to quickly locate a patient's financial account and medical records.

patient discharge status Field 17 of the Uniform Bill (UB-04) inpatient hospital billing claim form. A two-digit code in this field indicates the patient's disposition at the ending date of medical service for the period of care reported on the claim in Field 6. Also see *patient status* and *patient status code*.

patient discount Discount (5% to 20%) offered to self-pay patients if they pay the entire fee, in cash, at the time of service. For Medicare patients, the fee must not be lower than the Medicare fee schedule for the service. Also see *discount*.

patient eligibility Process of contacting the insurer or managed care plan to verify the patient's medical services will be covered by the insurance plan, the policy information is accurate, and the policy has not expired. Additional information may be necessary to discover the primary payer for the claim.

patient financial responsibility Portion of the medical bill that the patient is legally responsible for paying.

PATIENT FRIENDLY BILLING® Project Collaborative endeavor spearheaded by the Healthcare Financial Management Association (HFMA), with support from the American Hospital Association, the Medical Group Management Association, providers, and other interested parties to promote clear, concise, correct, patient-friendly financial communications.

patient information coordinator Gives service to patients on how to create and maintain accuracy and protect privacy of their personal health records via e-health websites.

patient liability Patient's legally obligated payment when medical services are received from a hospital, physician, or other provider.

patient lift Equipment used by a caregiver to move a patient from a bed or wheelchair using the patient's strength or a motor.

patient mix Numbers and types of patients who receive medical services at a specific hospital or health care program (e.g., classifications by homes, socioeconomic factors, diagnoses, or severity of illnesses).

patient origin study Hospital or health plan study to find out the geographical distribution of patients under various health programs. Such studies determine the effectiveness of programs or help when developing new health care services.

patient panel Members (patients) of a managed care plan who are assigned to a provider.

patient registration form Questionnaire designed to collect demographic data and essential facts about medical insurance coverage for each patient seen for professional services; also called *patient information form*.

patient safety Protection of health care recipients from being harmed or receiving damage from medical services.

patient service representative See *insurance counselor*.

patient service slip See *multipurpose billing form*.

patient services Medical and related health care, provided by a physician or health care facility, that is covered by an insurance policy or program.

patient status Patient's situation at the time of discharge or transfer when leaving an acute care hospital as an inpatient or outpatient. Also see *patient status code* and *patient discharge status*.

patient status code Two-digit number indicating the patient's disposition as of the ending date of service for the period of care reported on the claim being submitted (e.g., routine discharge, discharged to another facility, still a patient, expired). Patient status codes are inserted in Field 17 of the Uniform Bill (UB-04) inpatient hospital billing claim form. This information is also required for outpatient claims for Medicare billing purposes. Also see *patient status* and *patient discharge status*.

P

patient's account number Number with or without an alpha that is assigned to each patient's health and financial records for internal identification by the provider of health care. This identification number is inserted in Block 26 of the CMS-1500 claim form.

patient's bill of rights Document that lists the rights of patients to assure health care quality and protect consumers and workers in the health care system. Such documents have been created by a number of professional associations (e.g., American Cancer Society, American Hospital Association, Centers for Medicare and Medicaid Services).

pattern analysis Clinical and statistical analysis of data sets. Frequently used end-stage renal dialysis (ESRD) data sets include the Program Management and Medical Information System (PMMIS), United States Renal Data System (USRDS), the core indicators, network files, and Centers for Medicare and Medicaid Services analytical files.

pay-as-you-go financing Funding plan in which taxes are scheduled to produce as much income as required to pay current benefits, with trust fund assets built up only to the extent needed to prevent exhaustion of the fund by random fluctuations.

pay-as-you-go funding Payment that postpones the cost of coverage for a retired employee until after the person is actually retired.

pay-for-performance (P4P) Name of a Medicare reimbursement model.

pay-as-you-go plan See *current disbursement.*

payable Unpaid, but not necessarily overdue, financial account or bill.

payee 1. Individual to whom benefits are payable under a supplementary insurance contract. 2. Individual named on a draft or check as the receiver of the amount shown; also known as *bearer.*

payee number In workers' compensation cases, an identification number that is given to each medical provider that submits bills for services provided to the injured or ill worker.

payer 1. Organization or entity that pays for the patient's health care services and medical treatments (e.g., self-insured employer, managed care plan, federal government, commercial insurance company). Sometimes called *payer, indirect payer, insurance company,* or *insurer.* 2. Individual responsible for payment of the amount as shown on the face of a check.

payer ID See *NPLANID.*

PAYERID number Acronym that translates as payer identification number. The current acronym is NPLANID (national plan identifier). Medicare patients that have a Medigap supplemental insurance plan must show the PAYERID number (often called the *OCNA [Other Carrier Name and Address] key*) in Block 9d of the CMS-1500 insurance claim form. The Medicare fiscal intermediary transmits a Medigap claim electronically to the Medigap carrier after processing it for participating physicians. This is called a *crossover claim.* See *NPLANID.*

payer identification (PAYERID) number See *PAYERID number.*

payment (pmt) 1. Costs incurred for processing of data. 2. See *reimbursement.* 3. In Medicare fraud, deliberately applying for duplicate payment (e.g., to bill both Medicare and the beneficiary for the same service or to bill both Medicare and another insurance company to attempt to get paid twice). 4. Under the Health Insurance Portability and Accountability Act (HIPAA), use and disclosure of protected health information (PHI) is permissible for treatment, payment, and health care operations (TPO).

payment at time of service (PTOS) Collecting the amount or balance due directly from the patient at the conclusion of the patient's office visit.

payment error prevention program (PEPP) Program to assist in the reduction of Medicare prospective payment system (PPS) inpatient hospital reimbursement mistakes.

payment floor Minimum number of days that must pass before a Medicare administrative contractor can pay an insurance claim. Payment for manual claims is within 4 to 12 weeks and as little as 7 days when transmitted electronically. Prompt payment guidelines for clean claims transmitted by participating providers may be paid faster than for those submitted by non-participating providers.

payment in full Under Medicare guidelines, the amount that the provider must accept because of a contract or amount the provider voluntarily accepts as reimbursement in full from the insurer, meaning the patient's obligation has been met.

payment locality One of the many geographical pricing areas used by Medicare administrative contractors (MACs) to calculate physicians' customary and prevailing charges for payment. Localities are the basis for fee schedule payment areas and geographic adjustment factor (GAF) adjustments under the Medicare fee schedule (MFS).

payment mode System wherein the insured pays insurance premiums either monthly, quarterly, semiannually, or annually.

payment rate 1. Dollar amount to be paid to a provider for medical services given to a member of a managed care plan. 2. Total payment that a hospital or community mental health center gets when it provides outpatient services to Medicare patients. Also see *average payment rate (APR).*

payment safeguards Activities to prevent and recover inappropriate Medicare benefit payments including Medicare Secondary Payer (MSP), medical review/utilization review (MR/UR), provider audits, and fraud and abuse detection.

payment suspension See *suspension of payments.*

payment voucher See *check voucher.*

payor See *payer.*

payroll deduction plan Payment system in which an insurance premium is deducted by the employer from the employee's earnings and sent to the insurance company.

payroll taxes Taxes deducted from gross wages and salaries such as those for Social Security (Federal Insurance Contributions Act [FICA]) and unemployment insurance. Also called *contributions* and *taxes.*

PBGC See *Pension Benefit Guaranty Corporation (PBGC).*

PBM See *prescription benefit manager (PBM)* or *pharmacy benefit manager (PBM).*

PC See *professional component (PC).*

P/C Abbreviation that means property/casualty, such as independent property/casualty (P/C) brokers.

PCCM Abbreviation that means primary care case management. See *primary case management (PCM).*

PCCM provider See *primary care case management (PCCM) provider.*

PCM See *primary care manager (PCM)* and *primary case management (PCM).*

PCN See *primary care network (PCN).*

PCP Abbreviation for primary care provider, primary care physician, or primary care practitioner (PCP). See *primary care physician (PCP).*

PCPM Abbreviation that means per contract per month. See *per member per month (PMPM).*

PCS Abbreviation that means prescription medication coverage (PCS), personal communication system (PCS), and physician coding specialist (PCS).

PD See *peritoneal dialysis (PD).*

PDA See *personal digital assistant (PDA).*

PDP See *prescription drug plan (PDP).*

PDR See *Physicians' Desk Reference (PDR).*

PDX See *principal diagnosis (PDX).*

PE See *practice expense (PE)* and *physician extender (PE).*

peak Time of a business day in which wireless customers can expect to pay full-service rates.

PEC See *preexisting condition (PEC).*

pediatric oncology Study, diagnosis, and treatment of diseases and disorders of the blood and cancer in infants and children.

pediatric patient Individual who presents for medical services younger than 14 years of age.

pediatrician Physician specializing in the study, diagnosis, and treatment of disease and disorders of infants and children.

pediatrics Pertaining to preventive and primary health care and treatment of children and the study of childhood diseases.

peer review Review of a patient's case by one or more physicians using federal guidelines to evaluate another physician in regard to the quality and efficiency of medical care. This is done to discover overutilization or misutilization of a plan's benefits.

peer review committee See *peer review group.*

peer review group Several local physicians who come together to solve insurance claim disputes and support ethical medical practices in the community. Sometimes referred to as a *peer review committee.*

peer review organization (PRO) See *Quality Improvement Organization (QIO) program.*

pelvic examination Diagnostic procedure performed by a physician in which the external and internal genitalia are physically examined by inspection, palpation, percussion, and auscultation.

PEN See *parenteral nutrition (PEN).*

penalize To inflict a burden or penalty on an individual.

penalized claim Insurance claim submitted to an insurance carrier that did not pass the claim edits and a penalty was applied, thus reducing payment. Also see *downcoding.*

penalty 1. Punishment established by law. 2. Under Medicare, the amount added to the patient's monthly premium for Medicare Part B or for a Medicare drug plan if the individual does not join when first able. For Medicare Part D, this higher amount is deducted as long as the patient has Medicare.

pending claim Insurance claim held in suspense due to review or other reason. These claims may be cleared for payment or denied. See *delinquent claim.*

penetration rate Percentage rate at which eligible employees in a group select a system to provide their health coverage.

pension Funds payable monthly or annually to an individual who has retired.

Pension Benefit Guaranty Corporation (PBGC) Federal organization that was created by the Employee Retirement Income Security Act of 1974 (ERISA) to manage the Pension Plan Termination Insurance program. It insures benefits in qualified defined benefit pension plans (DBPP) and makes sure participants receive the benefits.

pension fund See *pension plan.*

pension plan Retirement program created to provide an individual with a monthly income payment for the remainder of his or her life.

Pension Reform Act See *Employee Retirement Income Security Act (ERISA).*

pension trust fund Fund that consists of money contributed by the employer and, in some cases, the employees to provide retirement benefits. Contributions are paid to a trustee who invests the money, collects the interest, and disburses the benefits under the terms of the trust agreement. Pension trusts can be either self-administered or partially insured with benefits purchased from an insurance company by the trustee. Also called *trust fund plan.*

people's court See *small claims court.*

PEPM Abbreviation that means per employee per month.

PEPP See *payment error prevention program (PEPP).*

PEPPER See *Program for Evaluating Payment Patterns Electronic Report (PEPPER).*

per capita See *capitation.*

per case payment System of reimbursement to providers in which payment is made by the type of case without regard to medical services given.

per-cause deductible Dollar amount that the insured must pay for each accident or illness before major medical benefits begin payment. Also called *per-disability deductible.*

per-cause maximum Greatest amount that a medical expense insurance policy will pay for medical benefits from any illness or injury.

per contract per month (PCPM) See *per member per month (PMPM).*

per-disability deductible See *per-cause deductible.*

per diem Single charge for a day in the hospital regardless of any actual charges or costs incurred. In some managed care plans, per diems can be created by type of care given (e.g., one per diem rate for general medical/surgical and a different rate for intensive care).

per diem cost Daily charge for hospital care that includes services and supplies given to the patient and excluding professional fees of nonstaff physicians.

per diem payment See *per diem reimbursement.*

per diem rate 1. Cost per day derived by dividing total costs by the number of inpatient days of care given. Per diem costs are an average and do not reflect the true cost for each patient. 2. Phrase used in managed care plan contracts that refers to reimbursement made to the hospital from which a patient is transferred for each day of stay. The formula for determining the per diem rate is to divide the full diagnosis-related group (DRG) payment by the geometric mean length of stay (GMLOS) for the DRG. The payment rate for the first day of stay is twice the per diem rate, and subsequent days are paid at the per diem rate up to the full DRG amount. 3. In a managed care plan, contracted amount paid for an inpatient that is calculated per day per type of stay.

per diem reimbursement Single charge for a day in the hospital regardless of actual charges or costs incurred (e.g., a plan that pays $800 for each day regardless of the actual cost of service). Some insurance plans may have separate categories of per diem (e.g., intensive care unit, medical, and surgical, each with a different reimbursement rate). Also called *per diem payment.*

per member per month (PMPM) Cost for each insurance plan's enrolled member for each month (each effective member for each month the member was effective). This is calculated by taking the number of units divided by member months. A variation is called *per contract per month (PCPM).*

per member per year (PMPY) Cost for each insurance plan's enrolled member for the year. Also see *per member per month (PMPM).*

per stirpes Distribution of a deceased member's share of the life insurance proceeds to the beneficiary's children.

per thousand members per year (PTMPY) Employed to report utilization for health plan members (e.g., hospital utilization shown in days PTMPY).

per visit fee Phrase used in managed care plan contracts that refers to the flat-rate payment made to a provider for one patient encounter.

percent of premium Fixed dollar amount that is calculated as a percentage of the average monthly premium paid by each member of a managed care plan. It is paid to the provider each month instead of another payment method. This phrase is used in managed care plan contracts and is one of two methods used to compute a capitation payment.

percentage contribution Amount of premium that a member pays in a contributory group insurance plan. Also called *employee contribution* or *member contribution.*

percentage of accrued charges Payment method that calculates reimbursement based on a percentage of total approved charges accrued during a hospital stay and submitted to the insurance plan.

percentage of revenue Fixed percentage of the collected premium rate that is paid to the hospital to cover services.

percentage participation See *coinsurance.*

percentile Number that corresponds to one of the equal divisions of the range of a variable in a given sample and that characterizes a value of the variable as not exceeded by a specified percentage of all the values in the sample (e.g., a score higher than 97 percent of those attained is said to be in the 97th percentile).

percutaneous skeletal fixation Treatment of a fracture in which the site is neither open nor closed. The fracture is not visualized, so fixation is placed across the fracture site using x-ray. Also called *percutaneous treatment.*

percutaneous treatment See *percutaneous skeletal fixation.*

performance The act of executing, accomplishing, or carrying out an important function or process by an individual, group, or organization.

performance assessment Analysis and interpretation of performance measurement data to transform it into useful information for purposes of continuous improvement.

performance goals See *performance standards.*

performance improvement program See *quality management (QM).*

performance improvement projects Schemes or plans that examine and seek to achieve enhancement in major areas of clinical and nonclinical services. These plans are usually based on utilization, diagnosis, and outcome information; data from surveys; and grievance and appeals processes. They measure performance at two periods of time to find out if improvement has occurred. These projects are required by the state and can be of the managed care organizations'/prepaid health plans' (MCOs'/PHPs') choosing or prescribed by the state.

performance management program See *quality management (QM).*

performance measure 1. Gauge used to assess the carrying out or execution of a process or function of any organization. 2. Quantitative or qualitative measure of the care and services delivered to enrollees (process) or the end result of that care and services (outcomes). Performance measures can be used to assess other aspects of an individual's or organization's performance such as access and availability of care, utilization of care, health plan stability, beneficiary characteristics, and other structural and operational aspects of health care services. Performance measures may include measures calculated by the state from encounter data or another data source, or measures submitted by the managed care organization or prepaid health plan. 3. Information that reveals how well a health plan provides a certain treatment, test, or other health care service to its members. For example, Medicare uses performance measures from National Committee for Quality Assurance's (NCQA's) Health Employer Data and Information Set (HEDIS) to get information on how well health plans perform in quality, how easy it is to get care, and members' satisfaction with the health plan and its doctors.

performance standards Quality of care goals that a medical provider is expected to meet such as office hours per week, office visits per month, on-call days, percentage of accounts receivable collected, and surgeries performed per year. Also called *performance goals.*

performing physician Provider who renders a service to a patient; also known as *treating physician.*

peril Certain specified risks covered by an insurance policy (e.g., fire, flood, hurricane, theft, windstorm).

perinatal period Interval from the 28th week of gestation to the 28th day after birth.

perinatal death Wide-ranging phrase that means both stillborn infants and neonatal deaths.

period certain 1. In an annuity, specific time during which the insurance company unconditionally guarantees benefit payments to continue. 2. In an insurance settlement, time period that the insurer assures payments of benefits.

periodic interim payment (PIP) 1. Phrase used in managed care plan contracts that refers to a reimbursement method that prepays providers for services based on their history of utilization by members. It is a much faster form of reimbursement than other arrangements. 2. Under the Medicare program, cost-based reimbursement method for hospitals before 1983 and the introduction of the prospective payment system (PPS).

period of disability Beginning and ending time when an insured is not able to perform regular job duties

or cannot perform normal activities of a healthy individual of the same age or sex.

periodic review of relative values Recalibration of Medicare's relative value scale for financial updating purposes. The Centers for Medicare and Medicaid Services (CMS) must conduct a periodic review every 5 years.

periods of care Set period of time that the patient can get hospice care after the physician says that the patient is eligible and still needs hospice care.

peritoneal dialysis (PD) Procedure that introduces dialysate into the abdominal cavity to remove waste products through the peritoneum (a membrane that surrounds the intestines and other organs in the abdominal cavity). It functions in a manner similar to that of the artificial semipermeable membrane in the hemodialysis machine. Three forms of peritoneal dialysis are continuous ambulatory peritoneal dialysis, continuous cycling peritoneal dialysis, and intermittent peritoneal dialysis. This treatment can be done at home, at work, or at another convenient location.

permanent and stationary (P & S) Phrase used when a workers' compensation patient has been on temporary disability and his or her condition has become stabilized within a reasonable period of time and no improvement is expected. It is only after this declaration that a case can be rated for a compromise and release. Also see *maximum medical improvement.*

permanent disability (PD) In workers' compensation cases, illness or injury (impairment of the normal use of a body part) expected to continue for the lifetime of the injured worker that prevents the person from performing the functions of his or her occupation, therefore, impairing his or her earning capacity. Permanent disability may be partial or total.

permanent disability compensation In workers' compensation cases, indemnity payments to compensate an injured worker for impairment from an industrial injury or illness that lessens the worker's ability to compete in the open labor market. It is not intended to replace wages or to compensate for pain and suffering.

permanent disability rating In workers' compensation cases, determination of the percentage of total disability of the injured worker. Considerations are the nature of the injury, occupation and age of the worker at the time of injury, and diminished ability to compete in the open labor market. The disability, not the pathological condition, is rated; thus a disease is not rated, but its permanent effect on the employee's working capability is.

permanent impairment In workers' compensation, a disability that has become stable during a time period that allows optimal tissue repair but is not likely to change regardless of further therapy or surgery.

P

permanent insurance Life insurance policy that is valid for the entire life of the insured.

permanent life insurance Any form of life insurance except term insurance (i.e., whole life or endowment).

permanent partial disability (PPD) 1. In workers' compensation cases, permanent disability with a rating of less than 100% permanent disability. 2. Disability that interferes with the injured worker's capability to compete in the open labor market in less than a total manner.

permanent total disability 1. Condition that prevents an insured from working because of injury or illness and presumably will last for a lifetime. 2. In workers' compensation cases, permanent disability with a rating of 100% permanent disability only.

persistency 1. Percentage of insurance policies that remain in force. 2. Percentage of insurance policies that have not lapsed. 3. Retention of business occurring when an insurance policy remains in force because of continued payment of the policy's premiums.

persistency fee Dollar amount paid above standard insurance commissions as long as a policy remains in force.

personal article floater Insurance policy or an addition to a policy that provides coverage for personal valuables (computer, furs, jewelry).

personal bond Insurance that provides coverage for those who handle large sums of money during business transactions.

personal care Nonskilled, personal services such as help with activities of daily living (bathing, dressing, eating, getting in and out of bed or chair, moving around, using the bathroom). It may also include care that most people do themselves such as inserting eye drops. The Medicare home health benefit does pay for some personal care services. In the Medicaid program, this is an optional benefit and varies state by state. Also see *custodial care.*

personal care aides See *home health aide.*

personal charges Hospital fees of a nonmedical nature such as telephone and television.

personal communication system (PCS) Electronic device that is capable of voice messaging, text messaging, Internet access, and data retrieval.

personal digital assistant (PDA) Palm-size or hand-held computer used for keeping a calendar, maintaining an address book, transmitting electronic mail (e-mail), word processing, and spreadsheet functions. In health care settings, this equipment is used for prescription writing, digital voice dictation or recognition for note taking, and access to patients' database.

personal health record (PHR) Lifelong resource of health data maintained and owned by the individual, which may be used for collecting, tracking, and sharing important, up-to-date information. Individuals may need it to make better health care decisions and improve quality of care. A PHR may be paper based, electronically based, or web based. An electronically based PHR must conform to nationally recognized interoperability standards.

personal health statement Health questionnaire filled in by an insurance applicant to obtain group insurance coverage; used as proof of insurability.

personal injury liability Insurance policy that protects the physician or his or her employees against claims of tangible personal physical injury suffered by others, as well as intangibles such as libel and slander.

personal injury protection (PIP) See *no-fault insurance.*

personal insurance Insurance plan issued to an individual (and/or his or her dependents). Also known as *individual contract, individual health insurance,* and *individual health plan.*

personal life insurance trust Trust agreement in which proceeds of the insured's life insurance policy go into a trust and the trustee is named as beneficiary of the policy. When the insured dies, the proceeds are paid to the trustee, who manages and disburses the funds according to the terms of the agreement.

personal lines Insurance products that are created for and purchased by individuals versus business or commercial lines.

personal physician In workers' compensation, a doctor of medicine or a doctor of osteopathy who, before a work injury, has directed medical treatment to an employee and keeps the employee's medical records and medical history. This can be a corporation, partnership, or association of physicians.

personal producing general agent (PPGA) Person appointed by the insurance company to act as an independent contractor, similar to a broker. A PPGA may be under contract to several insurance companies receiving a commission to sell insurance and overriding commissions on products sold by other agents.

personal protective equipment (PPE) Special clothing or equipment worn by an employee for protection against a hazard. Generally, uniforms are not considered personal protective equipment unless they function as protection against a hazardous condition at work.

personal qualifications Skill, education, and experience that makes an individual suited for a specific job or task.

personal selling distribution system Insurance system that employs commissioned or salaried sales agents to sell products by oral presentations to consumers.

personal supervision Direction and management of a medical procedure given by the physician and the doctor must be present during the procedure. Some medical procedures require personal supervision to bill for a specific level of service. This level of supervision is required when billing "incident-to" services outside the office setting. Also see *direct supervision* and *general supervision.*

person served In the Medicare program, enrollee to whom Medicare pays benefits for covered medical services if there are expenses beyond the deductible amount.

pertinent past, family, social history (PFSH) Review and documentation of the patient's past history, family history, and social history that are related to the history of present illness (HPI). When billing evaluation and management services for a new patient, at least one item must be documented from any of the three PFSH history areas directly related to the problem identified in the HPI.

pertinent PFSH See *pertinent past, family, social history (PFSH).*

petition 1. Formal written request commonly used to indicate an appeal. 2. Any request for relief, other than an application.

PFC See *potential fraud case (PFC).*

PFSH See *past, family, and social history (PFSH).*

phantom billing Billing for services not performed.

pharmaceutical care Practice in which the pharmaceutical care practitioner takes responsibility for all of a patient's drug-related needs and is held accountable for this commitment. It is care that a patient requires and receives, which ensures safe and rational drug usage.

pharmaceutical care practitioner Individual who renders beneficial drug therapy management services and creates a covenantal bond or therapeutic relationship between the patient and pharmacist.

pharmacoeconomics Study of cost effectiveness of drugs on patient care.

pharmacy 1. Study of preparing and dispensing drugs. 2. Place for preparing and dispensing drugs.

pharmacy and therapeutics committee (P & T) Panel of multispecialty physicians who advise the managed care plan on safe and effective prescription drugs and develop and maintain a drug formulary.

pharmacy benefit management organization See *pharmacy benefit manager (PBM).*

pharmacy benefit manager (PBM) Company under contract with managed care organizations, self-insured companies, and government programs to manage pharmacy network management, drug utilization review, outcomes management, and disease management. The goal is to save money. For example, a pharmacy benefit manager may fill drug prescriptions by mail order as part of a corporate health insurance plan. Also called a *pharmacy benefit management organization* or *prescription benefit manager (PBM).*

pharmacy claim Formal request for payment (bill) generated because of an insured's purchase of prescription drugs dispensed by a pharmacist from a physician's written instructions (prescription form).

pharmacy network See *pharmacy services administrative organization (PSAO).*

pharmacy services administrative organization (PSAO) Preferred provider organization (PPO) of community pharmacies that contracts either with employers or pharmacy benefit managers to give pharmacy services to members of the plan. Also known as *pharmacy network.*

PHARMD Abbreviation for Doctor of Pharmacy.

PhD Abbreviation for Doctor of Philosophy.

PHI See *protected health information (PHI).*

phishing Practice of masquerading as a legitimate company to con consumers into willingly giving up their personal information such as an e-mail stating that information must be resubmitted because records were lost or an account needs to be verified.

PHO Abbreviation for physician hospital organization. See *medical staff-hospital organization* and *physician hospital organization (PHO).*

PHP See *prepaid health plan (PHP).*

PHR See *personal health record (PHR).*

physical address 1. Actual street name and number, city, state, and zip code of where a patient lives and not a post office box number. 2. Actual location of a building and not a post office box number.

physical capacity evaluation See *functional capacity evaluation (FCE).*

physical examination (PE or PX) Objective inspection and/or testing of organ systems or body areas of a patient by a physician to obtain a diagnosis or, if necessary, referral to a specialist.

physical examination provision Clause in an insurance policy that gives the insurer the right to have the insured examined by a physician of the insurer's choice and paid by the insurer.

physical status modifier In CPT coding, a two-character alphanumeric add-on code placed after the usual anesthesia procedure code number to indicate the physical condition of the patient's health at the time of anesthesia delivery (e.g., normal, healthy patient; mild or severe systemic disease).

physical therapist (PT) Individual who is state licensed to practice in the examination, evaluation, and treatment of physical impairments through the use of special exercise, application of heat or cold, and other physical modalities.

physical therapy (PT) Treatment of injury and disease by mechanical means such as use of heat, light, exercise, and massage.

physical therapy modality Method of application of, or the employment of, a therapeutic agent or regimen to give treatment to assist in rehabilitating or restoring function to the body after an illness or injury.

physical therapy services Treatments for injuries and diseases consisting of cold, shortwave and microwave diathermy and ultrasonic heat, hydrotherapy, electric

P

stimulation, light, exercise, and massage to restore function to the body. Services also include evaluation and program planning.

physically clean claim Insurance claims with no staples or highlighted areas. The bar code area has not been deformed.

physician 1. Doctor of Medicine (MD) or Doctor of Osteopathy (DO) who, through education, training, and internship is licensed under state law to practice medicine and may diagnose and render treatment to individuals. 2. In workers' compensation cases, providers of care include state-licensed medical doctors, psychologists, optometrists, dentists, podiatrists, chiropractors, and acupuncturists.

physician advisor (PA) 1. In a medical center facility, doctor that is asked to do final decision-making in complicated or difficult cases by evaluating appropriateness of admission, judging efficiency of services for level of care and place of service, and in seeking appropriate care alternatives for selected patients. Additionally, a PA can act as a negotiator and educator with practicing physicians and as liaison between the utilization management company and the provider community in understanding and shaping more efficient and cost-effective medical practice. 2. Individual hired to improve the revenue cycle. Also called *business consultant*. 3. Individual who assists patients in selecting medical insurance and in choosing a physician.

physician agreement Legal contract between an insurance company or managed care plan and a physician (participating physician) to give medical services to the plan's members.

physician assistant (PA) Health care professional academically, clinically prepared, and licensed to practice medicine with supervision and guidance of a licensed doctor of medicine or osteopathy. Depending on state laws, PAs perform the following: take medical histories, diagnose and treat conditions, order and interpret laboratory tests, perform physical examinations, assist in surgery, counsel patients, and prescribe, administer, and dispense medications. Training programs average 25 to 27 months. National certification is available to graduates of approved training programs, a master's-degree level in most states. Also referred to as a *physician extender (PE)*.

physician associate (PA) group Partnership, association, or corporation composed of two or more physicians and/or nonphysician practitioners who wish to bill Medicare as a unit.

physician attestation Signed and dated verification by the attending physician of the accuracy, completeness, and description of the patient's principal and secondary diagnoses and procedures in a Medicare case. This document must be present in the patient's medical record for each Medicare inpatient admission. It is necessary for diagnosis-related groups (DRG) assignment.

Physician Coding Specialist (PCS) One type of certification earned by meeting the requirements of the American College of Medical Coding Specialists (ACMCS).

physician credentialing 1. Process of verifying a physician's medical education, training, and licenses so that a physician can be approved to practice in a hospital. 2. Process delegated by the board to the medical staff of medical staff appointment, reappointment, and delineation of clinical privileges. 3. From a health maintenance organization view, to credential physicians to ensure they have the right training and licensing and maintain information on their specialties.

physician-directed clinic Facility for diagnosis and treatment of outpatients where (1) a physician gives medical services at all times, (2) each patient is assigned to receive care from a clinic doctor, and (3) nonphysician services are under medical supervision.

physician extender (PE) Health care employee trained to provide medical care under the direct or indirect supervision of a physician (e.g., certified registered nurse practitioner, certified nurse midwife, physician assistant, occupational therapist, clinical psychologist, clinical social worker, clinical nurse specialist, physical therapist, certified registered nurse anesthetist). PEs might also include auxiliary personnel such as registered nurses, licensed practical nurses, technicians, medical assistants, and any other individual acting under a physician's supervision. Some states specify certain supervision requirements such as physician telephone or on-site access, chart review/sign-off, and conferencing. Further information via the Internet is available at the websites of the American Association of Physician Assistants and the American College of Nurse Practitioners. The Centers for Medicare and Medicaid Services (CMS) refers to PEs as *limited license practitioners (LLPs)*. Also referred to as *nonphysician practitioner (NPP), midlevel provider (MLP)*, or *midlevel practitioner (MLP)*.

physician group Partnership, association, corporation, individual practice association (IPA), or other group that distributes income from the practice among members. An IPA is considered to be a physician group only if it is composed of individual physicians and has no subcontracts with other physician groups.

physician hospital organization (PHO) Association between one or more hospitals and one or more physicians to assist in negotiation, contract development, administrative services, financial management services, and marketing of managed care plans for its members. The PHO may also undertake utilization review, credentialing, and quality assurance. Physicians have their own practices and continue their traditional business outside the PHO. Also called *medical staff-hospital organization*.

physician incentive plan (PIP) Any compensation arrangement at any contracting level between a managed care organization (MCO) and a physician or physician group that may directly or indirectly have the effect of reducing or limiting services furnished to Medicare or Medicaid enrollees in the MCO. MCOs must disclose physician incentive plans between groups or intermediate entities (e.g., certain individual practice associations [IPAs], physician-hospital organizations [PHOs]) and individual physicians and groups.

physician licensing board State organization responsible for issuing licenses, accreditation, or certification for a health care provider to practice. Also called *Board of Healing Arts, Board of Medical Examiners, Board of Medical Practice, Department of Business and Professional Regulation,* and *medical licensing board.*

physician management corporation (PMC) See *management services organization (MSO).*

physician organization (PO) Association of physicians who contract with managed care plans as an entity or represent the physician part in a physician hospital organization (PHO). Physician practice financials are linked to assist physicians in managing risk and capitation.

Physician Payment Review Commission (PPRC) See *Medicare Payment Advisory Commission (MedPAC or MedPac),* which replaced PPRC.

physician practice management company (PPMC) Business that is investor owned and purchases, partners, or manages physician practices and gives investment capital for development or expansion of a practice.

physician provider group (PPG) A physician-owned business that has the flexibility to deal with all forms of contract medicine and still offer its own packages to business groups, unions, and the general public.

physician profiling See *profiling.*

Physician Quality Reporting Initiative (PQRI) Voluntary program that provided a financial incentive to physicians and other eligible professionals who successfully reported quality information related to services provided under the Medicare Physician Fee Schedule between July 1 and December 31, 2007. It was established when President Bush signed the Tax Relief and Health Care Act of 2006 (TRHCA), Section 101 Title I.

physician services Medical services rendered by a physician to a patient. This may include surgery, consultation, home visit, office visit, hospital visits, and institutional visits. Physician services given while in the hospital that appear on the hospital bill are not included.

physician-sponsored health plan Type of managed care plan owned and controlled by large physician groups. These plans may offer enrollees a choice of programs with a financial incentive to use network physicians (e.g., exclusive provider organization [EPO], preferred provider organization [PPO], or point-of-service [POS] plan).

physician visits In-hospital, office, and home face-to-face visits by a physician. Most health plans provide insurance payment for visits when a patient is ill or has been injured.

physician work One of the three components used in the formula to develop relative value units (RVUs) for each medical service performed. This corresponds to the value of the physical skill, mental effort, judgment, and time required to perform a service. The other two components are practice expense and the cost of professional liability insurance. These three RVUs are then adjusted according to geographical area and used in a formula to determine the resource-based relative value scale (RBRVS) for the Medicare fees published annually in the *Federal Register.*

physicians at teaching hospitals (PATH) Initiative of the National Recovery Project via the Office of the Inspector General that established guidelines for payments for resident doctors that are employed at teaching facilities treating Medicare patients. Such services are performed under Medicare Part B but are paid for as part of Medicare Part A.

Physicians' Current Procedural Terminology (CPT) A reference procedural code book using a numerical system and description for procedures for reporting and billing medical services and procedures. It is established and owned by the American Medical Association.

Physicians' Desk Reference (PDR) Annual publication that lists prescription drugs and diagnostic products and is used by physicians as a reference tool.

physician's fee profile Compilation of each physician's charges for specific professional services and the payments made to the physician over a given period of time.

physician's profile Overall health condition of a patient as seen by the physician after a complete physical examination. Also see *physician's fee profile.*

physician's services In the Medicare program, medical care provided by an individual who has state licensure to practice medicine or osteopathy.

pigeonholing To use a brief list of diagnostic codes and use those codes for all patients whether or not the codes match their actual diagnoses.

PIM See *Medicare Program Integrity Manual (PIM).*

PIN Abbreviation for provider identification number (PIN). PINs are now referred to as *provider transaction access numbers (PTANs).* See *provider transaction access number (PTAN).*

ping-ponging Excessive referrals to other providers for unnecessary services. A physician or facility may use this technique to gain favor with colleagues.

PIP See *periodic interim payment (PIP), personal injury protection (PIP),* and *physician incentive plan (PIP).*

PIP-DCG model Principal inpatient diagnostic cost group model that was phased out in 2003 and replaced by the hierarchical condition categories (HCC) model. See *hierarchical condition categories (HCC) model.*

P

PL HCPCS Level II modifier that may be used with CPT or HCPCS Level II codes indicating progressive addition of lenses.

place of employment In workers' compensation, any place and adjacent premises where employment is carried out.

place of service (POS) Where a service is performed such as a hospital (inpatient or outpatient), doctor's office, or skilled nursing facility.

place of service (POS) code Two-digit standard codes used by providers to report the location where the medical service was provided (hospital, office, home). When the physician's office or an outpatient hospital is billing, the two-digit POS code is inserted in Block 24B of the CMS-1500 insurance claim form (e.g., 11 is doctor's office, 12 is patient's home).

plaintiff Individual who begins a civil legal action.

plan Referring to a managed care plan.

plan administration Department responsible for supervision of a managed care plan with job duties such as accounting, billing, legal services, marketing, personnel, purchasing, servicing of accounts, and underwriting.

plan administration functions Under the Health Insurance Portability and Accountability Act (HIPAA), management performed by the plan sponsor of a group health plan on behalf of the group health plan and excludes functions performed by the plan sponsor in connection with any other benefit or benefit plan of the plan sponsor.

plan age Amount of time, in years, that a managed care plan has operated.

plan area Region of a managed care plan's membership. Also may be referred to as *plan code*.

plan code See *plan area*.

plan document 1. Record that may be written in technical terms containing all provisions of the running of a managed care plan such as filing of claims, payment of claims, deductibles, copayment fees, prescription drug plan, and coordination of benefits. See also *benefit limitations* and *explanation of coverage (EOC)*. Also called *health plan document*. 2. Written agreement stating all of the benefits of an employer's pension plan for the employees and requirements they must have to qualify for those benefits.

plan ID See *national payer identifier* and *NPLANID*.

plan manager Payer employee who manages contracts and contract negotiations for one or more managed care plans.

plan of care Physician's written plan of the type of medical services and care to be given to the patient for a specific health problem.

plan of treatment 1. Written proposal by the patient's physician identifying the patient's medical care needs; therapy services to be provided; amount, frequency, and duration of the services; treatment goals; criteria for ending certain interventions; and documentation of the patient's progress in reaching the objectives. 2. Under the Medicare program, home health services must be given to beneficiaries under a proposal created and certified as needed by a qualified physician. The care plan must be reviewed by the physician every 60 days. Also called *care plan, plan of care (POC), service plan,* or *treatment plan*.

plan participant Employees who are covered under an employee benefit insurance plan or pension plan with contributions made on their behalf by either their employer, union, or trade or professional association.

plan sponsor 1. Employer or employee organization (union) or both that establishes and maintains an employee benefit plan (e.g., includes government health plans and church health plans). 2. In a 401(k) defined-contribution pension plan, an employer. 3. Under the Health Insurance Portability and Accountability Act (HIPAA), either an employer in case of an employee benefit plan, employee organization in case of a plan maintained by an employee organization, or if two or more employers, the association or committee that maintains the plan.

plan sponsorship Group that organizes the group health plan, oversees its facilities, and provides managerial authority.

plan valuation See *actuarial valuation*.

plan year Benefit year that the managed care or health insurance plan is in effect.

planning approval See *certificate of need (CON)*.

play or pay Health care financing approach requiring employers to provide private insurance coverage for their workers or pay a tax that would go into a public regional fund to cover the uninsured.

PLI Acronym that translates as professional liability insurance. See *malpractice insurance*.

plus sign (+) In the CPT code book, symbol that precedes a code number indicating the code may be reported in addition to the parent or primary procedure code number. Add-on codes are never reported for stand-alone services but are reported secondarily in addition to the primary procedure. Also see *add-on code*.

PM See *Program Management (PM)*.

PMC See *physician management corporation (PMC)*.

PMD See *power mobility device (PMD)*.

PMDC See *premajor diagnostic category (PMDC or Pre-MDC)*.

PMI See *mortgage insurance*.

PMMIS See *Program Management and Medical Information System (PMMIS)*.

PMPM Abbreviation for per member per month. See *member months*.

PMPY Abbreviation for per member per year. See *member months*.

pmt See *payment (pmt)*.

pneumococcal vaccine Preparation of killed microorganisms, living attenuated organisms, or living fully virulent organisms that is administered to produce or artificially increase immunity to pneumonia.

PO See *privacy officer (PO), postoperative (PO), and physician organization (PO).*

POA See *present on admission (POA).*

podiatrist See *Doctor of Podiatric Medicine (DPM).*

podiatry Diagnosis and treatment of diseases and other disorders of the feet. Also called *chiropody* in Canada.

POE See *proof of eligibility (POE).*

point-of-care technology Modern methodology in which medical personnel may electronically record findings, write orders, and review information from the location where care is provided such as telemedicine.

point of origin for admission or visit One-digit numerical code inserted in Field 15 on the Uniform Bill (UB-04) insurance claim form. This code indicates the source of the admission or outpatient service (e.g., emergency department, transfer from a skilled nursing facility [SNF], transfer from a hospital, transfer from a clinic).

point-of-sale (POS) device See *point-of-service (POS) device.*

point of service (POS) Location of where the particular heath care service is provided. POS often defines under what provisions of a health insurance policy the service will be paid. If a POS provision is added to a managed care plan, it allows a member to go outside the plan for services but the copayment varies in size depending on the level of benefit. Do not confuse this with *place of service (POS).* Also see *point-of-service (POS) plan.*

point-of-service (POS) device Piece of equipment interfaced with an analog telephone line used to identify a recipient's eligibility, obtain share of cost liability status, key in share of cost payment toward balance, reserve medical services, perform Family PACT (planning, access, care, and treatment) client eligibility transactions, and submit pharmacy or CMS-1500 insurance claims. Also referred to as *point-of-sale (POS) device* or *point-of-service (POS) network.*

point-of-service (POS) network See *point-of-service (POS) device.*

point-of-service (POS) option 1. Under a managed care plan or Medicare managed care plan, an opportunity for a member or beneficiary to choose doctors and hospitals outside the plan for an additional cost. 2. Option under TRICARE Prime that allows self-referral for any TRICARE-covered nonemergency services outside the prime network of providers.

point-of-service (POS) plan Managed care plan in which members are given a choice as to how to receive services, whether through an HMO, PPO, or fee-for-service plan. They may choose a nonparticipating provider (higher cost) or participating provider, with different levels associated with the use of participating providers, and with or without a referral. The decision

is made at the time the service is necessary (i.e., "at the point of service"); sometimes referred to as *open-ended HMOs, point-of-service (POS) program, swing-out HMOs, self-referral options,* or *multiple option plans.*

point-of-service (POS) program See *point-of-service (POS) plan.*

poisoning Condition resulting from a drug or chemical substance overdose or from the wrong drug or agent given or taken in error.

policy See *insurance policy.*

policy acquisition costs See *acquisition cost.*

policy administration department See *customer service department.*

policy advisory group Generic name for many work groups at Workgroup on Electronic Data Interchange (WEDI) and elsewhere. WEDI is a subgroup of the Accreditation Standards Committee X12 that has been involved in creating electronic data interchange standards for insurance billing transactions.

policy anniversary See *anniversary date.*

policy charge See *policy fee.*

policy dividend See *dividend.*

policy fee Dollar amount that an insurer adds to the basic premium rate to cover the insurer's cost of issuing a policy, setting up the required records, and sending premium notices. Also called *policy charge.*

policy filing Procedure of obtaining legal permission to sell an insurance product within a specific area.

policy issue Transmission of an insurance policy to an insured by the insurance company.

policy loan Amount of money (cash surrender value) that the policy owner of a life insurance policy may borrow at interest from the insurer.

policy number Identification number that is given to a group insurance contract. It contains the account number of the policy together with the policy code number.

policy owner See *enrollee.*

policy owner dividend See *dividend.*

policy owner service department See *customer service department.*

policy owner's equity See *cash value.*

policy period Amount of time an insurance contract is in force.

policy proceeds Amount of money that the beneficiary of a life insurance policy receives. Also called *net policy proceeds.*

policy provisions Words, sentences, and paragraphs that describe the benefits and nonbenefits of an insurance contract and its operation.

policy purchase rider See *guaranteed insurability (GI) rider.*

policy reserve 1. Amount of assets added to the future premiums to be received from insurance policies so that funds are sufficient to pay future claims on policies that are in force. 2. Assets that guarantee that the insurance company has funds sufficient to pay future claims.

P

policy summary Document that gives the legally required information of a specific insurance policy that is to be purchased by an applicant.

policy year Twelve-month period between an insurance policy's anniversaries.

policy year experience Twelve-month loss on an insurance policy or line of business.

policyholder See *enrollee.*

policyholder self-administration Type of self-management in which a group policyholder maintains the records and is responsible for the insureds covered under the insurance plan. They prepare the premium statements and submit them with the checks to the insurance company for each payment. The insurance company may audit the policyholder's records. Also called *self-administration.*

pool See *pooling* and *risk pool.*

pooled claims Insurance claims that apply to pooled risks that are excluded from individual case experience rating.

pooled rate See *community rating.*

pooling 1. In managed care contracts, amount of money retained from capitated payments or discounted fees to facilities and providers and held as an incentive or bonus if they meet the criteria of reducing health care costs by managing utilization. Also known as *withhold pool, bonus pool, risk pool,* or *at-risk contract.* 2. To put together premium claims and expenses (risks) for groups into one risk pool to spread the risk. See also *community rating.*

pooling charge Pooled risk cost included in an insurance premium. This amount is obtained by using an individual case experience rating refund formula.

POP See *population (POP).*

population (POP) Number or total number of people that live in a certain area, region, or country.

population-based care See *disease management.*

population-based care management See *disease management.*

POR See *problem-oriented record (POR).*

portable unit See *mobile facility.*

portable x-ray Radiological procedure performed outside of a permanent location (e.g., patient's home). It is done using portable radiological equipment by a licensed technician and under the general supervision of a physician.

portability Insurance plan provision that allows access to health care so that an insured does not lose insurance coverage because of a change in health, employment, marriage, or divorce. Insurance benefits may be transferred from one employer to another or from an employer to a personal policy.

portfolio 1. A compilation of items that represents a job applicant's skills. 2. Insurance company's total investments in financial securities. 3. All products offered by an insurance company.

portfolio method See *portfolio rate of return.*

portfolio rate of return System of accounting in insurance companies in which each policy owner receives a rate of interest equal to the average rate of interest earned on the entire insurance company's investments in stocks, bonds, and real estate. Also called *portfolio method.*

POS See *place of service* or *point-of-service (POS) plan.*

position-schedule bond Insurance that provides coverage for a designated job title rather than a named individual.

post 1. Record or transfer financial entries, debit or credit, to an account (e.g., day sheet, ledger, bank deposit slip, chest register, journal). 2. On the Internet, to send an e-mail message to a list server (distribution list), newsgroup, or blog site.

post notice Under the Fair Credit Reporting Act, document that an insurance company must send an applicant when an adverse decision has been made based on information in a report from a consumer reporting agency.

postacute care See *intermediate care.*

postclaims underwriting Investigation of an insurance applicant's data that is carried out by the insurance company after insurance coverage was already given. It is an illegal practice and may be triggered by medical bills that reach threshold costs.

posteroanterior (PA) Directional term from back to front. Also referred to as *posterior anterior (PA).* Some x-rays are taken in this direction.

posting date Date a fee entry or adjustment entry is inserted on a patient's financial account by the bookkeeper of the provider or facility. This may not be the same date as the actual date of service but may occur within 5 days of the actual date of service.

postoperative (PO) Pertaining to the period of time after surgery. It begins with the patient's emergence from anesthesia and continues through the time required for the acute effects of the anesthetic and surgical procedures to abate.

postpayment review Evaluation of an insurance claim after a determination and after payment has been made to the provider or beneficiary.

postservice appeal See *appeal.*

postservice float Period of time between a medical service provided and a provider's transmitted claim to the payer.

potential fraud case (PFC) Case developed after the program safeguard contractor (PSC) has substantiated an allegation of fraud.

potential payments Maximum anticipated total payments (based on the most recent year's utilization and experience and any current or anticipated factors that may affect payment amounts) that could be received if use or costs of referral services were low enough. These payments include amounts paid for services furnished or referred by the physician/group, plus amounts paid for administrative costs. Payments not included in potential payments include bonuses or other compensation not based on referrals (e.g., bonuses based on patient satisfaction or other quality of care factors).

power mobility device (PMD) Power wheelchair and power-operated vehicle such as a scooter. Medicare beneficiaries with a personal mobility deficit who meet criteria as noted in the *Medicare National Coverage Determinations Manual* are eligible to be provided with a PMD under the durable medical equipment (DME) benefit. The device must be ordered by a physician or treating provider.

power of agency Document that lets an agent act for an insurer. It is a contract drawn up between an insurance company and its agents.

power of attorney 1. Medical document that lets an individual appoint someone he or she trusts to make decisions about the individual's medical care. This type of advance directive also may be called a *health care proxy, appointment of health care agent,* or a *durable power of attorney for health care.* 2. Voluntary transfer of decision-making authority from one individual to another individual, both of whom are competent.

PPA Managed care plan that is similar to a preferred provider organization (PPO).

PPA See *Partnership for Prescription Assistance (PPA).*

PPAC See *Medicare Payment Advisory Commission (MedPAC or MedPac),* which replaced Prospective Payment Assessment Commission (PPAC).

PPE See *personal protective equipment (PPE).*

PPGA See *personal producing general agent (PPGA).*

PPMC See *physician practice management company (PPMC).*

PPN See *preferred provider network (PPN).*

PPO See *preferred provider organization (PPO).*

PPRC See *Medicare Payment Advisory Commission (MedPAC or MedPac),* which replaced the Physician Payment Review Commission (PPRC).

PPS See *prospective payment system (PPS).*

PQRI See *Physician Quality Reporting Initiative (PQRI).*

practical nurse See *licensed practical nurse (LPN).*

practice Frequently repeated process of an insurance company that constitutes a customary procedure.

practice expense (PE) One of three components used in the formula to develop relative value units (RVUs) for each medical service performed. PE consists of salaries, fringe benefits, and purchase and use of medical equipment and supplies. The other two components are (1) amount of physician work and (2) the cost of professional liability insurance. These three RVUs are then adjusted according to geographical area and used in a formula to determine the resource-based relative value scale (RBRVS) for the Medicare fees published annually in the *Federal Register.*

practice guidelines Suggested procedures and policies for patient management to help physicians in decisions about quality health care for certain medical conditions. Some managed care plans and professional organizations have guidelines to evaluate appropriateness and medical necessity of services such as the American Medical Association. Also called *critical pathways, practice options, practice parameters, practice policies, practice standards,* or *treatment protocols.*

practice options See *practice guidelines.*

practice parameters See *practice guidelines.*

practice policies See *practice guidelines.*

practice privileges See *clinical privileges.*

practice standards See *practice guidelines.*

practitioner Individual qualified to practice in a specialized professional field (e.g., family practitioner or nurse practitioner).

preadmission authorization See *preadmission certification (PAC).*

preadmission certification (PAC) Component of a managed care plan that reviews an inpatient hospital stay prospectively to determine coverage. Also called *preauthorization.* See *precertification.*

preadmission review (PAR) Review by a quality improvement organization (QIO) for specific surgical procedures and scheduled inpatient services that must be approved before being provided. Also called *preprocedure review.*

preadmission testing (PAT) Treatment, tests, and procedures done 48 to 72 hours before admission of a patient into the hospital. This is done to eliminate extra hospital days.

preauthorization Requirement in some health insurance plans for a physician or provider to obtain permission for a service or procedure before it is done and to see whether the insurance program agrees it is medically necessary. Factors determining authorization are eligibility, benefits of a specific plan, and setting of care. Also called *approval, authorization,* or *preapproval.* See also *precertification* and *predetermination.*

preauthorization of benefits provision See *predetermination of benefits provision.*

preauthorized checking See *automatic bill payment, check deposit billing, electronic funds transfer system (EFTS), preauthorized check system (PAC),* and *preauthorized payment.*

preauthorized check system (PAC) See *automatic bill payment, check deposit billing, electronic funds transfer (EFT),* and *preauthorized payment.*

preauthorized payment Bank service that permits a debtor to request funds to be transferred from the customer's bank deposit account to the account of a creditor. Also called *automatic bill payment, bank check plan, check-o-matic, check deposit billing, electronic funds transfer system (EFTS),* or *preauthorized checking.*

precertification To find out whether treatment (surgery, tests, hospitalization) is covered under a patient's health insurance policy. Also referred to as *preadmission certification (PAC)*.

precertification of benefits provision See *predetermination of benefits provision*.

predesignated chiropractor See *predesignated physician*.

predesignated physician In workers' compensation cases, doctor whom the employee has selected as his or her physician of choice by formally notifying the employer before the date of an industrial injury.

predetermination To determine before treatment the maximum dollar amount the insurance company will pay for surgery, consultations, postoperative care, and so forth.

predetermination of benefits provision In dental policies, a clause specifying that when dental care is expected to exceed a certain level, the dentist must submit a proposed treatment plan to the insurance company so that a determination can be made of how much the dental plan will pay. Also called *preauthorization of benefits provision, precertification of benefits provision,* or *pretreatment review provision*.

preemption analysis Comparison of state laws to the Health Insurance Portability and Accountability Act (HIPAA) by an organization (hospital facility), usually performed annually. State laws that are stricter supercede HIPAA privacy and security regulations. Areas in which state laws are typically more stringent include mental health and substance abuse, child abuse, elder abuse, domestic violence, AIDS/HIV, sexually transmitted diseases, genetics, and reproductive rights.

preestimate of cost See *predetermination*.

preexisting condition (PEC) Illness or injury acquired by the patient before enrollment in an insurance plan such as chronic illness, injury, and possible pregnancy. In some insurance plans, preexisting conditions are either excluded from coverage temporarily or permanently, may disqualify membership in the plan, or may cover them only after a waiting period. Federally qualified health maintenance organizations cannot limit coverage for preexisting conditions.

preexisting condition exclusion See *preexisting condition limitation*.

preexisting condition limitation Exclusion from insurance coverage or coverage after a waiting period of illness or injury received by the insured before enrollment in an insurance plan. Also called *preexisting condition exclusion*.

preexisting conditions provision Clause in an insurance contract that states until the insured has been covered under the policy for a certain period, the insurance company will not pay benefits for any preexisting conditions.

preference beneficiary clause In a life insurance policy, if no beneficiary is listed, the insurance company will pay the proceeds from the policy in a stated order to the individuals shown in the contract.

preferred-drug list (PDL) See *formulary* or *drug formulary*.

preferred plan Managed care plan that requires members to receive medical services from the network's physicians at a reduced cost instead of a doctor of their own choice at a larger cost.

preferred provider Any licensed health care professional who contracts with a managed care plan such as ambulatory surgical center, dentist, hospital, physician, and podiatrist.

preferred provider arrangement (PPA) System in managed care, in which a limited number of providers are selectively contracted at reduced rates of payment.

preferred provider network (PPN) Under the TRICARE program, group of civilian practitioners to supplement military direct care in TRICARE Prime and Extra. PPN members offer discounts, file patients' claims, and must meet the same professional standards as military treatment facility providers.

preferred provider organization (PPO) 1. Type of mixed health-plan model that combines managed care and traditional insurance. Enrollees receive the highest level of benefits when they obtain services from a physician, hospital, or other health provider designated by their program as a "preferred provider." They may receive substantial, though reduced, benefits or may have additional cost when they obtain care from a provider of their own choosing who is not designated as a "preferred provider" by their program. 2. A Medicare+Choice coordinated care plan that has a network of providers who have agreed to a contractually specified reimbursement for covered benefits with the organization offering the plan. It provides for payment for all covered benefits regardless of whether the benefits are given with the network of providers. It is offered by an organization that is not licensed or organized under state law as a health maintenance organization (HMO). 3. Type of Medicare Advantage Plan in which the patient uses doctors, hospitals, and providers that belong to the network. Patients can use doctors, hospitals, and providers outside of the network for an additional cost.

preferred risk class Category for an insured or applicant of insurance who has a lower expectation of incurring a loss and has greater life expectancy than a standard applicant and qualifies for a reduced premium rate (e.g., applicant who does not smoke, applicant who does not drink). Also called *superstandard risk class*.

prefunding System of financially supporting the cost of retirement coverage while employees are still working.

pregnancy care Federal legislation enacted in 1978 requiring employers with 15 or more employees who are engaged in interstate commerce and subject to

Title VII of the Civil Rights Act of 1964 to give the same benefits for pregnancy, childbirth, and related medical conditions as benefits for other illnesses or injuries.

pregnancy legislation See *pregnancy care.*

preinjury capacity In workers' compensation cases, an employee's capability to perform work before any work-related injury or illness.

preliminary inquiry form Application form used when the applicant might not be issued or will be issued with a high substandard rating that the premium will be unacceptable. Also called *trial application.*

preliminary report See *First Report of Injury.*

premajor diagnostic category (PMDC or Pre-MDC) Eight diagnosis-related groups (DRGs) to which cases are assigned that are based on procedure codes before classifying them to a major diagnostic category (MDC). The eight DRGs are one each for the heart, liver, bone marrow, simultaneous pancreas/kidney transplant, pancreas transplant, and lung transplant and two for tracheostomies.

premature delivery Infant, regardless of birth weight, born before 37 weeks of gestation.

premium Cost of insurance coverage paid by the insured person either monthly, quarterly, or annually, to Medicare, an insurance company, or a managed care plan that keeps the policy in force.

premium-delay arrangement See *deferred premium arrangement.*

premium deposits See *deposit premium.*

premium loan Loan made for the purpose of paying insurance policy premiums.

premium notice Billing statement to the insured requesting payment of the insurance premium on a specific due date.

premium payment mode Frequency in which premiums are payable in a policy year (e.g., monthly, semi-annually, annually).

premium rate 1. Cost of a unit of insurance coverage for an individual insurance policy. 2. Dollar amount for group insurance coverage that is stated in a master plan. Also called *contract rate.*

premium receipt Written document given to a policy owner by an insurance company or insurance agent as acknowledgment of an initial premium.

premium receipt book Book given to the insured when an insurance agent makes a policy sale during a home visit. It contains prenumbered receipts signed by the agent when the agent collects a premium.

premium refund Dollar amount returned to the insured because of favorable experience. Also called *dividend, experience refund, experience rating refund,* and *retroactive rate reduction.*

premium reduction option Stated choice in which life insurance policy dividends are applied to the payment of renewal premiums.

premium statement Invoice or bill from the insurance company that is sent to the insured for each premium due on an insurance plan.

premium surcharge Additional premium amount in which the standard Medicare Part B premium goes up 10% for each full 12-month period (beginning with the first month after the end of the beneficiary's initial enrollment period) in which the beneficiary could have had Medicare Part B but did not take it. There is also a surcharge for Medicare Part D.

premium tax Government- or state-imposed fee based on the net premium income collected in a jurisdiction by an insurance company.

prenotice Under the Fair Credit Reporting Act, advanced written statement to an insurance applicant from an insurance company that an investigative consumer report must be obtained on the applicant.

preop Abbreviation for preparation for operation or preoperative. See *preoperative (preop).*

preoperative (preop) Pertaining to the period before a surgical procedure. Commonly the preoperative period begins with the first preparation of the patient for surgery and ends with the induction of anesthesia in the operating suite.

prepaid group practice plan Managed care plan under which specified health services are rendered by participating physicians to an enrolled group of persons, with fixed periodic payments made in advance, by or on behalf of each person or family. If a health insurance carrier is involved, it contracts to pay in advance for the full range of health services to which the insured is entitled under the terms of the health insurance contract. Such a plan is one form of a *health maintenance organization.* Also called *prepaid group practice model* and *group model health maintenance organization (HMO).*

prepaid health care Managed care plan in which monthly premiums are paid before medical services are received by the patient.

prepaid health plan (PHP) Prepaid managed care program that either provides less than comprehensive services on an at-risk basis or one that provides any benefit package on a nonrisk basis or one in which a specified set of health benefits is provided in exchange for a yearly fee or fixed periodic payments. See *managed care.*

prepaid prescription drug program Insurance program that lets members of specific groups receive payment for prescription drugs.

prepayment System of paying for medical services before receiving them such as in the form of scheduled monthly insurance premiums or a budgeted basis, without regard to services rendered. In managed care plans, capitation is a form of prepayment.

prepayment health care plans Prepaid health care plans that meet federal legal standards for managed care plans (e.g., health maintenance organizations,

P

provider-sponsored organizations, preferred provider organizations, or other types of network plans except network medical savings account plans). They incorporate cost containment and emphasize preventive care to members of the plans. Also referred to as *coordinated care (CC) plans* or *managed care plans.*

prepayment review Evaluation of insurance claims before determination and payment.

preponderance of the evidence Legal phrase that means the greater the weight of the evidence when weighed with that opposed to it, has the most convincing force to assist with making a judgment. Also called *preponderance of proof.*

preponderance of proof See *preponderance of the evidence.*

preprinted claim form Insurance claim form in which the provider's name, address, and identification numbers have been reproduced on the form.

preprocedure review See *preadmission review (PAR).*

preretirement survivor annuity Provision in a pension plan that gives a benefit to the surviving spouse of a vested plan participant if the participant deceases before retiring. Qualified plans must include this provision.

prescribed drugs Medications that are available only with a written prescription from a licensed practitioner.

prescription Written order for medication, therapy, or therapeutic device given by a physician, dentist, or other licensed practitioner, which then goes to a person authorized to dispense the order.

prescription benefit manager (PBM) Management company or organization that monitors prescription claims for managed care plans and tracks the drugs and volume prescribed by the plan's participating providers of medical services. The PBM's sophisticated information systems help identify patients who have chronic diseases, drug utilization, compliance patterns, and physicians' prescribing patterns. Also called *pharmacy benefit manager (PBM).*

prescription drug Medication that can be dispensed to the public only with an order given by a properly authorized individual. The drug must be approved by the U.S. Food and Drug Administration (FDA) and only a licensed, registered pharmacist or physician may dispense the prescription.

prescription drug plan (PDP) Insurance plan for prescription drug expenses with deductible and copayments. Some plans allow the insured to obtain the medication at any pharmacy, and other plans have little or no copayment when going to specific pharmacies.

prescription medication See *prescription drug.*

present on admission (POA) Diagnosis present at the time of the inpatient admission. It can include conditions known at the time of admission, present at admission but not diagnosed until later, and conditions that develop during outpatient encounters such as emergency department, observation, or outpatient surgery. Also see *present-on-admission (POA) indicator.*

present-on-admission (POA) indicator Code, eighth digit, that is attached to the diagnostic code required for reporting Medicare inpatients' claims for specific types of conditions. It is to be reported on the UB-04 claim form in diagnostic coding fields 67 and 67A-Q. For electronically transmitted claims, the POA is reported in loop 2300, data element H101, which should contain the letters "POA" followed by the assigned value for the code. Also see *present on admission (POA).*

present value For future stream of payments, a lump sum amount that, if invested on a certain date (evaluation date), together with interest earnings, would be enough to meet each of the payments as they fell due. At the time of the last payment, the invested fund would be exactly zero.

present value factor Interest rate factor for determining the present value of a sum in the future. A formula is used to obtain this number.

presenting problem Reason for the patient's office visit such as complaints, condition, disease, findings, illness, injury, signs, or symptoms.

preservice appeal Appeal by a physician to a third-party payer for medical services not yet provided to the patient. Also see *appeal, postservice appeal,* and *expedited appeal.*

presumption Legal assumption that a fact exists.

presumptive disability Assumption of total disability when an insured is considered totally disabled (blindness, loss of hearing, speech, or limbs). The insurance company may pay a lump sum in addition to monthly payments for a maximum benefit period.

presumptive eligibility (PE) A federal/state program designed to ease access to prenatal care offering immediate temporary coverage to low-income women pending a formal Medi-Cal application.

presumptive father Possible biological father of a child but not necessarily the legal parent or the confirmed father. Also referred to as *alleged father.*

pretreatment review provision See *predetermination of benefits provision.*

prevailing charge Fee that is most frequently charged in an area by a specialty group of physicians. The top of this range establishes an overall limitation on the charges that a carrier, which considers prevailing charges in reimbursement, will accept as reasonable for a given service without special justification. In the Medicare program, this factor was previously used in determining payment.

prevalence Number of existing cases of a disease or condition in a defined population at a specific time. Calculation: Divide the number of persons with the disease by the total population of the defined group to obtain the prevalence rate of a disease.

prevention Action taken to diminish the onset of disease or an injury such as hand washing, refrigeration of foods, no smoking, little or no alcohol intake, prenatal care, and exercise.

preventive care Health care that focuses on disease prevention and maintaining good health such as annual physical examinations, mammograms, Pap smears, prostate and colorectal cancer screenings, and influenza and pneumonia vaccinations. This includes early diagnosis of disease, identification of individuals who are prone to certain illnesses, counseling, immunizations, regular exercise, avoidance of smoking, prudent diet, correction of congenital anomalies, and screening programs. Also called *disease prevention* and *health management.*

preventive medicine Services provided to prevent the occurrence of illness, injury, and disease such as vaccine immunizations, antiseptic measures, regular exercise, routine physical examinations, and screening programs for detection of signs of disorders.

preventive medicine codes CPT codes (99381-99397 and 99401-99429) used when billing for medical services provided to prevent the occurrence of illness or injury.

preventive services Health care to keep an individual healthy or to prevent illness (e.g., Papanicolaou tests, pelvic examinations, influenza shots, screening mammograms).

previous In the medical field, this relates to a patient who has had prior hospitalization, medical services, or surgery. This information is in a system that is used to check claims before approval is given to the provider of the service.

price controls Method of cost containment that freezes physician and hospital fees to try to curtail inflation.

pricer 1. Individual who reviews services, procedures, diagnoses, fee schedules, and other data and establishes the amount for a medical service or supply. Also called *repricer.* 2. Software package in an insurance claims processing system, specific to certain benefits, which analyzes specific data and determines the amount for a medical service or supply. Subsequently, other criteria are applied to establish the actual allowance or payment amount. It is most often used under prospective payment systems.

prima facie argument Principle that is presumed to be true unless there is evidence given to disprove the presumption.

prima facie rate Standard premium rate recommended by state government regulators for a contributory group creditor insurance policy.

primary beneficiary See *beneficiary.*

primary care 1. First time a patient seeks medical care from a provider. 2. Basic health care attention when a patient first contacts someone to care for simpler and more common illnesses and injuries. Primary care can be provided by a family practitioner, pediatrician, or internist and health professionals such as nurse practitioners or physician assistants.

primary care capitation Each primary care physician of a managed care plan receives a specific amount each

month for each member who selects that physician as his or her primary care physician. See *capitation (cap or CAP).*

primary care case management (PCCM) Managed care option under Section 1915(b) of the Social Security Act. In the Medicaid program, this lets states contract directly with primary care providers who agree to provide medical services to Medicaid recipients and authorize specialty care. In this system the state pays the primary care physician a monthly case management fee, as well as fee-for-service (FFS).

primary care case management (PCCM) provider Usually a physician, physician group practice, or an entity employing or having other arrangements with such physicians, but sometimes also including nurse practitioners, nurse midwives, or physician assistants who contract to locate, coordinate, and monitor covered primary care and sometimes additional services.

primary care center See *ambulatory care facility* and *free-standing surgical center.*

primary care doctor See *primary care physician (PCP).*

primary care manager (PCM) 1. In a managed care plan, individual who gives and coordinates members' health care and makes referrals to specialists when necessary. 2. In TRICARE, physician who is responsible for coordinating and managing all the beneficiary's health care unless there is an emergency.

primary care network (PCN) Panel of providers focused on giving primary care services to patients of a managed care plan.

primary care physician (PCP) Physician (e.g., family practitioner, general practitioner, pediatrician, obstetrician/gynecologist, general internist) who sees patients first for most health problems, who oversees the care of patients in a managed health care plan (HMO or PPO), and who refers patients to specialists (e.g., cardiologist, oncologists, surgeons) for services as needed. Also known as a *gatekeeper, primary care doctor,* or *primary care practitioner.*

primary care practitioner (PCP) See *primary care physician (PCP).*

primary care provider (PCP) See *primary care physician (PCP).*

primary carrier Health insurance company that pays on a claim as the first carrier before the second insurer pays when a patient has two policies and they are coordinating benefits.

primary case management (PCM) Program in which the state contracts directly with primary care providers who agree to be responsible for the provision and/or coordination of medical services to Medicaid recipients under their care. Most primary care case management (PCCM) programs pay the primary care physician a monthly case management fee in addition to reimbursing services on a fee-for-service basis. Also called *primary care case management (PCCM).*

P

primary coverage Provision in an insurance policy under the coordination of benefits clause in which the health plan pays without taking into account any other plans.

primary diagnosis 1. Initial identification of the condition, illness, injury, or chief complaint for which the patient is treated for medical care in a physician's office or as a hospital outpatient. Insurance claim forms must show the diagnostic code reflecting the primary diagnosis. 2. Underlying cause for the office visit or treatment.

primary insurer Insurance company that covers the initial payments for medical services when a person has more than one health insurance plan. The patient must pay the deductible and any copayment fee.

primary payer 1. Insurer obligated to pay losses first when two or more insurers may be responsible for paying the claim. 2. Medicare is a primary payer with respect to Medicaid; for a person eligible under both programs, Medicaid pays only for benefits not covered under Medicare or after Medicare benefits are exhausted. 3. An employer's health plan if a Medicare patient is covered by that plan, and then Medicare is the secondary payer. 4. Insurance carrier or managed care plan that has the first responsibility under the coordination of benefits clause between two or more insurers.

primary provider of benefits When coordinating benefits of two insurance plans, the medical expense plan pays benefits first before any benefits are paid by another medical expense plan.

primary site Site where the tumor began or originated.

principal Entity that authorizes another individual or representative to act on behalf of the principal in dealing with third parties.

principal diagnosis (PDX) Patient's condition established after study that is chiefly responsible for the admission of the patient to the hospital. The principal diagnosis may or may not be the same as the primary diagnosis. Also see *admitting diagnosis* and *major diagnosis.*

principal diagnosis code 1. Diagnostic code for a condition established after study that is responsible for the admission of the patient to the hospital. 2. When completing the Uniform Bill (UB-04) paper or electronic claim form, the principal diagnosis code including fourth and fifth digits should appear in Field 67.

principal procedure Most important medical service performed, usually for treatment, that is related to the chief diagnosis responsible for the admission of the patient to the hospital.

principal procedure code 1. ICD-9-CM procedure code for the most important medical service performed, usually for treatment, which is related to the chief diagnosis responsible for the admission of the patient to the hospital. If there are two procedures that are principal, then the one most related to the principal diagnosis should be the principal procedure.

2. When completing the Uniform Bill (UB-04) paper or electronic claim form, the principal procedure code should appear in Field 67. The electronic version requires an eight-character date listing year, month, and day (20XX0425).

principal sum Dollar amount paid in a lump sum by an insurance company for an accidental death or accidental dismemberment of the insured.

prior approval (PA) The evaluation of a provider request for a specific service to determine the medical necessity and appropriateness of the care requested for a patient. Also called *prior authorization* in some states.

prior authorization (PA) See *prior approval (PA).*

prior authorization number Group of figures assigned by a managed care plan or insurance program to a specific case after prior approval or precertification for treatment is completed.

prior coverage Insurance of an individual before the effective date of another policy and the subscriber has a different identification number.

prior service Insurance coverage of an individual who was covered under a previous employer and is now to be covered with the same insurance company under a new employer.

prior-stay dates The "from" and "through" dates of a patient's stay in a hospital, skilled nursing facility (SNF), or nursing home that ended within 60 days of the current hospital or SNF admission.

privacy 1. Confidentiality. 2. Free from observation such as closed doors, drawn curtains around a hospital bed. 3. Under the Health Insurance Portability and Accountability Act (HIPAA), use and disclosure of protected health information is permissible for treatment, payment, or health care operations (TPO).

Privacy Act of 1974 Federal legislation that became effective on September 27, 1975, and established an individual's right to review his or her medical records maintained by a federal medical care facility such as a VA medical center or U.S. Public Health Service facility and to contest inaccuracies in such records. This act also began to limit government use of the Social Security number. Some federal agencies or federally funded institutions may be regulated by both the Privacy Act and the HIPAA standards. Such entities are required to comply with both sets of regulations. Although the HIPAA standards generally provide more restrictive regulations, entities are advised to revise their policies and procedures to comply with both the HIPAA standards and the Privacy Act.

privacy notice See *Notice of Privacy Practices (NPP).*

privacy officer (PO) Under the Health Insurance Portability and Accountability Act (HIPAA), an individual designated to help the provider remain in compliance by setting policies and procedures (P & P) and by training and managing the staff regarding

HIPAA and patient rights. The PO is usually the contact person for questions and complaints. Also known as *privacy official (PO)*.

privacy official See *privacy officer (PO)*.

private contract Agreement between the patient and a doctor, podiatrist, dentist, or optometrist who has decided not to offer services through the Medicare program. This doctor cannot bill Medicare for any service or supplies given to the patient and all his or her other Medicare patients for at least 2 years. There are no limits on what the patient can be charged for the services under a private contract. The patient must pay the full amount of the bill and submit his or her own insurance claims for reimbursement. The GJ modifier must be used on all insurance claims for services rendered by an "opt out" provider for emergency/urgent services.

private duty nursing service Nursing services by a registered nurse (RN) or licensed practical nurse (LPN) who is not employed by an institution (hospital, home health care agency, skilled nursing facility, or hospice provider) but may work in an institution caring for a patient on a fee-for-service basis. Private duty care also may occur in the home.

private fee-for-service plan Medicare Advantage Plan in which the patient may go to any Medicare-approved physician or hospital that accepts the plan's payment. The insurance plan, rather than the Medicare program, decides how much it will pay and what the patient should pay for the medical services.

private hospital Medical facility that is privately owned and operated by an individual, several people, or a corporation.

private insurance Conventional health care coverage bought from an insurance company that allows the insured to select his or her physicians, hospitals, and other health care facilities.

private practice Work of a professional health care provider who is independent of financial or external policy control by professional peers, except for licensing and other legal restrictions.

privileged communications Verbal discussions that are confidential and not to be disclosed except by specific consent of the patient.

privileged information Data related to the treatment and progress of the patient that can be released only when written authorization of the patient or guardian is obtained.

PRO See *peer review organization (PRO), Professional Standards Review Organization (PSRO), Quality Improvement Organization (QIO) program,* and *Utilization and Quality Control Peer Review Organization (PRO)*.

probability (P value) Chance that an event will occur. The probability theory and statistics are the foundations of insurance.

probate Legal proceeding proving a will is genuine and allowing the carrying out of its provisions. Its purpose is to protect the heirs from fraud and embezzlement, ensure creditors of the deceased are paid for any outstanding debts, and oversee payment of federal, state, and local taxes by the estate.

probationary period See *eligibility waiting period*.

problem focused (PF) Phrase used to describe a type of medical decision-making when a patient is seen for an evaluation and management service.

problem-focused examination 1995 documentation guidelines: limited examination of the affected body area or organ system. The health record should describe only one body area or organ system. 1997 documentation guidelines for multisystem examination: performance and documentation of one to five elements identified by a bullet (•) in one or more body or system areas. 1997 documentation guidelines for single organ system examination: performance and documentation of one to five elements identified in a table by a bullet (•), whether in a shaded or unshaded box.

problem-focused history Documentation must include the chief complaint and a brief history of the presenting illness (HPI) or problem.

problem-oriented record (POR) System of medical recordkeeping that consists of flow sheets, charts, or graphs that allow a physician to quickly locate information and compare evaluations for data such as blood pressure readings, blood sugar levels for diabetic patients, weight for obese patients, medications, and immunizations.

problem-oriented V codes 1. ICD-9-CM diagnostic codes that are used when a person who is not currently sick encounters health services for some specific purpose such as to act as a donor of an organ or tissue, receive a vaccination, discuss a problem that is not in itself a disease or injury, seek consultation about family planning, request sterilization, or to obtain supervision of a normal pregnancy. In these situations the V code appears as a primary code and is placed first for the purpose of billing. 2. Codes used to identify a condition that might affect the patient at a future time but is not a current illness or injury. Use a V code to describe an existing situation that might influence potential medical care.

problem pertinent review of system (ROS) Documented report of an inquiry about the body system(s) directly related to the problem(s) identified in the history of present illness (HPI).

procedural codes See *procedure codes* or *CPT code*.

procedure Specific action, process, sequence of steps, or test performed on a patient either to establish a diagnosis or render a therapeutic service (e.g., minor or major surgery, laboratory tests, inserting an intravenous line).

procedure code See *procedure code numbers*.

procedure code numbers Five-digit numeric codes that describe each professional service the physician

P

renders to a patient and used to communicate medical service data to insurance companies or government programs. These codes are used on insurance claims submitted to insurance programs for payment. Also referred to as *CPT codes* or *procedural codes*.

procedure coding Standardized method used to transform written descriptions of procedures and professional services into numeric designations (code numbers).

procedure review Review of diagnostic and therapeutic procedures to determine appropriateness.

proceeds 1. Face value of an insurance policy or annuity and any additions payable at maturity or death. 2. Under Medicare Secondary Payer guidelines, money obtained as a result of a transaction that is in the possession of the party to whom it was intended.

process Goal-directed, interrelated series of actions, events, mechanisms, or steps.

process improvement Methodology used to make changes for the better to a procedure through the use of continuous quality enhancement and cost and productivity improvement standards or goals. Also referred to as *process management*.

process indicator Gauge that measures a goal-directed, interrelated series of actions, events, mechanisms, or steps.

process management See *process improvement*.

processing time Time period it takes an insurance carrier to process an insurance claim from when it is received by the carrier until it is approved for payment. Payment for manual claims is within 4 to 12 weeks and as little as 7 days when transmitted electronically.

procurement costs Under Medicare Secondary Payer guidelines, the attorney fees and other costs that are related to obtaining a settlement that are borne by the individual against which the Centers for Medicare and Medicaid Services (CMS) seeks to recover.

production credit New insurance policies (volume) or existing premiums that are ascribed to an insurance agent, broker, or group representative.

productivity Measurement of the increased or deceased rate of resources that an organization uses to produce a unit of output.

productivity investments Spending aimed at increasing contractor operational efficiency and production through improved work methods and application of technology.

profession Career that involves specialized training and requires individuals to study extensively to master a complex body of knowledge and have the ability to apply the knowledge.

professional activity study (PAS) Analysis and report performed regularly by the Commission on Professional and Hospital Activities and enumerated by average length of stay (ALOS) by region. Referred to as *PAS norms*. See also *Commission on Professional and Hospital Activities (CPHA)*.

Professional Association of Health Care Office Managers (PAHCOM) A nationwide organization dedicated to providing a strong professional network for health care office managers.

professional association plan Group insurance plan offered by a professional organization composed of self-employed professionals (e.g., accountants, attorneys, educators, physicians). This type of plan may provide more benefits and is less expensive than an individual plan.

professional component (PC) That portion of a test or procedure (containing both professional and technical components) for which the physician reads and interprets but does not perform the test (i.e., interpreting an electrocardiogram [ECG], reading an x-ray, or making an observation and determination using a microscope). In hospital billing, this component is billed separately from the inpatient hospital charges.

professional consultant Employee of the insurance carrier, generally a physician, who reviews and answers questions about complex or unusual medical claims.

professional corporation (PC) Physician or group of physicians who have incorporated, obtained a tax number, and filed articles of incorporation with the secretary of state's office where the practice is doing business.

professional courtesy Discount or exemption from charges for professional services given to certain people at the discretion of the physician rendering the service. Rarely used in current medicine.

professional liability See *malpractice*.

professional liability insurance (PLI) See *liability insurance* and *malpractice insurance*.

professional reinsurer Insurance company that specializes in selling and servicing proportional reinsurance and nonproportional reinsurance with the objective of making a profit.

professional review organizations (PROs) 1. Groups of licensed physicians and osteopaths engaged in the practice of medicine or surgery in a particular area, formed to ensure adequate review of the services provided by the various medical specialties and subspecialties in the area, as well as providing DRG validation. 2. A group of physicians working with the government to review cases for hospital admission and discharge under government guidelines. Under the Medicare program, PROs are known as *Quality Improvement Organization (QIO) programs*. See also *peer review* and *Quality Improvement Organization (QIO) program*.

Professional Standards Review Organization (PSRO) Replaced by Utilization and Quality Control Peer Review Organization (PRO) in 1982 and in 2003 called *Quality Improvement Organization (QIO) program*.

profile 1. Compilation of financial data maintained by an insurance carrier for reimbursement purposes. Also see *physician's fee profile*. 2. Data segregated by specific time period (e.g., quarterly, annually) and target area (e.g., facility or state) for the purpose of identifying patterns. This may include diagnoses, procedures, diagnosis-related groups, and so on.

profile analysis Examination and assessment of activities of patients and physicians to show trends and patterns of health care services.

profile year Twelve-month period that traditional indemnity insurance companies maintain to determine allowable charges.

profiling Evaluation of a physician's practice that includes demographics of patients, morbidity data, mortality rates, and treatment patterns. Also called *physician profiling*.

profit Dollar amount that remains from a payment after all expenses for the service have been paid.

profit-sharing plan Type of plan in which an employer pays a portion of the company's profits to the employees. Such plans can be used as retirement income or for short-term savings.

prognosis Prediction of a probable course of a disease or condition of injury and the chances of recovery.

program See *software*.

Program for Evaluating Payment Patterns Electronic Report (PEPPER) Electronic data report containing hospital-specific data for a number of problem areas identified by the Centers for Medicare and Medicaid Services (CMS) at high risk for payment errors such as specific DRGs and discharges. PEPPER data allow hospitals to compare their performance to other short-term, acute care prospective payment system hospitals as a means of reducing and preventing payment errors.

program integrity branch TRICARE central coordinating agency that investigates and reviews alleged cases of fraud and abuse committed against the Military Health System (MHS) TRICARE program, its beneficiaries, and U.S. taxpayers. Their active involvement investigating and prosecuting health care fraud cases has resulted in a return of millions of dollars to the federal government and Department of Defense (DoD).

Program Integrity Manual (PIM) See *Medicare Program Integrity Manual (PIM)*.

Program Management (PM) Centers for Medicare and Medicaid Services (CMS) operational account that supplies the agency with the resources to administer Medicare, the federal portion of Medicaid, and other agency responsibilities. The components of Program Management are Medicare contractors, survey and certification, research, and administrative costs.

Program Management and Medical Information System (PMMIS) Automated system of records, primarily those of current Medicare-eligible end-stage renal disease (ESRD) patients. The PMMIS also maintains historical information on people no longer

classified as ESRD patients because of death or successful transplantation or recovery of renal function. In addition, it contains information on all dialysis and kidney transplant patients, ESRD facilities, and facility payment. The PMMIS contains medical information on patients and the services that they received during the course of their therapy.

program memorandums Medicare program day-to-day operating instructions that as of October 1, 2003, are transmitted and incorporated into the applicable Medicare manuals. Archived memorandums are available on the Centers for Medicare and Medicaid Services' website.

program safeguard contractor (PSC) Contractor hired to investigate an allegation of fraud and establish a case after it is substantiated. Also called *contractor*. Also see *potential fraud case (PSC)*.

Program of All-Inclusive Care for the Elderly (PACE) Federal program that combines medical, social, and long-term care services for frail people. It is a provider under Medicare and available only in states that have chosen to offer it under the Medicaid program. An individual's eligibility requires that he or she be 55 years or older, live in the service area of the PACE program, be certified as eligible for nursing home care by the appropriate state agency, and be able to live safely in the community. PACE's goal is to help people stay independent and live in their community as long as possible while getting the high-quality care they need.

progress note Written notation, dated and signed, by a member of the health care team, that summarizes the facts about the medical care given and the patient's response during a specific period of time. Also called *chart note*.

progress report Written or dictated letter or chart note documenting details about subsequent examinations of the patient.

progressive care System of giving medically necessary health care at any given stage in illness or recovery (i.e., from acute care in a hospital through the recuperation phase).

progressive impairment A temporary or permanent increase in severity of impairment of a body part, organ, or system. This may be due to disease or injury (e.g., hearing loss going from bad to worse).

progressive rates System in which an insurance plan employs new rates either monthly, quarterly, or semiannually. Individuals who apply or renew policies are affected by the rates in effect.

project manager Supervises and administers the implementation of a data system that can support personal health records and website content.

project officer Appointed person who is responsible overall for a project. A departmental person is usually appointed.

projected costs Potential insurance claim costs that are expected for a specific group over a time period.

projection error Degree of variation between estimated and actual amounts.

projection factor Mathematical calculation applied to insurance claim costs so that adjustments can be made for possible increases in the costs from one time period to another.

prolonged physician services Extended preservices or postservices given to a patient by a doctor that go beyond the usual time allotted in either inpatient or outpatient settings.

prolonged services Services that go beyond the usual time allotted in either inpatient or outpatient settings.

prompt 1. List of items displayed on a CRT from which the typist can choose the function to be performed. Also known as *menu*. 2. In liability insurance cases, prompt or promptly means payment within 120 days after the earlier of the date a claim is filed with an insurer or a lien is filed against a potential liability settlement. It can also mean the date the service was furnished or, in the case of inpatient hospital services, the date of discharge. 3. In no-fault insurance and workers' compensation cases, prompt or promptly means payment within 120 days after receiving the insurance claim.

prompt payment laws State statutes designed to govern actions of insurers and third-party payers to pay insurance claims in a timely manner; also outlines actions collectors can take against insurance companies if statutes are not followed.

proof of age certificate Official document(s) that report the birthplace, date of birth, and parents' full names and home addresses such as a certified copy-of-birth record or a document supplied by a federal government agency during the census period that followed birth. This document may be required for a child participating in Little League in certain locations.

proof of eligibility (POE) Evidence or process to verify that a patient is entitled to medical benefits in an insurance plan or program.

proof of loss Documentation needed by the insurance company from the insured to prove that a claim is valid (e.g., death certificate for life insurance, completed insurance claim form, itemized bills for health services received, repair estimate from automobile body shop, police report).

proof of service In workers' compensation cases, evidence submitted by a process server that he or she has successfully delivered a legal document to a defendant in an action. Also called *return of service*.

ProPAC See *Prospective Payment Assessment Commission (PPAC or ProPAC)*.

proper care See *due care*.

proper claim Insurance claim that is submitted to the insurance carrier in a timely manner and meets all other claims filing requirements of the third-party payer (e.g., mandatory second opinion or prior authorization or approval before treatment).

property/casualty insurance See *casualty insurance*.

property insurance Insurance policy that provides benefits if something is damaged or lost and the cause is described in the policy (e.g., stolen, accident, destroyed by fire).

prophylactic restriction In workers' compensation cases, take preventive measures to guard against aggravation of an impairment (i.e., if the restrictions were exceeded, the injured worker may be at risk for additional injury).

proposal Formal suggested insurance plan offered by an insurance company to give insurance coverage to an employer, group, individual, or organization at stated premium rates. Also called *quotation* and *quote*.

proposed rule First draft of new regulations for legislation developed by the Secretary of Health and Human Services. After a public comment period, a final draft is created and adopted.

propriety hospital For-profit facility owned by individuals, partners, or a corporation. Also referred to as an *investor-owned hospital*.

prorate Proportionate reduction in the amount of insurance benefits payable as provided in the contract. Some examples for proration would be because the insured changed to a more perilous job, because benefits payable by all the insured's disability insurance are more than his or her current earnings over the preceding 2 years, or because the insured is actually older than stated in a life insurance application.

proration Act of modifying an insurance policy's benefits because of some type of change (e.g., insured's occupation).

pros and cons Good and bad parts of treatment for a health problem (e.g., a medicine may help the patient's pain [pro], but it may cause an upset stomach [con]).

prosecute To submit a charging document to a court; seek a grand jury indictment against person(s) accused of committing criminal offenses.

prospect Potential insurance client (individual or organization).

prospecting Aggressively searching for potential clients.

prospective payment See *prospective payment system (PPS)*.

Prospective Payment Assessment Commission (PPAC or ProPAC) Federal commission that was replaced by the Medicare Payment Advisory Commission (MedPAC). See *Medicare Payment Advisory Commission (MedPAC or MedPac)*.

prospective payment system (PPS) Method of payment mandated by the Balanced Budget Act of 1997 (BBA) that changed Medicare hospital payments from cost based to prospective, based on national average capital costs per case. Examples of PPS include Medicare's physician fee schedule and for inpatient diagnosis-related groups (DRGs) that set a predetermined, fixed dollar amount for a principal diagnosis. PPS helps Medicare control its spending by encouraging providers to furnish care that is efficient, appropriate, and typical of practice expenses for providers. Patients and resource needs are statistically grouped, and the system is adjusted for patient characteristics that affect the cost of providing care. A unit of service is then established, with a fixed, predetermined amount for payment. Sometimes called *prospective reimbursement.* Also see *outpatient prospective payment system (OPPS).*

prospective pricing To set a price before rendering a service (e.g., the Medicare prospective payment system [PPS]). The opposite of this would be the reimbursement system in which the medical service is given first and then the provider of the service receives payment.

prospective rating 1. To find out a future property or liability insurance rate. 2. Premium for a certain projected period of time based on the loss experience of a specific prior period of time. In such a contract, the carrier assumes the risk (inadequate or excessive) and the purchaser pays a fixed rate for the contract period. Other factors may be considered in adjusting the rates for renewal of insurance such as insurance industry trends or inflation.

prospective reimbursement See *prospective payment system (PPS).*

prospective review 1. Process of going over financial documents before billing is submitted to the insurance company to determine documentation deficiencies and errors. 2. Method of evaluating a case before admission to find out if hospitalization is necessary, the estimated length of stay, or alternate outpatient treatment.

prostate cancer screening test Procedure or test for the early detection of prostate cancer (e.g., digital rectal examination, prostate specific antigen [PSA] blood test).

prostate specific antigen (PSA) Blood test, detects marker for adenocarcinoma of the prostate.

prosthetics Design, construction, attachment, and use of artificial limbs or other substitutes to function for missing body parts.

protected health information (PHI) Under the Health Insurance Portability and Accountability Act (HIPAA), any data held by a covered entity or its business associate that identifies an individual and describes his or her health status, age, sex, ethnicity, or other demographical characteristics, whether or not that information is stored or transmitted electronically (see Box P-1). Additionally, PHI may include physician-patient interactions and conversations, physician-staff conversations, internal physician-physician conversations, external physician-physician conversations, staff-family communications, staff-staff conversations, physician dictation, and telephones in examination rooms.

Box P-1   PROTECTED HEALTH INFORMATION IN A MEDICAL OFFICE

Intake forms

Laboratory work requests

Physician-patient conversations

Conversations that refer to patients by name

Physician dictation tapes

Telephone conversations with patients

Encounter sheets

Physician's notes

Prescriptions

Insurance claim forms

X-rays

E-mail messages

Sometimes erroneously referred to as *private* health information or *personal* health information.

protocols See *clinical protocols.*

Prouty Word applied to women who are eligible for Social Security benefits based on federal legislation developed by Senator Prouty.

provider 1. Licensed physician or any qualified health care practitioner who provides health care services to the patient and is legally accountable for establishing patient diagnoses. If a medical doctor, the provider can be the attending, ordering, treating, performing, or referring physician. 2. Organization, institution, or individual that provides health care services to Medicare beneficiaries. Physicians, dentists, pharmacists, ambulatory surgical centers, home health care agencies, skilled nursing facilities, and outpatient clinics are some of the service providers covered under Medicare Part B. 3. In a 401(k) defined-contribution pension plan, a financial services company that offers the mutual funds and other investment choices.

provider complaint and grievance procedure Method the member of a managed care plan may use for the handling of dissatisfaction and unfair treatment against a provider.

provider contracting Process of negotiating and signing an agreement between a managed care plan and provider in which the provider agrees to give medical services to the plan's members.

provider customer service program (PCSP) Quality program that all Medicare contractors (fiscal intermediaries and regional carriers) are required to have. Contractors must have tools in place to assist physicians and their staff in understanding and complying with Medicare's operational processes, policies, and billing procedures.

provider directory Reference book for members of a managed care plan that alphabetically lists institutions, freestanding surgical centers, and providers who participate in the plan.

provider discounts Reduced fees for medical services that are negotiated with providers who participate in managed care programs.

provider excess Specific total stop loss coverage that is extended to a provider instead of a payer or employer.

provider fraud Type of medical insurance fraud that is committed by a provider on a patient's insurance claims so that he or she can obtain benefits in excess of their medical expenses. Also see *individual fraud* and *fraud*.

provider health plan See *provider-sponsored organization (PSO)*.

provider identification number (PIN) See *provider transaction access number (PTAN)*.

provider network 1. Groups of medical providers who give service to managed care plan members and deliver care inexpensively to control health care costs. 2. Providers with whom a Medicare+Choice organization contracts or makes arrangements with to furnish covered health care services to Medicare enrollees under a Medicare+Choice coordinated care or network medical savings account (MSA) plan.

provider number In Medicare fraud, to use another provider's Medicare number (e.g., a new physician who does not yet have a Medicare provider number and uses a provider number of another doctor to bill for services rendered until the new physician receives a provider number).

provider profiling See *economic credentialing*.

provider relations Department in an insurance company that helps providers solve claims problems and offers educational workshops about policies and procedures. Also called *provider services* or *relationship management*.

provider self-disclosure protocol Procedure that gives providers a chance to communicate any misconduct related to federal health care agencies whereby the provider may have lesser restitution than had the information not been revealed. Also called *voluntary disclosure protocol*.

provider services See *provider relations*.

provider-sponsored network (PSN) See *provider-sponsored organization (PSO)*.

provider-sponsored organization (PSO) Group of doctors, hospitals, and other health care providers that agree to give health care to Medicare beneficiaries for a set amount of money from Medicare every month. This type of managed care plan is run by the doctors and providers themselves and not by an insurance company. Also called *provider health plan* or *provider-sponsored network (PSN)*.

provider statistical and reimbursement (PS & R) report Document created by the facility that shows annual costs and expenses incurred in treating Medicare patients. Medicare gathers the reimbursement information from this report for Medicare services (e.g., ambulatory surgery, end-stage renal disease, laboratory, orthotics, outpatient diagnostic services, prosthetics, radiology). The Uniform Bill (UB-04) billing data must be accurate because it affects the facility's reimbursement received through the PS & R reporting system and cost-report settlement process.

provider-supplied information Manual claim information inserted in the bottom half of the CMS-1500 (08-05) claim form.

provider survey data Information collected through a survey or focus group of providers who participate in the Medicaid program and have provided services to enrolled Medicaid beneficiaries. The state or a contractor of the state may conduct the survey.

provider taxonomy codes See *taxonomy codes*.

provider telecommunications network (PTN) Automated voice-response system that allows the provider to use the telephone to obtain checkwrite, claim, and prior authorization information for services rendered through the Medi-Cal program and several other state programs.

provider tracking system (PTS) Method that identifies providers and follows all contacts made to correct problems (e.g., provider's eligibility, medical necessity issue, repeat billing abusers).

provider transaction access number (PTAN) Formerly known as *provider identification number (PIN)*. It is a carrier-assigned number that every facility, physician, clinic, or organization uses that renders services to patients when submitting insurance claims. It is issued to a provider by the insurance carrier or Medicare fiscal intermediary and allows the physician or patient to receive reimbursement for claims filed to the contractor. Also referred to as a *legacy number*. PINs have been replaced with the national provider identifiers (NPIs). See *national provider identifier (NPI)*.

provision Section of an insurance contract describing in detail a benefit, condition, feature, or requirement of the policy. Also called *clause, insurance clause,* or *insurance provision*.

provisional premium Premium requested by an insurance company for a type of policy that needs a premium adjustment. For example, a commercial property or liability insurance policy's final premium is determined at the end of the policy period based on an insured's loss experience and other factors.

provisional privileges Temporary or conditional rights that a physician is given at a medical facility for a specific length of time during which supervisors assess and validate his or her clinical performance.

proximate cause Legal term dealing with the concept of cause-and-effect relationships (e.g., would an injury have resulted from a particular accident?).

proximate cause of death Event(s) that are directly responsible for a person's demise.

proximate consequence Result that succeeds in the ordinary course of events. Also called *proximate result*.

proximate result See *proximate consequence*.

proxy Index of known values that likely approximates an index for which values are unavailable. The proxy is used as a stand-in for the unavailable index.

prudent expert rule Legal requirement that a manager of a pension plan have specific competence in accounting for assets and investing funds for the plan.

PSA See *prostate specific antigen (PSA)*.

PSAO See *pharmacy services administration organization (PSAO)*.

PSC See *program safeguard contractor (PSC)* and *potential fraud case (PFC)*.

PSN Acronym that means provider-sponsored network but is referred to as *provider-sponsored organization*. See *provider-sponsored organization (PSO)*.

PSO See *provider-sponsored organization (PSO)*.

PSPM Acronym that means per subscriber per month. See *per member per month (PMPM)*.

PSRO Acronym that means professional standards review organization. In 2003, called *Quality Improvement Organization (QIO) program*.

psychiatric counseling Interactive psychotherapy between provider and patient to understand, correct, or change communication, emotional, personality, or behavioral problems through a variety of methods. CPT codes from the Medicine Section, under Psychiatry, 90801-90899 are used for billing.

psychiatric facility Type of health care establishment for the diagnosis and treatment of mental illness on a 24-hour basis, by or under the supervision of a physician. Also see *partial hospitalization psychiatric facility*.

psychiatric information Handwritten, recorded, or transcribed typed data in the medical record that relate to a patient's psychiatric diagnosis and treatment and are kept as part of the patient's medical record.

psychiatric residential treatment center Health care facility or distinct part of a facility for care of patients exhibiting mental illness. The center provides a total 24-hour therapeutically planned and professionally staffed group living and learning environment.

psychiatrist Physician with additional medically qualified training and experience in the diagnosis, prevention, and treatment of mental and emotional disorders.

psychiatry Branch of medical science that deals with the causes, treatment, and prevention of mental, emotional, and behavioral disorders.

psychologist Licensed individual with a doctoral degree in psychology who specializes in the study of the structure and function of the brain and related mental processes of animals and humans. Two years of clinical experience in a health setting or meeting standards of the National Register of the Health Service Providers in Psychology is required. Also see *clinical psychologist*.

psychology 1. Study of behavior and of the functions and processes of the mind, especially as related to the social and physical environment. 2. Profession (clinical psychologist) that involves the practical applications of knowledge, skills, and techniques in the understanding of, prevention of, or solutions to individual or social problems, especially in regard to the interaction between the individual and the physical and social environment. 3. Mental, motivational, and behavioral characteristics and attitudes of an individual or group of individuals.

psychotherapy notes 1. Handwritten, recorded, or transcribed typed notes by a mental health clinician that document or analyze conversations between therapists and clients during individual, family, or group psychotherapy counseling sessions. These notes are retained separate and apart from the medical record. However, notes relative to therapy such as information shared in training in consultation with other clinicians, a summary of symptoms, a diagnosis, a treatment plan, or process of treatment are *not* psychotherapy notes and are known as *psychiatric information*. Billing for treatment of psychiatric disorders and psychotherapy falls under CPT codes 90804 through 90899 in the CPT Medicine Section. 2. Under the Health Insurance Portability and Accountability Act (HIPAA), notes recorded in any medium by a health care provider who is a mental health professional documenting or analyzing the contents of conversation during a private counseling session or a group, joint, or family counseling session and that are separated from the rest of the individual's medical record. Psychotherapy notes excludes medication prescription and monitoring, counseling session start and stop times, the modalities and frequencies of treatment furnished, results of clinical tests, and any summary of the following items: diagnosis, functional status, the treatment plan, symptoms, prognosis, and progress to date. Under HIPAA, a clinician is not required to disclose the original psychotherapy notes to the patient. Generally a summary of the notes is done to satisfy a patient's request.

pt See *patient (pt)*.

PT See *physical therapy (PT)* or *physical therapist (PT)*.

PTAN See *provider transaction access number (PTAN)*.

PTMPY Abbreviation that means per thousand members per year.

PTOS See *payment at time of service (PTOS)*.

PTS See *provider tracking system (PTS)*.

public health Science that deals with the protection and improvement of community health by organized community effort.

public health authority Under the Health Insurance Portability and Accountability Act (HIPAA), an agency or authority of the United States: a state; a territory; a political subdivision of a state, a territory, or an Indian tribe; or a person or entity acting under a grant of authority from or contract with such public agency including the employees or agents of such public agency or its contractors, persons, or entities to whom it has granted authority that is responsible for public health matters as part of its official mandate.

public health nurse (PHN) Registered nurse who works with families in the home, in schools, at the workplace, in government agencies, and at major health facilities. PHNs must complete a baccalaureate degree program approved by the National League for Nursing (NLN) or the American Association of Colleges of Nursing (AACN) for public health nursing preparation or after registered nurse study. A certification program sponsored by the Division of Community Health Nursing of the American Nurses Association is also available.

public use file Nonidentifiable data that are within the public domain.

pulmonary medicine Branch of medicine that relates to diseases of the respiratory system (i.e., lungs and aorta).

punitive damages Reimbursement (award by a court) for damages because of gross negligence in handling a claim by an insurance company.

purchase discount See *contractual allowance.*

purchase order Type of payment between two federal agencies.

purchased diagnostic test Test purchased from an outside supplier on behalf of the patient such as an electrocardiograph, x-ray, or ultrasound. The physician does not personally perform or supervise the test.

purchaser 1. Member of a managed care plan who pays the monthly insurance premium. 2. Managed care organization or insurance company that reimburses providers for the medical services that they provide ("purchase") for their members.

purchasing group See *alliance* and *consumer health alliances.*

pure endowment Life insurance policy in which the face value is paid only if the insured survives to the end of the stated endowment period; those who do not survive the endowment period receive nothing. Very few of these policies are sold.

pure premium See *pure premium rating method.*

pure premium rating method 1. Calculation of the cost of liability insurance protection without loadings for the insurance company's expenses, premium taxes, contingencies, and profit margins. 2. Average expected cost for insurance benefits.

pure risk Situation that involves a chance of a loss or no loss, with no chance of gain.

pursue and pay Phrase used to describe an insurance claim being processed for payment in which the coordination of benefits provision is investigated before the claim is paid.

pyramiding Situation in which a number of insurance policies that cover the same risk are in force. This results in higher limits of coverage than necessary for adequate insurance.

Q

Q2 HCPCS Level II modifier that may be used with CPT or HCPCS Level II codes indicating a service or procedure associated with a HCFA/ORD demonstration project.

Q3 HCPCS Level II modifier that may be used with CPT or HCPCS Level II codes indicating live kidney donor surgery and related services.

Q4 HCPCS Level II modifier that may be used with CPT or HCPCS Level II codes indicating a service for the ordering or referring physician that qualifies as a service exemption. The physician has a financial relationship with the entity performing the service that qualifies as one of the service-related exemptions.

Q5 HCPCS Level II modifier that may be used with CPT or HCPCS Level II codes indicating service furnished by a substitute physician under a reciprocal billing arrangement.

Q6 HCPCS Level II modifier that may be used with CPT or HCPCS Level II codes indicating a service furnished by a locum tenens physician.

Q7 HCPCS Level II modifier that may be used with CPT or HCPCS Level II codes indicating one class A finding on foot care procedures that indicates the severity of the patient's systemic condition without writing a narrative description. This is a nontraumatic amputation of foot or integral skeletal portions.

Q8 HCPCS Level II modifier that may be used with CPT or HCPCS Level II codes indicating two class B findings on foot care procedures that describe the severity of the patient's systemic condition without writing a narrative description. Class B findings: absent posterior tibial pulse, absent dorsalis pedis pulse, advanced trophic changes (i.e., hair growth [decrease, absence], nail changes [thickening], pigmentary changes [discoloration], skin texture [thin, shiny], and/or skin color [rubor, redness]).

Q9 HCPCS Level II modifier that may be used with CPT or HCPCS Level II codes indicating one class B and two class C findings on foot care procedures that describe the severity of the patient's systemic condition without writing a narrative description. Class C findings: claudication, temperature changes, edema, paresthesia, and burning.

QA 1. See *quality assurance (QA)*. 2. HCPCS Level II modifier that may be used with CPT or HCPCS Level II codes indicating Food and Drug Administration (FDA) investigational device exemption (IDE). The IDE project number must appear on the insurance claim form.

QARI See *Quality Assurance Reform Initiative (QARI)*.

QB HCPCS Level II modifier that was used with CPT or HCPCS Level II codes and indicated a physician provided a service in a rural health professional shortage area (HPSA). Modifier AQ, which became effective January 1, 2006, replaced the QU modifier.

QC HCPCS Level II modifier that may be used with CPT or HCPCS Level II codes indicating single channel monitoring.

QC Acronym that means quarters of coverage. See *credits, Social Security*.

QD HCPCS Level II modifier that may be used with CPT or HCPCS Level II codes indicating recording and storage in solid state memory by a digital recorder.

QDRO See *qualified domestic relations order (QDRO)*.

QE HCPCS Level II modifier that may be used with CPT or HCPCS Level II codes indicating the prescribed amount of oxygen is less than 1 L per minute (LPM). The Medicare allowed amount will decrease by 50%.

QF HCPCS Level II modifier that may be used with CPT or HCPCS Level II codes indicating the prescribed amount of oxygen exceeds 4 L per minute (LPM) and portable oxygen is prescribed. Monthly the Medicare allowed amount will increase by 50%.

QG HCPCS Level II modifier that may be used with CPT or HCPCS Level II codes indicating the prescribed amount of oxygen is greater than 4 L per minute (LPM).

QH HCPCS Level II modifier that may be used with CPT or HCPCS Level II codes indicating an oxygen-conserving device was used with an oxygen delivery system.

QHP See *qualified health care provider (QHP)*.

QI See *quality improvement (QI)*.

QI-1S See *qualifying individuals (1) (QI-1S)*.

QI-2S See *qualifying individuals (2) (QI-2S)*.

QIO See *Quality Improvement Organization (QIO) program*.

QISMC See *Quality Improvement System for Managed Care (QISMC)*.

QJ HCPCS Level II modifier that may be used with CPT or HCPCS Level II codes indicating services or items were provided to a prisoner or patient in state or local custody; however, the state or local government, as applicable, meets the requirements in 42 cfr 411.4 (b).

QJ&S See *qualified joint and survivor (QJ&S) annuity*.

QK HCPCS Level II modifier that may be used with CPT or HCPCS Level II codes indicating medical direction of two, three, or four concurrent anesthesia procedures involving qualified individuals.

QL HCPCS Level II modifier that may be used with CPT or HCPCS Level II codes indicating patient was pronounced dead after an ambulance was called.

QM 1. See *quality management (QM)*. 2. HCPCS Level II modifier that may be used with CPT or HCPCS Level II codes indicating an ambulance service was provided under arrangement by a provider of services. This modifier is payable under Medicare Part A but not Medicare Part B.

QMB See *qualified Medicare beneficiary (QMB)*.

QME See *qualified medical expense (QME)*.

QN HCPCS Level II modifier that may be used with CPT or HCPCS Level II codes indicating that a service provider directly furnished an ambulance service. This modifier is payable under Medicare Part A but not Medicare Part B.

QP HCPCS Level II modifier that may be used with CPT or HCPCS Level II codes indicating documentation is on file showing that the laboratory test(s) was ordered individually or ordered as a CPT-recognized panel other than automated profile codes 80002-80019, G0058, G0059, and G0060.

QQ HCPCS Level II modifier that may be used with CPT or HCPCS Level II codes indicating that a claim is being submitted with a written statement of intent (SOI).

QRR See *qualified rehabilitation representative (QRR)*.

QS HCPCS Level II modifier that may be used with CPT or HCPCS Level II codes indicating monitored anesthesia care service.

QT HCPCS Level II modifier that may be used with CPT or HCPCS Level II codes indicating recording and storage on tape by an analog tape recorder.

QU HCPCS Level II modifier that was used with CPT or HCPCS Level II codes and indicated a physician provided services in an urban health professional shortage area (HPSA). Modifier AQ, which became effective January 1, 2006, replaced the QU modifier.

qualification period Length of time that the insured must be totally disabled to be eligible for residual disability insurance benefits.

qualified annuity Type of annuity funded with money that is deductible, up to a maximum amount, from the depositor's gross income in the year that funds are deposited.

qualified domestic relations order (QDRO) Legal settlement that assigns all or a part of an individual's pension benefits to someone else (former spouse) for alimony, child support, or marital property rights.

qualified health care provider (QHP) Individual such as midwife, nurse practitioner, physician assistant, physician, and psychiatric clinical nurse specialist who may certify as to the inability of an individual to perform his or her regular or customary work due to

sickness under the state temporary disability insurance program in Rhode Island.

qualified injured worker In workers' compensation cases, an injured worker entitled to receive vocational rehabilitation services because the injury prevents return to his or her usual occupation or the job performed at the time of the injury. Thus the injured worker is considered medically eligible because he or she is expected to return to employment after undergoing vocational rehabilitation services.

qualified joint and survivor (QJ&S) annuity Qualified annuity plan that provides for pension benefits to a spouse of the retired plan participant after his or her death.

qualified medical evaluator (QME) Physician who has been appointed and certified by the Industrial Medical Council (IMC) and conducts medicolegal evaluations of injured workers in workers' compensation cases for insurance companies or workers' compensation appeals board. QMEs render an unbiased opinion about the degree of disability of an injured worker. May be referred to as *independent medical evaluator (IME)* or *agreed medical evaluator (AME)*.

qualified medical expense (QME) Medical expense that is primarily to alleviate or prevent a physical or mental defect or illness. This is defined by the Internal Revenue Service Code Section 213(d). Qualified medical expenses include medical, dental, and vision care deductibles, copayments, and coinsurance. Out-of-pocket costs not reimbursed by insurance (amounts above what insurance pays or amounts in excess of reasonable and customary charges). Expenses not covered by a health care policy (routine physical examinations or well-baby visits). Any other out-of-pocket medical expenses that are considered eligible as a tax deduction for federal income tax purposes.

qualified Medicare beneficiary (QMB) Medicaid program for beneficiaries who need help in paying for Medicare services. The beneficiary must have Medicare Part A and limited income and resources. For those who qualify, the Medicaid program pays Medicare Part A premiums, Part B premiums, and Medicare deductibles and coinsurance amounts for Medicare services.

qualified pension plan Retirement plan that conforms to the regulations contained in Section 401(a) of the Internal Revenue Code. It is established and maintained by an employer to provide for benefits to employees over a period of years after retirement. Qualified plans are approved by the Internal Revenue Service. The employer's contributions are considered a deduction in determining the employer's taxable income, not considered as employee earnings, and not taxable to the employee. Earnings of the pension plan are not subject to income tax.

qualified rehabilitation representative (QRR) In workers' compensation, a trained rehabilitation consultant who meets established criteria to administer vocational rehabilitation counseling and benefits to employees who have been injured at work.

qualified sick-pay plan Type of disability income insurance that gives benefits to employees when they are unable to work because of injury or illness that is not work related.

qualifying circumstances Particularly difficult situations such as extreme age, complication of total body hypothermia, controlled hypotension, or emergency condition for which a CPT add-on code (99100, 99116, 99135, or 99140) is used when an anesthesia service is provided.

qualifying individuals (1) (QI-1S) Medicaid program for beneficiaries who need help in paying for Medicare Part B premiums. The beneficiary must have Medicare Part A and limited income and resources and not be otherwise eligible for Medicaid. For those who qualify, the Medicaid program pays full Medicare Part B premiums only.

qualifying individuals (2) (QI-2S) Medicaid program for beneficiaries who need help in paying for Medicare Part B premiums. The beneficiary must have Medicare Part A and limited income and resources and not be otherwise eligible for Medicaid. For those who qualify, Medicaid pays a percentage of Medicare Part B premiums only.

qualitative Measuring the presence or absence of.

qualitative analysis Referring to a test that determines the presence of an agent within the body.

quality 1. For health plans, the general standard or grade of how well a plan keeps its members healthy or treats them when they are sick. Good-quality health care means doing the right thing at the right time, in the right way, for the right person, and getting the best possible results. 2. As defined by the Institute of Medicine, the degree to which health services for individuals and populations increase the likelihood of desired outcomes and are consistent with current professional knowledge. 3. Highest degree to which a product or service meets needs and expectations.

quality assurance (QA) 1. Process or activity of evaluating how well a medical service is provided. Now called *quality improvement (QI)*. This process may include formally reviewing health care given to a person or a group of persons, locating the problem, correcting the problem, and checking to see if the action taken worked or not. 2. Formal set of quality improvement organization (QIO) activities (formerly peer review organization [PRO]) designed to ensure the quality of medical services provided. See *quality improvement (QI)*.

quality assurance program Plan that continually assesses the effectiveness of inpatient and outpatient health care in managed care plans and federal programs such as TRICARE and CHAMPVA. Also see *quality assurance (QA)* and *quality improvement (QI)*.

Quality Assurance Reform Initiative (QARI) Created in 1993 by the Health Care Financing Administration to assist states in promoting a health care quality improvement system for Medicaid managed care plans.

quality compass Product developed by the National Committee for Quality Assurance (NCQA) that contains commercial, national, regional, and state averages and percentiles. The program contains information from all HEDIS (Health Plan Employer Data and Information Set) measures including utilization data in the Use of Services domain, as well as some selected consumer assessment of health plans survey (CAHPS) rates for plans publicly releasing data. Data are available for purchase in an online format.

quality improvement (QI) Programs to promote quality of health care such as peer review components to find and solve deficiencies in quality and assessment of effectiveness. Formerly known as *quality assurance (QA)*. Also referred to as *performance improvement (PI)* and *continuous performance improvement (CPI)*.

Quality Improvement Organization (QIO) program Program formerly known as *Utilization and Quality Control Peer Review Organization (PRO)* that is designed to review cases to determine appropriateness, medical necessity, and quality of care for Medicare beneficiaries. It consists of groups of practicing doctors and other health care experts. They are paid by the federal government to check and improve the care given to Medicare patients. They must review the patients' complaints about the quality of care given by inpatient hospitals, hospital outpatient departments, hospital emergency departments, skilled nursing facilities, home health agencies, private fee-for-service plans, and ambulatory surgical centers.

Quality Improvement System for Managed Care (QISMC) Centers for Medicare and Medicaid Services (CMS) program for health plans that participate in Medicare+Choice. This program features medical care quality measurement, reporting, and improvement requirements to improve health and satisfy Medicare and Medicaid recipients.

quality management (QM) Process to determine the quality of medical care, develop and monitor a standard of quality, introduce improvements, and maintain a desired level of excellence. Also referred to as *quality program, performance improvement program,* or *performance management program.*

quality of care Evaluation of health care services that meet established professional standards and judgments of value to the patient.

quality of life 1. Measure of the best possible energy that endows a person with the power to cope successfully with the full range of challenges faced in the real world such as personal security, degree of independence, and self-sufficient decision-making.

Q

2. Individual's expressed satisfaction with the current life situation.

quality program See *quality management (QM)*.

quality review organization (QRO) Group of practicing physicians and other health care practitioners who are under contract to the federal government to review medical care given to Medicare patients enrolled as members in managed care plans (e.g., health maintenance organizations [HMOs] and competitive medical plans [CMPs]).

quantitative Measuring the presence or absence and amount of.

quantitative analysis Referring to a test that determines the amount or percentage of an agent that is present within the body.

quantity limits (QL) Phrase related to prescription drug insurance plans indicating restriction of the amount of medication for which the Medicare beneficiary can obtain benefits during a specific period of time (most often set on a monthly basis).

quarters of coverage (QC) See *credits, Social Security*.

query Request from an insurance company for additional information about a patient.

questionable covered procedures Under the Medicare program, medical procedures that may be a benefit depending on the medical situation. When a procedure listed in Medicare's Outpatient Code Editor is billed, the insurance company must conduct a medical review of the claim to make a decision on payment. Formerly called *development needed procedures*.

qui tam **action** Action to recover a penalty, brought by an informer in a situation in which one portion of the recovery goes to the informer and the other portion to the state or government. Also see *qui tam provision* and *whistleblower*.

qui tam **provision** Federal statute of the False Claims Act that allows any person having knowledge of a false claim against the government to bring an action against the suspected wrongdoer on behalf of the U.S. government. A person who files a *qui tam* suit on behalf of the government is known as a "relator" and may share a percentage of the recovery realized from a successful action. Also referred to as "whistleblower." Also see *whistleblower*.

quinquennial military service determination and adjustments Estimates made once every 5 years of the costs arising from the granting of deemed wage credits for military service before 1957; annual reimbursements were made from the general fund of the U.S. Treasury to the health insurance (HI) trust fund for these costs. The Social Security Amendments of 1983 provided for (1) a lump-sum transfer in 1983 for (a) the costs arising from the pre-1957 wage credits and (b) amounts equivalent to the HI taxes that would have been paid on the deemed wage credits for military service for 1966 through 1983, inclusive, if such credits had been counted as covered earnings; (2) quinquennial adjustments to the pre-1957 portion of the 1983 lump-sum transfer; (3) general fund transfers equivalent to HI taxes on military deemed wage credits for 1984 and later, to be credited to the fund on July 1 of each year; and (4) adjustments as deemed necessary to any previously transferred amounts representing HI taxes on military deemed wage credits.

quota share reinsurance plan Automatic reinsurance plan wherein the assuming company reinsures a given percentage of certain types of risk that are insured by the ceding company.

quotation See *proposal*.

quote See *proposal*.

QV HCPCS Level II modifier that may be used with CPT or HCPCS Level II codes indicating an item or service provided as routine care in a Medicare-qualifying clinical trial. To be reported using ICD-9-CM diagnostic code V70.7 as the primary diagnosis for CMA-1500 claims and as a secondary diagnosis for Uniform Bill (UB-04) claims.

QW HCPCS Level II modifier that may be used with CPT or HCPCS Level II codes indicating a clinical laboratory improvement amendment (CLIA) waived test.

QX HCPCS Level II modifier that may be used with CPT or HCPCS Level II codes indicating a certified registered nurse anesthetist (CRNA) service with medical direction by a physician. Payment is up to 55% of the amount that would have been allowed if personally done by a physician.

QY HCPCS Level II modifier that may be used with CPT or HCPCS Level II codes indicating medical direction of one certified registered nurse anesthetist (CRNA) by an anesthesiologist.

QZ HCPCS Level II modifier that may be used with CPT or HCPCS Level II codes indicating a certified registered nurse anesthetist (CRNA) service without medical direction by a physician.

R

RA See *remittance advice (RA)*.

RAA See *retained asset account (RAA)*.

rabbi trust Legal document that was named by an Internal Revenue Service ruling that involved a trust created by a Jewish congregation on behalf of its rabbi. Such trusts require the employer to make contributions to the trust that are irrevocable. The trust is managed by an independent trustee who pays benefits in the event of death, disability, or retirement of the employee. The employer is not allowed to take tax deductions for its contributions to the trust until funds are actually distributed to the employee.

RAC See *recovery audit contractor (RAC)*.

radiation therapy Treatment of diseases and injuries using radioactive substances.

radiologist Doctor of Medicine who specializes in radiology and is concerned with the diagnostic and/or therapeutic use of x-rays and other imaging technologies.

radiology Branch of medicine that deals with radioactive substances and is concerned with the diagnosis and treatment of disease and injury by visualizing any of the various sources of radiant energy.

radiology including nuclear medicine and diagnostic ultrasound section Division of the *Current Procedural Terminology (CPT)* code book that contains information about radiographic, nuclear medicine, and diagnostic ultrasound procedures.

radiology report Written or dictated document of the findings after radiological films have been taken of an individual's body part or organ. Also referred to as *x-ray report*.

radiology services Three branches of radiology services include diagnostic radiology, which is imaging using external sources of radiation or no radiation; nuclear medicine, which is imaging radioactive materials that are placed in body organs; and therapeutic radiology, which is the treatment of cancer using radiation.

radionuclides Isotope that undergoes radioactive decay and is used for nuclear imaging or scanning and treating tumors and cancer.

RAI See *Resident Assessment Instrument (RAI)*.

Railroad Retirement Board (RRB) Organization that oversees and investigates medical insurance issues affecting Medicare Railroad Retirement beneficiaries. These individuals are entitled to Part A and/or Part B coverage based on the Railroad Retirement Act.

Railroad Retirement (RR) program Federal insurance program similar to Social Security designed for workers in the railroad industry. The provisions of the Railroad Retirement Act provide for a system of coordination and financial interchange between the Railroad Retirement program and the Social Security program.

random access memory (RAM) Allows data to be stored randomly and retrieved directly by specifying the address location.

random internal audit Type of audit of hospital patient records that occurs continually to verify charges in which blind charts are pulled and examined to maintain quality control. Also see *audit by request* and *defense audit*.

random sample Group of cases selected for study, which is drawn indiscriminately from the universe of cases by a statistically valid method.

RAP See *request for anticipated payment (RAP)*.

rate Price or cost of insurance per unit that is used as a means for determination of a premium amount.

rate making Establishing premium rates for an insurance company's policies by using a formula. In life insurance, important factors considered are mortality rates, interest rates, and loading.

rate method System used to bill for group health insurance based on type of contract or age/sex breaks.

rate of return method System of comparing costs of life insurance policies by using the following formula: 1. Determine pure cost of protection (mortality expectation). 2. Calculate amount of dividends paid. 3. Subtract the pure cost of protection plus dividends from the gross premiums paid into the policy (savings element). 4. Rate of return equals the interest rate at which the savings element must be accumulated to equal the cash value of the policy at a future specific time period. Also called *Linton yield method*.

rate request To ask for a set of insurance rates that are based on a specific list of benefits.

rate restriction System in health insurance for establishing premiums so that an insurance company's premium varies by not more than a fixed amount from other premiums for individuals in the same premium class within a certain geographical region.

rate review Advance evaluation of a health care facility's financial data by a government or private agency to determine the reasonableness of the hospital fees and assess a possible increase in the fees.

rate setting 1. System used to contain health care costs in which the government sets payment fees for all insurance payers for categories of medical services. 2. In the Medicare program, to determine and establish the cost of medical professional services provided to a patient by using historical cost data reported by providers.

rate stabilization reserve If a specific account's actual experience at the close of an insurance contract period results in excess funds, these can be applied toward the account's rate for the next year, which helps offset the rate increase.

rated policy Insurance contract issued to an individual in a greater-than-average likelihood of loss classification such as impaired health or a hazardous occupation. This type of policy may have an exclusion clause and/or higher premium rate than a standard policy. Sometimes called an *extra-risk policy*.

rating 1. Determining the value of risk of an individual or organization. 2. Establishing a year's cost of a specific unit of insurance.

rating classes Rate applied to risks of similar characteristics or a specific class of risk. For group life insurance the three rating classes for group premiums are (1) manually rated premiums, (2) experience-rated premiums, and (3) blended premiums. See also *blended rates, experience rating*, and *manual rate*.

rating manual Insurance handbook that includes suggested ratings and background information for each impairment shown.

rating period Time during which a set of health insurance rates is guaranteed.

RBNI See *reported but not incurred (RBNI)*.

RBRVS See *resource-based relative value scale (RBRVS)*.

RBRVU See *resource-based relative value unit (RBRVU)*.

RBS See *report of benefit savings (RBS)*.

RC HCPCS Level II modifier that may be used with CPT or HCPCS Level II codes indicating a specific vessel (right coronary artery) in a stent placement, balloon angioplasty, and/or atherectomy.

RD HCPCS Level II modifier that may be used with CPT or HCPCS Level II codes indicating drug given to beneficiary but not administered "incident-to."

read-only memory (ROM) Data stored in ROM can be read but not changed. It usually contains a permanent program.

readabililty standards Required criteria that insurance policies contain basic easy-to-understand English so that the average consumer can comprehend the meaning. A formula is used to determine the level of readability.

readmission review Review of patients readmitted to a hospital within 7 days with problems related to the first admission, to determine whether the first discharge was premature and/or the second admission is medically necessary.

real mother See *birth mother* and *biological mother*.

real time 1. Insurance claim processing that occurs immediately as opposed to batch processing (e.g., electronic claims transmission). 2. Immediate imaging to show movements.

real-wage differential Difference between the percentage increases before rounding in the average annual wage in covered employment and the average annual consumer price index (CPI).

reasonable accommodation In workers' compensation cases, any job adjustment or work environment modification that assists a disabled employee to perform essential job duties.

reasonable and customary See *usual, customary, and reasonable (UCR)*.

reasonable care See *due care*.

reasonable charge See *reasonable fee*.

reasonable cost Actual dollar amount of providing medical services or hospital services including direct and indirect costs to Medicare patients. Fiscal intermediaries and insurance carriers use the Centers for Medicare and Medicaid Services (CMS) guidelines to determine reasonable costs incurred by individual providers in furnishing covered services to enrollees.

reasonable cost basis Calculation to determine the reasonable cost incurred by individual providers when furnishing covered services to beneficiaries. Reasonable cost is based on the actual cost of providing such services including direct and indirect costs of providers, excluding any costs that are unnecessary in the efficient delivery of services covered by a health insurance program.

reasonable cost methodology System used by Medicare fiscal intermediaries under established guidelines from the Centers for Medicare and Medicaid Services (CMS) to find the reasonable cost incurred by the provider when rendering services to a Medicare patient. These guidelines try to exclude unnecessary medical costs.

reasonable-expectation doctrine See *doctrine of reasonable expectations*.

reasonable fee Amount on which payment is based for participating physicians in the Medicare program; a charge is considered reasonable if it is deemed acceptable after peer review even though it does not meet the *customary* or *prevailing* criteria. This would include unusual circumstances or complications requiring additional time, skill, or experience in connection with a particular service or procedure.

reasonable medical probability Legal phase used when proving the cause of an injury that means the injury was more likely than not caused by a certain agent or factor.

reauthorization Permission to extend an inpatient hospital stay beyond the number of days originally approved.

rebating See *antirebate law*.

rebill To send another request for payment for an overdue bill to either the insurance company or patient.

rebundling Procedure by an insurance company to regroup medical services that have been billed erroneously under different codes.

rebuttable presumptions In workers' compensation, this legal phrase exists for each case meaning that specific conditions are work related for certain groups of workers; thus the employer must prove the condition was not caused by work or the injury will be compensable.

recanvass See *resolicitation.*

receipt Document completed and given to a patient when the patient pays cash for professional services.

receivables See *accounts receivable (AR).*

receptionist Medical office employee who greets patients and obtains personal and financial information for the medical practice.

recertification 1. Renewal of certification after a specified time. 2. For home health plan recertification, physician receives, reviews, adjusts treatment; documents the plan in coordination with the care of the home health agency; and then bills for this subsequent plan adjustment. For initial certification, see *home health plan certification.*

recidivism Tendency of a patient to have a relapse or return to inpatient hospitalization with the same medical problem.

recipient 1. Person certified by the local welfare department to receive the benefits of Medicaid under one of the specific aid categories. Also referred to as a *client.* 2. Individual certified to receive Medicare benefits. Also referred to as a *beneficiary, dependents, enrollee, member, participant,* or *subscriber.*

reciprocity 1. Mutual exchange of privileges or services. 2. In the Medicaid program, it applies to an individual who obtains medical services while out of the state in which he or she receives benefits. 3. In managed care plans, a member may receive treatment for illness or injuries from another prepaid plan while out of state.

recon See *reconsideration (recon).*

reconsideration (recon) 1. In the Medicare program, after payment or denial of an insurance claim, this is the second level of appeal. 2. First level of appeal process for an individual applying for SSDI or SSI. It is a complete review of the claim by a medical or psychological consultant/disability examiner team who did not take part in the original disability determination.

reconstructive surgery Plastic surgery performed to improve physical function and lessen disfigurement from an accident or injury, birth defect, burn, or disease. Difference between reconstructive surgery and cosmetic surgery is that the latter is considered elective and done for aesthetic reasons. See *cosmetic surgery.*

record card See *register.*

records retention Keeping medical records based on state and/or federal statutes. The federal minimum for records retention is at least 6 years after the patient is last seen. Each state has different laws but usually mandate longer than 6 years. State law has more authority than federal statutes. The American Health Information Management Association (AHIMA) recommends retaining medical records for 10 years after the date the patient was last seen regardless of whether the state regulation says 7 to 10 years. Records of children must be kept a certain amount of time after the patient becomes an adult, which can be anywhere from age 18 to 21 depending on the state law.

recoupment Recovery by Medicare of any Medicare debt by reducing present or future Medicare payments and applying the amount withheld to the indebtedness.

recovery audit contractor (RAC) Demonstration project developed from the Medicare Prescription Drug Improvement and Modernization Act. States that participated in this project for three years (2006-2008) have been California, Florida, and New York.

recovery of funds Monies obtained from a successful judgment, settlement, erroneous, or conditional payment. Also called *recovery of money.*

recurrence In workers' compensation cases, refers to symptoms that occur or may have been expected to occur of a previous industrial injury or illness without relationship to the current employment. This would not constitute a new injury.

recurrent disability clause Provision in an insurance policy that details the benefits payable if an insured becomes disabled again by the same illness or condition when benefits previously were paid.

recurring claim provision See *recurring clause.*

recurring clause Provision in a health insurance policy that states the time period that must elapse between a prior illness and a current one. Benefits might be available if the current illness occurs beyond the elapsed time period. Also called *recurring claim provision.*

recurring outpatient services See *repetitive outpatient services.*

redacted Identifying information replaced with _____ or XXX, or blacked out with a permanent marker throughout a patient's medical documentation such as patient's name, Social Security number, insurance number, city, facility's name, or physician's name.

redetermination process In the Medicare program, this was formerly referred to as the *appeal process.* If a patient disagrees with any decision about health care services or if Medicare does not pay for an item or service, the initial Medicare decision may be reviewed again using this process. It has five levels: (1) redetermination (telephone, letter, or CMS-20027 form); (2) hearing officer (HO) hearing or reconsideration; (3) administrative law judge (ALJ) hearing; (4) Departmental Appeal Board review; and (5) judicial review in U.S. District Court.

redlining Civil rights issue wherein an insurance company denies coverage to questionable or high risks in a given geographical area.

reduced paid-up insurance option See *nonforfeiture reduced paid-up benefit.*

reduction See *fracture manipulation.*

R

reduction formula Provision in an insurance policy that reduces the level of life insurance to another amount of coverage. This situation can occur when the insured reaches a specific age or retires.

reenroll Inactive membership in an insurance plan that is reestablished using the same subscriber identification number and may be in the same group or a new group.

referenced diagnostic laboratory services Diagnostic laboratory tests performed on samples that are referred to the hospital laboratory.

referral 1. Transfer of the total or specific care of a patient from one physician to another. 2. In managed care, a request by the primary care physician for authorization for a member to receive care from a specialist or hospital or get certain services. In some managed care plans, a member may need an approval from the primary care physician to a specialist for insurance coverage. 3. Document obtained from a provider or plan-approved caregiver so that a plan enrollee may receive additional medical services from a specific place/person.

referral authorization Verbal or formal written document that gives approval to a managed care plan member to obtain medical services outside of the network of participating providers (e.g., primary care physician approves a plan member to see a specialist).

referral center Telephone service staffed by nonclinical personnel that directs patients to approved hospital facilities and physicians and may also perform triage. Managed care plans use these call centers to communicate with patients and providers and sometimes to precertify or preapprove care. Usually the center has a toll-free 800 number for easy access and no charge to health plan members. Also known as *call center, 24-hour certification,* or *triage.*

referral pool Funds put aside for noncapitated medical services given by a primary care physician (PCP), referral specialist, or emergency services.

referral provider See *gatekeeper.*

referral services Any specialty, inpatient, outpatient, or laboratory services that are ordered or arranged but not furnished directly. Certain situations may exist that should be considered referral services for purposes of determining if a physician/group is at substantial financial risk (see Box R-1).

referred outpatient Patient who is sent from a physician to a diagnostic or therapeutic outpatient facility or to a specific hospital outpatient department for the diagnosis and treatment of an illness or injury.

referring physician 1. Doctor who sends the patient for testing or treatment noted on the insurance claim when submitted by the physician performing the service. 2. When completing the CMS-1500, the referring physician's complete name and degree is inserted in Block 17 and his or her national provider identifier (NPI) is placed in Block 17a of the paper claim form.

Box R-1   REFERRAL SERVICES

Example 1: A managed care organization (MCO) may require a physician group/physician to authorize retroactive referral for emergency care received outside the MCO's network. If the physician group/physician's payment from the MCO can be affected by the use of emergency care such as a bonus if emergency referrals are low, then these emergency services are considered services and must be included in the calculation of substantial financial risk.

Example 2: If a physician group contracts with an individual physician or another group to provide services that the initial group cannot provide itself, any services referred to the contracted physician group/physician should be considered referral services.

---

refund Money returned by an insurance company to a group or individual.

refund annuity Type of annuity that gives back premiums plus interest to a beneficiary if the annuitant dies during the accumulation period.

refund life income option See *life income option with refund.*

Regenstrief Institute Internationally recognized informatics and health care research organization dedicated to the improvement of health through research that enhances the quality and cost-effectiveness of health care. The institute offers education and training opportunities in academic and research careers. It maintains the logical observation identifiers, names, and codes (LOINC) system that is being considered for use as part of the HIPAA claim attachments standard.

regional health alliances See *consumer health alliances.*

regional health information organization (RHIO) Health information organization that brings together health care associations in a specific geographical area and governs health information exchange between them to improve health and care in that community.

regional home health intermediary (RHHI) Four national Medicare fiscal intermediaries contracted to process Medicare home health and hospice claims, audit home health physicians, and check on the quality of home health care. Also called *contractor.*

regional medical center Location where comprehensive medical services are provided to serve a large area. Not a tertiary care center.

regional office (RO) 1. Social Security state office. 2. Centers for Medicare and Medicaid Services (CMS) has 10 ROs that work closely together with Medicare contractors in their assigned geographical areas on a day-to-day basis. Four of these ROs monitor network contractor performance, negotiate contractor budgets, distribute administrative monies to contractors, work with contractors when corrective actions are needed, and provide a variety of other liaison services to the contractors in their respective regions.

register Electronic data file used by the insurance company or administrator of a group insurance plan that lists the insured, insurance coverage, amounts of insurance, beneficiary, and other information. Also called *record card* or *insurance register*.

Registered Health Information Administrator (RHIA) American Health Information Management Association (AHIMA) certification describing medical record administrators; formerly known as *registered records administrator (RRA)*.

Registered Health Information Technician (RHIT) American Health Information Management Association (AHIMA) certification describing medical records practitioners; formerly known as *accredited records technician (ART)*.

Registered Medical Assistant (RMA) Professional title earned by completing appropriate training and by passing a registry examination administered by the American Medical Technologists (AMT). Education places emphasis on administrative and clinical procedures performed in a medical office.

Registered Medical Coder (RMC) Professional title awarded after completion of coursework given by the Medical Management Institute (MMI) with recertification requirements.

registered nurse (RN) Individual who has graduated from a course of study at a state-approved school of nursing, passed the National Council Licensure Examination (NCLEX-RN), and been licensed by appropriate state authority. RNs are the most highly educated of nurses with the widest scope of responsibility including, at least potentially, all aspects of nursing care. RNs work in a variety of settings (e.g., hospital facilities, medical offices and clinics, public health departments, schools).

registration Entry in an official registry or record that lists names of persons in an occupation who have satisfied specific requirements or attained a certain level of education and paid a registration fee.

regulation Rule or guideline published by the federal government and administrative agencies implementing a law.

rehab See *rehabilitation (rehab)*.

rehabilitation (rehab) Restoring an individual or part of the body to normal or almost normal function after a disease, injury, addiction, or incarceration (e.g., working with a physical therapist to walk better or with an occupational therapist to get dressed). Rehabilitation services are ordered by the attending physician for the patient. These services are given by nurses and physical, occupational, and speech therapists. Also referred to as *rehabilitation care*.

rehabilitation care See *rehabilitation (rehab)*.

rehabilitation center Facility that provides treatment, training, and assists in restoring an individual who is disabled to maximum independence and productivity. It may offer occupational therapy, physical therapy, speech therapy, and vocational therapy.

rehabilitation facility See *rehabilitation hospital* or *rehabilitation center*.

rehabilitation hospital Institution or facility that gives health-related services to disabled individuals such as rehabilitative services and social or vocational services to help him or her obtain maximum function. For example, some conditions might be amputation, brain or spinal cord injuries, neurological disorders, and stroke. Also called *rehabilitation facility*.

reimbursement 1. Payment made because of accident or illness by an insurance company to a provider or facility that rendered medical services to patients covered by a managed care plan or insurance contract. 2. Repayment. 3. Term used when insurance payment is pending. Also known as *payment*.

reimbursement decision tree Billing tool used for choosing the action to take after receiving an explanation of benefits document from a third-party payer.

reimbursement manager Individual who designs systems to assure generation of accurate clinical documentation to substantiate billing and develops and puts into action systems to assure the secure transmission of data to billing centers, clearinghouses, or third-party payers.

reimbursement specialist See *insurance billing specialist*.

reinstate To place an insurance policy in force again without any probationary period that has lapsed or terminated.

reinstated benefits Insurance policy that restores the lifetime maximum according to a specified schedule during periods when the insured is not drawing benefits.

reinstatement To restore an insured to an active status that has been canceled for insurance coverage. This may be with or without continuation of medical benefits. Also see *automatic reinstatement clause*.

reinstatement provision Clause in an insurance agreement that describes the conditions an insured must meet for the insurance company to restore the policy if it is terminated because of nonpayment of a renewal premium.

reinsurance 1. Insurance agreement in which an insurance company pays a premium into a pool fund and any insurance claims paid by the insurer above a specific dollar amount are covered partially or totally by the pool. 2. Practice of one insurance company purchasing insurance from a second company for the purpose of protecting itself against part or all of the losses it might incur in the process of honoring the claims of its policyholders (e.g., catastrophic care). The original company is called the *ceding company;* the second is the *assuming company* or *reinsurer.* Reinsurance may be sought by the ceding company to protect itself against losses in individual cases beyond a certain amount, where competition requires it to offer policies providing coverage in excess of these amounts; to offer protection against catastrophic losses in a certain line of insurance such as aviation accident; or to protect against mistakes in rating and underwriting in entering a new line of insurance such as major medical. Also called *risk-control insurance* or *stop-loss insurance.*

reinsurance treaty Insurance agreement between a reinsurer and a ceding company that states the way the insurance on many different risks is to be shared.

reinsurer Insurance company that accepts all or part of an insurance policy from the primary insurance company. Also called *assuming company.*

reject status Insurance claim encounter data that did not pass the front-end edit process and the data need to be corrected and resubmitted.

rejected claim Insurance claim submitted to insurance carrier that is discarded by the system due to a technical error (omission of erroneous information) or because it does not follow Medicare instructions. It is returned to the provider for correction or change so that it may be processed properly for payment. It cannot be appealed. Also called *soft denial.*

rejection 1. Refusal by an insurance company to insure an applicant. 2. Refusal by an insurance company to pay an insurance claim. This can occur when a medical service is not a benefit of the health insurance plan.

related cases Clinical cases that have medical procedures with the same diagnosis, same operative area, and same indication.

relation of earnings to insurance clause Provision in some policies that limits the amount of benefits in which the insurance company will participate when the total amount of disability benefits from all insurers is beyond the insured's usual earnings. Also known as *participation limit.*

relationship code Code that identifies the gender and association of a member to the subscriber.

relationship management See *provider relations.*

relative value scale (RVS) See *relative value studies (RVS).*

relative value studies (RVS) Compiled list of particular rating or rank of medical services based on the intensity of the procedure performed. Each professional service listed by procedure code is given a relative value unit (RVU) and that is multiplied by a dollar conversion factor to show the monetary value for each procedure. The study becomes a fee schedule when dollar conversion factors are applied. RVS is published as a guide book to show the relative value of one procedure over another. Also called *relative value scale (RVS).*

relative value unit (RVU) Monetary value assigned to each service based on the amount of physician work, practice expenses, and the cost of professional liability insurance. These three RVUs are then adjusted according to geographical area and used in a formula to determine Medicare fees.

relative weight (RW) Assigned weight calculated by the Centers for Medicare and Medicaid Services (CMS) that reflects the resource consumption of each diagnosis-related group (DRG). The higher the relative weight, the larger the payment to the facility. Relative weights are published in the final prospective payment system rule.

relative weighted product (RWP) Measure used in health care cost accounting and data analysis that links the amount of personnel time, medical resources, and cost to care for a diagnosis-related group (DRG). If the RWP is higher, then more hospital resources are needed to care for that disease or injury. Also called *ambulatory weighted unit.*

relative work value (RWV) Monetary dollar amount that indicates the average work of a physician of average efficiency relative to a given standard.

relator Person who files a *qui tam* suit on behalf of the U.S. government. See *qui tam action, qui tam provision,* and *whistleblower.*

release of information (ROI) To disclose a patient's protected health information (PHI). See *authorization form* and *consent form* for mandates required by the Health Insurance Portability and Accountability Act (HIPAA).

reliable information Data that include truthful written or oral allegations or other material facts that might cause a noninterested third party to think there is reason to believe a specific set of data exists (e.g., false claims submitted for noncovered or miscoded services).

remittance advice (RA) Document detailing services billed and describing payment determination (paid or denied) for one or more beneficiaries issued to providers of managed care or federal programs (Medicare or Medicaid) for a specific payment period; formerly known as *Explanation of Medicare Benefits (EOMB).* Sometimes a payment check is attached to the form. Also known in some programs as an *explanation of benefits, remittance notice,* or *standard paper remittance (SPR).*

remittance advice details (RAD) Document that accompanies all Medi-Cal payment vouchers (checks) sent to providers of medical services.

remittance notice See *remittance advice (RA).*

remuneration Act of paying or compensating for medical services given to a patient.

renal transplant center Hospital unit that is approved to furnish transplantation and other medical and surgical specialty services directly for the care of end-stage renal disease (ESRD) transplant patients including inpatient dialysis furnished directly or under arrangement.

renewable and convertible term insurance Type of life insurance that offers the insured the option to renew the coverage at the end of the term period and the option to convert to a permanent basis.

renewable at company option Provision in an insurance policy that gives the insurance company the right to stop insuring the individual. If the insured is receiving benefits under the policy, he or she cannot be cut off in the midst of an illness or accident.

renewable term insurance Type of life insurance under which the insured has the right to continue the insurance for another term of the same length without submitting evidence of insurability. Premium rates increase at each renewal as the age of the insured increases.

renewal Automatic continuance of an insurance policy for a specific time period by payment of the premium for a new policy term.

renewal commissions Commissions paid to the insurance agent for a specific number of years after the first policy year and are only for those policies that remain in force.

renewal date Month, day, and year when an insurance policy must be reestablished for another time period. Insurance rates may possibly be increased. An option is to obtain other coverage or decrease insurance benefits.

renewal premiums Monthly, semiannual, or annual premium payment after the initial premium has been paid.

renewal provision Clause in an insurance policy that either gives the insured the right to continue insurance coverage or allows the insurance company to refuse to renew coverage, cancel coverage, or increase the premium.

renewal rating Insurance company's evaluation of the premium and claim expense for a group plan to determine if a rate change needs to be made.

renewal service call Visit made by the insurance company's insurance agent to the insured to discuss an existing policy and give any additional service that may be warranted.

renewal underwriting Evaluation of the premium and claim expense of an existing policy to set renewal premium rates and create terms for the next year of insurance.

renter's insurance Insurance policy that gives coverage for a dwelling occupied by a renter that gives coverage against explosion, fire, hail, riot/civil commotion, theft, vandalism, volcanic eruption, windstorm, and accidental discharge of steam from a heater.

reopen Term that refers to informal revisiting of a claim payment decision that has been made by a

Medicare fiscal intermediary. Situations for reopening are (1) after appeal rights are exhausted, (2) after the time limit for requesting an appeal has expired, (3) 12 months to 4 years after the date of the initial decision, (4) when a decision is unfavorable, (5) to correct a clerical error for fraud, or (6) in response to a court order. Also called *revisit*.

reopening 1. Remedial action taken after all appeal rights of a denied insurance claim are exhausted, to reexamine or question the correctness of a determination, a decision, or cost report otherwise final. 2. To resolicit an insurance plan to an employer for enrollment of his or her employees who were not previously enrolled.

repeat claims Insurance claims in which information has been changed, corrected, and resubmitted and is not the same as a duplicate claim.

repetitive outpatient services Medicare Part B recurring services billed monthly or at the conclusion of outpatient treatment such as cardiac rehabilitation services; home health visits; kidney dialysis treatments; psychological services; rental of durable medical equipment; therapeutic nuclear medicine; therapeutic radiology; respiratory, physical, and occupational therapy; and speech pathology. Also called *recurring outpatient services* or *series outpatient services*.

replacement To replace insurance coverage under one health insurance policy for coverage under another policy.

replacement cost insurance (contents) Type of insurance coverage that protects personal possessions and, if damaged, will replace those items without depreciation.

replacement cost insurance (dwelling) Insurance coverage that protects property and, if damaged, will replace it without deducting for depreciation. However, usually there is a limit to the amount that is stated in the insurance agreement.

report card System used to check the quality of care delivered by health plans. Report cards provide information on how well a health plan treats its members, keeps them healthy, and gives access to needed care. Report cards can be published by states, private health organizations, consumer groups, or health plans. The Health Plan Employee Data and Information Set (HEDIS) is regarded as a report card by some insurance companies.

report of benefit savings (RBS) Mandated medical review document that outlines savings realized each quarter as a direct result of medical review activities by Medicare administrative contractors.

report of eligibility (ROE) List of a health insurance plan's categories for eligible individuals and their dependents.

reportable event Situation that indicates a deteriorating financial condition of a retirement plan that needs to be reported to the Pension Benefit Guaranty Corporation (PBGC).

R

reported but not incurred (RBNI) Health plan benefit that is planned, has been reported to the insurance company, but has not yet occurred (e.g., scheduled surgery).

reports See *results/testing/reports.*

representations Written statements by an individual applying for insurance about health history, family health history, occupation, and other personal information that must be substantially correct. Such representations are fraud only if they pertain to an insurance risk and were made with the intent to deceive.

representative payee Individual appointed to represent someone who receives Social Security or Supplemental Security Income (SSI) and cannot handle his or her own financial affairs. A representative payee is required to maintain complete accounting records and periodically provide reports to Social Security.

represented employee In a workers' compensation case, an injured worker who is represented by an attorney.

repricer See *pricer.*

request for anticipated payment (RAP) Formal request submitted for processing at the beginning of a 60-day home health episode after a physician evaluates a Medicare beneficiary's condition and assigns him or her to a case-mix group. The RAP payment is the first of the two payments required during an episode under the home health prospective payment system.

requestor Entity who formally requests access to the Centers for Medicare and Medicaid Services (CMS) data.

required by law Under the Health Insurance Portability and Accountability Act (HIPAA), mandate contained in law that compels a covered entity to make use or disclosure of protected health information and that is enforceable in a court of law such as court orders and subpoenas.

rerelease Situation when a requestor formally requests permission to rerelease Centers for Medicare and Medicaid Services (CMS) data that has been formatted into statistical or aggregated information by the recipient. CMS is responsible for reviewing the files and reports to ensure that they contain no data elements or combination of data elements that could allow for the disclosure of the identity of the Medicare beneficiary or a physician and that the level of cell size aggregation meets the stated requirement.

res ipsa loquitur Latin for "the thing speaks for itself."

rescission Act of voiding an insurance contract because of misrepresentation on the insurance application.

research data assistance center Centers for Medicare and Medicaid Services (CMS) contractor who provides free assistance to academic and nonprofit research interested in using Medicare and Medicaid data for research.

research protocol Document that outlines a strong research design, which clearly states the objectives, background, methods, and significance of the study being proposed.

reserve Funds set aside and designated for future financial liabilities for life or health insurance such as to meet the difference between future benefits and future premiums. Also called *prospective reserve* or *policy reserve.* See *policy reserve.*

reserve days See *lifetime reserve days (LRDs).*

reserve for future contingent benefits In health insurance, funds set aside for deferred maternity benefits and for other claims that have happened but are contingent on a future event.

reserve strengthening Process of creating additional policy reserves.

resident For Medicare, a physician who is participating in an approved graduate medical education (GME) training program or one who is not in an approved program but who is authorized to practice only in a hospital setting. This includes interns and fellows where direct GME payments are made by the fiscal intermediary.

Resident Assessment Instrument (RAI) System that provides a comprehensive, accurate, standardized, reproducible evaluation of each long-term care facility resident's functional capabilities and helps staff to identify health problems. This assessment is performed on every resident in a Medicare and/or Medicaid-certified long-term care facility including private pay.

residential care See *assisted living center (ALC).*

residential substance abuse treatment facility Facility that provides treatment for substance (alcohol and drug) abuse to live-in residents who do not require acute medical care. Services include individual and group therapy and counseling, family counseling, laboratory tests, drugs and supplies, psychological testing, and room and board.

residential treatment center (RTC) Health care facility that provides treatment for alcoholism, drug abuse, and psychiatric problems. These facilities are usually accredited by The Joint Commission and must be licensed by the state.

residual Temporary or permanent medical condition that results after treatment for an illness or injury.

residual benefits Term used in disability income insurance for disability that is not work related. It is the payment of partial benefits when the insured is not totally disabled.

residual disability Inability to perform one or more job duties or inability to do usual work for the time period of partial disability that follows a period of total disability.

residual disability benefit Payment for an individual with a residual disability. Amount may vary depending on the percentage of income loss that is attributed to the disability. See *partial disability benefit.*

residual factors Factors other than price including volume of services, intensity of services, and age/sex changes.

residual subscriber Dependent of the insured who has a different type of insurance coverage and identification number from the insured. They are billed separately as a residual member.

resisted claim Insurance claim that an insurance company refused to pay but may pay in the future.

resolicitation Sales drive carried out to enroll eligible individuals who are not covered into an existing group insurance plan. Also called *recanvass.*

resource-based relative value scale (RBRVS) System of national uniform relative values for all physicians' services. It ranks physician services and procedures by units that provide a formula to determine an annual Medicare fee schedule. Relative value units (RVUs) are based on the physicians' work RVU, practice expense RVU, and cost of professional liability insurance RVU (see Figure R-1). RVUs are adjusted for each Medicare local fiscal agent by geographical practice cost indices. A conversion factor is used to convert a geographically adjusted relative value into a payment amount. Also called *resource-based relative value unit (RBRVU)* and synonymous with *Medicare fee schedule.*

resource-based relative value unit (RBRVU) See *resource-based relative value scale (RBRVS).*

resource costs Expense used by a physician to render a service or procedure that includes the doctor's time and effort and the expenses of nonphysician time and effort.

resource management Administration of the health care product in a cost-effective manner and maintaining quality of health care and contributing to the goals of the organization.

resource utilization group (RUG-III) Patient classification system that obtains patients' medical data and health status information from the minimum data set (MDS) to assign each patient to a resource group for Medicare reimbursement. The RUG-III system has seven major categories of patient types: rehabilitation, extensive services, special care, clinically complex, impaired cognition, behavior problems, and reduced physical function. These categories are further broken down into 44 specific patient groupings.

respiratory system Body structures involved consist of the nose, pharynx, larynx, trachea, bronchi, bronchioles, and lungs.

respite care Short-term hospice inpatient stay that may be necessary to give temporary relief to the person (primary health care giver) who regularly assists with home care of a patient. This temporary or periodic care may be provided in a nursing home, assisted living residence, or other type of long-term care program. Also known as *short-term assisted living care.*

respondeat superior Latin for "let the master answer." Refers to a physician's liability in certain cases for the wrongful acts of his or her assistant(s) or employee(s). Also referred to as *vicarious liability.*

responsibility statement See *Advance Beneficiary Notice (ABN).*

restitution Court-ordered giving back or returning of funds.

restraint Any manual method or physical or mechanical device, material, or equipment attached to or adjacent to a client's or patient's body that the individual cannot remove easily and that restricts freedom of movement or normal access to one's body. Chemical restraints are any drug used for discipline or convenience and not required to treat medical symptoms.

restricted formulary List of drugs covered by a benefit plan in which there are some limitations or restrictions about which medications may be chosen for the members of the managed care plan. See also *closed formulary* and *open formulary.*

resubmission turnaround document (RTD) Document that the Medi-Cal fiscal intermediary sends to providers when a claim form has questionable or missing information.

R

		PRACTICE	
HCPCS/CPT	WORK	EXPENSE	MALPRACTICE
CODE	RVUs	RVUs	RVUs

91000 RVUs   1.04   0.70   0.06
    GPCI* ×1.028   +   ×1.258   +   × 1.370   = Total adjusted
        1.07   0.88   0.08   RVUs, 2.03

For 2009, the conversion factor for nonsurgical care is
$36.06 × 2.03 = Allowed amount $73.20

*The GPCI for the medical practice whose location in the example is Oakland, California.

Figure R-1 Formula used to calculate the fee for a specific procedure using the resource-based relative value scale system. *CPT,* Current Procedural Terminology; *GPCI,* geographical practice cost indices; *HCPCS,* Healthcare Common Procedure Coding System; *RVUs,* relative value units.

result clause Type of war hazard exclusion that does not pay benefits for losses from acts of war.

results/testing/reports Terms seen in CPT 2008. *Results* are the technical component of a service; *testing* leads to results; results lead to interpretation; and *reports* are the work product of the interpretation of test results.

retail outlet distribution system See *location-selling distribution system.*

retaliation laws State legislation that taxes out-of-state insurance companies that do business in the state with the same tax rate as their home state.

retained asset account (RAA) Money market checking account for the beneficiary that is set up by the insurance company into which the life insurance policy's death benefits are deposited.

retention 1. Act of keeping a portion of the premiums by the insurance company to cover administrative expenses, commissions, contributions to contingency reserves, risk charges, and taxes. See *records retention.* 2. In reinsurance, amount the ceding company retains.

retention charge Dollar amount of the premium to cover expenses (not claims) and to allow the insurance company to make a profit for a group insurance contract.

retention limit Largest amount of insurance that an insurance company will write at its risk on an individual without ceding part of the risk to a reinsurer.

retired lives reserve (RLR) Fund established by an employer to provide a retired employee with life insurance. The employer's premium payments are tax deductible. If the employee ends service before retirement, funds remain in the employee's account and are used to fund benefits of the remaining employees.

retiree Individual who has retired and is no longer at work or in a business.

retirees, family members, and survivors (RFMS) Spouse and dependents of a retired member or veteran of the U.S. government military services (e.g., Army, Navy, Air Force, Marines, Coast Guard). This phrase is used more frequently in the TRICARE and CHAMPVA health care programs.

retirement age Age when an employee ceases work; age when pension benefits begin to be paid. The Age Discrimination in Employment Act states that minimum mandatory retirement is 70 years of age.

retirement date Date an elderly patient or the patient's spouse retired from active employment. For Medicare patients, this date is important when ascertaining the primary and secondary insurance coverage.

retro See *retrospective rating (retro).*

retro premium Premium rate that the insurance company and the insured agree at the beginning of the pay period, but it is paid at the end of the period only if the group's claim experience justifies it. The insurance company obtains a lower base premium at the beginning of the period and charges a retro premium retroactively at the end of the period.

retroactive Made effective to an earlier date.

retroactive disability benefit Insurance benefit paid from the date of disability after the insurance policy's stated elimination period.

retroactive Medicaid eligibility Qualified for the Medicaid program, which may begin as early as the first day of the third month before the month of application provided all appropriate factors are met in those months.

retroactive rate credit Funds from the premiums that the insurance company returns to a group insurance policyholder after analyzing the claims incurred, expenses, risk charges, changes in reserves, and profit.

retroactive rate reduction See *dividend, experience refund,* and *experience rating refund.*

retroactive reimbursement See *retrospective reimbursement.*

retrospective coding Process in which coding for medical services occurs after the patient is discharged from the hospital.

retrospective payment audit See *retrospective review.*

retrospective premium agreement Contract in which the policyholder pays the insurance company for any deficiencies incurred when the insurer agrees to continue coverage at a premium rate that eliminates any rise and fall in claims.

retrospective rate derivation See *retrospective rating (retro).*

retrospective rating (retro) System of establishing rates in which the current year's insurance premium is calculated to give the actual current year's loss experience (usage of health care). Gains may be returned by rate credits or increase of benefits or cash, and deficiencies are obtained through a recovery factor in the rates or cash. Also called *retrospective rate derivation.*

retrospective reimbursement Payment made to a provider by the insurance company for actual costs or charges incurred by the insured during the previous time period. Also called *retroactive reimbursement.*

retrospective reimbursement system Method that sets the payment rate for hospital services after services have been provided.

retrospective review 1. In external auditing, process of going over financial documents after billing an insurance carrier to determine documentation deficiencies and errors. Also called *retrospective payment audit.* 2. In utilization review, evaluation of medical services given to a patient to make sure the insurance claims are paid for appropriate care (i.e., medical necessity, quality of care, physicians' practice patterns, hospitals' average length of stay, and reasonableness of services given).

return of service See *proof of service.*

reuse In reference to Centers for Medicare and Medicaid Services (CMS) data, a situation that occurs when a requestor from the same or different organization requests permission to use CMS data already obtained for a prior approved project.

revenue Recognition of income earned and the use of appropriated capital from the rendering of services in the current period.

revenue code Four-digit number in the hospital's chargemaster that identifies a specific accommodation, ancillary service, or billing calculation related to the claim being submitted. These payment codes are inserted in Field 42 in ascending order on the Uniform Bill (UB-04) inpatient hospital billing claim form. Billing guidelines for revenue codes are extensive, so refer to the UB-04 manual for detailed information. Revenue codes are important because some managed care plans base payment on diagnosis, procedure, and revenue codes. All revenue codes from 001 to 999 must be preceded with a "0." The leading "0" is added automatically for electronic claims. Basic revenue codes end in "0." Detailed revenue codes end in 1 through 9. Do not repeat revenue codes on the same claim except when required by field or for coding more than one HCPCS code for the same revenue code item.

revenue share Proportion of a medical practice's total income allocated for a specific type of expense (e.g., practice expense profit share is that proportion of income used to pay for practice expense).

reverse capitation Payment method in which subspecialists are paid a capitated rate and primary care physicians are paid on a fee-for-service (FFS) basis. This is considered reverse because most managed care plans pay the primary care physician capitated payments and pay subspecialists on an FFS basis.

reverse membership In a managed care plan, membership established in the name of a member, who was not previously the subscriber, who is given a new identification number.

review 1. Independent, critical examination of an insurance claim made by the insurance carrier personnel not involved in the initial claim determination. 2. Request for a redetermination to the local Medicare carrier by telephone or in writing. 3. Brief note or a provider's initials appended to a test report is considered a review; when billing, it is included in evaluation and management services.

review committee Group of individuals who evaluate insurance claims that have been denied payment by the insurance carrier and appealed by the provider of the medical services. In the Medicare program, this process is called *redetermination* and was formerly known as *review*.

review of claims Evaluation of information on an insurance claim or other information requested to support the medical services billed and to make a determination regarding payment to the provider.

review of systems (ROS) Inventory of body systems obtained through a series of questions that is used to identify signs and/or symptoms that the patient might be experiencing or has experienced. ROS may clarify the differential diagnosis or identify needed tests. A documented report of the body system directly related to the problem must be identified in the history of present illness (HPI) plus all additional body systems (at least 10) for comprehensive assessments. Also called *system review*.

review period See *experience period*.

revisit See *reopen*.

revocable beneficiary See *beneficiary*.

REVS Acronym that means recipient eligibility verification system. See *Medicaid eligibility verification system (MEVS)*.

RFI Abbreviation that means request for information.

RFMS Abbreviation in the TRICARE program that means retirees, family members, and survivors.

RFP Abbreviation that means request for proposal.

RHC Abbreviation for rural health center or rural health clinic. See *rural health clinic (RHC)*.

RHCA See *Rural Health Clinics Act (RHCA)*.

rheumatology Study of disorders characterized by inflammation, degeneration, or metabolic derangement of connective tissue and related structures of the body such as arthritis and rheumatic disorders.

RHHI See *regional home health intermediary (RHHI)*.

RHIA See *Registered Health Information Administrator (RHIA)*.

RHIO See *regional health information organization (RHIO)*.

RHIT See *Registered Health Information Technician (RHIT)*.

rider See *endorsement, amendment,* and *waiver*.

right of subrogation See *subrogation*.

right of survivorship Clause in a life insurance policy that refers to ownership of property by two or more people in which the survivors automatically gain ownership of a decedent's interest.

rights of individuals In the Medicare program, a beneficiary is entitled to receive notice of information practices; see and copy his or her own records; request corrections; obtain accounting of disclosures; request restrictions and confidential communications; and file complaints.

risk 1. Possibility that revenues of the insurance company will not be sufficient to cover expenditures incurred in delivery of medical services. 2. Probability of loss in a given population.

risk adjuster See *risk adjustment*.

risk adjustment System of changing capitation rates paid to providers of medical services given to a group of members whose medical care has higher medical costs than average. This may be due to medical condition, geographical location, age, gender, ethnicity, or race. Also called *risk load* or *risk adjuster*.

risk-based health maintenance organization (HMO)/ competitive medical plan Type of managed care

R

organization. After any applicable deductible or copayment, all of an enrollee's or member's medical care costs are paid for in return for a monthly premium. However, due to the lock-in provision, all of the enrollee's or member's services (except for out-of-area emergency services) must be arranged for by the risk-HMO. Should the Medicare enrollee or member choose to obtain service not arranged for by the plan, he or she will be liable for the costs. Neither the HMO nor the Medicare program will pay for services from providers who are not part of the HMO's health care system or network.

risk-bearing entity Health plan, health insurer, or self-funded employer that takes on financial responsibility for a provision that lists specific benefits and accepts prepayment for the cost of the medical care.

risk class Group of insured individuals who have a similar risk to the insurance company. Common risk classes are standard, preferred, nonsmoker, substandard, and uninsurable.

risk contract 1. Provider's agreement with a managed care plan to deliver medical services to members for a determined, fixed payment without knowing the cost of the services. The provider is responsible for managing the medical care and risks losing money if total expenses are more than the predetermined amount of funds. 2. In a Medicare risk contract, the federal government sends monthly fixed payments to the managed care plan for services given to Medicare beneficiaries who join the plan and agree to receive all medical care through the plan. The plan is at risk for services regardless of the extent, expense, or intensity of services rendered. Sometimes an additional fee may be paid by each enrollee. Medicaid beneficiaries enrolled in risk contracts are not required to pay monthly premiums.

risk distribution System to redistribute premium income with many insurance companies to diminish the risk when selecting people to insure.

risk factors Situations that influence an individual's health and may cause illness including heredity, sex, race, age, biological factors, environmental factors, and behavioral factors (smoking, inactivity, response to stress).

risk factor reduction In a managed care plan, this phrase refers to a decrease of a risk (loss foreseen) in the group of members.

risk load See *risk adjustment.*

risk management For financial aspects of health care benefits, administrative procedures to reduce the bad effects of financial loss by recognizing possible sources of loss, measuring the consequences if a loss takes place, and adopting controls to cut down actual loss or their effects.

risk manager Individual responsible for clinical and administrative procedures used to identify, evaluate, and reduce the risk of injury to patients, staff, and visitors and the risk of loss to the facility or organization.

risk of complications Risks are based on documentation of the presenting problem(s), the procedure(s) performed, treatments ordered, and other possible management options.

risk of morbidity or mortality See *risk of complications.*

risk pool 1. Individuals who comprise an insured group based on health status, age, sex, and future health. Also called *risk spread.* 2. State program that groups those who cannot obtain insurance coverage. Funds for these programs come from either the state or an assessment on insurers. 3. In managed care plans, a collection of funds established by a managed care plan that uses a risk-sharing system (i.e., capitation) with providers of medical services. Funds are taken from withholding a portion of provider fees or capitation payments to make up the reserve to cover unforeseen use of services. Funds that remain at the end of a year are distributed among the providers. Also called *pool.* 4. Financial account to which a managed care plan's specific income and expenses are posted.

risk rating Classification system used by the insurance industry to set premiums for health plans. Insured individuals who have a high risk pay more than others who are insured because of their health-related behaviors.

risk score Measurement of the costs of an enrollee who has specific risks compared with the cost of care for the average beneficiary in a managed care plan.

risk selection See *cherry picking.*

risk sharing In managed care plans, methods used in which the plan and contracted providers share the financial risks and benefits to care for the plan members in a cost-effective manner (e.g., capitation, risk pools, per diem contracts). It is a system used to control health care costs.

risk spread See *risk pool.*

RLR See *retired lives reserve (RLR).*

RN See *registered nurse (RN).*

ROE See *report of eligibility (ROE).*

ROI See *release of information (ROI).*

ROS See *review of systems (ROS).*

routine In medical care, physical examination performed on an annual (regular) basis.

routine disclosure Under the Health Insurance Portability and Accountability Act (HIPAA), release of protected health information for treatment, payment, or other health care operations that does not require the patient to sign a consent form.

routine home care days Days in which a hospice patient and member of an insurance plan who is not receiving continuous medical care has chosen to receive hospice care at home.

routine newborn services First inpatient examination of a newborn infant done by a doctor but not done by the physician who delivered the baby or the doctor who gave anesthetics during delivery.

routine physical examination Annual physical examination made in the absence of definite symptoms of disease or injury. Sometimes an electrocardiogram, laboratory tests, and a chest x-ray may be done. Also see *physical examination (PE or PX)*.

routine use With respect to individually identifiable health information, the sharing, employment, application, utilization, examination, or analysis of such information within an entity that maintains such information.

routing form See *multipurpose billing form*.

RP HCPCS Level II modifier that may be used with CPT or HCPCS Level II codes indicating replacement and repair of durable medical equipment, prosthetics, orthotics, and supplies (DMEPOS).

RPCH See *rural primary care hospital (RPCH)*.

RR HCPCS Level II modifier that may be used with CPT or HCPCS Level II codes indicating rental of durable medical equipment (DME). Should be used with other rental modifiers: KH, KI, and KJ. List the RR modifier first.

RRA Acronym for Registered Records Administrator. See *Registered Health Information Administrator (RHIA)*.

RRB See *Railroad Retirement Board (RRB)*.

RT HCPCS Level II modifier that may be used with CPT or HCPCS Level II codes indicating a procedure performed on the right side of the body.

RTC See *residential treatment center (RTC)*.

RTD See *resubmission turnaround document (RTD)*.

rubric 1. Group of similar conditions. 2. In ICD-10-CM, a three-character category or a four-character subcategory.

running balance Amount owed on a credit transaction; also known as *outstanding* or *unpaid balance*.

RUG-III See *resource utilization group (RUG-III)*.

rule of nines Measurement system for assessing burn injury to the total body surface area (TBSA). The body is divided into segments as multiples of 9%. Adults: The external genitals are 1%; each arm is 9%; front and back of the trunk and each leg is counted as 18%; and head is 9%. Children and infants: The head is 18% (larger surface area in proportion to the body) and legs 14% each. See Figure R-2.

ruling Legal judicial decision.

rural health center (RHC) See *rural health clinic (RHC)*.

rural health clinic (RHC) Public or private outpatient health care facility located where there is a shortage of health services and staffed by a nurse practitioner, physician assistant, or certified nurse midwife under the direction of a physician. It gives routine diagnostic services, laboratory services, drugs, and biologicals. It has access to other diagnostic services from facilities that meet federal guidelines and must be licensed by the state. Also called *rural health center (RHC)*.

Rural Health Clinics Act (RHCA) Legislation enacted by Congress in 1977 and implemented in 1978 to increase access to primary health care services for Medicare and Medicaid beneficiaries living in rural areas. The RHCA also created a cost-based payment

R

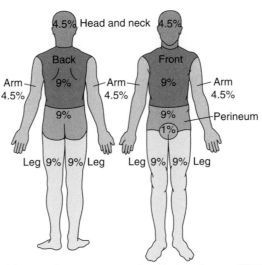

Figure R-2 The rule of nines estimation of total body surface area (TBSA) burned.

mechanism to ensure the financial viability of rural health clinics and encouraged the use of midlevel practitioners by providing payment for their services, even in the absence of a full-time physician.

rural primary care hospital (RPCH) Limited-service rural hospitals that provide outpatient and short-term inpatient hospital care on an urgent or emergency basis, then release patients or transfer them to an Essential Access Community Hospital (EACH) or other full-service hospital. To be designated as RPCHs, hospitals have to meet certain criteria including requirements that they not have more than six inpatient beds for acute (hospital-level) care and maintain an average inpatient length of stay of no more than 72 hours.

rush charge Billed amount for quick test results report. Also see *stat charge.*

RVS See *relative value studies (RVS).*

RVU See *relative value unit (RVU).*

RW See *relative weight (RW).*

RWP See *relative weighted product (RWP).*

RWV See *relative work value (RWV).*

Rx Symbol for the Latin *recipe* (meaning "to take prescription drugs").

S

S codes HCPCS codes that are temporary codes used by the private sector to report drugs and services.

SA HCPCS Level II modifier that may be used with CPT or HCPCS Level II codes indicating a nurse practitioner's rendering service together with a physician. It is required by some Medicaid programs, so check with your state guidelines.

safe harbor 1. Area or means of protection. 2. Business arrangement that is legal under a specific law but in other circumstances might be considered illegal. 3. Categories defined by the Department of Health and Human Services for practices that technically violate either the antireferral or antikickback statutes but have been exempted from penalty because they are not likely to bring harm to the federal health care programs.

safe harbor regulation 1. Provision that affords protection from liability or penalty. 2. Protected business arrangement between a managed care plan and physicians in which the arrangement would not violate Medicare fraud and abuse laws. This statute can be found in the *Code of Federal Regulations* 1001.952.

safety margin Degree by which actuaries increase the probability of mortality for each age group in a mortality table for life insurance. This protects the insurance company from adverse experience.

salaried sales agents Insurance sales representatives who are paid hourly instead of by commissions. Also known as *salaried sales representatives*.

salaried sales distribution system Method that uses an insurance company's salaried employees to sell and service insurance policies. They may work independently or with other sales agents.

salaried sales representatives See *salaried sales agents.*

salary continuation plan Type of sick leave plan that allows employees to receive 100% of their salary for a specific number of days if they become ill or disabled. The number of days may increase as the worker's length of service increases. Also called *sick leave plan.*

salary reduction plan Employer-sponsored retirement savings program in which the employee invests pretax dollars that may be matched by the employer. Also referred to as *Section 401(k) plan.*

same-day surgery See *ambulatory surgery.*

same-day transfer Patient admitted as an inpatient to a hospital and then transferred the same day to another acute care or skilled nursing facility.

sanction 1. Official approval or authorization. 2. Penalty that results from failure to comply with a law. 3. In the Medicare or Medicaid programs, a penalty or exclu-sion from the program for fraud or other violation such as soliciting or receiving a kickback for referring patients for other medical services, using substandard treatments, or doing procedures that harm patients.

sanction action To impose civil monetary penalties or exclusion of a provider from participation in the Medicare and Medicaid programs for a specific period of time due to conviction of a Medicare- or Medicaid-related crime.

sanctioned provider list Office of Inspector General (OIG) record of providers, individuals, and entities that are excluded from Medicare reimbursement. This list includes identifying information about the sanctioned party, specialty, notice date, sanction period, and sections of the Social Security Act used in arriving at the determination to impose a sanction. It is titled *List of Excluded Individuals/Entities (LEIE)* and may be found at http://oig.hhs.gov/fraud/exclusions.asp. Also called *exclusion list.*

sanitizing See *obliterate.*

SAP See *statutory accounting practices (SAP).*

saturation Act of a managed care plan that has reached its maximum penetration either in a specific subscriber group or in the commercial market. Also see *penetration.*

savings plan Voluntary program offered by an employer that gives workers a system for investing funds for retirement. In some plans the employer matches employees' contributions. Also called a *thrift plan.*

SB HCPCS Level II modifier that may be used with CPT or HCPCS Level II codes indicating a service or supply provided by a nurse midwife. It is required by some Medicaid programs, so check with your state guidelines.

SC HCPCS Level II modifier that may be used with CPT or HCPCS Level II codes indicating medically necessary service or supply.

SCH See *sole community hospital (SCH).*

schedule 1. List of appointments of patients to be seen in the medical practice for the day. Also known as *appointment schedule.* 2. List of CPT codes with amounts payable for certain medical procedures and tests. Also known as *fee schedule.*

schedule of allowances List of specified dollar amounts payable as certain benefits in an indemnity-type health insurance plan. Also called *indemnity schedule.* See *indemnity plan.*

schedule of benefits See *benefit payment schedule, benefit schedule,* and *fee schedule.*

schedule of eligibility Portion contained in the insurance policy that states the categories of eligible individuals and eligible dependents.

scheduled dental plan Dental insurance that pays for specific procedures listed on a fee schedule.

scheduler Medical assistant who schedules patient appointments for a physician's medical practice.

SCI See *surrender cost index (SCI)* and *surrender cost index (SCI) method.*

SCHIP See *State Children's Health Insurance Program (SCHIP), Children's Special Health Care Services (CSHCS),* or *Maternal and Child Health Program (MCHP).*

scope of practice Professional activities that a state-licensed health care professional may perform under state laws.

SCR See *standard class rate (SCR).*

screening Use of a quick procedure to differentiate well persons from individuals who have a disease or a high risk of disease from those who do not have the disease.

screening mammography Radiographic images taken of the breast(s) for early unsuspected detection of cancer. It usually consists of two views of each breast.

screening mammography service Procedure in which radiographic images (two views) are taken of the breast(s) for early unsuspected detection of cancer. Under the Medicare program, this radiological benefit was added for early detection of breast cancer and became effective January 1, 1991. No symptoms need to be present for this procedure to be covered.

screening Pap (Papanicolaou) smear Diagnostic laboratory test of a sample of exfoliative material obtained during a routine pelvic examination. It is done for the purpose of detecting cervical dysplasia (a precursor to cancer), carcinoma in situ, invasive cervical and uterine carcinoma, herpes or trichomonad infections, and human papillomavirus. The test is named after George Papanicolaou (1883-1962), an American anatomist who developed it. Generally, the Bethesda System has replaced the Pap cervical cancer staging-class system.

screening test Examination performed for early detection of a specific disease before symptoms develop; Medicare pays for specific routine screenings such as Pap smears, mammograms, prostate cancer screenings, and colorectal cancer screenings.

screens In the Medicare program, preestablished limits for certain medical services (e.g., one Papanicolaou test every 3 years). Medical necessity of the procedure must be documented.

scribe Person who assists with the clerical aspects of patient encounters and writes what the physician dictates such as a nurse or nonphysician practitioner (e.g., premed student, physician assistant, nurse practitioner). This information may be the patient's history, discharge summary, or any entry in the medical record. A scribe may also compile follow-up instructions for patients. The note should state, "written by XXX, acting as a scribe for Dr. XXX." Also called *medical scribe.*

scripting Concise canned responses by a receptionist to a patient's questions delivered via telephone.

SD HCPCS Level II modifier that may be used with CPT or HCPCS Level II codes indicating services provided by a registered nurse with specialized, highly technical home infusion training.

SDP See *single drug pricer (SDP).*

SE HCPCS Level II modifier that may be used with CPT or HCPCS Level II codes indicating state and/or federally funded programs or services.

SECA See *Self-Employment Contribution Act (SECA) payroll tax.*

second-injury fund Special fund that assumes all or part of the liability for benefits provided to a worker because of the combined effect of a work-related impairment and a preexisting condition; also known as *subsequent injury fund (SIF).*

second opinion Consulting physician's evaluation and assessment of a patient's condition to assist in determining whether a proposed elective surgical procedure recommended by the first physician is necessary. Some insurance plans mandate a second opinion before the surgery is done, and if not performed, reimbursement may be reduced or denied. A voluntary program informs the patient that a second opinion will be reimbursed by the plan. Some plans have a list of surgical procedures that require a second opinion. Also called *second surgical opinion (SSO).*

second surgical opinion (SSO) Consultation with a second physician about a proposed elective operative procedure after surgery has been recommended by a first physician.

second-to-die life insurance See *survivorship life insurance.*

secondary Second in order of time, place, or importance such as that seen during the course of another disease or condition.

secondary beneficiary See *alternate beneficiary* or *contingent beneficiary.*

secondary care Medical services provided by medical specialists who generally do not have first contact with patients (e.g., cardiologists, urologists, dermatologists). In managed care plans, the patient is seen by the primary care physician and then may be referred to secondary and/or tertiary providers as needed.

secondary carrier See *secondary insurer.*

secondary condition Medical situation that exists with the primary diagnosis and does not affect the treatment or results of the primary diagnosis.

secondary coverage Health insurance plan that pays for expenses not covered by primary coverage under the coordination of benefits provision.

secondary diagnosis Reason subsequent to the primary diagnosis for an office or hospital encounter that may contribute to the condition or define the need for a higher level of care but is not the underlying cause.

There may be more than one secondary diagnosis. See *other diagnoses.*

secondary health condition Patient's medical problem resulting from the location of his or her work environment, but the condition does not originate from the job.

secondary insurance See *secondary insurer.*

secondary insurer Second insurance plan identified through coordination of benefits (COB) that has the responsibility to pay if there are benefits pending after the first insurance company has sent the provider or patient reimbursement for the medical services. Also called *secondary carrier or secondary insurance.*

secondary payer 1. Insurance carrier that reimburses the residual balance of the insurance claim after the primary insurance has paid its benefits. 2. When Medicare is the secondary payer (MSP), the primary insurance plan of a Medicare beneficiary must pay for any medical care or services first before Medicare is sent a claim. MSP may involve aged or disabled patients who are under group health plans and cases related to workers' compensation, automobile accident, medical no-fault, and liability insurance. For a Medicare patient suffering from end-stage renal disease (ESRD), MSP is the payer for the first 30 months that the beneficiary is entitled to benefits.

section 1. In the diagnostic code book, ICD-9-CM, related groups of codes within a chapter and the major divisions within a chapter in Volume 1, Tabular List. 2. Major division or part of the *Current Procedural Terminology (CPT)* code book.

Section 79 of the Internal Revenue Code Group whole life insurance plan in which the employer's contributions help with income tax exemptions. This federal statute lists specifications that a plan must meet.

Section 101 (a) (1) of the Internal Revenue Code Federal statute that qualifies the death benefit paid under a life insurance policy is received by the beneficiary of the policy income-tax free.

Section 105 of the Internal Revenue Code Federal statute that permits the self-employed a 100% tax deduction for the family health care expenses to include premiums related to health insurance, disability income insurance, and long-term care insurance. A 100% deductible is also allowed for noninsured medical, dental, and vision care expenses.

Section 105 Medical Reimbursement Plan Federal statute that employers receive a 100% tax deduction for reimbursement to eligible employees for health care expenses paid by those employees and reimbursed by the employer (e.g., premiums and noninsured medical expenses).

Section 125 of the Internal Revenue Code Federal statute that an employer may maintain a separate written plan for employees that meets specific requirements and regulations and provides participants an opportunity to receive certain benefits on a pretax basis. Also known as *cafeteria plan.* Participants in a cafeteria plan must be permitted to choose among at least one taxable benefit (such as cash) and one qualified benefit. A qualified benefit is a benefit that does not defer compensation and is excludable from an employee's gross income under a specific provision of the Code, without being subject to the principles of constructive receipt. Qualified benefits include accident and health benefits (but not Archer medical savings accounts or long-term care insurance); adoption assistance; dependent care assistance; group-term life insurance coverage; health savings accounts including distributions to pay long-term care services. The written plan must specifically describe all benefits and establish rules for eligibility and elections. A section 125 plan is the only means by which an employer can offer employees a choice between taxable and nontaxable benefits without the choice causing the benefits to become taxable. A plan offering only a choice between taxable benefits is not a section 125 plan. Employer contributions to the cafeteria plan are usually made pursuant to salary reduction agreements between the employer and the employee in which the employee agrees to contribute a portion of his or her salary on a pretax basis to pay for the qualified benefits. Salary reduction contributions are not actually or constructively received by the participant. Therefore those contributions are not considered wages for federal income tax purposes. In addition, those sums generally are not subject to FICA and FUTA.

Section 401(h) pension plan trust Under the Internal Revenue Code federal statutes, allows employees to set up a retirement plan (trust) within the employer's defined benefit pension plan from which the employees' life insurance and medical expense costs are paid. Contributions are tax deductible and earnings accumulated are not taxable until the funds are withdrawn.

Section 401(k) plan Under the Internal Revenue Code federal statutes, employer-sponsored retirement savings program. Employees contribute and employers may match contributions that are not taxable until the funds are withdrawn. Referred to as a *cash or deferred arrangement (CODA).* See *salary reduction plan.*

Section 401(k) plan switchback Under the Internal Revenue Code federal statutes, allows an employee in an employee stock ownership plan (ESOP) trust to reinvest dividends into their Section 401(k) plans (a switchback approach). Participants may reinvest their dividends into this "KSOP" on a tax-deferred basis or obtain the dividends in cash and pay income tax. If reinvested, the contribution is reduced by the amount of the dividend. Also referred to by the acronym KSOP or 401k.

Section 402(b) of the Internal Revenue Code Federal legislation allows establishment of a secular trust that is a nonqualified plan of deferred compensation and is irrevocable. It compensates key employees but does

S

not give similar benefits to rank and file employees. The company may take an income tax deduction for the contributed funds even though they have not been given to the employee during the current taxable income period. When the funds are paid out, the employee is taxed only to the extent that these funds are from earnings of the trust or from current trust income. This allows the employee to pay taxes owed as the result of the company's contributions to the trust. The employer is not taxed on the trust income and the employee pays all taxes on this income. Also called a *nonexempt trust*.

Section 403(b) of the Internal Revenue Code Federal statute allows retirement plans to be offered by public employers and tax-exempt organizations (e.g., charities, churches, hospitals, public school systems). The employer pays into the retirement annuity policy for employees, and payments may be excluded from the employees' gross income for tax reasons. Also called *tax-deferred annuity (TDA) plan* or *tax-sheltered annuity (TSA) plan*.

Section 404(c) of the Employee Retirement Income Security Act of 1974 Federal act that requires employers to offer employees at least three investment choices and each with different risk and return features. Individuals who participate must be able to switch quarterly from one fund to another. The Act requires that sufficient information must be provided so that employees can make wise financial investment decisions.

Section 408(k) of the Internal Revenue Code Federal regulation for establishing an individual retirement account or a simplified employee pension (SEP); also known as a *SEP-IRA*. Funds are vested immediately, and the employee owns the IRA and has control of the investments. The maximum annual contribution is limited. If funds are withdrawn, then income taxes must be paid. SEPs may also be established by self-employed individuals.

Section 415 of the Internal Revenue Code Federal regulation that limits the amount of annual contributions made to a defined contribution plan on behalf of a participant or benefits paid to a participant.

Section 457 of the Internal Revenue Code Federal statute that allows a deferred retirement savings plan sponsored by a public employer (e.g., university, state, county, municipality). By mutual agreement, it lets the employer reduce the employee's salary by a certain amount and invest this, with pretax dollars, in various financial instruments. At the end of employment, the principal amount invested and any earnings are given to the employee or to the employee's estate.

Section 501(c)(9) Voluntary Employees Beneficiary Association (VEBA) Federal legislation that allows employers to establish a trust that may be used to provide accident and illness benefits to employees who are members.

Section 1035 Exchange See *Section 1035 of the Internal Revenue Code*.

Section 1035 of the Internal Revenue Code Federal statute allows taking proceeds from one life insurance policy or annuity and reinvesting the funds immediately in another life insurance policy or annuity of the same type without having to pay tax on any profit. Sometimes referred to as a *Section 1035 Exchange*.

Section 2503(c) of the Internal Revenue Code Federal regulation allows the establishment of a trust for minors so that income can be collected until the minor reaches age 21. Then the income can be paid out and the $10,000 annual gift tax exclusion for each beneficiary can be applied.

Section 4958 of the Internal Revenue Code Federal statute imposes a penalty excise tax on an excess benefit transaction of 25% of the excess benefit on the individual from inside the organization (disqualified person) receiving the benefit. Also imposes a penalty excise tax of 10% of the excess benefit on the manager in the organization awarding the excess benefit. If the excess benefit is not repaid to the tax-exempt organization in a reasonable time, the disqualified individual is assessed an additional tax penalty of 200% of the excess benefit received.

section guidelines Instructions that precede the major divisions or parts of the *Current Procedural Terminology (CPT)* code book providing information for accurate coding.

secured debt Debt (an amount owed) in which a debtor pledges certain property (collateral), in a written security agreement, to the repayment of the debt.

security officer Under the Health Insurance Portability and Accountability Act (HIPAA), individual who protects the computer and networking systems within the medical practice or hospital facility and implements protocols such as password assignment, backup procedures, firewalls, virus protection, and contingency planning for emergencies.

security regulations See *security rules*.

security rules Under the Health Insurance Portability and Accountability Act (HIPAA), regulations related to the security of electronic protected health information (ePHI) that, along with regulations related to electronic transactions and code sets, privacy, and enforcement, compose the Administrative Simplification provisions. Also called *security regulations*.

security standards for health information See *Health Insurance Portability and Accountability Act of 1996 (HIPAA)*.

see Cross-reference word used in ICD-9-CM that is a mandatory instruction following a main term in the index, indicating that another term should be referenced and to look elsewhere for the correct diagnostic code.

see also Cross-reference phrase used in ICD-9-CM that is a suggestion following a main term in the index, indicating that there is another main term that may also be referenced that may provide additional, useful index entries.

see condition Cross-reference phrase used in ICD-9-CM that is an instruction note found in the Alphabetic Index to Diseases. It instructs the coder to refer to a main term for the condition.

see/see also Cross-reference word/phrase used in *Current Procedural Terminology (CPT)* that directs the coder to look at other sections or codes.

SEER Medicare database Data that link the clinical data collected by the Surveillance Epidemiology and End Results (SEER) registries with insurance claims for health services collected by Medicare for its beneficiaries.

SEER program Acronym for Surveillance Epidemiology and End Results that is a program of the National Cancer Institute. It is the most authoritative source of information on cancer incidence and survival in the United States. Website: http://seer.cancer.gov.

segment Under HIPAA, a collection of interrelated data elements in a batch of claims (transaction) that are to be electronically transmitted.

segmentation 1. Act of creating a group health benefits program for coverage to a limited number of eligible employees or to give different types of benefits to different categories of workers (e.g., exempt or nonexempt, union or nonunion, hourly or salaried). 2. Act of an insurance company dividing its general account investments into separate parts that match each of the insurer's major lines of business (e.g., account for group life insurance investments, account for individual life insurance investments).

select drug list See *drug formulary* or *formulary.*

selection of risks See *underwriting.*

selective contracting Under the Social Security Act, Section 1915(B), state may create a competitive contract system for services (e.g., inpatient hospital care).

self-administration See *policyholder self-administration.*

self-dialysis Dialysis performed with little or no professional assistance except in an emergency situation by an end-stage renal disease patient who has completed an appropriate course of training in a dialysis facility or at home.

self-disclosure Act of admission or to give information about one's own appropriate, inappropriate, lawful, or unlawful action.

self-employment To work for oneself, with direct control over work, services, and fees. This may be the operation of a trade or business by either an individual or by a partnership in which an individual is a member.

Self-Employment Contribution Act (SECA) payroll tax Federal law that provides for the obligation of the self-employment tax by a self-employed worker. Medicare's share of SECA is used to fund the health insurance trust fund. Also referred to as SECA.

self-funding See *self-insurance.*

self-insurance System or program of insurance for employees and their dependents in which employers (generally companies with 500 or more employees) establish a plan and assume the functions, responsibilities, and liabilities of an insurer. Health care expenses are paid through a special fund established by the employer. Such plans may be self-administered or the employer may contract with a third-party administrator (TPA) for administrative services only (ASO). Self-insured plans are exempted by the Employee Retirement Income Security Act (ERISA) from state insurance laws, state-mandated requirements for employer health benefit programs, state taxes on insurance premiums, and participation in state risk pools or uncompensated care plans. Also called *self-funding, self-insured, employer self-insured program,* or *partially self-funded.*

self-insured Individual or organization that assumes the financial risk of paying for health care. Also see *self-insurance.*

self-insured employer Employer that offers health insurance coverage to its employees and pays for the medical expenses directly instead of contracting with an insurance company.

self-insured group insurance Type of group insurance in which a group sponsor, not an insurance company, pays the claims made by group insureds. It may be partially or fully self-insured.

self-insured health plan Health insurance in which the employer and not an insurance company is at risk for the employees' medical expenses.

self-limited or minor In CPT coding of a service or procedure, problem that runs a definite and prescribed course, is transient in nature, and is not likely to permanently alter health status or has a good prognosis with management/compliance.

self-pay patient Individual (self) or patient's family who pays out of pocket for the medical services instead of a third-party payer (insurance company). Self-pay patients may not have health insurance coverage.

self-procured care In workers' compensation, health care obtained by an injured worker either before determination of eligibility or after rejection or delay of benefits by the insurance company.

self-referral Patient in a managed care plan that refers himself or herself to a specialist, outpatient clinic, emergency department, or hospital outpatient department. The patient may be required to inform the primary care physician.

semicolon (;) Punctuation sign used to identify the common part or main entry and is placed at the end of the phrase followed by indented modifying terms or descriptions in the *Current Procedural Terminology (CPT)* code book.

senility General state of decline in mental and physical functioning associated with the aging process.

senior center Facility that provides a variety of on-site programs and information for older adults including recreation, socialization, congregate meals, and some health services.

Senior Advantage Plans Health care programs offered by a managed care plan or insurance company to individuals who are eligible for Medicare Parts A and B. Also see *Medicare Part C, Medicare Plus (+) Choice (M+C) plan,* and *managed care.*

senior plan Health care program offered by a managed care plan or insurance company to individuals who are eligible for Medicare Parts A and B. Also see *Medicare Part C, Medicare Plus (+) Choice (M+C) plan.*

sensitive information Medical record data related to diagnoses of sexually transmitted diseases, HIV/AIDS data, mental health problems, and treatment for drug and alcohol abuse. Additional examples of information that could be considered sensitive include data about minors, reproductive health information, communicable disease data, chemical dependency data, genetic information, prescription drug information that may lead to disclosure of a sensitive condition, abuse and neglect exposure, and social and family history.

SEP See *special enrollment period (SEP).* Acronym for simplified employee pension; see *Section 408(k) of the Internal Revenue Code.*

separate account Asset account established by a life insurance company detached from other funds and used primarily for investments for a retirement plan.

separate account contract Type of agreement for funding a pension plan in which a pension's assets are invested through an insurance company's separate account. This agreement does not guarantee investment performance. Also called *investment facility contract.*

separate account guaranteed investment contract (GIC) Type of guaranteed investment agreement in which funds for the agreement are placed in the insurance company's separate account.

separate procedure Procedure that is an integral part of a larger procedure and does not need a separate code, unless performed independently and not immediately related to other services. The phrase (separate procedure) appears at the end of the specific description of codes listed in the *Current Procedural Terminology (CPT)* code book. See also *complete procedure* to learn the difference between separate and complete. See also *partial procedure.*

sequelae Diseased conditions following, and usually resulting from, a previous disease.

sequencing codes 1. Code numbers inserted on claim forms by order, level, or rank. 2. In diagnostic coding for the outpatient setting, first list the primary diagnosis, which is the main reason for the encounter. The secondary diagnosis, listed subsequently, may contribute to the condition or define the need for a higher level of care but is not the underlying cause. Always code the underlying disease first, which is referred to

as the *etiology.* In the inpatient setting, first list the principal diagnosis, which is obtained after the study that prompted the hospitalization. 3. In procedural coding, code the primary surgical procedure and then list secondary or adjunct procedures.

sequester Reduction of funds to be used for benefits or administrative costs from a federal account based on the requirements specified in the Gramm-Rudman-Hollings Act.

serious illness See *serious injury.*

serious injury In workers' compensation cases, any injury or illness that occurs in a place of employment or in connection with any employment requiring inpatient hospitalization for a period in excess of 24 hours for other than medical observation or in which an employee suffers a loss of any member of the body or suffers any serious degree of permanent disfigurement.

SERP See *supplemental executive retirement plan (SERP).*

service (svc) Medical care and items such as medical diagnosis and treatment, drugs and biologicals, supplies, appliances, and equipment, medical social services, and use of rural primary care hospital (RPCH) or skilled nursing facilities (SNFs).

service agreement 1. Contract between any two parties. 2. Under the Health Insurance Portability and Accountability Act (HIPAA), basic agreement between a business associate and a covered entity that describes the business relationship (e.g., a transcription business and a health care provider).

service and claim department See *customer service department.*

service area 1. Geographical area defined by a managed care plan such as a health maintenance organization (HMO) as the locale in which it will provide health care services to its members directly through its own resources or through arrangements with other providers in the area. Members may be disenrolled if they move out of the plan's service area. 2. Area where a Medicare private fee-for-service plan accepts members.

service benefit program Program (e.g., TRICARE) that provides benefits without a contract guaranteeing the indemnification of an insured party against a specific loss; there are no premiums.

service benefits Health insurance coverage and/or medical and surgical services without cost limitations to the insured.

service bureau Organization that offers data processing of insurance claims and time-sharing services for hospital facilities and physicians.

service category definition General description of the types of service provided under the service and/or characteristics that define the service category.

service-connected disability Disability incurred by a service member while on active duty.

service-connected injury Injury incurred by a service member while on active duty or incurred during reserve duty with a military unit.

service date 1. Month, day, and year a patient receives a medical service. Dates of service are inserted in Block 24A Lines 1 through 6 of the CMS-1500 insurance claim form. Service date is inserted in Field 45 of the Uniform Bill (UB-04) inpatient hospital billing claim form. The electronic version requires an eight-character date listing year, month, and day: 20XX0328. 2. For health insurance, the effective date of membership. 3. For employment, the effective date of full-time employment.

service fee Special dollar amount given to insurance consultants or brokers who may perform many functions of group representatives or home offices. This occurs when commissions paid to the servicing agent have ceased.

service plan 1. Health insurance plan that directly contracts with providers such as Blue Cross and Blue Shield. The providers directly bill the plan and the plan pays directly to the providers. The providers agree to certain fees and payment in full with no balance billing to the patient. The patient (member or insured) is responsible for the deductible and copayments. 2. Written document that outlines the types and frequency of long-term care services that a client receives. It may include treatment goals for a specified time period. 3. See *plan of treatment*.

service provider Any individual who gives medical services or conducts a medical procedure.

service retiree Individual who is retired from a career in the armed forces; also known as *military retiree*.

service-oriented V codes ICD-9-CM diagnostic codes that are used when a person who is not currently sick encounters health services for some specific purpose such as identify or define a physical examination, aftercare, ancillary service, or therapy. In these situations the V code appears as a primary code and is placed first for the purpose of billing outpatient services.

service plan Insurance coverage that has contracts with providers and in which health care benefits are given to individuals instead of monetary payment. Sometimes a Blue Cross and Blue Shield plan may be referred to as a *service plan*.

set up bed See *bed, set up*.

settlement See *financial settlement*.

settlement agreement Arrangement between an insurance company and an insured about the method of payment of the insurance proceeds to the beneficiary.

settlement option Method in which a policyholder or beneficiary may choose to have an insurance policy's proceeds paid.

settlement option payments Periodic payments of life insurance policy proceeds to the insured by an insurance company instead of a lump-sum payment.

settlement options Methods of payments of life insurance policy proceeds to the beneficiary by an insurance company such as a lump sum or periodic payments.

settlement option table Table showing amounts the insurance company will pay as periodic payments in settling a life insurance policy.

settlor See *trustor*.

72/24-hour rule See *72-hour rule*.

72-hour rule Medicare policy that states if a patient receives diagnostic tests and hospital outpatient services within 72 hours of admission to a hospital, then all such tests and services are combined (bundled) with inpatient services only if services are related to the admission. However, unrelated therapeutic service is paid. Also called the *3-day payment window* because it is 3 calendar days rather than 72 hours. Sometimes referred to as the *72/24-hour rule*.

severe pain In workers' compensation cases, pain that would preclude the activity precipitating the pain.

severity Word used to describe the level of seriousness of a patient's medical condition.

severity modifier Adjustment that shows the effect of patient factors on the work needed to deliver a medical service such as severity of illness, comorbidity, and risk of complications.

severity of illness (SOI) 1. Degree of disease or loss of function and mortality that a patient is experiencing before treatment. Severity of illness is used in the interpretation of performance data of facilities. 2. Variation in patients classified to the same diagnosis related group that includes age, systems involved in illness, stage of disease, complications, and response to treatment.

sex distribution Percentage analysis of genders (male or female) of insureds within a group.

SF 1. HCPCS Level II modifier that may be used with CPT or HCPCS Level II codes indicating a second opinion ordered by a quality improvement organization (QIO), eligible for reimbursement at 100%. The usual Medicare deductible and/or coinsurance amounts are not applied. 2. See *straightforward (SF)*.

SFR See *substantial financial risk (SFR)*.

SG HCPCS Level II modifier that may be used with CPT or HCPCS Level II codes indicating an ambulatory surgery center (ASC) facility service. Physicians who provide ASC facility services do not need to append this modifier to their insurance claim forms.

SH HCPCS Level II modifier that may be used with CPT or HCPCS Level II codes indicating a second concurrently administered infusion therapy.

shadow claims See *encounter data*.

shadow pricing 1. Policy of setting fees equal or slightly below a competitor's fees. This may tend to maximize profits but will raise medical costs and is generally considered to be unethical. 2. In an employer group's managed care plan, to price premiums based on the cost of indemnity insurance instead of following community or experience rating standards.

S

shadow record Duplicate of an original medical record in hard copy, scanned for an electronic file, or downloaded from primary information systems. It is retained for the convenience of a department or health care provider.

shadowing Practice used to improve clinical documentation in a facility in which a nonphysician clinician/documentation expert is paired with a physician for 1 day of patient care. At the end of the day, the two practitioners compare notes on what should have been documented based on what the physician did for each patient.

share of cost (SOC) The amount the patient must pay each month before he or she can be eligible for Medicaid. Also known as *liability* or *spend down*.

shared office visit See *split/shared office visit*.

shared risk Arrangement in a managed care plan in which the provider and health plan share the risk for excessive utilization and/or excessive costs of plan members. It is used to give financial incentive to managed care providers for giving cost-effective, high-quality care. Also called *risk sharing* or *risk pool*.

shared savings Insurance provision of managed care plans in which a portion of the providers' income is linked to the financial performance of the plan. When costs are lower than predicted, a percentage of the savings is given to providers.

shareholder See *stockholder*.

SHMO See *social health maintenance organization (SHMO)*.

shock claim See *large claim*.

shortfall Difference between the billed charge for a hospital service and the actual payment the hospital receives from a third-party payer.

short-form reinstatement application Document completed for reinstatement of an insurance policy 30 to 90 days after the end of a grace period. To safeguard against reinsuring someone whose conditions may have changed, the insured must answer some questions.

short range The next 10 years.

short-stay hospital Medical facility with patients who have an average length of stay less than 30 days.

short-stay patient Hospital inpatient admitted for 48 hours or less, or hospital outpatient who stays 24 hours or less.

short-term assisted living care See *respite care*.

short-term disability In disability income insurance (nonoccupational accident or illness), an employee cannot perform the duties of his or her occupation for a short period of time.

short-term disability income insurance Insurance provision to pay benefits to a covered disabled person as long as he or she remains disabled, up to a specified period not exceeding 2 years.

sick baby Infant who has medical complications that are not the result of a premature birth.

sick leave plan See *salary continuation plan*.

sickness insurance Type of health insurance that covers only loss from illness or disease and excludes loss from accidents or injuries.

side effect Problem caused by treatment (e.g., medicine the patient takes for high blood pressure that makes the patient feel sleepy). Most treatments have side effects.

side fund See *conversion fund*.

SIF See *subsequent injury fund (SIF)*.

sigmoidoscopy Process of using a sigmoidoscope to examine the sigmoid colon to identify disorders or early signs of cancer.

sign Objective symptom of a disease from a normal condition or that which is observed by an examiner.

signature log List of all staff members' names, job titles, signatures, and initials (see Figure S-1).

signature on file (SOF) Brief statement that contains the patient's signature authorization retained in an office file for future use when mailing claims or transmitting electronic claims. It allows the provider to submit assigned and nonassigned insurance claims on the beneficiary's behalf.

SIGNATURE LOG

Name	Position	Signature or Initials	
Ann M. Arch	Receptionist	Ann M. Arch	AMA
John Bortolonni	Office manager	John Bortolonni	JB
Gerald Practon, MD	Provider	Gerald Practon, MD	GP
Rachel Vasquez, CPC	Insurance billing specialist	Rachel Vasquez, CPC	RV
Mary Ann Worth	Clinical medical assistant	Mary Ann Worth	MAW

Figure S-1 Example of a signature log.

significant finding Sign or symptom from a normal condition or important normal observation that assists in making a diagnosis of the patient's problem.

silent PPO See *silent preferred provider organization (silent PPO).*

silent preferred provider organization (silent PPO) Type of managed care plan that has a contract with a clause that allows the plan to assign the contract, or parts of it, to another third party. These contracts are considered legal in most states. If an explanation of benefits document has "network discount applied," then investigate further into the claim to determine if a silent PPO is operating. Always precertify procedures and look at patients' insurance cards even if the patients are established because this may help discover silent PPOs. Also called *blind PPO, phantom PPO, discounted indemnity plans, nondirected PPO,* or *wraparound PPO.*

simple repair Physical restoration of damaged tissue when the wound is superficial (e.g., involving primarily epidermis or dermis or subcutaneous tissues without significant involvement of deeper structures, requiring one-layer closure).

simplified employee pension (SEP) See *Section 408(k) of the Internal Revenue Code.*

simultaneous death act State law that if the insured and beneficiary of a life insurance policy both die and determination of who died first cannot be made, then the insured is presumed to be the primary beneficiary unless there is an insurance clause stating otherwise.

single component code See *component code.*

single drug pricer (SDP) Drug pricing file containing the allowable price for each drug covered that is incident to a physician's service, drugs furnished by independent dialysis facilities that are separately billable from the composite rate, and clotting factors to inpatients. The SDP is, in effect, a fee schedule, similar to other Centers for Medicare and Medicaid Services (CMS) fee schedules.

single organ system examination 1997 guidelines Examinations other than eye or psychiatric examinations should include performance and documentation of at least 12 elements identified in a table by a bullet (•), whether in a shaded or unshaded box. Eye and psychiatric examinations should include the performance and documentation of at least nine elements identified in a table by a bullet (•), whether in a shaded or unshaded box.

single-payer health care system Centralized system in which one organization, usually the government, sets reimbursement rates and pays all of the bills for health care to the providers (e.g., Canada, Germany, Great Britain). Individuals are not restricted as to which physicians or hospitals they can visit for medical services. Also known as *socialized medicine* and *single-payer system.*

single-payer system See *single-payer health care system.*

single practitioner Physician or provider who does not practice in a group and does not share personnel, facilities, or equipment with another business. Also called *solo practitioner.*

single-premium annuity Deferred or immediate annuity purchased with one premium payment. Also see *annuity.*

single-premium deferred annuity (SPDA) See *single-premium annuity.*

single-premium method Group creditor insurance purchased either at the beginning of the loan, with the entire premium lump-sum amount being paid, or by adding the premium to the principal of the loan.

single-purchase annuity contract Group annuity agreement where one premium is used to purchase for the participants in a retirement plan that is terminating (i.e., immediate annuities for current retirees and deferred annuities for those who are not yet of retirement age).

single service plan (SSP) See *carve-out plan.*

single sign-on (SSO) Password security method that enables computer users to enter one password and gain access to a range of applications instead of having to enter unique codes for each application.

single stage agency State organization that administers and manages the state's Medicaid program, a requirement of the Social Security Act.

SIR See *Society of Interventional Radiology (SIR).*

site-of-service (SOS) differential Difference in the amount paid when the same medical service is provided in different medical practice settings (e.g., outpatient visit in a physician's office or a hospital clinic).

site visit Evaluation of a place of business (e.g., under the Health Care Financing Administration's Medicare contracting program, health maintenance organizations and competitive medical plans are reviewed and monitored to see if they are complying with federal requirements).

situs See *state of issue.*

six and six exclusion Provision in a credit disability policy for a preexisting condition that states an insured's disability is not covered if he or she was treated for the condition within 6 months before the effective date of coverage and becomes disabled from that same condition within 6 months after the effective date of coverage.

size discount Fee reduction based on the initial gross monthly premium to groups that have a self-administered health insurance plan.

SJ HCPCS Level II modifier that may be used with CPT or HCPCS Level II codes indicating a third or more concurrently administered infusion therapy.

SK HCPCS Level II modifier that may be used with CPT or HCPCS Level II codes indicating a member of high-risk population (use only with codes for immunization).

S

skeletal traction One of two basic types of traction used in orthopedics to treat fractured bones and correct orthopedic abnormalities. It is applied to the structure by metal pins, clamps, screws, or wires inserted into the affected structure and attached to traction ropes. It allows for continuous traction keeping the bones aligned and immobilized during the initial healing process.

skilled care Type of health care given when a patient needs skilled nursing or rehabilitation staff to manage, observe, and evaluate the care such as injections, catheterizations, and dressing changes.

skilled nursing care Inpatient 24-hour nursing care, rehabilitative services, and related health services for patients who need continuous medical care but do not need acute nursing care. This care can only be performed safely and correctly by either a licensed registered nurse or a licensed practical nurse. Procedures and treatments include injections, administration of medications, changing of dressings, and observation and monitoring of a patient's condition including taking vital signs.

skilled nursing facility (SNF) Commonly pronounced "sniff." 1. Setting, either part of a facility or distinct from it, that provides inpatient 24-hour nursing and related health services for patients who need continuous medical care or rehabilitation services. Patients in need of SNF care may have a condition that is acute, chronic, or terminal and it makes no difference. It is considered to be more cost-effective than an extended hospital stay. Formerly called *extended care facility (ECF)* before 1972 when the Social Security statute was amended and SNF was introduced. 2. Under the Medicaid program, this is known as a *nursing facility (NF)*. Medicaid also has a separate category of intermediate care facility for the mentally retarded. 3. Under the Medicare program, a SNF is staffed and equipped to give intensive nursing and rehabilitative care by registered and licensed nurses or licensed therapists under the supervision of a physician. SNFs must be certified by Medicare and there are specific requirements for admission, certain covered benefits, and a period of coverage. Inpatient SNF, known as *extended care services*, is given to a patient in a SNF up to 100 days of each spell of illness, depending on the patient's condition.

skilled nursing facility care Level of care that requires the daily involvement of skilled nursing or rehabilitation staff and cannot be provided on an outpatient basis such as intravenous injections and physical therapy.

skilled nursing facility (SNF) coinsurance In Medicare, for the 21st through 100th day of extended care services in a benefit period, a daily amount for which the beneficiary is responsible, equal to one eighth of the inpatient hospital deductible. Also called *SNF coinsurance*.

skilled nursing facility services Alternate name for *extended care services*.

skimming the cream Slang expression that means the practice of removing the youngest and healthiest people from a pool of insurance applicants so that they get coverage at the best rates. The remaining group of older, sicker patients and those of questionable health status will be denied coverage or must pay higher rates.

skin traction One of two basic types of traction used in orthopedics for the treatment of fractured bones and to correct orthopedic abnormalities. Felt or adhesive and nonadhesive straps are applied directly to the skin, and traction is used to pull the skin surrounding the structure.

skip Debtor who has moved and neglected to give a forwarding address (i.e., skipped town).

SL HCPCS Level II modifier that may be used with CPT or HCPCS Level II codes indicating state-supplied vaccine.

slanted brackets Symbol used with a diagnostic code in ICD-9-CM, Volume 2, Alphabetic Index, indicating the code may never be sequenced as the principal diagnosis.

slight pain In workers' compensation cases, pain could be tolerated but would cause some handicap in the performance of the activity precipitating the pain.

SLMB See *specified low-income Medicare beneficiaries (SLMB)*.

SM HCPCS Level II modifier that may be used with CPT or HCPCS Level II codes indicating second surgical opinion.

small claims court Court that allows lay people to have access to a court system without the use of an attorney to informally and quickly adjudicate claims below a specific dollar amount. The monetary amount varies from state to state. Claims are usually for collecting small accounts or debts. Also called *conciliation court, common pleas, general session, justice court*, or *people's court*.

small estates statutes State laws enabling an insurance company to pay small amounts of insurance policy proceeds to an estate without complicated court proceedings.

small group About 3 to 99 employees, but state statutes may vary on the numbers.

small group insurance plan Type of group life insurance plan uses simplified individual underwriting combined with group underwriting techniques and covers groups 2 to 25 individuals. Also called *baby group plan*.

small health plan Under the Health Insurance Portability and Accountability Act (HIPAA), this is a health plan with annual receipts of $5 million or less.

small subscriber group aggregate Combination of professional associations, small businesses, or other entities formed and considered as a single, large subscriber group of a health insurance plan.

smart card Plastic card embedded with a microprocessor chip, which can contain health insurance coverage, personal information, and basic recent medical history. It can be written on and updated.

SMI See *supplementary medical insurance (SMI)*.

SMI premium See *supplementary medical insurance (SMI) premium*.

SMS See *socioeconomic monitoring system (SMS)*.

SN HCPCS Level II modifier that may be used with CPT or HCPCS Level II codes indicating third surgical opinion.

SNF See *skilled nursing facility (SNF)*.

SNF coinsurance See *skilled nursing facility (SNF) coinsurance*.

SNOMED See *Systematized Nomenclature of Human and Veterinary Medicine (SNOMED International)*.

SNOMED CT See *Systematized Nomenclature of Medicine for Clinical Terminology (SNOMED CT)*.

SOAP One of a standard style of charting (documenting) procedures for progress notes in patient's medical records; the acronym means subjective, objective, assessment, plan. Subjective = statements of symptoms and chief complaints (CC) in the patient's own words, which is the reason for the encounter. Objective = facts and findings from the physical examination, x-rays, laboratory, and other diagnostic tests. Assessment = evaluation of subjective and objective findings, which is medical decision-making by putting all the facts together to obtain a diagnosis. Plan of treatment = documentation of a strategy for care to be put into action and list of recommendations, instructions, further testing, and medication. Also see *CHEDDAR*.

social health maintenance organization (SHMO) Special type of health plan that provides the full range of Medicare benefits offered by standard Medicare HMOs, plus other services that include prescription drug and chronic care benefits, respite care, and short-term nursing home care; homemaker, personal care services, and medical transportation; and eyeglasses, hearing aids, and dental benefits.

social history (SH) Age-appropriate review of a patient's past and current activities (e.g., marital status, employment history, sexual history, level of education, smoking, diet intake, alcohol use). Depending on the category of evaluation and management (E/M) service, documented review of two or all three past, family, and/or social history (PFSH) is required. For comprehensive assessments, all three areas are required.

social insurance Type of insurance plan that is compulsory under an employee benefit plan. By law, participants have certain benefits. It is administered by a federal or state government agency.

social insurance supplement policy 1. Additional medical insurance coverage to protect against losses when the insured wage earner's income is interrupted or terminated because of illness or accident and the loss is not covered by workers' compensation, disability income benefits, or Social Security Disability Insurance (SSDI). 2. Insurance plan that complements the benefits from a specified government health insurance program.

Social Security Concept in which an individual works, the worker pays taxes into the system, and when the worker retires or becomes disabled, the worker, his or her spouse, and his or her dependent children receive monthly benefits based on the reported earnings. Also, the worker's survivors can collect benefits if the worker dies.

Social Security Act Public Law 74-271, enacted on August 14, 1935, with subsequent amendments. The Social Security Act consists of 20 titles, four of which have been repealed. The health insurance (HI) and supplementary medical insurance (SMI) programs are authorized by Title XVIII of the Social Security Act.

Social Security Administration (SSA) Federal agency that administers Social Security Disability Insurance (SSDI) and Supplemental Security Income (SSI) programs for disabled persons and determines initial entitlement to and eligibility for Medicare benefits.

Social Security benefits Five major categories of benefits are (1) retirement, (2) disability, (3) dependent (family), (4) survivors, and (5) Medicare. The retirement, dependent (family), survivor, and disability programs provide monthly cash benefits and Medicare provides medical coverage.

Social Security Disability Insurance (SSDI) Federal long-term disability income program that gives benefits to disabled workers who are younger than age 65 and paid Social Security tax for a specific number of quarter-year periods.

Social Security number (SSN) Nine-digit number assigned to each individual by the federal government for identification purposes; used as a tax identification number to maintain an accurate record of each person's wages or self-employment earnings.

Social Services Block Grant services Grants given to states under the Social Security Act that fund limited amounts of social services for people of all ages (includes some in-home services and abuse prevention services). Formerly known as *Title XX services*.

social worker Individual who has obtained a degree in social work, has met the requirements of being supervised in the clinical social work, has obtained state licensure or certification, and provides a wide variety of social services in many types of health care settings. The National Association of Social Workers (NASW) classifies several levels of social work positions in two groups: preprofessional and professional. Some types of social workers are caseworkers, child welfare caseworker, clinical social worker, eligibility worker, family counselor, industrial social worker, licensed social worker, medical social worker, psychiatric social worker, public health social worker, registered social worker, school social worker, social group worker, social service caseworker, and social welfare administrator.

socialized medicine This term made its appearance in the 1940s and is a type of coverage for health care expenses provided by a federal government. Also called *statutory health insurance*. See also *national health insurance* and *universal coverage*.

Society of Interventional Radiology (SIR) Professional society for physicians who specialize in interventional or minimally invasive procedures. SIR is a nonprofit, national scientific organization deeply committed to its mission to improve health and the quality of life through the practice of cardiovascular and interventional radiology. The society promotes education, research, and communication in the field while providing strong leadership in the development of health care policy. Formerly known as the *Society of Cardiovascular and Interventional Radiology (SCVIR)*.

socioeconomic monitoring system (SMS) Annual survey of physicians by the American Medical Association that provides information about physicians' earnings, expense, work patterns, and fees.

SOF See *signature on file (SOF)*.

soft copy That which is displayed on a computer screen.

soft denial See *rejected claim*.

software Instructions (programs) required to make hardware perform a specific task.

SOI See *severity of illness*.

sole community hospital (SCH) Under guidelines of the Centers for Medicare and Medicaid Services (CMS), facility that is located more than 35 miles from other like hospitals. It may be classified as an SCH if it is located in a rural area and meets one of the following three conditions: (1) located between 25 and 35 miles from other like hospitals and meets one of three criteria; (2) located between 15 and 25 miles from other like hospitals but because of local topography or periods of prolonged severe weather conditions, the other like hospital are inaccessible for at least 30 days in each of 2 out of 3 years; or (3) because of distance, posted speed limits, and predictable weather conditions, the travel time between the hospital and the nearest like hospital is at least 45 minutes.

sole proprietorship insurance Life insurance coverage for the owner of a business. This type of insurance is used to pay the salary of someone who runs the business after the owner's death or disability or to help the owner's family for loss of income due to failure of the business after the owner's death or disability.

soliciting agent See *agent*.

solo practitioner See *single practitioner*.

solvency Ability of an individual or organization to pay all legal debts.

SOR See *source-oriented record (SOR) system*.

SOS See *site-of-service (SOS) differential*.

source document 1. Financial draft that is the initial point of entry to an accounting system (e.g., invoice, bill, check, deposit slip). 2. In insurance billing, a multipurpose billing form that is also called a *charge document, charge slip, communicator, encounter form, fee ticket, patient service slip, routing form, superbill*, or *transaction slip*. See multipurpose billing form.

source of admission See *point of origin for admission or visit*.

source-oriented record (SOR) system Method of medical recordkeeping in which documents are arranged according to sections (e.g., history and physical section, progress notes, laboratory tests, radiology reports, surgical operations).

spam Unsolicited e-mail message, commercial or political, transmitted to many people at the same time.

SPD See *summary plan description (SPD)*.

SPDA See *single-premium deferred annuity (SPDA)*.

special benefit networks Particular association of providers for a specific type of service (e.g., mental health, prescription drugs, substance abuse).

special care unit Long-term care facility units with services specifically for persons with Alzheimer's disease, dementia, head injuries, or other disorders. Also see *intensive care unit (ICU)*.

special election period Time in which an individual is given a special election period to change Medicare+Choice plans or return to Original Medicare in certain situations. Situations in which this occurs include (1) when a person makes a permanent move outside the service area, (2) when the Medicare+Choice organization breaks its contract with the insured or does not renew its contract with the Centers for Medicare and Medicaid Services (CMS), or (3) when other exceptional conditions determined by CMS apply. The special election period is different from the special enrollment period (SEP). See *election period*.

special enrollment period (SEP) One of four periods during which an individual can enroll in Medicare Part A. SEP is for people who did not take Medicare Part A during their initial enrollment period (IEP) because they currently work and have group health plan coverage through their employer or union. He or she can sign up for Medicare Part A at any time they are covered under the group health plan based on current employment. If the employment or group health coverage ends, the individual has 8 months to sign up. The 8 months start the month after the employment ends or the group health coverage ends, whichever comes first. See also *initial enrollment period (IEP), general enrollment period (GEP)*, and *transfer enrollment period (TEP)*.

special needs plan Under Medicare, type of plan that provides more focused health care for specific groups of individuals such as those who have both Medicare and Medicaid or those who reside in a nursing home.

special public-debt obligation Securities of the U.S. government issued exclusively to the Old Age, Survivors, and Disability Insurance (OASDI); Disability Insurance (DI); Health Insurance (HI); and Supplementary Medical Insurance (SMI) trust funds and other federal trust funds. Section 1841(a) of the Social Security Act provides that the public-debt obligations issued for purchase by the SMI trust fund shall have maturities fixed with due regard for the needs of the funds. The usual practice in the past has been to spread the holdings of special issues, as of every June 30, so that the amounts maturing in each of the next 15 years are approximately equal. Special public-debt obligations are redeemable at par at any time.

special report Document that gives the details of an unusual or infrequently performed medical procedure and supports the necessity for providing services. It is submitted with an insurance claim.

specialist physician Medical doctor who has received training in a specific area of medicine and who treats only certain parts of the body, certain health problems, or certain age groups such as cardiovascular surgeon, dermatologist, and endocrinologist. These doctors are board certified by doing additional advanced residency training followed by several years of practice in the specialty and then passing a specialty board examination. Members of managed care plans usually need approval from their primary care physician to see a specialist.

specialist referral authorization See *referral authorization.*

specialty capitation System of payment used by a managed care plan in which a specialist provider is paid a fixed, capitated fee for giving medical services.

specialty care Health care services that a medical specialist provides (e.g., cardiologist, dermatologist, orthopedic surgeon).

specialty case rate Flat fee paid to a medical specialist for all medical services or procedures.

specialty codes See *taxonomy codes.*

specialty contractor Medicare contractor who performs a limited Medicare function such as coordination of benefits and statistical analysis.

specialty hospital Medical facility that provides health care services for specific illnesses or diseases (e.g., psychiatric hospital, rehabilitation hospital, long-term care hospital [LTCH]).

specialty plan Type of Medicare Advantage Plan that provides more focused health care for some people. These plans give all the Medicare health care, as well as more focused care to manage a disease or condition such as congestive heart failure, diabetes, or end-stage renal disease (ESRD).

specific injury In a workers' compensation case, injury occurring as the result of one incident or exposure that causes disability or need for medical treatment.

specific stop loss insurance Medical insurance plan that pays when an individual's claim reaches a certain threshold chosen by the employer. After the threshold is attained, the stop-loss insurance policy pays claims up to the lifetime limit per employee.

specifications List of qualifying factors of a specific group of individuals, insurance coverage, and services that an insurance company assembles to administer and manage a group insurance program.

specified disease insurance Type of insurance that pays benefits for only a single disease such as cancer or end-stage renal disease or for a group of diseases. It does not fill gaps in Medicare coverage.

specified expense coverage Health insurance that provides benefits for certain medical supplies or treatments or for specific illnesses (e.g., dental, vision care, prescription drugs, long-term care, dread disease).

specified low-income Medicare beneficiaries (SLMB) Medicaid program that pays for Medicare Part B premiums for individuals who have Medicare Part A, a low monthly income, and limited resources.

specimen Small sample of tissue, intended to show the nature of the whole, for pathological diagnosis (e.g., a urine specimen).

speech-language pathologist (SLP) Individual who has a certificate of clinical competence from the American Speech and Hearing Association, has completed the equivalent educational requirements and work experience necessary for the certificate, or has completed the academic program and is acquiring supervised work experience to qualify for the certificate. SLPs specialize in the measurement and evaluation of language abilities, auditory processes, speech production, and swallowing problems.

speech-language therapy Treatment to regain and strengthen speech skills.

speech recognition system Computerized voice recognition system that makes it possible for a computer system to respond to spoken words. Two basic categories are *navigation* or *command control,* which allows an individual to launch and operate software applications with spoken directions, and *dictation software,* which makes it possible for a computer system to recognize spoken words and automatically convert them into text.

speech therapy (ST) Treatment designed to help restore speech through exercises. May be a benefit covered by the Medicare program.

spell of illness See *benefit period.*

spend down In the Medicaid program, process of using up assets or income until an individual reaches the eligibility level because of the need for confinement in a nursing home or for long-term care. Also referred to as *spending down.*

S

spending down See *spend down.*

spendthrift trust clause Provision in a life insurance policy that protects its proceeds from being seized by the beneficiary's creditors.

split billing In Medicare fraud, to use a separated or divided billing scheme such as billing procedures over a period of days when all treatment occurred during one visit.

split-dollar insurance coverage 1. In disability income insurance, employer and employee each pay a portion of the premium. The employer pays for coverage for sick pay or paid disability leave as an employee benefit. The employee pays for disability coverage beyond what the employer provides. 2. In life insurance, premiums, ownership, and death proceeds are paid jointly by an employer and an employee. The employer may elect to pay part or all of the premium. If the employee dies, a beneficiary receives the difference between the cash value and the amount paid to the employer, whichever is greater. Two types of split-dollar life insurance policies are endorsement and collateral.

split funded plan Type of retirement plan in which contributions are shared between the insured and an uninsured plan to have advantages of guaranteed income and investment flexibility.

split funding System of funding a retirement plan in which part of the total contributions are used to purchase a permanent life insurance policy and the remainder of the funds are used to purchase another fund held and invested by a trustee.

split/shared office visit Medically necessary patient encounter in which the physician and a qualified nonphysician practitioner each personally perform a substantive part of an evaluation and management visit (e.g., all or a part of the history, examination, or medical decision-making), face to face with the same patient on the same date of service.

sponsor 1. For the TRICARE program, the service person, either active duty, retired, or deceased, whose relationship makes the patient (dependent) eligible for TRICARE. 2. In managed care, large business that purchases health insurance directly from the accountable health partnerships (AHPs).

sponsor identification card See *military identification card.*

sponsored dependent Family member who is financially supported by the insured and relies on the insured for more than half of his or her support as per the Internal Revenue Service definition.

spousal impoverishment In the Medicaid program, preserve some income and assets for the spouse of a nursing home resident who is on Medicaid.

spousal IRA Trust account established for an individual who is not covered by a qualified employee retirement plan. This account may be created by purchasing individual retirement annuities from an insurance company.

spouse and children's insurance rider Endorsement to an insurance policy that provides insurance coverage for dependents (spouse and children).

SQ HCPCS Level II modifier that may be used with CPT or HCPCS Level II codes indicating an item ordered by home health.

SS-5 Application form used to obtain a Social Security number and card or a replacement card through the Social Security Administration.

SSA See *Social Security Administration (SSA).*

SSDI See *Social Security Disability Insurance (SSDI).*

SSI See *Supplemental Security Income (SSI).*

SSN See *Social Security number (SSN).*

SSO See *second surgical opinion (SSO), single sign-on (SSO),* and *standard setting organization (SSO).*

SSP Acronym for single service plan. See *carve-out plan.*

ST HCPCS Level II modifier that may be used with CPT or HCPCS Level II codes indicating trauma or injury.

ST See *speech therapy (ST).*

stabilization Act of remaining stable and no deterioration of an emergency medical condition is likely to occur within reasonable medical probability.

stacking 1. Situation in which an insurance policy covers two scheduled items of real or personal property and the coverage should be twice the stated limit in the policy. 2. In a retirement plan, when no effort is made to put together benefits from a public and a private pension plan—the plans are "stacked."

staff-assisted dialysis Kidney dialysis performed by the staff of the renal dialysis center or facility.

staff model Type of health maintenance organization (HMO) in which the health plan hires physicians, nurses, and other medical professionals directly and pays them a salary. They provide services at plan-owned facilities. Patients pay low premiums and have few out-of-pocket expenses but must choose doctors within the plan. Also see *group model health maintenance organization (HMO).*

staging Find out the distinct phases in the course of a disease or the life history of an organism or biological process (e.g., in cancer to ascertain whether the disease process is at the primary site or has spread [metastasized]). Also called *disease staging* or *staging of disease.*

stand-alone code Procedure code that has a full description.

standard 1. Under the Health Insurance Portability and Accountability Act (HIPAA), rule, condition, or requirement that describes products, systems, services, or practices with respect to the privacy of individually identifiable health information. 2. In a workers' compensation case, permanent disability (PD) rating before adjustment for age or occupation (e.g., "the rating was 30% standard" or "we settled for the standard PD").

standard anesthesia formula Payment equation that is made up of base units plus time units plus modifying units (e.g., physical status and qualifying circumstances) plus additional (other) allowed units or charges and then multiplied by a conversion factor:

$$B + T + M \text{ (basic + time + modifying}$$
$$\text{circumstances)} + O \text{ (other)}$$
$$\times \text{ conversion factor = payment}$$

standard benefit package 1. Stated set of health insurance benefits that all insurance plans are required to offer. 2. In managed care plans, package of medical services that must be provided to individuals, small businesses, and large businesses at competitive rates (e.g., preventive care, hospital and physician services, prescription medications).

standard claim Insurance claim submitted to a third-party payer that is not accompanied by unnecessary attachments.

standard claims processing system Standard computer system used by insurance carriers and fiscal intermediaries to process Medicare insurance claims.

standard class rate (SCR) Monthly insurance premium for an insurance company's policy applied per member to risks with similar characteristics or to a specified class of risk. A formula is used by multiplying group demographic information to obtain the monthly rate. Also called *class rate.*

standard error In statistics, standard deviation of an estimate—multiple measurements of a given value will generally group around the mean (or average) value in a normal distribution. The shape of this distribution is known as the *standard error.*

standard Medicare drug coverage Model insurance plan that was designed as the minimum drug coverage required by law. It is the standard to which all offered plans are compared. Most plans offer better coverage than the minimum required.

standard nonforfeiture law Legislation that is uniform in all states and requires annuity and whole-life contracts to have certain minimum cash values that are not forfeited by policyholders even if a policy is canceled. A formula is given for computing the present value, cash surrender value, and paid-up annuity benefits. The model requires insurers to state clearly if an annuity has limited or no death benefits.

standard of care 1. Written statement that describes the rules, actions, or conditions that direct proper treatment of patients. 2. Specific guidelines that direct medical practice and can be used to evaluate performance. Also see *standards of care protocols.*

standard paper remittance (SPR) Document detailing services billed and describing payment determination (paid or denied) issued to providers of the Medicare or Medicaid program. Providers that electronically

transmit Medicare claims receive an electronic remittance advice (ERA). Beginning June 1, 2006, they were no longer mailed an SPR. Also known in some programs as an *explanation of benefits.*

standard plan termination Process of ending a retirement or employee-benefit plan that has enough funds to cover all benefit amounts to which the plan's participants are entitled.

standard premium rate See *basic premium.*

standard provisions Elements common to life and health insurance policies stating coverage and benefits and obligations of the insured and insurance company in basic contract language.

standard risk Future probability that is considered normal and insurable at standard rates without an additional premium or restrictions.

standard risk class Insurance category composed of individuals whose loss is considered normal or average. This class pays basic or standard premium rates. Other classifications are given credits or debits depending on their difference from the standard.

standard setting organization (SSO) Association accredited by the American National Standards Institute that develops and maintains standards for information transactions or data elements or any other standard under the Health Insurance Portability and Accountability Act (HIPAA).

standard transaction format 837P Electronic claims transmittal format of the CMS-1500 insurance claim.

standard transaction format compliance system (STFCS) An Electronic Healthcare Network Accreditation Commission (EHNAC)-sponsored Washington Publishing Company (WPC)-hosted Health Insurance Portability and Accountability Act (HIPAA) compliance certification service.

standard transactions 1. Under the Health Insurance Portability and Accountability Act (HIPAA), the electronic files in which medical data are compiled to produce a specific format. 2. Under HIPAA, a transaction that complies with the applicable HIPAA standard.

standard valuation law Legislation that is uniform in all states and stipulates the minimum standards for calculating or valuing insurance reserves that a life insurance company must maintain for its life insurance policies and annuity contracts. It was first developed by the National Association of Insurance Commissioners.

standardization Act of making charges or costs more comparable among medical providers, plans, and geographical areas. This is accomplished by adjusting specific services or bundles of services to remove differences that result from geographical variation in prices and beneficiary health risk.

standards of care protocols Set of guidelines for medical tests and procedures that are considered covered services for specific predetermined diagnoses.

S

Standards of Ethical Coding Code of conduct developed by the American Health Information Management Association to provide a basis for ethical decision-making in coding practice.

standby anesthesia service Backup anesthetist requested by another physician for a case that involves prolonged attendance without direct patient contact. If the physician does the procedure, this service would not be billable.

standing order Written direction given for ongoing treatment or medical care until it is overridden by another written direction (e.g., vital signs every hour).

star procedure Beginning in CPT 2004, the star (*) symbol was deleted.

star symbol This symbol (*) was deleted beginning in CPT 2004.

Stark I Regulations [42 U.S.C.A. § 1395nn (1989)] Legislation introduced by U.S. Representative Pete Stark and passed as part of the Omnibus Budget Reconciliation Act (OBRA) of 1993. Its purpose was to save Medicare dollars by preventing overuse of medical services. Stark I prohibits physicians from referring a patient to a clinical laboratory in which the doctor or a member of his or her family has a financial interest, except in specific situations. This differs from anti-kickback laws because it has to do with self-referral instead of referring to another physician. Sometimes referred to as *antikickback act* or *antikickback statute*.

Stark II Regulations [42 U.S.C.A. § 1395nn(h)(6) (1993)] Amendment to Stark I as part of the Omnibus Budget Reconciliation Act (OBRA) of 1993. Its purpose was to prevent a physician from referring a Medicare or Medicaid patient to a facility in which the physician has a financial interest. It prohibits any payment paid directly or indirectly to providers. A facility might have services such as physical therapy, occupational therapy, radiology and other diagnostic services, radiation therapy, durable medical equipment, parenteral and enteral nutrition, equipment and supplies, prosthetics and orthotics, home health services, outpatient prescription drugs, and inpatient or outpatient hospital services. This law encouraged doctors to form groups and join health systems as employees. Sometimes referred to as *antikickback act* or *antikickback statute*.

stat Medical term derived from the Latin word *statim*. It is commonly used and means "immediately."

stat charge Fee for immediate test results. Also called *rush charge*.

state certification In Medicare, inspections of Medicare provider facilities to ensure compliance with federal health, safety, and program standards.

State Children's Health Insurance Program (SCHIP) Free or low-cost state child health program that operates with federal grant support under Titles V and XXI of the Social Security Act. It is for uninsured children younger than age 19 whose families earn too much to qualify for Medicaid but do not have enough resources to get private coverage. In some states this program may be known as *Maternal and Child Health Program (MCHP)* or *Children's Special Health Care Services (CSHCS)*. In California it is called *Healthy Families in California*.

state compensation board or commission See *workers' compensation agency*.

state compensation fund Type of workers' compensation program in which the state appoints an agency to act as the insurance company to cover industrial claims.

State Disability Insurance (SDI) Insurance that covers off-the-job injury or sickness and is paid for by deductions from a person's paycheck. This program is administered by a state agency and is sometimes known as *Unemployment Compensation Disability (UCD)*. Six states have compulsory state disability plans: California, Hawaii, New Jersey, New York, Puerto Rico, and Rhode Island.

state fund Insurer established and operated by a state government that is a mandatory insurance program such as workers' compensation insurance.

state fund employer Employer or corporation who pays premiums into the state insurance fund for workers' compensation insurance coverage.

state health insurance assistance program State program that receives monies from the federal government to give free local health insurance counseling to people with Medicare.

state insurance commission Official state group charged with regulating, administering, licensing insurance companies, and enforcing laws pertaining to insurance business in the state and providing public information on insurance. Also known as *State Insurance Department* or *Department of Insurance (DOI)*.

state insurance department See *state insurance commission*.

state law Under the Health Insurance Portability and Accountability Act (HIPAA), constitution, statute, regulation, rule, common law, or any other state action that has the force and effect of law.

state legislated benefits See *mandated benefits*.

state license number Number issued to a physician who has passed the state medical examination indicating his or her right to practice medicine in the state where issued.

state licensure agency State agency that has the authority to terminate, sanction, or prosecute fraudulent providers under state laws.

state medical assistance office State agency that is in charge of the state's Medicaid program and can give information about programs to help pay medical bills for people with low incomes. It also provides help with prescription drug coverage.

state of issue Region where group insurance contract is delivered or issued. Also called *situs*.

state practice acts State medical licensing statutes for physicians, nurses, and other health care professionals that list each recognized health care profession and its legal scope of practice.

state public health clinic Health facility maintained by either state or local health departments that provides ambulatory primary medical care under the general direction of a physician. Also called *local public health clinic*.

state survey Under §1864 of the Act, Centers for Medicare and Medicaid Services (CMS) has entered into agreements with agencies of state governments, typically the agency that licenses health facilities within the state health departments, to conduct surveys of Medicare participating providers and suppliers for purposes of determining compliance with Medicare requirements for participation in the Medicare program.

state survey agency State agency that inspects renal dialysis facilities and makes sure that Medicare standards are met.

State Uniform Billing Committee State-specific affiliate of the National Uniform Billing Committee (NUBC) that developed the Uniform Bill (UB-92) insurance claim form for hospital inpatient billing and payment transactions in use from 1994. It replaced the Uniform Bill (UB-82) claim form that was also referred to as *HCFA-1450 claim form*. The Uniform Bill (UB-92) was replaced by the Uniform Bill (UB-04) claim form in 2008.

state unit on aging State office authorized by the Older Americans Act that administers the plan for service to the aged and coordinates programs for the aged with other state offices.

statistical fluctuation Deviations from the predicted future of occurrences that was based on past numerical data.

statistics Accumulation of numbers recorded and then to analyze information (e.g., occurrences of injuries and accidents, causes of death, losses). The information is used to predict future occurrences and calculate insurance premium rates.

status clause Insurance policy provision that excludes payment of benefits for loss that occurs when an insured is in active military service.

status location Indicator on an insurance claim record that describes the queue (line or file) where the claim is situated and the action that needs to be performed on the claim.

status modifier See *physical status modifier*.

statute Law passed by a legislative body including administrative boards, municipal courts, and legislatures (e.g., legislative branch of the federal government). See *act*. Also called *act* or *law*.

statute of limitations 1. Time limit established for filing lawsuits; may vary from state to state. 2. Specific period of time after a patient receives medical services in which a claim must be filed and after which lapse of time the claim may no longer be enforced.

statutory accounting practices (SAP) Guidelines that insurance companies are required to follow when filing an annual financial statement (convention blank) with state insurance regulatory authorities. Statutory accounting is more conservative than generally accepted accounting principles (GAAP) because it overstates expenses and liabilities and understates income and assets. Also see *generally accepted accounting principles (GAAP)*.

statutory health insurance See *national health insurance*.

statutory reserves Funds (reserves) set aside and designated for future financial liabilities for life or health insurance that are required by state regulations. Also called *legal reserve*.

stay outlier See *outlier*.

steering Financial incentives for managed care plan members to use a panel of preferred providers. This may be done through benefits applied to the deductible, coinsurance, and coinsurance limits.

stent 1. Compound used in making dental impressions and medical molds. 2. Mold or device made of stent, used in anchoring skin grafts. 3. Rod or threadlike device for supporting tubular structures during surgical anastomosis or for holding arteries open during angioplasty.

step therapy In Medicare Part D plans, requirement that a certain drug be tried before another drug is covered by an insurance plan.

step-down unit See *intermediate unit*.

step-rate premium Type of insurance rating structure in which premiums may be increased at predetermined times (e.g., at renewal, policy years, or insured's age).

STFCS See *standard transaction format compliance system (STFCS)*.

stochastic model Analysis involving a random variable. For example, a stochastic model may include a frequency distribution for one assumption. From the frequency distribution, possible outcomes for the assumption are selected randomly for use in an illustration.

stock bonus plan Employee-benefit plan in which a portion of the employees' salary is in the form of the employer's stock.

stock company In insurance, this is a business owned and operated by a group of stockholders whose investments provide the safety margin necessary for the issuance of guaranteed, fixed premium, nonparticipating insurance policies. The stockholders share in the profits and losses of the company. Also referred to as *stock insurance company, stock insurer*, or *stock life insurance company*.

S

stock insurance company See *stock company*.

stock insurer See *stock company*.

stock life insurance company See *stock company*.

stock option incentive Type of motivation plan in which an employer offers to sell the company's stock to a company executive at a specific price on a specific date. If the stock's value increases, the executive may exercise the stock option and buy the company's stock at a price below the stock market's value.

stock repurchase insurance Type of life insurance for financing the purchase of stock from the estate of a deceased stockholder by other stockholders in the same company.

stockholder Individual who owns shares of stock in a corporation. Also called *shareholder*.

stocks Shares of capital bought and held as certificates by an individual investor.

stop loss 1. An agreement between a managed care company and a reinsurer in which absorption of prepaid patient expenses is limited; or limiting losses on an individual expensive hospital claim or professional services claim. 2. Form of reinsurance by which the managed care program limits the losses of an individual expensive hospital claim. See *excess risk*.

stop-loss attachment point Place where the stop-loss insurance company assumes liability.

stop-loss insurance Type of insurance coverage purchased by an employer to limit the losses under a self-insurance medical plan. Two types are specific stop loss and aggregate stop loss.

stop-loss provision Clause in a health insurance policy that states the insurance company will pay 100% of the insured's eligible medical expenses after the insured has met a certain amount of expense (coinsurance).

stop-loss reinsurance Reinsurance purchased to protect an insurance company (cedent) against an aggregate amount of insurance claims over a specific time period. This type of plan does not cover individual claims.

straight bankruptcy See *straight petition in bankruptcy*.

straight life annuity Type of annuity policy that makes periodic payments to the annuitant as long as the annuitant is alive but no benefits after death.

straight life income option Life insurance policy settlement where payments to the beneficiary continue until the beneficiary's death.

straight life insurance See *continuous-premium whole life insurance*.

straight petition in bankruptcy All nonexempt assets of the bankrupt person are liquidated and are distributed according to the law to the creditors. Secured creditors are first in line for payment of all secured debt. Unsecured creditors are last. Also called Chapter 7 *bankruptcy* or *absolute bankruptcy*.

straightforward (SF) Minimal type of medical decision-making.

straightforward (SF) medical decision-making One of four types of medical decision-making that indicates a minimal number of diagnoses, zero to minimal data or complexity of data to be reviewed, and minimal risk of complications and/or morbidity or mortality.

strategic national implementation process Workgroup on Electronic Data Interchange's (WEDI's) national effort for helping the health care industry identify and resolve any Health Insurance Portability and Accountability Act (HIPAA) implementation issues.

structured settlement Agreement to pay a specific amount at regular intervals instead of a lump sum payment.

student See *medical student*.

SU HCPCS Level II modifier that may be used with CPT or HCPCS Level II codes indicating procedure performed in a physician's office (to denote use of facility and equipment).

sub rosa films Videotapes made without the knowledge of the subject; used to investigate suspicious claims in workers' compensation cases.

subacute care See *intermediate care*.

subcapitation Situation in which an organization using a capitated method of payment contracts with other providers on a capitated basis and shares a part of the original capitated premium (e.g., carve out services).

subcategory 1. Fourth digit of a diagnostic code in ICD-9-CM that further defines a three-digit category such as site, cause, or other characteristics. 2. Division under a category in the *Current Procedural Terminology (CPT)* code book.

subclassification Fifth digit of a diagnostic code in ICD-9-CM that gives further specificity and makes a distinction between a code in a four-digit subcategory.

subgroup number Additional alpha characters or numbers assigned to a group number for the purpose of identification (e.g., two characters separated by a dash [SA-12345]).

subjective Perceived by the individual only and not evident to the examiner (e.g., pain).

subjective factors of disability In a workers' compensation case, symptoms that interfere with the injured worker's ability to work that cannot be objectively measured and are obtained from the injured worker's description of symptoms (e.g., pain or emotional symptoms that limit specific activities).

subjective information Data that cannot be measured, typically referred to as "symptoms."

submitted charge Bill sent by a health care provider to the third-party payer or to the patient.

subpoena Latin-derived term meaning "under penalty." Legal document that commands a witness to appear at a trial or other proceeding and give testimony.

subpoena duces tecum Latin-derived term meaning "in his possession." Legal document (subpoena) that requires the appearance of a witness with his or her records. Sometimes the judge permits the mailing of records, and the physician is not required to appear in court.

subrogation 1. Legal right of an insurance company to recover monies or benefits from a third party who was at fault and is liable for the payment. When compared with coordination of benefits (COB), in which liability is shared between third parties, subrogation differs because it assigns the rights to another party. Also called *right of subrogation*. 2. Insurance policy provision requiring an insured to turn over rights he or she may have to recover damages from another party to the insurer, to the extent to which he or she has received reimbursement by the insurer.

subrogation clause See *subrogation*.

subrogation of benefits Process to identify the party responsible for payment of an accident claim.

subscriber Contract holder who either has insurance coverage through his or her place of employment or has purchased coverage directly from the plan or affiliate. This term is used primarily in Blue Cross and Blue Shield programs. Also referred to as *policyholder* or *insured*.

subscriber agreement See *certificate of coverage (COC)*.

subscriber certificate See *certificate of coverage (COC)*.

subscriber contract See *certificate of coverage (COC)*.

subscriber database Collection of information stored on an insurance company's computer system that pertains to insureds covered by insurance policies.

subscriber maintenance To update, correct, add, and delete any information made to the database of insureds.

subsection One division of the *Current Procedural Terminology (CPT)* code book. The book is divided into seven code sections and appendices. Within each of the main sections are subsections and categories divided according to anatomical body system, organ, or site; procedure or service; condition; and specialty.

subsequent injury fund (SIF) A special fund that assumes all or part of the liability for benefits provided to a worker because of the combined effect of a work-related impairment and a preexisting condition.

subsidiary codes CPT code numbers for services that are not part of the primary procedure and are not performed alone. These may be listed as each additional or list-in-addition-to services. Key phrases used throughout the CPT code book to identify subsidiary codes are *each additional, list in addition to*, and *done at time of other major procedure(s)*.

subsidized senior housing Type of program available through the Federal Department of Housing and Urban Development and some states to help people with low or moderate incomes pay for housing.

substance abuse Overindulgence in and dependence on alcohol or drugs (stimulants, depressants, or other chemical substances) that lead to effects that are detrimental to the individual's physical or mental health or the safety or welfare of others. Also called *chemical dependency*.

substandard broker Agent who runs a brokerage that specializes in locating coverage for substandard cases or sells products of several insurers that underwrite substandard risks.

substandard premium rate Insurance premium charged for an insured that is classified as a greater than average possibility of loss, usually a higher rate than a standard premium rate.

substandard risk See *modified risk*.

substandard risk class Insured classification of individuals whose physical conditions are less than standard or who have a dangerous occupation or hobby. An additional premium is required because of the likelihood of loss from an impairment.

substantial comorbidity Medical condition that coexists with the primary cause for hospitalization (principal diagnosis) and affects the patient's treatment and length of stay by at least 1 day in approximately 75% of the cases.

substantial complication Condition that occurs during the hospitalization and prolongs the length of stay by at least 1 day in approximately 75% of the cases.

substantial financial risk (SFR) Incentive arrangement that places the physician or physician group at risk for amounts beyond the risk threshold, if the risk is based on the use or costs of referral services. The risk threshold is 25%. However, if the patient panel is greater than 25,000 patients, then the physician group is not considered to be at substantial financial risk because the risk is spread over the large number of patients. Stop loss and beneficiary surveys would not be required.

subterms 1. In the ICD-9-CM diagnostic code book, words or phrases that appear under a main term and identify site, type, or etiology for diseases, conditions, or injuries. 2. See *modifying terms*.

subtraction Act of removing an overlying structure to better visualize the structure being examined (i.e., imposing one x-ray on top of another).

successor beneficiary See *contingent beneficiary*.

successor owner Individual chosen to be the owner of the life insurance policy if the owner dies before the person insured by the policy dies.

successor payee See *contingent payee*.

suicide clause Life insurance policy provision that states if the insured takes his or her own life, then the proceeds of the policy will not be paid.

suit See *lawsuit*.

summarized cost rate Ratio of the present value of expenditures to the present value of the taxable payroll for the years in a given period. In this context the expenditures are on an incurred basis and exclude costs for those uninsured persons for whom payments are reimbursed from the general fund of the U.S. Treasury and for voluntary enrollees, who pay a premium in order to be enrolled. The summarized cost rate includes the cost of reaching and maintaining a target trust fund level known as a *contingency fund ratio*. Because a trust fund level of about 1 year's expenditures is considered to be an adequate reserve for unforeseen contingencies, the targeted contingency fund ratio used in determining summarized cost rates is 100% of annual expenditures. Accordingly, the summarized cost rate is equal to the ratio of (1) the sum of the present value of the outgo during the period, plus the present value of the targeted ending trust fund level, plus the beginning trust fund level, to (2) the present value of the taxable payroll during the period.

summarized income rate Ratio of (1) the present value of the tax revenues incurred during a given period (from both payroll taxes and taxation of Old Age, Survivors, and Disability Insurance [OASDI] Program benefits), to (2) the present value of the taxable payroll for the years in the period.

summary health information Under the Health Insurance Portability and Accountability Act (HIPAA), data that may be individually identifiable health information and summarizes the claims history, claims expenses, or types of claims experienced by individuals for whom a plan sponsor has provided health benefits under a group health plan.

summary of charges See *itemized billing statement*.

summary payment voucher Document the fiscal agent sends to the provider and/or beneficiary, showing the service or supplies received, allowable charges, amount billed, the amount TRICARE paid, how much deductible has been paid, and the patient's cost-share.

summary plan description (SPD) 1. Document containing all provisions of the managed care plan that must be written in layman's language, which is a requirement of the Employee Retirement Income Security Act (ERISA). 2. Description of a group insurance plan that must be given to all plan participants and to the Department of Labor. See *benefit limitations, explanation of coverage (EOC)*, and *plan document*.

superbill See *multipurpose billing form*.

superimposed major medical plan Health insurance plan that has basic medical expense coverage plus benefits for expenses that go above this coverage.

Superintendent of Insurance See *Commissioner of Insurance*.

superstandard risk class See *preferred risk class*.

supervision Defined by Medicare, situation whenever there are more than four cases concurrently directed by one physician, certified registered nurse anesthetist (CRNA), anesthesiology assistant (AA), or resident or a combination of those providers.

supervision and interpretation *Supervision* means performing the radiological procedure, and *interpretation* means reading or analyzing the film and preparing a report. This phrase is considered when choosing a CPT code for a radiological procedure (70010 to 79999).

When the radiological procedure is performed by two physicians, the radiological portion of the procedure is designated as "radiological supervision and interpretation." When a physician performs the procedure and provides imaging supervision and interpretation, a combination of procedure codes outside the 70000 series and imaging supervision and interpretation codes is used.

supplemental accident Type of health insurance that offers first dollar coverage (no deductible or copayments) or a fixed dollar amount when a loss is due to an accident.

supplemental benefits 1. Disability insurance provisions that allow benefits to the insured to increase the monthly indemnity or to receive a percentage of the policy premiums if an individual keeps a policy in force for 5 or 10 years or does not file any claims. 2. Medical benefits for an employer group in addition to the basic health plan.

supplemental billing Additional invoicing of a specific time period for additional members or for changes to an insurance plan.

supplemental edit software System that is outside the Standard Claims Processing System, which allows further automation of claim reviews. It may be designed using the logic, or expertise, of a medical professional.

supplemental executive retirement plan (SERP) Nonqualified deferred compensation retirement plan that gives benefits for a group of company executives regardless of benefits provided under a qualified retirement plan.

supplemental group life insurance Additional life insurance beyond basic coverage provided by a group policy such as additional amount of the same or a different type of insurance.

supplemental health insurance See *Medigap (MG) policy*.

supplemental health services Optional medical services that may be available for insurance coverage in addition to basic health benefits such as chiropractic, podiatric, dental, or vision care.

supplemental hospital plan Insurance agreement designed to meet a substantial part of out-of-pocket medical expenses from other health care finance plans.

supplemental insurance Secondary insurance policy that covers only what the primary insurance does not cover. For Medicare beneficiaries, see *Medigap (MG) policy*.

supplemental major medical insurance Health insurance that provides benefits above the benefits in a basic hospital-surgical insurance policy.

supplemental medical-legal evaluation In a workers' compensation case, evaluation that (1) does not involve an examination of the patient; (2) is based on the physician's review of records, test results, or other medically relevant information that was not available to the physician at the time of the initial examination; (3) results in the preparation of a narrative medical report prepared and attested to in accordance with specific sections of the labor code; and (4) is performed by a qualified medical evaluator or primary treating physician following the evaluator's completion of a comprehensive medical-legal evaluation.

Supplemental Security Income (SSI) Federal program of income support for low-income aged, blind, and disabled persons established by Title XVI of the Social Security Act in 1972. SSI provides monthly cash payments to meet basic needs for food, clothing, and shelter.

supplemental services Additional or optional medical services that a health insurance plan covers besides basic health benefits.

supplementary benefit rider Endorsement to an insurance policy that gives additional benefits (e.g., accidental death coverage, guaranteed insurance option, waiver of premium).

Supplementary Classification of External Causes of Injury and Poisoning (E800-E999) See *E codes*.

supplementary contract Agreement between a life insurance company and a policyholder by which the company keeps the cash sum payable under an insurance policy and makes payments in agreement with the settlement option selected.

supplementary contract with life contingencies (WLC) Additional agreement in which the payment period is based on the lifetime of the beneficiary.

supplementary contract without life contingencies (WOLC) Additional agreement in which proceeds of a life insurance policy are either held at interest or paid periodically over a specific time period.

supplementary medical insurance (SMI) Medicare program that pays for a portion of the costs of physicians' services, outpatient hospital services, and other related medical and health services for voluntarily insured aged and disabled individuals. Also known as *Medicare Part B*—medical benefits of Medicare program.

supplementary medical insurance (SMI) premium In Medicare, the monthly premium paid by those individuals who have enrolled in the voluntary SMI program. Also called *SMI premium*.

supplementary notice Written announcement required by the Fair Credit Reporting Act sent to a consumer about the scope of investigation stated in a prenotice form that an insurance company has previously sent to the consumer.

supplementary statement Under the National Association of Insurance Commissioners Model Privacy Act, written notice to correct erroneous information made by an individual who has been investigated. This statement is kept in the person's file and is available to anyone reviewing the disputed information.

supplier 1. Institution, company, individual, or agency that furnishes a medical item or service such as a wheelchair or walker. 2. In Medicare, suppliers are distinguished from providers including hospitals and skilled nursing facilities. Institutions classified as providers are reimbursed by fiscal intermediaries and suppliers including physicians, durable medical equipment companies, medical-surgical supplies, nonhospital laboratories, and ambulance companies are paid by insurance carriers.

support groups Three or more individuals who share a common bond and come together on a regular basis to share problems and experiences. These groups may be sponsored by social service agencies, senior centers, religious organizations, hospital facilities, and charitable nonprofit organizations.

supportive data Information that substantiates and authenticates an incident such as author of the document, creation date, accessed date, and modified date. Also called *metadata*.

surety Individual who undertakes to fulfill the obligation of another.

surgeon Physician who is specially trained in operative procedures and treats injuries, deformities, and diseases by operative methods.

surgery Branch of medicine that deals with diseases and trauma requiring invasive operative procedures.

surgery section Division of the *Current Procedural Terminology (CPT)* code book that contains information about surgical procedures.

surgical hierarchy Sequencing of operative cases from those most to those least resource intensive (e.g., if a patient needs to have multiple surgical procedures, each of which occurs by itself, and the procedures could result in assignments to different diagnosis-related groups [DRGs]). A patient must be assigned to only one DRG per hospital admit.

surgical package In CPT coding, this is a surgical procedure code that includes the operation, local infiltration, digital block, or topical anesthesia, and normal, uncomplicated postoperative care. This is referred to as a "package," and one fee covers the whole package. See also *global surgery policy (GSP)*.

surgical schedule Fee schedule in an insurance policy that lists the maximum amounts payable for various operative procedures.

surgical team Situation in which several surgeons are present during the operation. A five-digit CPT code number is used with an attached modifier -66 to list the procedure. If listing more than one modifier, the appropriate sequence is to list -66 first and any one of these modifiers in the next position (-54, -55).

surgicenter See *ambulatory surgery center (ASC)*.

surplus Dollar amount that shows an insurance company's assets exceed its liabilities and capital.

surplus account Account that shows the insurance company's assets minus its liabilities.

S

surplus lines Special property liability insurance coverage by an insurer not licensed to transact business in the state where the risk is located. Also referred to as *excess-surplus lines*.

surrender charge 1. Dollar amount deducted from an insurance policy's reserves to obtain the policy's cash value. 2. Fee requested from a policy owner when the owner surrenders the policy for its cash value.

surrender cost index (SCI) See *interest-adjusted cost*.

surrender cost index (SCI) method See *interest-adjusted net cost (IANC) method*.

surrogate Court officer who administers matters of estate probate, guardianships, and adoptions.

surrogate UPIN Originally used if no unique physician identification number (UPIN) had been assigned to the ordering/referring physician; it was temporary, except for retired physicians, and only used until an individual UPIN was assigned. UPINs have been replaced by national provider identifiers (NPIs). See *national provider identifier (NPI)*.

surveillance Systematic collection of information that pertains to the occurrence of specific diseases, the analysis and interpretation of the data, and the dissemination of the results within government, to the public, and to other interested parties.

Surveillance and Utilization Review System (SURS) One of the systems approved by the Centers for Medicare and Medicaid Services (CMS) that supports the operation of the Medicaid program. The SURS safeguards against unnecessary or inappropriate use of Medicaid services or excess payments and assesses the quality of those services.

Surveillance Epidemiology and End Results (SEER) See *SEER program* and *SEER Medicare database*.

survey Investigation in which information is systematically collected for research.

survey and certification process Activity conducted by state survey agencies or other Centers for Medicare and Medicaid Services (CMS) agents under the direction of CMS and within the scope of applicable regulations and operating instructions and under the provisions of §1864 of the Social Security Act whereby surveyors determine compliance or noncompliance of Medicare providers and suppliers with applicable Medicare requirements for participation. The survey and certification process for each provider and supplier is outlined in detail in the state operations and regional office manuals published by CMS.

surviving spouse 1. Wife or husband of a deceased worker who is eligible for group insurance coverage through the spouse's company. 2. For TRICARE or a veteran's program, individual who is married to the service member or veteran at the time of death.

survivor income benefit insurance Type of group life insurance providing income benefits if the insured is survived by a qualified survivor (spouse and children).

survivorship clause Life insurance policy provision stating the beneficiary must survive the insured by a specific number of days to receive the death benefit. This clause is usually inserted at the request of the insured. Also referred to as a *delay clause* or a *time clause*.

survivorship life insurance Type of whole life insurance for two people that pays benefits only when the second person dies. This type of insurance is usually obtained to help pay estate taxes. Also called *second-to-die life insurance*.

suspect procedure Medical or surgical procedure that may be obsolete or of doubtful value. Such procedures or tests are usually marked to be manually reviewed by a managed care plan's utilization review committee for appropriateness of care.

suspended claim Insurance claim held by the insurance carrier as pending either due to an error or the need for additional information.

suspense 1. Processed insurance claim held as pending either due to an error or the need for additional information. 2. Reminder method used to track pending or resubmitted insurance claims and to telephone or send inquiries about nonpayment. Also called a *follow-up file*, *tickler file*, or *tracing file*. Also see *tracing file* or *tickler file*.

suspense period Time span or hold period following discharge of a hospitalized patient in which the patient's financial account remains available for charges and services before it drops into the claim-submission queue. Once this period passes, the account is deemed "unbilled." This hold period is established by the hospital's finance department.

suspension Preparation of a liquid drug in which the particles are undissolved and must be mixed by stirring or shaking before administration.

suspension of payments Withholding of payment by a fiscal intermediary or insurance carrier from a provider or supplier of an approved Medicare payment amount before a determination of the amount of the overpayment exists. Also called *managed care payment suspension*.

sustainable growth rate System for establishing goals for the rate of growth in expenditures for physicians' services.

SV HCPCS Level II modifier that may be used with CPT or HCPCS Level II codes indicating pharmaceuticals delivered to the patient's home but not used.

svc See *service (svc)*.

SW HCPCS Level II modifier that may be used with CPT or HCPCS Level II codes indicating services provided by a certified diabetic educator.

swing bed Bed used for acute or long-term care facilities usually located in small and rural hospitals. A patient in a swing bed in an acute care setting may be discharged and readmitted to a swing bed and receive skilled or intermediate levels of care. A patient may remain in the swing bed while changes occur in medical care, charges, and payment.

swing-bed hospital Facility usually in small and rural hospitals that provides skilled nursing care and other services comparable with those of a skilled nursing facility (SNF).

SY HCPCS Level II modifier that may be used with CPT or HCPCS Level II codes indicating persons who are in close contact with members of a high-risk population (use only with codes for immunization).

symptom Change in normal bodily function, appearance, or sensation; any indication of disease perceived by the patient.

syntax Rules and conventions that one needs to know or follow in order to validly record information, or interpret previously recorded information, for a specific purpose. Thus a syntax is sentence structure and language rules—grammar. Such rules and conventions may be either explicit or implicit. In X12 transactions the data-element separators, subelement separators, segment terminators, segment identifiers, loops, loop identifiers (when present), repetition factors, and so on are all aspects of the X12 syntax. When explicit, such syntactical elements tend to be the structural, or format-related, data elements that are not required when a direct data entry architecture is used. Ultimately, though, there is not a perfectly clear division between the syntactical elements and the business data content.

system notice Document published in the *Federal Register* notifying the public of a new or revised system of records.

system of records Collection of records from which an agency retrieves information by reference to an individual identifier.

systematic Pursuing a defined objective(s) in a planned, step-by-step manner.

Systematized Nomenclature of Human and Veterinary Medicine (SNOMED International) Comprehensive multilingual clinical terminology book Volumes I through IV used by institutions (within a facility), pathologists, and those involved with generating medical reports and billing for laboratory medicine procedures. In addition, this system is used for managing patient records, teaching medical information science (informatics), and indexing and managing research data. SNOMED is also used to compare terminology context or classification description principles with the ICD-9-CM system; also known as *mapping*.

Systematized Nomenclature of Medicine for Clinical Terminology (SNOMED CT) Reference medical terminology classification system designed and created by the College of American Pathologists that is used to code text data after they are captured by an electronic health record (EHR) system. It assists in the standardization of clinical medical terminology used in EHRs. It is designed to obtain the most detailed, complete, and accurate clinical data possible.

system review See *review of systems (ROS)*.

system security Situation in which all electronic files and folders that contain protected health information are secure from any unauthorized access.

S

T1 HCPCS Level II modifier that may be used with CPT or HCPCS Level II codes indicating the second digit of the left foot.

T2 HCPCS Level II modifier that may be used with CPT or HCPCS Level II codes indicating the third digit of the left foot.

T3 HCPCS Level II modifier that may be used with CPT or HCPCS Level II codes indicating the fourth digit of the left foot.

T4 HCPCS Level II modifier that may be used with CPT or HCPCS Level II codes indicating the fifth digit of the left foot.

T5 HCPCS Level II modifier that may be used with CPT or HCPCS Level II codes indicating the great toe of the right foot.

T6 HCPCS Level II modifier that may be used with CPT or HCPCS Level II codes indicating the second digit of the right foot.

T7 HCPCS Level II modifier that may be used with CPT or HCPCS Level II codes indicating the third digit of the right foot.

T8 HCPCS Level II modifier that may be used with CPT or HCPCS Level II codes indicating the fourth digit of the right foot.

T9 HCPCS Level II modifier that may be used with CPT or HCPCS Level II codes indicating the fifth digit of the right foot.

TA 1. HCPCS Level II modifier that may be used with CPT or HCPCS Level II codes indicating the great toe of the left foot. 2. See *technology assessment (TA).*

table of allowances See *fee schedule.*

Table of Drugs and Chemicals Table that lists three- to five-digit code numbers with descriptions to identify classifications of drugs and other chemical substances for poisoning states and external causes of adverse effects (see Table T-1). It is found after the Alphabetical Index in Volume 2, Section 2 of the *International Classification of Diseases, Ninth Revision, Clinical Modification (ICD-9-CM)* code book.

table rates See *age/sex rates (ASR).*

Tabular List Series of three- to five-digit code numbers with descriptions for disease classifications listed in Volume 1 of the *International Classification of Diseases, Ninth Revision, Clinical Modification (ICD-9-CM)* code book.

Taft-Hartley Trust See *negotiated trusteeship.*

TAR See *treatment authorization request (TAR).*

target benefit plan Type of retirement plan for an individual in which contributions are put into variable annuities or mutual funds to reach a specific level. Performance of investments may exceed or fall below the goals of the plan. Annual contributions are subject to the same rules as those for money purchase plans. When the employee retires, the funds may be paid in a lump sum or used to purchase an annuity.

task force Under the Health Insurance Portability and Accountability Act (HIPAA), representatives from all hospital departments plus legal counsel formed to assist in HIPAA compliance.

TAT See *turnaround time (TAT).*

tax Amount of money charged on an individual's property or activity for the support of state or federal government (e.g., income tax, sales tax, school tax, state tax, use tax).

tax and donations State programs under which funds collected by the state through certain health care–related taxes and provider-related donations were used to effectively increase the amount of federal Medicaid reimbursement without a comparable increase in state Medicaid funding or provider payment levels.

tax cap Limit on income tax deductions for health insurance.

tax-deferred annuity (TDA) See *Section 403(b) of the Internal Revenue Code.*

Tax Equity and Fiscal Responsibility Act (TEFRA) Federal legislation passed in 1982 that raised tax revenue, instituted many provisions for managed care plans, set up Medicare payment limits, and added Medicare coverage for hospice care. It established that an employee or spouse age 65 to 69 years is entitled to the same health insurance benefits offered under the same conditions to younger employees and their spouses. TEFRA applies to employers with at least 20 full- or part-time employees. A TEFRA provision allowed states to extend Medicaid coverage to certain disabled children.

tax identification number (TIN) See *employer identification number (EIN).*

tax-qualified policies See *long-term care insurance.*

tax rate Percentage of taxable earnings, up to the maximum tax base, that is paid for the health insurance tax.

Tax Reform Act of 1976 Allowed states to use the Social Security number in the administration of any tax, general public assistance, and driver's license or motor vehicle registration laws.

Tax Reform Act of 1986 Required individuals who filed tax returns to include the taxpayer identification

Table T-1	TABLE OF DRUGS AND CHEMICALS					
		External Cause (E Code)				
Substance	Poisoning	Accident	Therapeutic Use	Suicide Attempt	Assault	Undetermined
Acetylsalicylic acid...	965.1	E850.3	E935.3	E950.0	E962.0	E980.0

number, usually the Social Security number, of each dependent age 5 or older. The Act defined a highly compensated or key employee as follows: (1) directly or indirectly owns more than 5% interest in the company, (2) receives compensation from the company of more than $75,000, (3) is paid more than $50,000 and was among the top 20% of employees ranked by compensation, or (4) is at any time an officer and receives compensation that was more than 150% of the Section 415 defined-contribution dollar amount.

tax saver See *dependent-care spending account.*

tax-sheltered annuity (TSA) plan See *Section 403(b) of the Internal Revenue Code.*

taxable earnings Taxable wages and/or self-employment income under the prevailing annual maximum taxable limit.

taxable payroll Weighted average of taxable wages and taxable self-employment income. When multiplied by the combined employee-employer tax rate, it yields the total amount of taxes incurred by employees, employers, and the self-employed for work during the period.

taxable self-employment income Net earnings from self-employment, generally above $400 and below the annual maximum taxable amount for a calendar or other taxable year, less any taxable wages in the same taxable year.

taxable wages Salaries paid for services rendered in covered employment up to the annual maximum taxable amount.

taxation of benefits Beginning in 1994, up to 85% of an individual's or a couple's OASDI benefits is potentially subject to federal income taxation under certain circumstances. The revenue derived from taxation of benefits in excess of 50%, up to 85%, is allocated to the health insurance trust fund.

taxes See *payroll taxes.*

taxonomy codes Ten-character alphanumeric provider *specialty* codes that are assigned and classify each health care provider (e.g., general practice 208D0000X). These codes are maintained and distributed by the Centers for Medicare and Medicaid Services (CMS) and used when transmitting electronic insurance claims. A given provider can have several provider taxonomy codes. This code set is used in the X12 278 Referral Certification and Authorization and the X12 837 claim transactions and is maintained by the National Uniform Claim Committee (NUCC).

TC 1. HCPCS Level II modifier that may be used with CPT or HCPCS Level II codes indicating the technical component only of a procedure or service. Technical component services are only institutional and should not be billed separately by the physician. 2. Abbreviation for technical component. See *technical component (TC).*

TCC See *transitional care center (TCC).*

TD HCPCS Level II modifier that may be used with CPT or HCPCS Level II codes indicating services provided by a registered nurse (RN). It is required by some Medicaid and state health departments, so check with your state guidelines.

TDA Acronym for tax-deferred annuity. See *Section 403(b) of the Internal Revenue Code.*

TE HCPCS Level II modifier that may be used with CPT or HCPCS Level II codes indicating services provided by a licensed practical nurse (LPN) or licensed visiting nurse (LVN). It is required by some Medicaid and state health departments, so check with your state guidelines.

teaching hospital Medical facility that is associated with a university and has an accredited program in various specialties of medical practice. It gives clinical experience to medical students while they deliver supervised medical care to patients.

technical component (TC) Portion of a test or procedure (containing both a technical and a professional component) that pertains to the use of the equipment, supplies, materials, and the operator (technician) that performs it but does not interpret the results (i.e., electrocardiograph [ECG] machine and technician, radiography machine and technician, microscope and technician). When billing using CPT codes, a service that is TC only should not be billed with a two-digit modifier. See also *professional component (PC).*

technical qualifications Skills that may be acquired through education and experience and make an individual suitable for a job or activity.

technology assessment (TA) Multidisciplinary field of policy analysis that studies the medical, social, ethical, and economic implications of the development, diffusion, and use of technologies. In support of national coverage determinations (NCDs), TA often focuses

T

on the safety and efficacy of technologies. Each NCD includes a comprehensive TA process. For some NCDs, external TAs are requested through the Agency for Health Research and Quality (AHRQ). Also referred to as *health care technology assessment (HTA)*.

TEFRA See *Tax Equity and Fiscal Responsibility Act (TEFRA)*.

TEFRA 134 Provision of the Tax Equity and Fiscal Responsibility Act of 1982 that allows states to give Medicaid coverage to certain disabled children. Also referred to as the *Katie Beckett option*.

TEFRA corridor See *corridor*.

telemedicine 1. Use of telecommunication systems in real-time or near real-time to transmit medical images and information to distant professionals for purposes of diagnosis and medical care (e.g., scanned images, direct digital capture [DDC], interactive television [IATV], and high-definition television [HDTV]). 2. Professional services given to a patient through an interactive telecommunications system by a practitioner at a distant site.

telemetry bed Bed that is able produce wireless or wired electronic transmission to a remote location for continuous monitoring of the patient's condition.

telemetry unit Section in a hospital facility that has telemetry beds such as intensive care unit.

telephone triage system See *nurse triage*.

teletypewriter (TTY) Communication device used by people who are deaf, hard of hearing, or have a severe speech impairment. A TTY consists of a keyboard, display screen, and modem. Messages travel over regular telephone lines. Individuals who do not have a TTY can communicate with a TTY user through a message relay center (MRC). An MRC has TTY operators available to send and interpret TTY messages.

Temporary Assistance to Needy Families (TANF) Established by the Social Security Act of 1965 and formerly known as *Aid to Families with Dependent Children (AFDC)*, this is a Medicaid category of certain needy and low-income people with dependent children who are deprived of the support of at least one parent and are financially eligible on the basis of income and resources. TANF provides financial assistance to children and families and to pregnant women who meet specific income and resource requirements specified by the state.

temporary codes HCPCS Level II codes that begin with the letters C, G, H, K, Q, S, and T and are established to meet a pressing, urgent operation need and are frequently based on new policy. Frequently, these codes are only effective until the annual update of the coding books.

temporary disability (TD) 1. Recovery period following a work-related injury during which the employee is unable to work and the condition has not stabilized. TD can be overcome by medical treatment or rehabilitation. 2. Schedule of benefits payable for the temporary disability based on the earnings of the injured worker at the time of injury with statutory minimum and maximum rates; temporary compensation (e.g., "TD was paid."). 3. In a workers' compensation case, situation when the worker is unable to perform usual duties for a limited period of time but is expected to recover and return to work. A worker with a TD collects TD payments as partial wage replacement during the time period he or she is unable to work.

temporary disability insurance (TDI) See *unemployment compensation disability*.

temporary insurance agreement (TIA) Form given with an insurance application that acts as a receipt when the individual applying pays the first premium to the insurance agent. Under a TIA, the insurance company promises to provide coverage between the date of prepayment and the date it notifies the applicant of its underwriting decision. Also called *binding receipt, interim insurance agreement*, and *temporary insurance receipts*.

temporary insurance receipt See *temporary insurance agreement (TIA)*.

temporary life annuity Annuity plan that provides a specified number of income payments while the annuitant is alive but stops at death.

temporary partial disability (TPD) In a workers' compensation case, disability that prevents an injured worker, whose condition is not yet permanent and stationary, from performing all or part of his or her work duties but does not completely prevent the worker from working and earning some money. Partial TPD payments are based on a calculation of a percentage of the portion of earnings lost.

temporary total disability (TTD) Situation in which an individual, whose condition is not yet permanent and stationary, is unable to perform his or her usual work duties for a limited period of time. It is anticipated that he or she will fully recover from the condition and be capable of returning to work.

ten-day free look See *free examination period*.

TEP See *transfer enrollment period (TEP)*.

term insurance Type of insurance that is in force and provides protection for a specified period of time (the term). It does not build cash value and if the insured survives the stated period, it expires without value. Insurance is payable to a beneficiary at the death of the insured provided death occurs within a specified period or before a specified age. Also called *term life insurance*.

term life insurance See *term insurance*.

term rider Additional insurance coverage that may be purchased when a permanent life insurance policy is bought. Both types of insurance are included in one contract.

terminal dividend Extra dividend paid to a life insurance policyholder between the last policy anniversary date and the termination date of the policy. Also called *terminal policy dividend*.

terminal policy dividend See *terminal dividend*.

termination Cancellation of an insurance policy by an insurance company when premium is not paid, if insured dies, or a dependent is no longer eligible for coverage. Health insurance benefits are not paid for medical services received after the date of termination.

termination date Month, day, and year a health insurance policy's coverage ends.

termination expenses Dollar amount costs of processing death benefit claims and cash surrenders of a life insurance policy.

termination reason Cause for cancellation of an insurance policy.

territory Geographical region in which an insurance agent has exclusive sales.

tertiary Third in frequency, rank, order, formation, or stage.

tertiary beneficiary Individual entitled to the proceeds of a life insurance policy if no primary or secondary beneficiaries are living when the insured dies. Also called *contingent beneficiary* or *alternate beneficiary*.

tertiary care Health care services requested by a specialist from another specialist (e.g., hand surgeon, neurosurgeon, pediatric endocrinologist, thoracic surgeon, intensive care unit). It usually requires sophisticated technologies located in a teaching hospital or university-affiliated facility that are not available elsewhere (e.g., complex cancer procedures, transplants, neonatal intensive care).

tertiary care center Medical facility that receives referred patients from primary and secondary care levels because of severe injury or illness. It provides tests, treatments, and procedures that are not available elsewhere. Also called *tertiary care facility* or *tertiary care hospital*.

tertiary care facility See *tertiary care center*.

tertiary care hospital See *tertiary care center*.

tertiary payer Third-party payer that is responsible for reimbursement of an insurance claim after the primary and secondary payers have paid their share.

test of long-range close actuarial balance Summarized income rates and cost rates are calculated for each of 66 valuation periods within the full 75-year long-range projection period under the intermediate assumptions. The first of these periods consists of the next 10 years. Each succeeding period becomes longer by 1 year, culminating with the period consisting of the next 75 years. The long-range test is met if, for each of the 66 time periods, the actuarial balance is not less than zero or is negative by, at most, a specified percentage of the summarized cost rate for the same time period. The

percentage allowed for a negative actuarial balance is 5% for the full 75-year period and is reduced uniformly for shorter periods, approaching zero as the duration of the time periods approaches the first 10 years. The criterion for meeting the test is less stringent for the longer periods in recognition of the greater uncertainty associated with estimates for more distant years. This test is applied to trust fund projections made under the intermediate assumptions.

test of short-range financial adequacy Conditions required to meet this test as follows: (1) If the trust fund ratio for a fund exceeds 100% at the beginning of the projection period, then it must be projected to remain at or about 100% throughout the 10-year projection period; (2) alternatively, if the fund ratio is initially less than 100%, it must be projected to reach a level of at least 100% within 5 years (and not be depleted at any time during this period) and then remain at or above 100% throughout the rest of the 10-year period. This test is applied to trust fund projections made under the intermediate assumptions.

test panel Grouping of a number of laboratory tests (represented by individual codes) that are usually performed together and reported using one CPT code. The most common tests done to investigate a specific disease or organ have been included in test panels.

testamentary deposition Use of a will to legally state to whom the proceeds of a life insurance policy will be transferred.

testamentary trust Trust that is created as a result of the death of a person whose will provides for the creation of the trust after his or her death.

testator Individual who makes a will.

testimony Sworn statement used for legal evidence or proof.

testing See *results/testing/reports*.

testing facility In the Medicare program, provider or supplier that furnishes diagnostic tests such as a physician, group of physicians (e.g., radiologist, pathologist), laboratory, or independent diagnostic testing facility (IDTF).

text messaging Electronic written messages transmitted over a wireless network.

TF HCPCS Level II modifier that may be used with CPT or HCPCS Level II codes indicating intermediate level of care. It is required by some Medicaid and state health departments, so check with your state guidelines.

TFL See *TRICARE for Life (TFL)*.

TG HCPCS Level II modifier that may be used with CPT or HCPCS Level II codes indicating a complex or highly technical level of care. It is required by some Medicaid and state health departments, so check with your state guidelines.

T

302   TH

TH HCPCS Level II modifier that may be used with CPT or HCPCS Level II codes indicating obstetrical treatment or service, prenatal or postpartum. When submitting insurance claims, it is required by some Medicaid and state health departments, so check with your state guidelines.

The gap See *doughnut hole.*

therapeutic 1. Pertaining to a treatment. 2. Beneficial.

therapeutic procedure Treatment of a disease or injury with the use of a modality by someone clinically trained and skilled to effect change and improve function and physical condition of the patient.

therapeutic service Medical treatment provided for a certain diagnosis (i.e., carrying out the procedure, other ancillary elements, and normal follow-up care related to the medical problem).

therapeutic substitution Act of replacing one drug in a therapeutic class for another drug in the same category of drugs but with a different chemical ingredient. It is expected to have similar beneficial effects. Also see *generic substitution.*

therapeutic treatment Treatment of disease or injury of a patient seeking to relieve symptoms or produce a cure.

therapy care Health care treatment of any illness or injury to encourage the recovery of the patient (e.g., cardiac rehabilitation, kidney dialysis, occupational therapy, physical therapy, radiation therapy, respiratory therapy, shock therapy, speech therapy).

third party Entity that processes insurance claims for patients (e.g., private insurance companies, Medicare fiscal intermediaries).

third-party administrator (TPA) Independent organization or individual, other than the insurance company or health care provider, that processes and pays insurance claims to providers, provides administrative services for self-insured employer groups or managed care plans (e.g., collects insurance premiums, maintains records, handles routine underwriting but does not assume the risk). A TPA is recognized as a third party because it is separate from the employee participants and employer sponsoring the insurance plan. Also known as a *clearinghouse.*

third-party application Insurance application submitted by an individual other than the person being insured.

third-party endorsement System of marketing individual insurance to groups in which the insurance company formally agrees with an organization to sell individual insurance to members of the organization.

third-party insurance Insurance coverage bought by the insured (first party) from an insurance company (second party) for coverage to protect against lawsuits by another (third party).

third-party liability 1. Third-party liability exists if an entity (not connected with the employer) is the cause and is liable to pay the medical cost for injury, disease, or disability of a person hurt during the performance of his or her occupation and the injury is caused by an entity not connected with the employer. 2. Entity that is responsible for the cost of an illness or injury (e.g., automobile, homeowner insurer). Also referred to as *third-party payer liable.*

third-party payer Private insurance company or government fiscal intermediary (third party) that insures and/or pays provider (second party) for health care benefits of members or beneficiaries (first parties) (e.g., Blue Cross, Medicare, Medicaid, commercial insurance companies). Also known as *indirect payer, insurance company, insurer,* or *payer.*

third-party payer liable (TPL) Private insurance company or government fiscal intermediary (third party) legally responsible under a contract to pay providers who rendered health care benefits to its members or beneficiaries.

third-party payment Reimbursement sent to the provider (second party) of health care services by an insurance carrier or government program (third party) on behalf of the patient (first party). Also called *third-party reimbursement (TPR).*

third-party reimbursement (TPR) See *third-party payment.*

third-party subrogation The legal process by which an insurance company seeks from a third party, who has caused a loss, recovery of the amount paid to the policyholder.

third-party use Situation in which a third party from another organization is given permission to use data originally obtained from the Centers for Medicare and Medicaid Services (CMS) by the original requestor.

three-character category See *category.*

three-day payment window See *72-hour rule.*

three-digit diagnostic codes Diagnostic codes consisting of three numbers with descriptions that appear in ICD-9-CM code books and are used only when no fourth or fifth digits are available. Approximately 100 codes are at the highest level of specificity in the three-digit characters. Third-party payers, as well as Medicare fiscal intermediaries, do not accept three-digit codes if a higher level of specificity is available.

three-factor contribution method System of calculating insurance policy dividends and distributing excess funds above the amount needed for legal reserves. Excess funds come from mortality savings, interest earned on investments, and expense savings.

thrift plan See *savings plan.*

tickler file Manual reminder method used to track pending or resubmitted insurance claims and to telephone or send inquiries about nonpayment. Also called a *suspense, follow-up file,* or *tracing file.* Also see *tracing file.*

tier In Medicare Part D plans, a drug formulary is divided into tiers, with each representing a different level of cost-sharing by the insured. Some plans may have more tiers and some may have less (e.g., tiers 1, 2, 3 and/or a specialty tier).

Tier, A Under the Medicare Part D prescription drug plan, this is a specific list of drugs. A plan may have several tiers, and the patient's copayment amount depends on which tier the drug is listed in. The plans are variable because patients can choose their own tiers. Each plan benefit booklet contains the list of drugs pertinent to a specific plan.

time 1. Measure of duration. 2. Interval separating two points in a continuum between the past and future events.

time clause See *survivorship clause.*

time limit 1. In a managed care or insurance contract, the amount of time from the date of service to the date the insurance claim or a proof of loss can be filed with the insurance carrier. 2. Under the Medicare program, payments for Part B insurance claims must be submitted within 15 months from the date of the procedure or service. 3. Under the TRICARE program, claims must be filed within 1 year from the date a service is provided or (for inpatient care) within 1 year from the patient's date of discharge from the inpatient facility. 4. Time period (2 to 3 years) in which an insurance company cannot deny a claim or cancel an insurance policy because of a preexisting condition or statement in an application.

TIN See *tax identification number (TIN).*

Title III of the Older Americans Act Statutory authority that provides services to individuals age 60 and older such as congregate and home-delivered meals, supportive services (transportation, information and referral, legal assistance), in-home services (homemaker services, personal care, chore services), and health promotion and disease prevention services (health screenings and exercise programs).

Title XVIII of the Social Security Act Statutory authority for federal health insurance for persons age 65 and older and certain disabled persons younger than age 65 called the *Medicare program.* Also see *Social Security Act, Medicare Part A, Medicare Part B, Medicare Part C,* and *Medicare Part D.*

Title XIX of the Social Security Act Statutory authority for state and federal funded programs of medical assistance to low-income individuals of all ages called the *Medicaid program.* See *Medicaid (MCD).*

Title XX services See *Social Services Block Grant services.*

Titles V and XXI of the Social Security Act Statutory authority that allows states to create health insurance programs for children of low-income, working families known as the *Children's Health Insurance Program (CHIP).* See *Children's Special Health Care Services (CSHCS).*

TJ HCPCS Level II modifier that may be used with CPT or HCPCS Level II codes indicating a child and/or adolescent program group.

TK HCPCS Level II modifier that may be used with CPT or HCPCS Level II codes indicating an extra patient or passenger in a nonambulance transport. When submitting insurance claims, it is required by some Medicaid and state health departments, so check with your state guidelines.

TL HCPCS Level II modifier that may be used with CPT or HCPCS Level II codes indicating early intervention or individualized family service plan (FSP). When submitting insurance claims, it is required by some Medicaid and state health departments, so check with your state guidelines.

TM HCPCS Level II modifier that may be used with CPT or HCPCS Level II codes indicating an individualized education program (IEP). When submitting insurance claims, it is required by some Medicaid and state health departments, so check with your state guidelines.

TMA See *TRICARE Management Agency (TMA).*

TN HCPCS Level II modifier that may be used with CPT or HCPCS Level II codes indicating a service provided in a rural area or outside a providers' customary service area. When submitting insurance claims, it is required by some Medicaid and state health departments, so check with your state guidelines.

TNC See *total net cost (TNC) method.*

TOB See *type of bill (TOB).*

toileting Ability of an individual to go to and from the toilet unassisted. Also see *activities of daily living (ADLs).*

token payment Small reimbursement for a medical service or supply item. Also called *hesitation payment* or *nominal payment.*

tomograph Special type of x-ray imaging apparatus that makes a record (tomogram) of slices through a body structure to obliterate overlying structures (e.g., study of the kidneys or temporomandibular joints).

tomography Recording of internal body images at a predetermined plane (sectional imaging) by means of the tomography. Also called *body section radiography.*

top-heavy plan Employee benefit or retirement plan that provides 60% or more of its accrued benefits to the owners, executives, and key employees and specific minimum benefits to non–key employees.

tort Legal wrong committed to an individual or to property that results in injury or damage on which a civil action can be based.

tort reform Changes in the law pertaining to medical professional liability (malpractice).

TOS code See *type of service (TOS) code.*

total budget See *global budget.*

total certificate membership benefit maximum See *lifetime maximum benefit.*

total cost of drugs Under a Medicare Part D plan, this phrase means the sum total the insured pays plus the dollar amount that the insurance plan pays for the drugs.

total disability 1. Phrase that varies in meaning from one disability insurance policy to another. An example of a liberal definition might read, "The insured must be unable to perform the major duties of his or her specific occupation." Also called *full disability.* 2. In nonoccupational injury or illness, unable to perform ordinary activities like someone of the same age. 3. In a workers' compensation case, unable to perform substantial duties of his or her occupation. Also see *permanent disability (PD)*.

total-needs programming See *financial planning*.

total net cost (TNC) method Insurance policy cost comparison system that adds a policy's premiums and subtracts dividends and cash value. TNC is not allowed by the National Association of Insurance Commissioners (NAIC) Model Life Insurance Solicitation Regulation because it does not consider the time value of money.

total, permanent service-connected disability Total permanent disability incurred by a service member while on active duty.

total quality management (TQM) Operations management philosophy to continually improve performance, quality, and cost effectiveness by putting into operation employee involvement programs, self-directed work teams, flexible service delivery processes, quick changeover and adaptability, customer focus, supplier integration, and production cycle time reduction. Some health care organizations adopt TQM programs to meet competition. Also called *continuous quality improvement (CQI)*.

total value Sum of the three components (physician work, physician expense, malpractice costs), used in the formula to develop relative value units under the resource-based relative value scale for each medical service performed. These three relative value units (RVUs) are then adjusted according to geographical area and used in a formula to determine the resource-based relative value scale (RBRVS) for the Medicare fees published annually in the *Federal Register*.

TP HCPCS Level II modifier that may be used with CPT or HCPCS Level II codes indicating medical transport, unloaded vehicle. When submitting insurance claims, it is required by some Medicaid and state health departments, so check with your state guidelines.

TPA See *third-party administrator (TPA)* or *trading partner agreement (TPA)*.

TPD See *temporary partial disability (TPD)*.

TPL See *third-party payer liable (TPL)*.

TPO See *treatment, payment, or health care operations (TPO)*.

TPR Acronym for TRICARE Prime Remote and third-party reimbursement. See *third-party payment* and *TRICARE Prime Remote (TPR)*.

TQ HCPCS Level II modifier that may be used with CPT or HCPCS Level II codes indicating basic life support transport by a volunteer ambulance provider. When submitting insurance claims, it is required by some Medicaid and state health departments, so check with your state guidelines.

TQM See *total quality management (TQM)*.

TR HCPCS Level II modifier that may be used with CPT or HCPCS Level II codes indicating school-based

individualized education program (IEP) services provided outside the public school district responsible for the student. When submitting insurance claims, it is required by some Medicaid and state health departments, so check with your state guidelines.

tracer Written request made to an insurance company to locate the status of an insurance claim (i.e., claim in review, claim never received, clarification about something related to the member's health plan) or general information such as deductible or entitlement. Also called *inquiry*. An inquiry is not a complaint.

tracer methodology Review system in hospital facilities used by The Joint Commission surveyors in which they randomly select patients, obtain their medical records, and then trace the path of the patients by visiting the units, sites, or departments in the exact sequence, when possible, that the patients experienced. The surveyor talks to the direct caregivers who provided care and treatment to the patient. The Joint Commission assesses care and compliance with relevant standards related to operational systems and processes based on actual experience of the patients.

tracing file Electronic reminder method used to track pending or resubmitted insurance claims and to telephone or send inquiries about nonpayment. Also called a *suspense, follow-up file*, or *tickler file*. Also see *tickler file*.

trade name See *brand name drugs*.

trading partner 1. External entity with whom business is conducted (i.e., customer). This relationship can be formalized via a trading partner agreement. A trading partner of an entity for some purposes; may be a business associate of that same entity for other purposes. 2. Company that agrees to exchange information electronically with another company.

trading partner agreement (TPA) 1. Any contract (manual, bulletin, or memorandum) between the provider and the claim transmission receiver that details the electronic data interchange requirements between the parties. 2. Under the Health Insurance Portability and Accountability Act (HIPAA), a TPA may not include any agreement to use the codes, segments, or transactions published in an implementation guide in a manner different from that prescribed in the applicable guide.

traditional insurance See *indemnity plan*.

transaction Under the Health Insurance Portability and Accountability Act (HIPAA), transmission or exchange of information between two parties to carry out financial or administrative activities related to health care.

transaction change request system Electronic method established under the Health Insurance Portability and Accountability Act (HIPAA) for accepting and tracking change requests for any of the adopted HIPAA transaction standards via a single website.

transaction set 1. Under the Health Insurance Portability and Accountability Act (HIPAA), a complete batch of claims that includes the header, trailer, and claim data. 2. Series of blocks that compose a business transaction (e.g., patient admission form).

transaction slip See *multipurpose billing form.*

transaction standards Under the Health Insurance Portability and Accountability Act (HIPAA), specific rules and guidelines for the transmission of electronic insurance claims.

transcription See *medical transcription.*

transfer 1. Relocating or moving a patient from one health care facility or inpatient unit to another for additional treatment. Under the Medicare prospective payment system, the transferring hospital is paid based on a per diem rate and the patient's length of stay. The diagnosis-related group (DRG) payment is made to the final discharging facility. 2. Move membership from one health insurance to another.

transfer enrollment period (TEP) One of four periods during which an individual can enroll in Medicare Part A. TEP is for people age 65 or older who have Part B only and are enrolled in a Medicare managed care plan. They can sign up for Medicare Part A during any month they leave the plan or if the plan coverage ends, they have 8 months to sign up. The 8 months start the month after the month they leave the plan or the plan coverage ends. If they enroll in Part B or Part A during the general enrollment period (GEP), the coverage starts on July 1. Also see *initial enrollment period (IEP), general enrollment period (GEP),* and *special enrollment period (SEP).*

transfer review Review of transfers to different areas of the same hospital that are exempted from prospective payment.

transferable skills Proficiency obtained through work by the insured that he or she can apply to another job using similar physical or mental limitations caused by a disability.

transferred business Group insurance plan that is changed from one insurance company to another.

transferred business analysis (TBA) Assessment of an insurance risk and establishment of a rate for a specific level of benefits that is competitive and matches with the current experience rating system.

transferring Ability of an individual to move in and out of a bed or chair. Also see *activities of daily living (ADLs).*

transient patients 1. Patients who receive treatment on an episodic basis and are not part of a facility's regular caseload (i.e., patients who have not been permanently transferred to a facility for ongoing treatment). 2. Patients who temporarily live in a locale but continually move from one region to another. These types of patients may cause collection problems, so initially gathering comprehensive and accurate demographic data is important.

transitional bed Bed in a skilled nursing facility for a patient who does not need intense observation as in an acute care unit. Also see *intermediate care.*

transitional care See *intermediate care.*

transitional care center (TCC) Facility used instead of or before discharge to an extended care facility.

transitional pass-through payment Under the Medicare outpatient prospective payment system (OPPS), certain drugs, biologicals, and devices are eligible for payments in addition to the ambulatory payment classification (APC) payment (i.e., the costs are passed through [around] the APC system).

translator Under the Health Insurance Portability and Accountability Act (HIPAA), a software tool for accepting an electronic data interchange (EDI) transmission and converting the information into another format or for converting a non-EDI data file into an EDI format for transmission. Also known as *EDI translator.*

transplant Surgical procedure that involves removing tissue or a functional organ from either a deceased or living individual (donor) and implanting it in a patient (recipient) that needs a functional organ to replace their nonfunctional one. Also called *transplant surgery.*

transplant surgery See *transplant.*

transportation services Escort service that provides carrying usually older adults from one place to another such as appointments for medical services. These services accommodate persons in wheelchairs and persons with other special needs. Such services include buses, shuttle vans, taxis, and volunteer drivers.

trauma 1. Physical injury caused by violent or disruptive action or by the introduction into the body of a toxic substance (e.g., penetrating or blunt serious trauma, drowning, poisoning, burns). 2. Psychic injury resulting from a severe emotional shock.

trauma center Medical facility that gives emergency and specialized intensive care to critically ill and severely injured patients due to a major catastrophic event with services provided 24 hours a day, 7 days a week. Generally an emergency department does not have the specialized capabilities and critical patients may need to be transferred to a trauma center for a higher level of care.

trauma code development Medicare Secondary Payer (MSP) investigative process triggered by receipt of a Medicare claim with a diagnosis indicating traumatic injury.

travel accident insurance Type of health insurance coverage for accidents that occur while an insured is on a trip. Individual or employee policies are available for one specific trip or type of travel or may cover all trips taken during a year.

travel insurance Type of insurance that covers trip cancellation, trip interruption, lost luggage, and default protection (trip cancellation because an airline or tour company is no longer in business).

treating physician 1. Provider that renders a service to a patient; also known as *performing physician*. 2. Defined in the Social Security Act §1861, physician who furnishes a consultation or treats a beneficiary for a specific medical problem, and who uses the result of a diagnostic test in the management of the beneficiary's specific medical problem.

treating practitioner See *nonphysician practitioner (NPP)*.

treatment 1. Care and management of a patient to combat, ameliorate, or prevent a disease, disorder, or injury. 2. Method of combating, ameliorating, or preventing a disease, disorder, or injury. Active or curative treatment is designed to cure; palliative treatment is directed to relieve pain and distress; prophylactic treatment is for the prevention of a disease or disorder; and causal treatment focuses on the cause of a disorder. Treatment may be pharmacological, using drugs; surgical, involving operative procedures; or supportive, building the patient's strength.

treatment authorization request (TAR) form Medi-Cal form that must be completed by a provider for certain procedures and services that require prior approval.

treatment episode Time period between admission and discharge from specific section of a facility (e.g., inpatient, partial hospitalization, outpatient, residential).

treatment options Choices the patient may have when there is more than one method to treat a health problem or an illness.

treatment, payment, or health care operations (TPO) Under the Health Insurance Portability and Accountability Act, covered entities may disclose protected health information for TPO but must receive written consent from a patient for other situations.

treatment plan See *plan of treatment*.

treatment protocols See *practice guidelines*.

treaty See *automatic reinsurance*.

trend factor Annual adjustment amount applied to total claim costs to represent the change in level of the costs from one period of time to another because of inflation and increase in use.

trended See *trending*.

trending System of estimating costs of health care services by reviewing past trends in cost and use of the services. Also called *trended*.

triage 1. Process of sorting a group of sick or injured patients according to their need for medical care. 2. Fee charged by health care facilities for emergency and other patients.

trial application See *preliminary inquiry form*.

triangle (▲) Symbol used in the procedure code book titled *Current Procedural Terminology (CPT)* to indicate a revised code with an altered procedure descriptor that is new to that specific annual edition.

triangles See *facing triangles*.

TRICARE Three-option managed health care program offered to spouses and dependents of service personnel with uniform benefits and fees implemented nationwide by the federal government. It also covers retirees, reservists on active duty after 30 days, widows, and widowers. Formerly known as *Civilian Health and Medical Program of the Uniformed Services (CHAMPUS)*. 2. In the Medicare Secondary Payer guidelines, TRICARE is considered a group health plan.

TRICARE contractor Civilian health care organization selected by the U.S. federal government to serve as Managed Care Support Contractor (MCSC) for TRICARE in a specific region. This contractor supplements all military direct care for TRICARE beneficiaries in the region. The contractor also provides health services and support to TRICARE Prime members and organizes the preferred provider network (PPN).

TRICARE Extra Preferred provider organization type of TRICARE option in which the individual does not have to enroll or pay an annual fee. On a visit-by-visit basis, the individual may seek care from an authorized network provider and receive a discount on services and reduced cost-share (copayment).

TRICARE for Life (TFL) Health care program that offers additional TRICARE benefits as a supplementary payer to Medicare for uniformed service retirees, their spouses, survivors age 65 or older, and certain former spouses. TFL became effective October 1, 2001. Also known as *TRICARE Senior Prime*.

TRICARE identification cards See *United States Uniformed Services identification cards*.

TRICARE Management Agency (TMA) Organization that administers the TRICARE program; formerly known as the *Office of Civilian Health and Medical Programs of the Uniformed Services (OCHAMPUS)*.

TRICARE Prime Voluntary health maintenance organization–type option for TRICARE beneficiaries. TRICARE Prime works like a civilian health maintenance organization (HMO) to control costs. Beneficiaries are assigned a primary care manager (PCM) at a military treatment facility (MTF). (In some areas, PCMs are civilian network providers.) The PCM handles all routine health care. If the beneficiary needs care that the PCM does not offer, he or she will give the beneficiary a referral. Then the managed care support contractor (MCSC) finds the most appropriate provider and location for additional care. With TRICARE Prime, beneficiaries have expanded health care benefits in addition to the core benefits and freedom to choose civilian providers (at a higher cost) when they use the point-of-service (POS) option.

TRICARE Prime Remote (TPR) Program designed for active duty service members who work and live more than 50 miles or 1 hour from military treatment facilities (military hospitals and clinics).

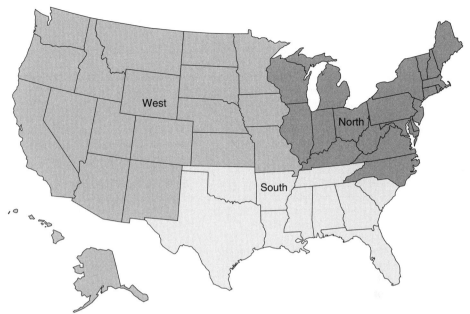

Figure T-1 Map of TRICARE West Region, North Region, and South Region, which shows states that have been merged into each of the regions.

TRICARE regions Large geographical sections in the United States in which states are merged. Figure T-1 shows the locations of the states in these regions. Also see *fiscal intermediary (FI)*.

TRICARE Senior Prime See *TRICARE for Life (TFL)*.

TRICARE Service Center Office staffed by TRI-CARE Health Care Finders and beneficiary service representatives that has information for beneficiaries about TRICARE Prime enrollment, Health Care Finder (HCF) services, and more.

TRICARE Standard Health care program offered to spouses and dependents of service personnel with uniform core health care benefits and fees implemented nationwide by the federal government; also known as "the old CHAMPUS program." Standard allows beneficiaries to see any TRICARE-certified (authorized), non-network civilian providers. Beneficiaries pay an annual deductible and a 25% cost share of covered treatment and services.

TRICARE supplemental insurance Health insurance that generally pays what is left over after TRICARE Standard pays a beneficiary's covered benefits. Such a policy may cover certain cost-share amounts.

trigger point Particular level when an insurance company is responsible for payment of benefits with a stated minimum premium.

triple indemnity In a life insurance policy, provision that pays an amount (three times the face value) in addition to the policy's basic death benefit if death is due to an accident. There are exclusions for the type of accident and time and age limits (e.g., the insured must die within a specific number of days of the accident and be of a certain age or younger).

triple-option plan Type of managed care plan that allows a member a choice of one of three service alternatives (health maintenance organization [HMO], preferred provider organization [PPO], or traditional indemnity plan) each time he or she requires medical care. Scope of covered services is the same for each option, but the level of cost shared by the enrollee is different among the options. Also called *point-of-service (POS) program*.

true negatives Eligible members or enrollees who have not received any medical services through a managed care plan as evidenced by the absence of a medical record and any encounter data. True negatives signify potential access problems and should be investigated by the managed care plan.

truncated code Invalid diagnostic code in which an extra digit has been added to a four-digit code to make it five digits. Medicare payers return such claims as unprocessable.

trust Legal entity (trustee) in which property and funds are held and managed by either a person or third party for a beneficiary. Two types are living trust and testamentary trust.

T

trust agreement Legal document that sets up a trust fund, allocates specific assets contained in the trust, and states rules for carrying out the duties and responsibilities of the trustee for investing and administration.

trust fund 1. Type of employer's funding instrument for retirement accounts and employee benefits. The other types are an *insured plan* or *combination plan*. 2. Separate account in the U.S. Treasury, mandated by Congress, whose assets may be used only for a specified purpose. For the supplementary medical insurance (SMI) trust fund, monies not withdrawn for current benefit payments and administrative expenses are invested in interest-bearing federal securities, as required by law; the interest earned is also deposited in the trust fund.

trust fund plan Type of retirement plan in which employer and employee contributions are given to a trustee (individual or institution) who invests the funds and may make benefit payments to the participants.

trust fund ratio Short-range measure of the adequacy of the trust fund level; defined as the assets at the beginning of the year expressed as a percentage of the outgo during the year.

trustee Appointed individual to administer a trust that must manage and safeguard the property according to the conditions stated in the trust. Also called *grantee*.

trusteed pension plan See *pension trust fund*.

trustor Individual who creates a trust that grants the contents of the trust to another person (grantee). Also called *grantor* or *settlor*.

TS HCPCS Level II modifier that may be used with CPT or HCPCS Level II codes indicating follow-up service. When submitting insurance claims, it is required by some Medicaid and state health departments, so check with your state guidelines.

TSA Acronym for tax-sheltered annuity plan. See *Section 403(b) of the Internal Revenue Code*.

TT HCPCS Level II modifier that may be used with CPT or HCPCS Level II codes indicating individualized service provided to more than one patient in the same setting. When submitting insurance claims, it is required by some Medicaid and state health departments, so check with your state guidelines.

TTD See *temporary total disability (TTD)*.

TTY See *teletypewriter (TTY)*.

TU HCPCS Level II modifier that may be used with CPT or HCPCS Level II codes indicating special overtime payment rate. When submitting insurance claims, it is required by some Medicaid and state health departments, so check with your state guidelines.

turfing Transferring the sickest, high-cost patients to other physicians so that the provider appears as a low-utilizer in a managed care setting.

turnaround time (TAT) 1. Period from the date a transaction is received to the date completed. 2. For insurance claims, the number of days from the date a claim is received by the insurance company to the date it is paid.

turnover rate Number of times employees terminate employment other than by death (i.e., they're fired, they resign, or they retire) and are replaced. This is a factor that affects the cost of a retirement plan.

TV HCPCS Level II modifier that may be used with CPT or HCPCS Level II codes indicating special holiday or weekend payment rates. When submitting insurance claims, it is required by some Medicaid and state health departments, so check with your state guidelines.

TW HCPCS Level II modifier that may be used with CPT or HCPCS Level II codes indicating back-up equipment. When submitting insurance claims, it is required by some Medicaid and state health departments, so check with your state guidelines.

twenty-four-hour coverage 1. Insurance coverage of medical and disability benefits for the insured regardless of employment or financial status. 2. Insurance coverage for an employee under the correct insurance policy (e.g., workers' compensation, group health, disability).

twisting Insurance agent or broker encourages a policyholder to cancel a policy and purchase another policy but neglects to state the differences between the two policies or the financial consequences of replacement. This practice is prohibited in the insurance industry.

two-party check Check that is made out to the physician and the patient by the maker.

two-person membership Insured or subscriber and one dependent of an insurance contract.

two surgeons Situation when more than two surgeons are present at the time of the operation. A five-digit CPT code number is used with an attached modifier -62 to list the procedure. If listing more than one modifier, the appropriate sequence is to list -62 first and any one of these modifiers in the next position (-54, -55).

type of bill (TOB) Field 4 of the Uniform Bill (UB-04) claim form that requires the facility code preceded by a leading zero as specified in the *UB-04 (CMS-1450) Manual Billing Procedures*.

type of contract Classification of an insurance agreement (e.g., one person, two persons, or family membership; group or individual policy).

type of service (TOS) code Numeric or alpha code that indicates the medical service. When the physician's office or an outpatient hospital is billing, the code is inserted in Block 24C of the CMS-1500 insurance claim form (e.g., 1 is medical care, 2 is surgery, D is hospice).

U

U1 HCPCS Level II modifier that may be used with CPT or HCPCS Level II codes indicating Medicaid level of care 1, as defined by each state. When submitting insurance claims, it is required by some Medicaid and state health departments, so check with your state guidelines.

U2 HCPCS Level II modifier that may be used with CPT or HCPCS Level II codes indicating Medicaid level of care 2, as defined by each state. When submitting insurance claims, it is required by some Medicaid and state health departments, so check with your state guidelines.

U3 HCPCS Level II modifier that may be used with CPT or HCPCS Level II codes indicating Medicaid level of care 3, as defined by each state. When submitting insurance claims, it is required by some Medicaid and state health departments, so check with your state guidelines.

U4 HCPCS Level II modifier that may be used with CPT or HCPCS Level II codes indicating Medicaid level of care 4, as defined by each state. When submitting insurance claims, it is required by some Medicaid and state health departments, so check with your state guidelines.

U5 HCPCS Level II modifier that may be used with CPT or HCPCS Level II codes indicating Medicaid level of care 5, as defined by each state. When submitting insurance claims, it is required by some Medicaid and state health departments, so check with your state guidelines.

U6 HCPCS Level II modifier that may be used with CPT or HCPCS Level II codes indicating Medicaid level of care 6, as defined by each state. When submitting insurance claims, it is required by some Medicaid and state health departments, so check with your state guidelines.

U7 HCPCS Level II modifier that may be used with CPT or HCPCS Level II codes indicating Medicaid level of care 7, as defined by each state. When submitting insurance claims, it is required by some Medicaid and state health departments, so check with your state guidelines.

U8 HCPCS Level II modifier that may be used with CPT or HCPCS Level II codes indicating Medicaid level of care 8, as defined by each state. When submitting insurance claims, it is required by some Medicaid and state health departments, so check with your state guidelines.

U9 HCPCS Level II modifier that may be used with CPT or HCPCS Level II codes indicating Medicaid level of care 9, as defined by each state. When submitting insurance claims, it is required by some Medicaid and state health departments, so check with your state guidelines.

UA HCPCS Level II modifier that may be used with CPT or HCPCS Level II codes indicating Medicaid level of care 10, as defined by each state. When submitting insurance claims, it is required by some Medicaid and state health departments, so check with your state guidelines.

UB HCPCS Level II modifier that may be used with CPT or HCPCS Level II codes indicating Medicaid level of care 11, as defined by each state. When submitting insurance claims, it is required by some Medicaid and state health departments, so check with your state guidelines.

UB-04 See *Uniform Bill (UB-04) claim form.*

UB-82 See *Uniform Bill (UB-82) claim form.*

UB-92 See *Uniform Bill (UB-92) claim form.*

UC HCPCS Level II modifier that may be used with CPT or HCPCS Level II codes indicating Medicaid level of care 12, as defined by each state. When submitting insurance claims, it is required by some Medicaid and state health departments, so check with your state guidelines.

UCD See *unemployment compensation disability (UCD).*

UCF-1500 Acronym for uniform claim form 1500. See *health insurance claim form (CMS-1500).*

UCR See *usual, customary, and reasonable (UCR).*

UD HCPCS Level II modifier that may be used with CPT or HCPCS Level II codes indicating Medicaid level of care 13, as defined by each state. When submitting insurance claims, it is required by some Medicaid and state health departments, so check with your state guidelines.

UDC Acronym for unemployment disability compensation. See *unemployment compensation disability (UCD).*

UE HCPCS Level II modifier that may be used with CPT or HCPCS Level II codes indicating used durable medical equipment (DME).

UF HCPCS Level II modifier that may be used with CPT or HCPCS Level II codes indicating services provided in the morning.

UG HCPCS Level II modifier that may be used with CPT or HCPCS Level II codes indicating services provided in the afternoon.

UH HCPCS Level II modifier that may be used with CPT or HCPCS Level II codes indicating services provided in the evening.

UHDDS See *uniform hospital discharge data set (UHDDS)*.

UJ HCPCS Level II modifier that may be used with CPT or HCPCS Level II codes indicating services provided at night.

UK HCPCS Level II modifier that may be used with CPT or HCPCS Level II codes indicating services provided on behalf of the client to someone other than the client (collateral relationship).

ultimate cost Total net dollar amount of benefits and expenses incurred by a retirement plan over the life span of the plan.

ultrasound Sound waves that create high frequency of vibrations per second. Medical applications include fetal monitoring, imaging of internal organs, and cleaning of dental and surgical instruments.

UM See *utilization management (UM)*.

umbrella coverage Insurance protection for losses beyond the policy limits, for example, in homeowner's insurance.

UMGA Acronym for Unified Medical Group Association. See *American Medical Group Association (AMGA)*.

UMLS See *Unified Medical Language System (UMLS)*.

UN HCPCS Level II modifier that may be used with CPT or HCPCS Level II codes indicating two patients served.

unallocated benefits Insurance benefits in which payment is made up to a maximum amount but does not list a specific dollar amount for each service provided.

unallocated funding System of funding a retirement plan in which funds are put into a retirement plan but are not set aside to purchase retirement benefits. When a participant retires, the funding agency may either purchase an annuity or pay benefits from the fund. The funding agency does not make contract promises on specific benefit amounts.

unassigned claim In Medicare and TRICARE programs, insurance claim submitted for a medical service or supply by a provider who does not accept assignment. The provider must bill the fiscal intermediary and the beneficiary must pay the provider for the service. Also see *nonparticipating physician (nonpar)* and *nonparticipating provider (nonpar)*.

unbundled life insurance policy See *universal life insurance*.

unbundling 1. Practice of billing using numerous CPT codes to identify procedures normally covered by a single code; also known as *itemizing, fragmented billing, fragmentation, exploding*, or *a la carte medicine*. 2. Billing under Medicare Part B for nonphysician services to hospital inpatients furnished to the hospital by an outside supplier or another provider. Under the new law, unbundling is prohibited, and all nonphysician services provided in an inpatient setting will be paid as hospital services.

unclaimed benefits Insurance policy benefits when no payee can be located. When this situation occurs, the insurer holds the unclaimed benefits for 7 years and then turns them over to the state. The beneficiary's last known address or state of domicile, whichever is known, applies.

unclaimed property statutes State laws that regulate the disposition of funds when the owner cannot be located. When this situation occurs, the insurer holds the unclaimed benefits for 7 years and then turns them over to the state. Also known as *escheat laws*. See also *unclaimed benefits*.

uncompensated care Billed medical services provided to patients by physicians and hospital facilities for which no payment is received from third-party payers or patients (e.g., charity care, bad debtors).

under bill Type of hospital invoice (patient's financial accounting statement) assessed by someone auditing a hospital bill that has services that have been provided and not billed. Also see *clean bill* and *over bill*.

underbilled services Uncoded or undercoded services and procedures that are due to poor medical documentation and not enough information in the patients' medical records to code at levels of full payment.

undercoding See *downcoding*.

undergraduate medical education Medical training provided to students in medical school.

underinsured Individual whose insurance policies do not cover all necessary health care services and he or she cannot pay the entire balance due.

underinsured motorist insurance Under Medicare Secondary Payer guidelines, this is described as an optional liability insurance available in some regions under which the policyholder's level of protection against losses caused by another is extended to compensate for inadequate coverage in the other party's policy.

underpayment Third-party payment paid to the provider at less than negotiated contract rate.

underutilization Act of a provider withholding necessary medical services because of cost constraints.

underwriter 1. Individual who works for an insurance company and performs the service of underwriting. 2. Individual or organization (insurance company) that guarantees availability of funds to pay for losses that are covered under an insurance contract.

underwriting 1. In insurance, the process of selecting, classifying, evaluating, and assuming risks according to their insurability so that appropriate rates may be assigned. Its fundamental purpose is to make sure that the group insured has the same probability of loss and probable amount of loss, within reasonable limits, as the universe on which premium rates were based. Because premium rates are based on an expectation of loss, the underwriting process must classify risks into classes with about the same expectation of loss. Also called *selection of risks*. 2. Individual or organization (insurance company) that guarantees availability of funds to pay for losses covered under an insurance contract.

underwriting department Section in an insurance company that chooses the risks that the company will insure and verifies that the mortality and morbidity rates of the company's insureds do not exceed the rates adopted when premium rates were calculated. This division also negotiates and manages reinsurance agreements. Also called the *new business department.*

underwriting gain Profit that remains as a surplus of health insurance premium income over claims and administrative expenses.

underwriting impairments Factors that may increase an individual's risk greater than that which is normal for his or her age.

underwriting loss After health insurance premium income, the deficiency that remains after payment of insurance claims and administrative expenses.

underwriting manual Procedure and policy book that summarizes methods used by a specific insurance company to evaluate and rate risks. Underwriters use this as a reference book to research background information on underwriting impairments. It gives suggestions for underwriting actions to take when various impairments are present.

underwriting profit Insurance company's income from its operations as distinct from its investment earnings.

underwriting requirements Instructions giving information on data required for insurability for a given situation and optional information sources needed to provide underwriters with needed information about the insured (e.g., medical records or physical examination report). These requirements are graduated based on the insured's age and the amount of insurance coverage.

undocumented service A service that has been billed on an insurance claim for which there is either insufficient or no supporting documentation to validate the service or procedure in the patient's medical record.

unearned premium See *unearned premium reserve.*

unearned premium reserve Fund that holds a part of the insurance premium that has been paid in advance for which the protection of the policy has not yet been provided. Also called *unearned premium.*

unemployment compensation disability (UCD) Insurance that covers off-the-job injury or sickness and is paid for by deductions from a person's paycheck. This program is administered by a state agency and is sometimes also known as *state disability insurance (SDI)* and *unemployment disability compensation (UDC).*

unemployment disability compensation (UDC) See *unemployment compensation disability (UCD).*

unethical Wrong, not in accordance with professional rules of behavior.

Unfair Trade Practices Act Regulatory model created by the National Association of Insurance Commissioners (NAIC) that established standards to prevent fraudulent or unethical practices in the

insurance industry (e.g., misrepresentation, false advertising, misappropriation of policyholder's money, twisting). States that have adopted the NAIC model may impose fines or revoke licenses of agents or brokers.

Unified Medical Group Association (UMGA) See *American Medical Group Association (AMGA).*

Unified Medical Language System (UMLS) Database created by the National Library of Medicine (NLM) to assist the development of computer systems that behave as if they "understand" the meaning of the language of biomedicine and health. It is divided into three components termed *Knowledge Sources* (UMLS Metathesaurus, the SPECIALIST Lexicon, and the UMLS Semantic Network). NLM produces and distributes the UMLS Knowledge Sources (databases) and associated software tools (programs) for use by system developers in building or enhancing electronic information systems that create, process, retrieve, integrate, and/or aggregate biomedical and health data and information, as well as in informatics research.

Uniform Bill (UB-04) claim form Insurance claim form developed by the National Uniform Billing Committee for hospital inpatient billing and payment transactions put into use by 2008. It replaces the Uniform Bill (UB-92) claim form. In the Medicare program, this is known as the *CMS-1450 Medicare Uniform Institutional Provider Bill claim form.* See *CMS-1450.* For electronically transmitted institutional claims, the 837i replaces the paper UB-04.

Uniform Bill (UB-82) claim form Uniform Bill insurance claim form developed by the National Uniform Billing Committee for hospital inpatient billing and payment transactions in use from 1983 to 1993. It was replaced with the Uniform Bill (UB-92) claim form.

Uniform Bill (UB-92) claim form Institutional uniform claim form developed by the National Uniform Billing Committee for hospital inpatient billing and payment transactions in use from 1994. The Centers for Medicare and Medicaid Services (CMS) refers to this as the CMS-1450 claim form. The UB-92 replaced the Uniform Bill (UB-82) claim form that was also referred to as *HCFA-1450.* The UB-92 will be replaced with the Uniform Bill (UB-04) claim form in 2008. For electronically transmitted institutional claims, the 837i replaces the paper UB-92.

Uniform Billing Code of 1982 (UB-82) Code system for institutional providers developed by the National Uniform Billing Committee for hospital inpatient billing and payment transactions in use from 1983 to 1993. Also see *Uniform Bill (UB-82) claim form.*

Uniform Billing Code of 1992 (UB-92) Code system for institutional providers developed by the National Uniform Billing Committee for hospital inpatient billing and payment transactions in use from 1994. Also see *Uniform Bill (UB-92) claim form.*

U

Uniform Billing Code of 2004 (UB-04) Code system for institutional providers developed by the National Uniform Billing Committee for hospital inpatient billing and payment transactions put into use by 2008. Also see *Uniform Bill (UB-04) claim form.*

uniform billing format Under a federal directive, standard billing style that requires hospitals and other Part A providers to itemize medical services on each billing statement. For electronically transmitted institutional claims, the uniform billing format is the 837i, which replaces the paper UB-04.

uniform claim task force Organization that developed the initial HCFA-1500, now known as the *CMS-1500*, professional claim form. The maintenance responsibilities were later assumed by the National Uniform Claim Committee (NUCC).

uniform hospital discharge data set (UHDDS) Collection of consistently defined, classified data that describe the medical content of a patient's bill. For acute-care and short-term facilities, UHDDS is required by the federal government for Medicare and Medicaid discharged patients. UHDDS contains the patient's age, sex, and ICD-9-CM diagnoses and procedures. The Uniform Hospital Discharge Abstract is used to collect the UHDDS. Assignment to a diagnosis-related group (DRG) is made from this data set by a fiscal intermediary.

Uniform Individual Accident and Sickness Policy Provisions Act Insurance policy regulations created by the National Association of Insurance Commissioners establishing provisions required in all individual health insurance policies. These provisions have been adopted by all 50 states and the District of Columbia. They include use of basic contract language, situations in which changes can be made to the policy, guidelines on how a beneficiary can be changed, submission of proof of loss, reinstatement of the policy, and grace period.

uniform policy provisions (UPP) Health insurance contract conditions that require the use of basic contract language. The Uniform Individual Accident and Sickness Policy Provisions Act lists these provisions required by laws of all 50 states and the District of Columbia.

uniform premium Type of rating system in which one premium is applicable for all insureds regardless of age, sex, or occupation.

uniform rate See *flat rate.*

Uniform Simultaneous Death Act Federal legislation passed by some states in the United States to alleviate problems of simultaneous death unless the will specifies what to do under simultaneous death. If the insured and beneficiary die together, the insurance company pays the secondary or contingent beneficiary. If the policy owner has not named a secondary beneficiary, the payment goes to the insured's estate.

uniformed services Government and international organizations (e.g., U.S. Air Force, U.S. Army, U.S. Coast Guard, U.S. Marines, U.S. Navy, U.S. Public Health Service, National Oceanic and Atmospheric Administration, North Atlantic Treaty Organization).

unilateral Involving only one side.

unilateral contract Type of agreement in which only one of the parties is legally required to carry out the terms. Insurance contracts are unilateral because the insurance company promises benefits and only the insurer can be charged with breach of contract.

uninsurable Entity that fails to meet the requirements of an insurable risk and falls outside the parameters of risk coverage using standard underwriting practices (e.g., high-risk individuals).

uninsurable risk class Category of individuals who have such a high risk of loss that an insurance company will not insure them.

uninsured Individuals who have no health insurance coverage either privately or via state or government programs.

uninsured motorist insurance 1. Insurance coverage for damages as a result of an accident involving a hit-and-run driver or a driver who does not have insurance. 2. Under Medicare Secondary Payer guidelines, this is described as liability insurance under which the policyholder's insurer pays for damages caused by a motorist who has no automobile liability insurance, carries less than the amount of insurance required by law, or is underinsured.

union welfare fund Financial account created by a union and one or more employers to which employers may contribute so that group benefits are available to the members of the union. Also called *union welfare trust.*

union welfare trust See *union welfare fund.*

unique physician/practitioner identification number (UPIN) Six-character, alphanumeric number issued by the Medicare fiscal intermediary to each physician who rendered medical services to Medicare recipients; required for identification purposes on the CMS-1500 claim form. It tracked payments and utilization information of each provider. UPINs have been replaced by national provider identifiers (NPIs). See *national provider identifier (NPI).*

unit benefit formula Method for calculating benefits for a defined benefit pension plan based on either years of service or years of service and earnings.

unit benefit plan Retirement plan in which a specific period of retirement income (dollar amount or percentage) is credited to an employer for each year of service with the employer.

unit input intensity allowance Amount added to, or subtracted from, the hospital input price index to yield the prospective payment system (PPS) update factor.

unit per day (unit/day) Standard measurement of medical care on a referral (e.g., inpatient hospital stays are measured in days, mental health or office visits are measured in units).

unit time See *floor time.*

United Nations Centre for Facilitation of Procedures and Practices for Administration, Commerce, and Transport International organization dedicated to the elimination or simplification of procedural barriers to international commerce.

United Nations Rules for Electronic Data Interchange for Administration, Commerce, and Transport (EDIFACT) International electronic data interchange (EDI) format. Interactive X12 transactions use the EDIFACT message syntax. Also see *Electronic Data Interchange for Administration, Commerce and Transport (EDIFACT).*

United States For Medicare coverage, this includes the 50 states, District of Columbia, Puerto Rico, Virgin Islands, Guam, Northern Mariana Islands, and America Samoa. Medical services provided on a ship would include the territorial waters that adjoin the land areas of the United States.

United States per capita cost (USPCC) National average fee-for-service dollar amount expense for each Medicare beneficiary that is calculated yearly by the Centers for Medicare and Medicaid Services (CMS) Office of the Actuary.

United States Pharmacopeia (USP) Legally recognized compendium of standards for drugs, published by the United States Pharmacopeia Convention, Inc., and revised periodically. It includes assays and tests for the determination of strength, quality, and purity. Another book that has information not in the USP is the *National Formulary (NF)*. Also see *compendium* and *Homeopathic Pharmacopoeia of the United States.*

United States Public Health Service (USPHS) Federal government agency founded in 1798 that is in charge of the control of all people and immigrants arriving from foreign countries and products that might affect the health of people in America. It sets standards for domestic handling and processing of food and manufacture of serums, vaccines, cosmetics, and drugs. It is the uniformed service of the U.S. Department of Health and Human Services. USPHS-commissioned officers serve their country by controlling the spread of contagious diseases such as smallpox and yellow fever, conducting important biomedical research, regulating the food and drug supply, providing health care to underserved groups, and supplying medical assistance in the aftermath of disasters.

United States Uniformed Services identification cards Insurance card issued to dependents of active duty military members and retirees who are beneficiaries of the TRICARE government program (see Figure U-1). Essential information is included on front and back sides of the card.

universal access Condition of a health benefits system indicating the right of all individuals to receive basic medical services in a health care setting.

universal coverage System of health care in which every citizen of the United States is covered and may receive medical services, even those who cannot pay for coverage. The United Kingdom and Canada have universal coverage. Also called *socialized medicine* and *statutory health insurance.* Also see *national health insurance.*

universal life insurance Type of whole life insurance with flexible premiums, adjustable protection, and company expenses disclosed in the policy to the purchaser. They are separated so that each can be analyzed for premium rates and cash value. Also called *unbundled life insurance.*

universal precautions Protective safety measures used by medical personnel to avoid and minimize infection when exposed to bloodborne pathogens, infectious materials, and viruses.

universal resource locator (URL) String of characters that identifies the location of a document on the Internet (World Wide Web).

unlisted procedure code *Current Procedural Terminology (CPT)* code that identifies and has a description of a procedure that is rarely provided, unusual, variable, or new and for which a code does not appear in the code book. Such a code typically ends in 99. A report or documentation needs to be submitted with the insurance claim form to explain the procedure in more detail when using an unlisted procedure code.

unlisted service See *unlisted procedure code.*

unmarried In a managed care contract, a hospital facility and a managed care plan that work with each other but are not exclusive to each other. Also see *married.*

unpaid balance See *beginning balance.*

unprocessable claim Insurance claim transmitted to an insurance carrier that cannot be processed due to missing, certain incomplete, or incorrect information.

unproved procedures See *experimental procedures.*

unreplaced blood In the Medicare program, a beneficiary who receives blood may either restore the blood or pay the provider's charges for the unrestored blood. Blood is replaced on a pint-for-pint or unit-for-unit basis.

unreported claims See *incurred but not reported (IBNR).*

unrepresented employee In a workers' compensation case, injured worker who is not represented by an attorney.

unsecured debt Obligation (amount owed) that is not secured or backed by any form of collateral.

unspecified See *not otherwise specified (NOS)* and *nonspecific code.*

unusual procedural service Procedure or service that is unique or an atypical finding that affects the patient's treatment. When billing for an unusual procedural service, a -22 modifier is appended to the usual five-digit CPT procedure code when the service provided

U

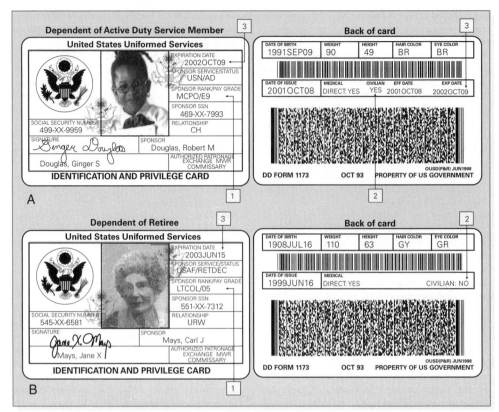

Figure U-1 A, TRICARE Standard active duty dependent's identification card (DD Form 1173) from which essential information must be abstracted. **B,** Sample identification card (DD Form 1173) for a retiree's widowed spouse. Cards indicate *1*, sponsor's status and rank; *2*, authorization status for treatment by a civilian provider; and *3*, expiration date.

is greater than that usually required for the listed procedure.

UP HCPCS Level II modifier that may be used with CPT or HCPCS Level II codes indicating three patients served.

upcode See *upcoding*.

upcoding Deliberate manipulation of *Current Procedural Terminology (CPT)* codes for increased payment by using a code for a higher payment than the code for the service performed (e.g., a podiatrist who performs a simple nail clip service but bills for foot surgery). Under the False Claims Act, providers who are caught upcoding face a civil monetary penalty of $5,000 to $10,000 per service. In addition, the federal government can make an assessment against a provider of up to three times the service claim amount as repayment for a Medicare case. Also called *code creep* or *overcoding*.

update Annual adjustment of the Medicare fee schedule to raise or lower base payment amounts to allow for changes in cost of living by determining the relative values of new and revised procedure codes. See *Medicare economic index (MEI)* and *Medicare Volume Performance Standard (MVPS)*.

UPIN See *unique physician/practitioner identifier number (UPIN)*.

UPPL See *uniform policy provisions (UPP)*.

UQ HCPCS Level II modifier that may be used with CPT or HCPCS Level II codes indicating four patients served.

UR See *utilization review (UR)*.

URAC See *Utilization Review Accreditation Commission (URAC)*.

urgent Inpatient hospital admission category. Patients in this category need to be admitted as soon as a bed is available, within 24 to 48 hours. See *urgent admission*.

urgent admission Inpatient hospital or facility acceptance of a patient who requires immediate medical or psychiatric care because of life-threatening, serious, and possible disabling conditions.

urgent care Medically necessary treatment required for illness or injury that is not a serious threat and would not result in further disability or death if not treated immediately (e.g., ear infection, ear wax removal, small laceration).

urgent care center See *emergency center*. Also see *ambulatory care facility*.

urgent care clinic Health care facility whose primary purpose is to provide immediate, short-term medical care for minor, but urgent, medical conditions.

urgently needed care Medical care a patient receives for a sudden illness or injury that needs care right away but is not life threatening. The patient's primary care doctor generally provides urgently needed care if the patient is in a Medicare health plan other than the Original Medicare Plan. If the patient is out of the plan's service area for a short time and cannot wait until he or she returns home, then the health plan must pay for urgently needed care.

urgi-center See *emergency center*.

URL See *universal resource locator (URL)*.

URO See *utilization review organization (URO)*.

urology Branch of medicine concerned with the study of the anatomy, physiology, disorders, and medical or surgical treatment of the genitourinary tract in men and women and of the male genital tract.

US HCPCS Level II modifier that may be used with CPT or HCPCS Level II codes indicating six or more patients served.

use Under the Health Insurance Portability and Accountability Act (HIPAA), means the sharing, employment, application, utilization, examination, or analysis of individually identifiable health information within an entity that maintains such information.

use additional code Cross-reference phrase used in ICD-9-CM, Volume 1, Tabular List, that follows a main term description indicating that an additional code should be used if the information is available to provide a more complete picture of the diagnosis.

use and disclosure Under the Health Insurance Portability and Accountability Act (HIPAA), disclosure is when a patient's medical information is released to an individual or entity outside of the medical practice's organization and use is when information is shared within the medical office to facilitate patient treatment.

USPCC See *United States per capita cost (USPCC)*.

USPHS See *United States Public Health Service (USPHS)*.

usual, customary, and reasonable (UCR) Method used by insurance companies and managed care plans to establish their fee schedules in which three fees are considered in calculating payment: (1) The usual fee is the fee typically submitted by the physician, (2) the customary fee falls within the range of usual fees charged by providers of similar training in a geographical area, and (3) the reasonable fee meets the aforementioned criteria or is considered justifiable because of special circumstances.

USP See *United States Pharmacopeia*.

Utah Health Information Network Public-private coalition for reducing health care administrative costs through the standardization and electronic exchange of health care data.

utilitarianism Philosophical view or doctrine of ethics that the purpose of all action should be to bring about the greatest happiness for the greatest number of people and that the value of anything is determined by its utility.

utilization Measurement of the frequency that members of a health insurance group use the services or procedures of a particular benefit plan, stated by average number of claims per insured over a specific time period.

Utilization and Quality Control Peer Review Organization (PRO) Program that replaced the Professional Standards Review Organization (PSRO) program. See *Quality Improvement Organization (QIO) program*.

utilization management (UM) Process and procedures implemented to administer the use of health care services in the hospital by evaluating quality of care and establishing appropriateness and medical necessity for services. It ensures maximum medical care resource use and helps reduce health care spending. Examples of UM are preadmission certifications, admission reviews, concurrent reviews, focused reviews, individual case management, discharge planning, retrospective reviews, provider profiling, and second surgical opinions.

utilization or management control See *utilization review (UR)* and *medical review (MR)*.

utilization review (UR) Process, based on established criteria, of evaluating and controlling the medical necessity for services and providers' use of medical care resources. Reviews are carried out by allied health personnel at predetermined times during the hospital stay to assess the need for the full facilities of an acute care hospital. In managed care systems such as an HMO, reviews are done to establish medical necessity and appropriateness or efficiency of health care services, thus curbing costs. UR is also monitored by both insurers and employers. Also called *medical review, continued stay review, utilization*, and *management control*.

Utilization Review Accreditation Commission (URAC) Independent, nonprofit organization established in 1990 that promotes health care quality through its accreditation and certification programs. URAC offers a wide range of quality programs and services that keep pace with the rapid changes in the health care system and provide

U

a symbol of excellence for organizations to validate their commitment to quality and accountability.

utilization review nurse Registered nurse who evaluates medical cases for appropriateness of care and length of service and plans services required after discharge from a health facility.

utilization review organization (URO) 1. In the insurance industry, state association that conducts utilization reviews for property and casualty insurers. 2. In health care, entity that has established one or more utilization review programs, which evaluates the medical necessity, appropriateness, and efficiency of the use of health care services, procedures, and facilities.

utilization summary data Information that is aggregated by the capitated managed care entity (e.g., the number of primary care visits provided by the plan during the calendar year).

V

V codes Numeric designation preceded by the letter "V" that is a subclassification of ICD-9-CM coding known as *The Supplementary Classification of Factors Influencing Health Status and Contact with Health Services (V01-V85)*. For hospital inpatients, V codes are used to identify health care encounters that occur for reasons other than illness or injury and to identify patients whose injury or illness is influenced by special circumstances or problems such as chemotherapy, consultation, renal dialysis, or organ donor. For hospital outpatients, V codes are used to classify patient encounters for treatment of a current or resolving disease or injury. For ancillary diagnostic or therapeutic services, list the V code first followed by the code for the diagnosis that prompted the outpatient encounter.

VA Abbreviation for Veterans Affairs. See *Department of Veterans Affairs (VA)*.

valid Legally binding.

validation Process by which the integrity and correctness of data are established. Validation processes can occur immediately after a data item is collected or after a complete set of data is collected.

valuation mortality table Table showing number of deaths that is used to calculate the legal reserve and life insurance policy cash surrender values. It has wide margins of safety and indicates much higher rates of mortality than the tables that insurance companies use for calculating premiums.

valuation period Period of years that is considered as a unit for purposes of calculating the status of a trust fund.

valuation premium Annual net premium used to calculate reserves by insurance companies (e.g., to describe the generally accepted accounting principles [GAAP] net premium).

value Accepted principle, standard, or quality regarded as worthwhile or desirable.

value added network (VAN) Vendor that facilitates transmission of electronic data interchange (EDI) data communications and translation services among multiple trading partners.

value added tax (VAT) Amount of money levied on the increment of value that is added to a product at each stage of the production process. It is similar to a sales tax and is sometimes referred to as a *consumption tax*.

value codes Two-digit codes that have related dollar amounts that identify monetary data required for processing insurance claims. Value codes represent payments received, laboratory readings, newborn weights, outlier amount, patient liability amount, and other types of data. Value codes are inserted in Fields 39, 40, and 41 of the Uniform Bill (UB-04) inpatient hospital billing claim form.

value health care purchasing Providers and buyers work together and use available information to buy and sell medical care based on cost and outcome (value).

valued contract Life insurance policy in which the amount of the benefit is established in advance.

VAN See *value added network (VAN)*.

vandalism Willful injury, malicious mischief, and deliberate destruction of property (e.g., shooting BBs or tossing stones at window panes of a home, painting grafiti on a homeowner's property, damaging house furnishings).

vandalism insurance Type of insurance coverage that protects an individual against loss and damage to property caused by a willful act.

variable annuity See *annuity*.

variable life insurance Type of whole life insurance in which benefits relate to the value of assets in the investment portfolio of the contract at the time the benefit is paid. Premiums are fixed and there is a minimum death benefit.

variable premium life insurance See *indeterminate premium life insurance*.

variable universal life insurance Type of whole life insurance that combines the premium and death benefit flexibility of universal life insurance with the flexible investment and risk of variable life insurance. Such policies are considered securities contracts and must be registered with the Securities and Exchange Commission (SEC). Agents who have passed the National Association of Securities Dealers (NASD) may sell this type of insurance.

VAT See *value added tax (VAT)*.

VEBA Acronym for Voluntary Employees Beneficiary Association. See *Section 501(c)(9) Voluntary Employees Beneficiary Association (VEBA)*.

vendor Individual or entity that sells and provides hardware, software, and/or ongoing support services for providers to file claims electronically to private insurance carriers, Medicare administrative contractors, and Medicaid fiscal agents.

verbal referral Referral carried out via a telephone call from the primary care physician to the referring physician.

verification See *eligibility verification*.

vertical integration Health care system that includes the entire range of medical services from outpatient to hospital and long-term care. Integrated delivery systems are an example of vertical integration. See *integrated delivery systems (IDS)* and *horizontal integration*.

vertically integrated network (VIN) Alliance of various health care providers whose intention is to service all the needs of managed care contracts.

vested benefit Retirement benefit payment that does not depend on whether a participant continued in specific employment. A plan participant may receive payment if he or she leaves the plan.

vested commissions Renewal insurance commissions paid to insurance agents or their estates regardless of whether the agents stay with the issuing insurance company.

vested reserves Funds (reserves) that remain owned (vested) by the insured and which cannot be used by the insurance company except for paying refunds or claims.

vesting requirements Terms set down in an employment agreement stating the time period and dollar amount when retirement or other benefits will begin and the rate of increase.

veteran Any person who has served in the armed forces of the United States, especially in time of war; is no longer in the service; and has received an honorable discharge.

Veterans Affairs (VA) Disability program Program for honorably discharged veterans who file claim for a service-connected disability.

Veterans Affairs (VA) Outpatient Clinic A clinic where medical and dental services are rendered to veterans who have service-related disabilities.

vicarious liability See *respondeat superior*.

video conferencing Multimedia communications equipment that permits real-time communication between the distant site practitioner (i.e., where the expert physician or practitioner is located at the time the service is provided) and the patient.

video display terminal (VDT) A television-like screen attached to a computer or word processing terminal; also known as a *cathode ray tube (CRT)*.

VIN See *vertically integrated network (VIN)*.

virtual integrated delivery system Method of purchasing group medical practices and linking them together with information technology so that they can exchange clinical and financial data.

virtual private network Technical strategy for creating secure connections or tunnels over the Internet.

virtual visit Online medical advice (electronic mail and live chat) for a patient who is already under the care of a medical provider for treatment of minor ailments and follow-up consultations (e.g., medication questions, colds and influenza, laboratory test results, cough and sore throat, headache and migraine, fever, asthma). Some insurance plans pay doctors for online visits.

virus Destructive program that attaches and copies itself to other programs in a computer system. Some

viruses destroy programs or operating systems and data after a precise lapse of time.

vision care Insurance coverage that provides benefits for preventive and corrective eye care and is usually offered with basic coverage (e.g., surgical and/or medical benefits).

vision examination Inspection of the eye by an optometrist or ophthalmologist that includes the case history, external examination, ophthalmoscopic examination, refractive status, binocular balance testing, glaucoma testing, and prescription for corrective lenses.

visit See *encounter*.

visit crosswalk Cross-reference connection between discontinued CPT codes and new codes that replace them. Also see *crosswalk* and *crosswalking*.

Visiting Nurse Association (VNA) Nonprofit agency serving the community since 1888, committed to the belief that every individual deserves care and support to preserve independence, dignity, and quality of life. VNA dedicates itself to this belief by providing professional and compassionate health care solutions to people touched by disease, disability, or death. Basic services available throughout each state include health supervision, education, and counseling; bedside care; and carrying out physicians' orders. Personnel include nurses and home health aides.

Visiting Nurse Associations of America (VNAA) Official national association created in 1983 for not-for-profit, community-based home health organizations known as *Visiting Nurse Associations (VNAs)*. VNAA's mission is to bring compassionate, high-quality, and cost-effective home care to individuals in their respective communities by promoting community-based home health care through business development, national public imaging, member services, and government advocacy.

visits per 1000 See *days per thousand (DPT)*.

visual integration tools Tools developed for access, extraction, and integration of patient-specific information from disparate clinical information systems and visually presenting it to the user.

vital statistics Collection of information of individuals in regions that relates to births (natality), deaths (mortality), marriages, health, and disease (morbidity). In the United States, these statistics are published by the National Center for Health Statistics.

VNA See *visiting nurse association (VNA)*.

vocational feasibility In workers' compensation cases, phrase used when an employee meets the requirement that he or she is expected to return to gainful employment after undergoing vocational rehabilitation services.

vocational nurse See *licensed practical nurse (LPN)*.

vocational rehabilitation 1. Process of facilitating an individual in the choice of or return to a suitable profession because of permanent or temporary disability.

When necessary, assisting the patient to obtain training for such a career. 2. Preparing an individual regardless of age, status (whether U.S. citizen or immigrant), or physical condition (disability other than end-stage renal disease) to cope emotionally, psychologically, and physically with changing circumstances in life including remaining at school or returning to school, work, or work equivalent (homemaker).

vocational rehabilitation plan In a workers' compensation case, written document that describes the program designed to give assistance in returning the injured workers to the labor market and provides income while a worker completes a course of study such as academic instruction, formal training, on-the-job training, job placement assistance, or self-employment.

voice drug TAR system (VDTS) A Medi-Cal telecommunication system for processing urgent and initial drug treatment authorization requests (TARs), to inquire about the status of previously entered drug TARs, or to inquire whether a patient is receiving continual care with a drug.

voice recognition system See *speech recognition system.*

voidable contract Insurance agreement that is no longer valid because it was canceled by one or more parties (insured or insurance company).

void contract Insurance agreement that is not a valid agreement.

volcanic insurance coverage See *catastrophe insurance policy.*

volume 1. Amount of space taken by a body as stated in cubic units. 2. Number of services, procedures, or tests performed. 3. Number of patients seen in a medical office or hospital facility. 4. Number of patients in a diagnosis-related group (DRG) during a certain period of time.

volume and intensity of services In the Medicare program, quantity of medical services per beneficiary, taking into account the number and complexity of the services provided.

volume behavioral offset Change factor in the volume of services that occurs in reaction to a change in fees. It is used in the annual setting of the Medicare volume performance standard (VPS), resulting in higher annual payments than would otherwise be expected.

volume discount Reduction in premium rate applied to new group insurance coverage based on total case premium for specific coverage or total premium and premium per employee certificate.

volume loading Increase in premium rate applied to new group insurance coverage based on total case premium for specific coverage or total premium and premium per employee certificate.

volume performance standard (VPS) Method for updating and adjusting fees based on annual increase in actual expenditures compared with previously determined VPS rates of increase. It is the desired growth rate for spending on Medicare Part B physician services that is set each year by Congress.

voluntary agreement Contracts between the Centers for Medicare and Medicaid Services (CMS) and various insurers and employers to exchange Medicare information and group health plan eligibility information for the purpose of coordinating health benefit payments.

voluntary controls Measures that providers have agreed to establish to assist in keeping medical costs down.

voluntary disability insurance Self-insured disability insurance plan used in lieu of a state plan, in which a majority of employees voluntarily consent to be covered.

voluntary disclosure protocol Procedure that providers follow to self-disclose claims presented to the government that are asserted to be mistaken or fraudulent. Also referred to as *provider self-disclosure protocol.*

voluntary employees' beneficiary association (VEBA) See *501(c)(9) trust.*

voluntary enrollee Certain individuals aged 65 or older or disabled, who are not otherwise entitled to Medicare and who opt to obtain coverage under Part A by paying a monthly premium.

voluntary plan termination Act of ending a retirement plan with the cancellation initiated by the plan sponsor.

voucher See *check voucher* and *payment voucher.*

VP HCPCS Level II modifier that may be used with CPT or HCPCS Level II codes indicating an aphakic patient.

VPS See *volume performance standard (VPS).*

V

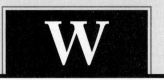

wage earner Individual who earns Social Security credits while working for wages or self-employment income. Also referred to as *number holder* and *worker*.

wage earner's bankruptcy See *Chapter 13 bankruptcy*.

wage loss In a workers' compensation case, the difference between the average weekly wages and the injured worker's actual earnings while he or she is still temporarily partially disabled but is working at modified work or a reduced work schedule.

wage replacement ratio In disability insurance, the percentage of the insured's working wages that a policy will pay, usually 50% to 80% and not 100%.

waiting period (WP) 1. In individual or group health insurance, time between enrollment and the date an individual is eligible for insurance coverage. Usually WPs last from 14 to 30 days after issue of a policy and apply to medical expenses from illness, not from accidents. 2. For a hospital indemnity policy, the time in which benefits may not be paid for the first several days of hospitalization. Elimination periods vary from policy to policy and from company to company. The longer the WP, the lower the cost of insurance. 3. For disability income insurance, the initial period of time when a disabled individual is not eligible to receive benefits even though unable to work. 4. For workers' compensation, the days that must elapse before workers' compensation weekly income benefits become payable. Also called *eligibility waiting period*, *elimination period*, or *probationary period*. 5. Time between when an individual signs up with a Medigap insurance company or Medicare health plan and when the coverage starts. 6. In a group health plan, it is the time that must pass before a new employee becomes eligible for plan benefits. The WP usually begins on the date of hire.

waiver 1. Agreement attached to an insurance contract eliminating a specific preexisting condition or certain hazard from coverage. Also known as *exclusion amendment*, *endorsement*, or *rider*. 2. Exception to the usual requirements of Medicaid in which state Medicaid agencies must apply and receive permission to provide a service not usually covered by Medicaid.

waiver of deductible Provision in a health insurance policy in which the insured does not have to pay the initial deductible if medical expenses result from an accidental injury.

waiver of liability 1. Provision of the Social Security Act, Sections 1842(1) and 1879, that protects the patient from financial liability when Medicare denies or reduces payment for a service or item based on it being considered as 'not reasonable and necessary'; under this provision, the patient may not be required to pay the provider for a service, if certain conditions are met. 2. In the Medicare program, provision that a beneficiary is not responsible to pay for a medical service if he or she was not informed that the service would not be covered by Medicare. Also see *Advance Beneficiary Notice (ABN)*.

waiver of liability agreement See *Advance Beneficiary Notice (ABN)*.

waiver of premium (WP) 1. Provision in an insurance policy that states under certain situations the insured's coverage will continue without further payment of premiums (e.g., occurrence of permanent or total disability or unable to work due to an accident or injury). 2. Disability insurance policy provision that an employee does not have to pay any premiums while disabled. Also known as *elimination period* or *waiver of premium for disability benefit*.

waiver of premium for disability benefit See *waiver of premium (WP)*.

waiver of premium for payer benefit Provision in an insurance policy that states the insurance company will not collect the policy's premiums if the policyholder, not the insured child, dies or becomes disabled. This rider is often seen in juvenile policies.

waiver tests Laboratory tests that are exempt from Clinical Laboratory Improvement Amendments (CLIA) regulations and may be performed by medical assistants who are not certified medical laboratory technicians.

war exclusion clause Provision in a life insurance policy that limits the insurance company's liability to pay a death benefit if the insured's death is associated with war or military service.

warranty Guarantee of a true statement and, if proven to be false, would make an insurance policy void (e.g., insured states he or she has or does not have a specific condition).

Washington Publishing Company Business firm that publishes the *X12N HIPAA Implementation Guides* and the *X12N HIPAA Data Dictionary*. It developed the X12 Data Dictionary. It hosts the Electronic Healthcare Network Accreditation Commission (EHNAC) standard transaction format compliance system (STFCS) testing program.

WC See *workers' compensation (WC)*.

weblogs See *blogs* and *medical blogging*.

WEDI See *Workgroup on Electronic Data Interchange (WEDI)*.

weekly indemnity plan Type of short-term disability income insurance that pays weekly a stated dollar amount or a percentage of the insured's individual's earnings.

weekly treatment management services When a patient is receiving radiation therapy, treatment visits are paid increments of weekly time periods. For example, five sessions (fractions) of radiation therapy comprise a week of service and two radiation treatments in one day equal two fractions. When multiple sites are treated in a session, this is classified as one fraction.

weight (wt) In statistics, awarding more value (weight) to a fee based on the number of times it is billed. This term is used when weighting the resource-based relative value fees for a region.

weighting 1. To assign greater value to a factor or variable. 2. Procedure of giving more value to a fee based on the number of times it is charged such as weighting the resource-based relative value scale (RBRVS) fees for a region.

well-baby care Preventive medical services for an infant to 1 year of age (e.g., immunization, physical examination).

wellness State of health in which a person progresses to a higher level of functioning and achieves optimum physical and mental health. Wellness programs or classes include cholesterol tracking, diet, exercise, smoking cessation, and weight reduction.

wellness programs Community service or health facility programs to reduce health risks, reduce absenteeism, and prevent health problems that include cholesterol tracking, diet, exercise, smoking cessation, and weight reduction.

whistleblower Informant who reports a physician for financial misconduct and may be suspected of defrauding the federal government. Also see *qui tam action* and *qui tam provision*.

whistleblower provision *Qui tam* provision that allows any person having knowledge of a false claim against the U.S. government to bring an action against the suspected wrongdoer on behalf of the federal government. A person who files a *qui tam* suit on behalf of the government is known as a 'relator' and may share a percentage of the recovery realized from a successful action.

WHO See *World Health Organization (WHO)*.

whole life annuity See *annuity*.

whole life insurance Type of life insurance policy that continues during the whole of the insured's life and provides for the payment of amount insured at death or at a specific age. Premiums may be paid for a specific number of years (limited payment life) or for life (straight life). See also *continuous-premium whole life insurance*. Also called *ordinary life insurance, straight life insurance*, or *continuous-premium whole life insurance*.

wholesale life insurance Type of term life insurance for a small group employed by the same company. Each employee applies for, is given a special rate, and owns his or her own policy. Also called *franchise, blanket,* or *employee life plan* or *wholesale plan*.

wholesale plan See *wholesale life insurance*.

wholesaling System of marketing in which an insurance company allows a product to be sold by a third party, which adds its own commission and fees and resells the product to its clients.

wide area network (WAN) Interconnected computers that cover a large geographical area (e.g., America Online).

withdrawal 1. Pertaining to voluntary ending of an insurance agreement by the insured (policyholder). 2. Related to a provider withdrawing from treating a patient.

withdrawal provision Clause in a universal life insurance or annuity policy that allows the policy owner to reduce the amount in the policy's cash value by taking that amount in cash. Also known as *partial surrender provision*.

withhold 1. Portion of the monthly capitation payment to physicians retained by the health maintenance organization (HMO) until the end of the year to create an incentive for efficient care. If the physician exceeds utilization norms, he or she will not receive it. Also called *withhold incentive*. 2. Percentage of payment or set dollar amounts that are deducted from the payment to the physician group/physician that may or may not be returned depending on specific predetermined factors.

withhold fund Account established to cover use of medical services that exceed the managed care plan budget. The funds are given to participating providers when medical services do not exceed the budget.

withhold incentive See *withhold*.

withhold pool Total amount that a health maintenance organization (HMO) retains from the providers' payments until the end of the year. Cost of referrals and medical services that are considered excessive are held back by the HMO.

witness Individual who has personal knowledge of a situation and can give testimony on it in a court of law.

WLC See *supplementary contract with life contingencies (WLC)*.

WOLC See *supplementary contract without life contingencies (WOLC)*.

work capacity evaluation See *functional capacity evaluation (FCE)*.

work conditioning Program that focuses on the restoration of musculoskeletal, cardiovascular, and safe work demand performance for individuals who have suffered an industrial injury. Circuit training and work simulation are included in the program.

W

work force Under the Health Insurance Portability and Accountability Act (HIPAA), this means employees, volunteers, trainees, and other persons under the direct control of a covered entity, whether or not they are paid by the covered entity.

work hardening 1. Individualized program of therapy using simulated or real job duties to build up strength and improve the worker's endurance to be able to work up to 8 hours per day. Sometimes work site modifications are instituted to get the employee back to gainful employment. 2. In a workers' compensation case, program that uses conditioning tasks with real or simulated work activities that are graded to progressively improve the biomechanical, neuromuscular, cardiovascular, metabolic, and psychosocial functioning of the injured worker to maximize the ability to return to work (e.g, in vocational rehabilitation). It incorporates psychomedical counseling, ergonomics, job coaching, and transitional work development.

work practice controls Policies and procedures that reduce the possibility of employee exposure to hazards by changing the manner in which a task is done (e.g., to handwash after removal of gloves, to prohibit mouth pipetting for a laboratory test, to recap needles using the two-handed method).

work rehabilitation Structured and supervised program of physical conditioning, exercise, strengthening, and functional task performance with real and simulated job activities for workers recovering from industrial injuries. Its purpose is to return people back to work and prevent future injury risk.

work restrictions In a workers' compensation case, temporary or permanent prohibitions of certain activities, body positions, motions, exposure and time limitations that have been placed on the injured worker by the treating or consulting physician to expedite recovery from the injury or on a permanent basis because of the effects of the injury. Restrictions can be actual because of inability to perform the activity or prophylactic to prevent further injury. Permanent work restrictions are rated disabilities.

worker See *wage earner.*

workers' compensation (WC) See *workers' compensation (WC) insurance* and *workers' compensation (WC) program.*

workers' compensation agency Federal entity that administers a federal or state workers' compensation law such as workers' compensation commission, industrial commissions, industrial boards, workers' compensation insurance funds, workers' compensation courts, and U.S. Department of Labor. Also referred to as *state compensation board* or *commission.*

Workers' Compensation Appeals Board (WCAB) Board that handles workers' compensation liens and appeals.

workers' compensation carrier 1. Insurance company that writes workers' compensation insurance under state or federal law. 2. State compensation fund where the state administers the workers' compensation program. 3. Beneficiary's employer where the employer is self-insured.

workers' compensation injury See *industrial accident.*

workers' compensation (WC) insurance Formal legal contract that insures an employee against on-the-job injury or illness and provides death benefits to dependents. It pays for medical treatment, physical rehabilitation, permanent disability, and through temporary disability benefits covers lost wages while off the job. Federal and state regulations require that the employer have this coverage and pay the premiums for his or her employees.

workers' compensation (WC) program Federal and state government-mandated system that requires employers to furnish insurance and cash benefits for employees who suffer work-related injuries, illnesses, or death. Employers pay the insurance premiums. workers' compensation insurance does not usually cover agricultural employees, interstate railroad employees, employees of small businesses, domestic employees, casual employees, and self-employed individuals. Also called *workers' comp.*

Workgroup for Electronic Data Interchange (WEDI) 1. Health care industry group that has a formal consultative role under the Health Insurance Portability and Accountability Act (HIPAA) legislation (also sponsors Strategic National Implementation Process [SNIP], a workgroup for electronic data interchange that improves health care through electronic commerce). 2. Policy advisory subgroup of the Accreditation Standards Committee X12 that has been involved in creating electronic data interchange standards for insurance billing transactions. Also see *policy advisory group.*

working aged See *Medicare/employer supplemental insurance.*

World Health Organization (WHO) United Nations specialized agency for health that was established in April 1948. WHO's objective, as set out in its Constitution, is the attainment by all peoples of the highest possible level of health. Health is defined in WHO's Constitution as a state of complete physical, mental, and social well-being and not merely the absence of disease or infirmity. WHO is governed by 192 Member States through the World Health Assembly. The Health Assembly is composed of representatives from WHO's member states. The main tasks of the World Health Assembly are to approve the WHO program and the budget for the following biennium and to decide major policy questions. WHO maintains the International Classification of Diseases (ICD) medical code set.

WP See *waiting period (WP)* and *waiver of premium (WP)*.

wrap-around plan Supplemental health benefit plan that pays for medical costs such as copayments and deductibles not covered by a primary benefit plan such as Medicare or TRICARE. Also called *Medigap (MG) policy, gap fill, Medifill,* and *Medicare supplement policy.*

wrap-around services In the Medicaid program, medical services not usually covered by managed care plans but covered either by referral or direct access to fee-for-service providers.

writ Order issued in writing by a court of law (e.g., subpoena).

writ of mandamus Legal order by a court compelling a regulatory officer (insurance commissioner) to perform a specific act.

write-off 1. Assets or debts that have been determined to be uncollectable and are therefore adjusted off the accounting books as a loss. This does not represent a discount. 2. Difference between the total fee the provider billed for a medical service and the insurance company's allowed fee for the service.

wrongful adoption Misrepresentation or to withhold crucial facts in an adoption case (e.g., withholding medical or mental health history about a child when the parents expect to have a healthy child).

wrongful death Termination of a life caused by a wrongful act, neglect, or fault (liability situation).

W

X

x-ray report See *radiology report*.

X12 American National Standards Institute (ANSI)-accredited group that defines electronic date interchange standards for many American industries including health care insurance. Most of the electronic transaction standards mandated or proposed under Health Insurance Portability and Accountability Act (HIPAA) are X12 standards. Also see *Accredited Standards Committee X12 (ASC X12).*

X12 148 X12 First Report of Injury, Illness or Incident transaction. This standard could eventually be included in the Health Insurance Portability and Accountability Act (HIPAA) mandate.

X12 270 X12 Health Care Eligibility & Benefit Inquiry transaction. Version 4010 of this transaction has been included in the Health Insurance Portability and Accountability Act (HIPAA) mandates.

X12 271 X12 Health Care Eligibility & Benefit Response transaction. Version 4010 of the transaction has been included in the Health Insurance Portability and Accountability Act (HIPAA) mandates.

X12 274 X12 Provider Information transaction.

X12 275 X12 Patient Information transaction. This transaction is expected to be part of the Health Insurance Portability and Accountability Act (HIPAA) claim attachments standard.

X12 276 X12 Health Care Claims Status Inquiry transaction. Version 4010 of this transaction has been included in the Health Insurance Portability and Accountability Act (HIPAA) mandates.

X12 277 X12 HealthCare Claim Status Response transaction. Version 4010 of this transaction has been included in the Health Insurance Portability and Accountability Act (HIPAA) mandates. This transaction is also expected to be part of the HIPAA claim attachments standard.

X12 278 X12 Referral Certification and Authorization transaction. Version 4010 of this transaction has been included in the Health Insurance Portability and Accountability Act (HIPAA) mandates.

X12 811 X12 Consolidated Service Invoice & Statement transaction.

X12 820 X12 Payment Order & Remittance Advice transaction. Version 4010 of this transaction has been included in the Health Insurance Portability and Accountability Act (HIPAA) mandates.

X12 831 X12 Application Control Totals transaction.

X12 834 X12 Benefit Enrollment & Maintenance transaction. Version 4010 of this transaction has been included in the Health Insurance Portability and Accountability Act (HIPAA) mandates.

X12 835 X12 Health Care Claim Payment & Remittance Advice transaction. Version 4010 of this transaction has been included in the Health Insurance Portability and Accountability Act (HIPAA) mandates.

X12 837 X12 Health Care Claim or Encounter transaction. This transaction can be used for institutional, professional, dental, or drug claims. Version 4010 of this transaction has been included in the Health Insurance Portability and Accountability Act (HIPAA) mandates.

X12 997 X12 Functional Acknowledgement transaction.

X12 IHCEBI & IHCEBR X12 Interactive Healthcare Eligibility & Benefits Inquiry (IHCEBI) and Response (IHCEBR) transactions. These are being combined and converted to UN/EDIFACT Version 5 syntax.

X12 IHCLME X12 Interactive Healthcare Claim transaction.

X12 Standard Term currently used for any X12 standard that has been approved since the most recent release of X12 American National Standards. Because a full set of X12 American National Standards is only released about once every 5 years, it is the X12 standards that are most likely to be in active use. These standards were previously called Draft Standards for Trial Use.

X12/PRB X12 Procedures Review Board.

X12F Subcommittee of X12 that defines electronic date interchange standards for the financial industry. This group maintains the X12 811 [generic] Invoice and the X12 820 [generic] Payment & Remittance Advice transactions, although X12N maintains the associated Health Insurance Portability and Accountability Act (HIPAA) implementation guides.

X12J Subcommittee of X12 that reviews X12 work products for compliance with the X12 design rules.

X12N Subcommittee of X12 that defines electronic date interchange (EDI) standards for the insurance industry including health care insurance.

X12N/SPTG4 HIPAA Liaison Special Task Group of the Insurance Subcommittee (N) of X12. This group's responsibilities have been assumed by X12N/TG3/WG3.

X12N/TG1 Property & Casualty Task Group (TG1) of the Insurance Subcommittee (N) of X12.

X12N/TG2 Health Care Task Group (TG2) of the Insurance Subcommittee (N) of X12.

X12N/TG2/WG1 Health Care Eligibility Work Group (WG1) of the Health Care Task Group (TG2) of the Insurance Subcommittee (N) of X12. This group maintains the X12 270 Health Care Eligibility & Benefit Inquiry and the X12 271 Health Care Eligibility & Benefit Response transactions. It is also responsible for maintaining the Interactive Healthcare Eligibility & Benefits Inquiry (IHCEBI) and Response (IHCEBR) transactions.

X12N/TG2/WG10 Health Care Services Review Work Group (WG10) of the Health Care Task Group (TG2) of the Insurance Subcommittee (N) of X12. This group maintains the X12 278 Referral Certification and Authorization transaction.

X12N/TG2/WG12 Interactive Health Care Claims Work Group (WG12) of the Health Care Task Group (TG2) of the Insurance Subcommittee (N) of X12. This group maintains the IHCLME Interactive Claims transaction.

X12N/TG2/WG15 Health Care Provider Information Work Group (WG15) of the Health Care Task Group (TG2) of the Insurance Subcommittee (N) of X12. This group maintains the X12 274 Provider Information transaction.

X12N/TG2/WG19 Health Care Implementation Coordination Work Group (WG19) of the Health Care Task Group (TG2) of the Insurance Subcommittee (N) of X12. This is now X12N/TG3/WG3.

X12N/TG2/WG2 Health Care Claims Work Group (WG2) of the Health Care Task Group (TG2) of the Insurance Subcommittee (N) of X12. This group maintains the X12 837 Health Care Claim or Encounter transaction.

X12N/TG2/WG3 Health Care Claim Payments Work Group (WG3) of the Health Care Task Group (TG2) of the Insurance Subcommittee (N) of X12. This group maintains the X12 835 Health Care Claim Payment & Remittance Advice transaction.

X12N/TG2/WG4 Health Care Enrollments Work Group (WG4) of the Health Care Task Group (TG2) of the Insurance Subcommittee (N) of X12. This group maintains the X12 834 Benefit Enrollment & Maintenance transaction.

X12N/TG2/WG5 Health Care Claims Status Work Group (WG5) of the Health Care Task Group (TG2) of the Insurance Subcommittee (N) of X12. This group maintains the X12 276 Health Care Claims Status Inquiry and the X12 277 Health Care Claim Status Response transactions.

X12N/TG2/WG9 Health Care Patient Information Work Group (WG9) of the Health Care Task Group (TG2) of the Insurance Subcommittee (N) of X12. This group maintains the X12 275 Patient Information transaction.

X12N/TG3 Business Transaction Coordination and Modeling Task Group (TG3) of the Insurance Subcommittee (N) of X12. TG3 maintains the X12N Business and Data Models and the HIPAA Dictionary. This was formerly X12N/TG2/WG11.

X12N/TG3/WG1 Property & Casualty Work Group (WG1) of the Business Transaction Coordination and Modeling Task Group (TG3) of the Insurance Subcommittee (N) of X12.

X12N/TG3/WG2 Healthcare Business & Information Modeling Work Group (WG2) of the Business Transaction Coordination and Modeling Task Group (TG3) of the Insurance Subcommittee (N) of X12.

X12N/TG3/WG3 HIPAA Implementation Coordination Work Group (WG3) of the Business Transaction Coordination and Modeling Task Group (TG3) of the Insurance Subcommittee (N) of X12. This was formerly X12N/TG2/WG19 and X12N/SPTG4.

X12N/TG3/WG4 Object-oriented Modeling and XML Liaison Work Group (WG4) of the Business Transaction Coordination and Modeling Task Group (TG3) of the Insurance Subcommittee (N) of X12.

X12N/TG4 Implementation Guide Task Group (TG4) of the Insurance Subcommittee (N) of X12. This group supports the development and maintenance of X12 Implementation Guides including the Health Insurance Portability and Accountability Act (HIPAA) X12 IGs.

X12N/TG8 Architecture Task Group (TG8) of the Insurance Subcommittee (N) of X12.

X

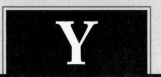

year Twelve months that a health insurance policy is in force.

year of exhaustion First year in which a trust fund is unable to pay benefits when due because the assets of the fund are exhausted.

year of service Defined by Employee Retirement Income Security Act (ERISA), a 12-month period during which an employee completes 1000 hours of service to the employer.

yearly renewable term (YRT) insurance Type of term life insurance in which the policy owner may continue the coverage at the end of each year. This arrangement continues either for a specified number of years or until the insured attains a specific age. Also called *annually renewable term (ART) insurance*.

years of service Length of employment of an individual that is used to determine eligibility, vesting, and benefits for employees in retirement plans. Sometimes years of service must be continuous.

yo-yoing Calling patients back for repeated and unnecessary follow-up visits.

YRT See *yearly renewable term (YRT) insurance*.

Z

ZBA See *zero-balance account (ZBA)*.

ZEBRA See *zero balanced reimbursement account (ZEBRA)*.

zero-balance account (ZBA) See *deposit-only bank account*.

zero balanced reimbursement account (ZEBRA) Type of health benefit plan used by self-insured employers that pays for medical services as they are received by the employee.

zero premium plan Type of insurance in which there is no additional health plan premium above the monthly Medicare Part B premium for an enrollee. Plans may include health maintenance organizations (HMOs), fee-for-service plans, preferred provider organizations (PPOs), point-of-service (POS) plans, provider-sponsored organizations (PSOs), religious fraternal benefit society plans (RFPs), and Medicare medical savings accounts (MSAs). Also see *Medicare Part C* and *Medicare Plus (+) Choice (M+C) plan*.

zone 1 Surgical field on the palm side of the hand indicating from the distal interphalangeal crease to the ends of each digit.

zone 2 Surgical field on the palm side of the hand from the crease in the wrist to the distal interphalangeal crease in the finger. Also referred to as "no man's land."

zone system Method developed by the National Association of Insurance Commissioners (NAIC) to examine the solvency of insurers. The examination is conducted every 3 years by teams of examiners. These teams are formed by four geographical areas. Results of NAIC examinations are usually accepted by states where insurers are licensed so that each state does not have to conduct its own examinations.

zoonosis Diseases and infections that are naturally transmitted between vertebrates and humans (e.g., anthrax, bovine spongiform encephalitis [mad cow disease], brucellosis, Q fever, Lyme disease, plague, psittacosis (parrot fever), rabies). Several of these diseases that are caused by prions, viruses, bacteria, fungi, protozoa, and helminths (worms) are spread by aerosols or ticks together with many related invertebrate animals known as *arthropods*.

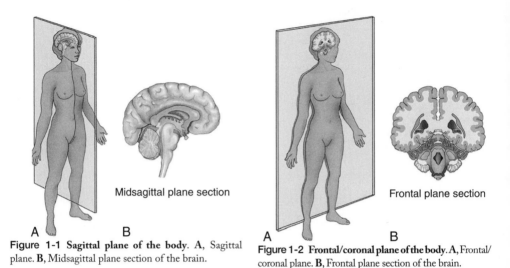

Midsagittal plane section

Frontal plane section

A   B
Figure 1-1 Sagittal plane of the body. A, Sagittal plane. **B,** Midsagittal plane section of the brain.

A   B
Figure 1-2 Frontal/coronal plane of the body. A, Frontal/coronal plane. **B,** Frontal plane section of the brain.

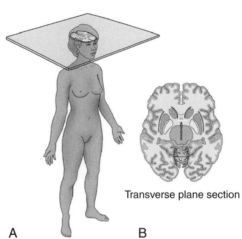

Transverse plane section

A   B
Figure 1-3 Transverse plane of the body. A, Transverse plane. **B,** Transverse plane section of the brain.

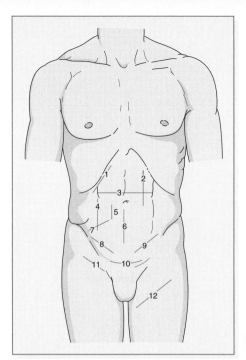

Figure 1-4 Operational incisions. Anterior (front) view: *1*, subcostal incicion; *2*, paramedian incision; *3*, tranverse incision; *4*, upper right rectus incision; *5*, midrectus incision; *6*, midline incision; *7*, lower right rectus incision; *8*, McBurney or right iliac incision; *9*, left iliac incision; *10*, suprapubic incision; *11*, hernia incision; *12*, femoral incision.

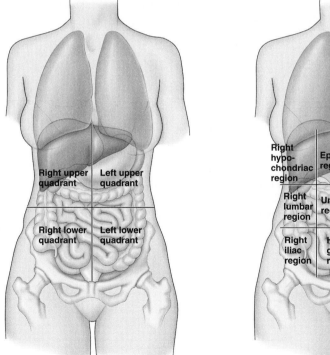

Figure 1-5 Quadrants of the abdomen.

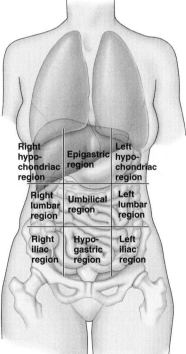

Figure 1-6 Regions of the abdomen.

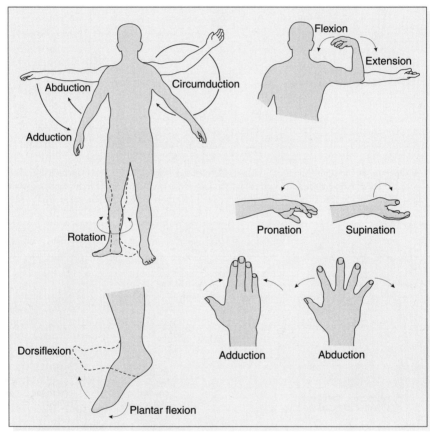

Figure 1-7 Directional terms.

Anterior (anter/o),
Ventral (ventr/o)
Front or belly side

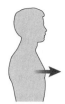

Posterior (poster/o),
Dorsal (dors/o)
Back of body

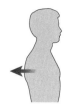

Superior (super/o),
Cephalad (cephal/o)
Toward the head, up

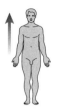

Inferior (infer/o),
Caudad (caud/o)
Toward the tail, down

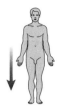

Medial (medi/o)
Toward the midline

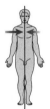

Lateral (later/o)
Toward the side

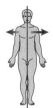

Ipsilateral (ipsi-)
On the same side
Unilateral (uni-)
On one side
Superficial
Toward the surface
Proximal (proxim/o)
Close or nearer to the
    point of attachment/
    origin

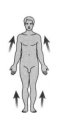

Contralateral (contra-)
On the opposite side
Bilateral (bi-)
On two (both) sides
Deep
Away from the surface
Distal (dist/o)
Far or farther from the
    point of attachment/
    origin

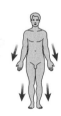

Supine
Lying on one's
    back
Supinate
Turn the palm upward
Palmar
Pertaining to the palm of the hand
Dextrad (dextr/o)
To the right
Afferent
Toward an organ

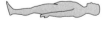

Prone
Lying on one's
    belly
Pronate
Turn the palm downward
Plantar
Pertaining to the sole of the foot
Sinistrad (sinistr/o, levo-)
To the left
Efferent
Away from an organ

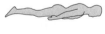

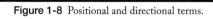

Figure 1-8 Positional and directional terms.

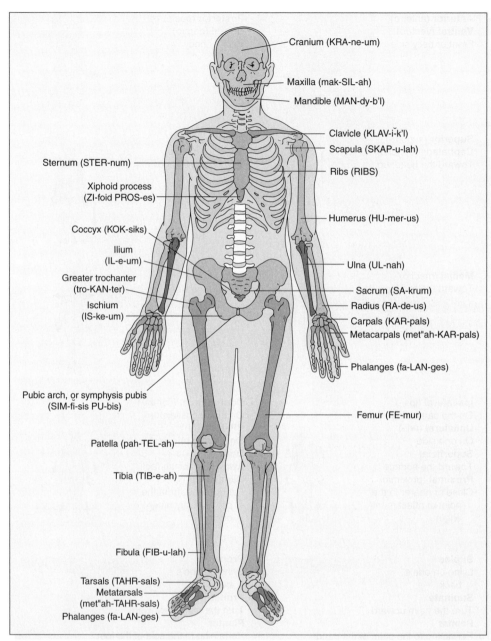

Figure 1-9 The skeleton (anterior view). Terminology pertinent to the skeletal anatomy commonly used in reports on injury cases.

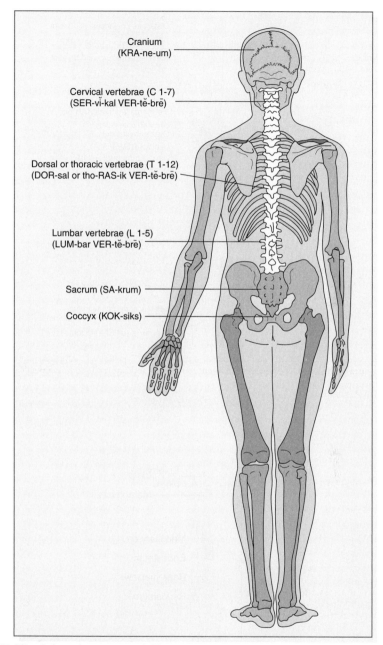

Figure 1-10 The skeleton (posterior view). Terminology pertinent to the skeletal anatomy commonly used in reports on injury cases.

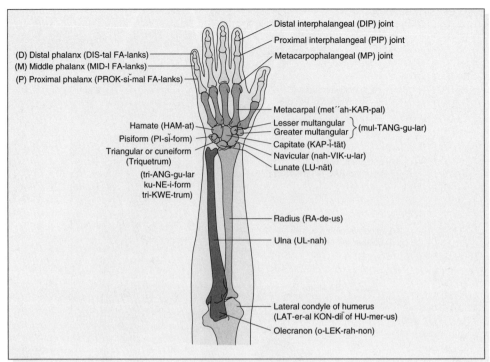

Figure 1-11 Bones of the hand. Terminology pertinent to the hand indicating the common medical terms seen in reports on injury cases.

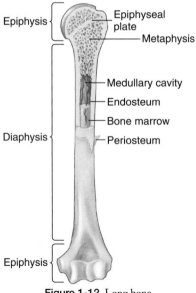

Figure 1-12 Long bone.

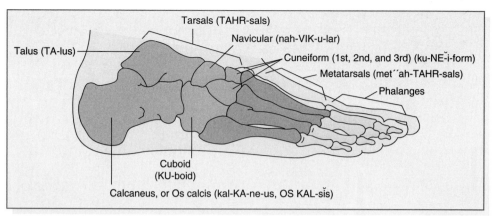

Figure 1-13 Bones of the foot. Terminology pertinent to the foot indicating the common medical terms seen in reports on injury cases.

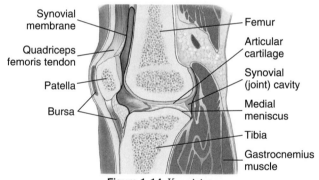

Figure 1-14 Knee joint.

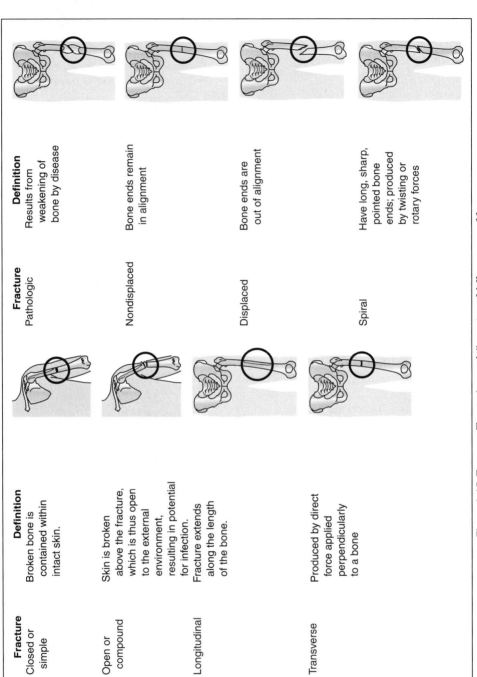

Figure 1-15 Fractures. Terminology and illustration of different types of fractures.

Oblique — Produced by a twisting force with an upward thrust; fracture ends are short and run at an oblique angle across the bone

Greenstick — Produced by compression or angulation forces in long bones of children younger than 10. Bone is cracked on one side and intact on the other due to softness.

Comminuted — Has multiple fragments and is produced by severe direct violence

Impacted — Produced by strong forces that drive bone fragments firmly together

Compression — Produced by transmitted forces that drive bones together

Avulsion — Produced by forceful contraction of a muscle against resistance, with a bone fragment tearing at the site of muscle insertion

Depression — Bone fragments of the skull are driven inward.

Figure 1-15, cont'd

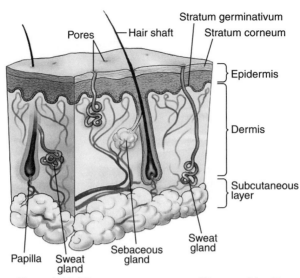

Figure 1-16 **The integumentary system**. Diagram of the skin.

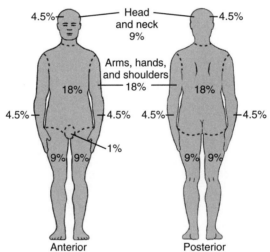

Figure 1-17 **Estimation of total body surface area (TBSA)**. Rule of nines estimating extent of burns.

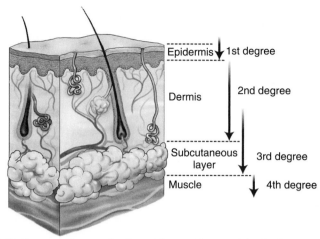

Figure 1-18 **Degrees of burn to skin layers**. Degree of burns and depth of tissue involvement.

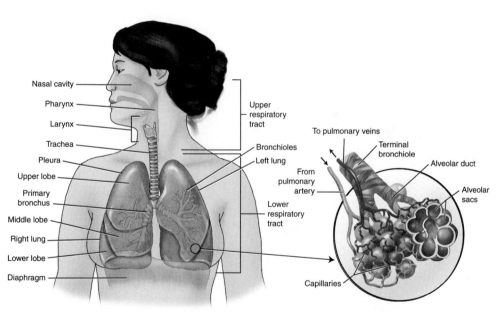

Figure 1-19 **The respiratory system**. The respiratory systems showing a bronchial tree *(insert)*.

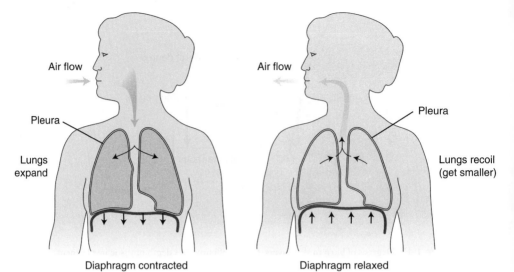

Diaphragm contracted   Diaphragm relaxed

Figure 1-20 Inspiration and expiration.

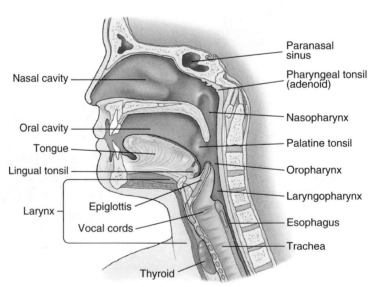

Figure 1-21 The upper respiratory system.

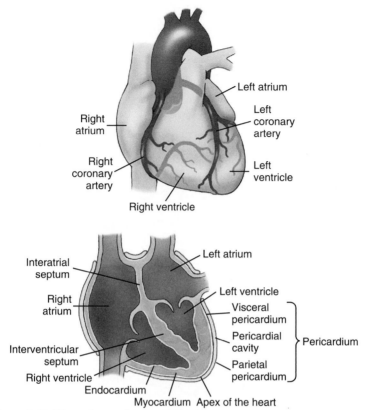

Figure 1-22 **The cardiovascular system**. *Top*, Coronary arteries. *Bottom*, Heart chambers.

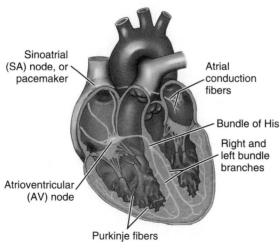

Figure 1-23 Electrical conduction pathways of the heart.

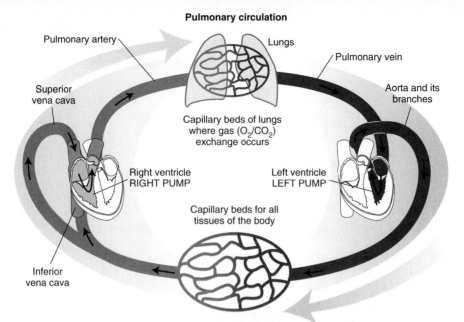

Pulmonary circulation

Pulmonary artery

Lungs

Pulmonary vein

Superior vena cava

Aorta and its branches

Capillary beds of lungs where gas (O_2/CO_2) exchange occurs

Right ventricle RIGHT PUMP

Left ventricle LEFT PUMP

Capillary beds for all tissues of the body

Inferior vena cava

Systemic circulation

Figure 1-24 Pulmonary and systemic circulation.

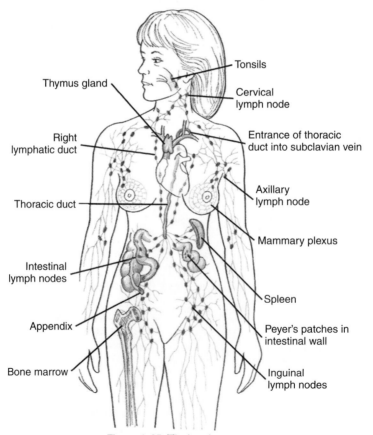

Thymus gland

Tonsils

Cervical lymph node

Right lymphatic duct

Entrance of thoracic duct into subclavian vein

Thoracic duct

Axillary lymph node

Mammary plexus

Intestinal lymph nodes

Spleen

Appendix

Peyer's patches in intestinal wall

Bone marrow

Inguinal lymph nodes

Figure 1-25 The lymphatic system.

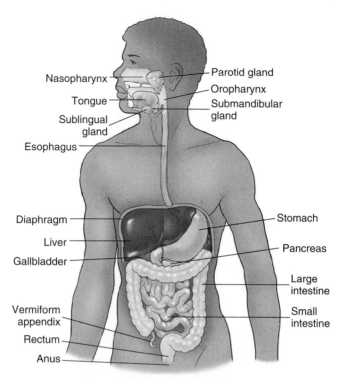

Nasopharynx
Tongue
Sublingual gland
Esophagus
Parotid gland
Oropharynx
Submandibular gland

Diaphragm
Liver
Gallbladder
Stomach
Pancreas
Large intestine
Small intestine

Vermiform appendix
Rectum
Anus

Figure 1-26 The gastrointestinal system.

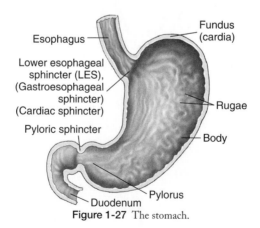

Esophagus
Lower esophageal sphincter (LES), (Gastroesophageal sphincter) (Cardiac sphincter)
Pyloric sphincter
Fundus (cardia)
Rugae
Body
Duodenum
Pylorus

Figure 1-27 The stomach.

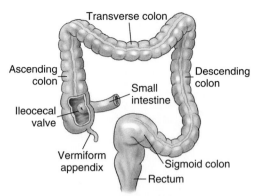

Figure 1-28 The large intestine.

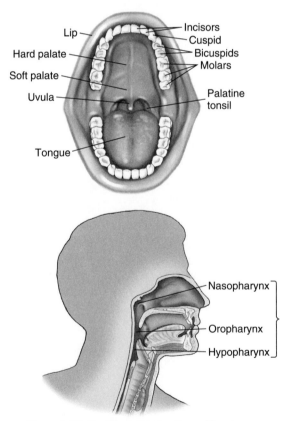

Figure 1-29 *Top*, The oral cavity. *Bottom*, The pharynx.

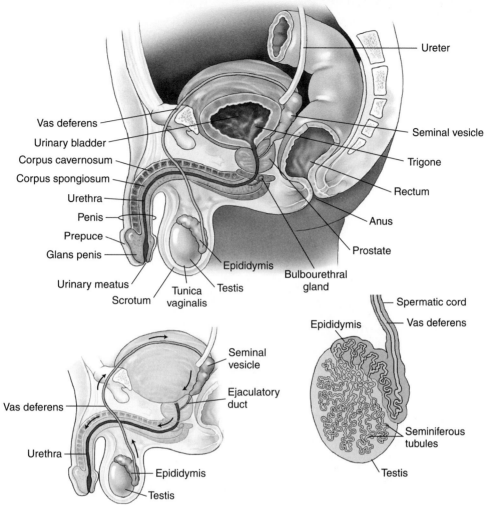

Figure 1-30 The urinary system, male genital system. Male reproductive system with inset of sperm production.

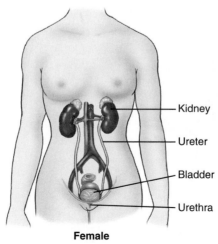

Female
Figure 1-31 The female urinary system.

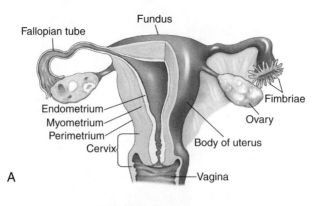

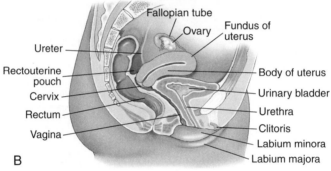

Figure 1-32 **The female genital system**. Female reproductive organs. **A**, Front view. **B**, Sagittal view.

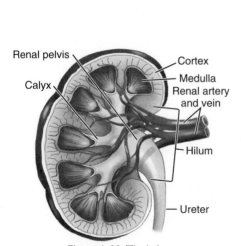

Figure 1-33 The kidney.

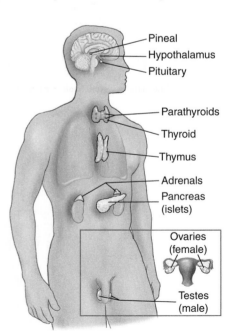

Figure 1-34 **The endocrine system**. Location of the endocrine glands.

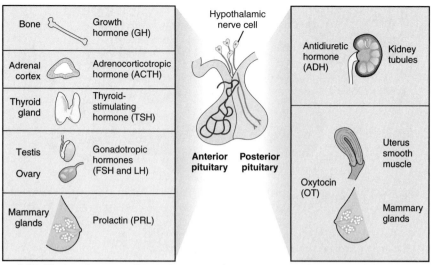

Figure 1-35 **Pituitary hormones**. Principal anterior and posterior pituitary hormones and their target organs.

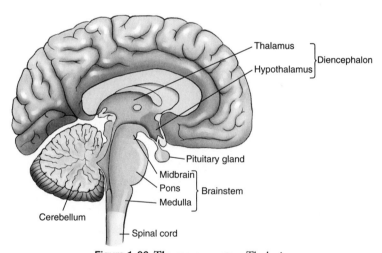

Figure 1-36 **The nervous system**. The brain.

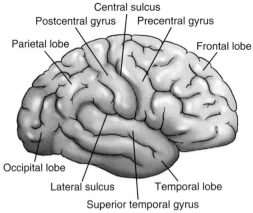

Figure 1-37 The cerebrum.

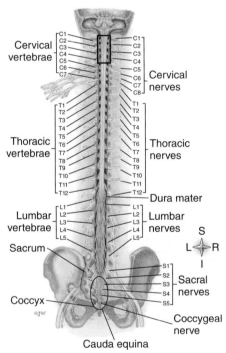

Figure 1-38 The spinal cord.

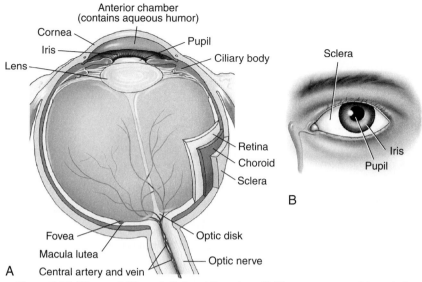

Figure 1-39 **The eye. A,** The eyeball viewed from above. **B,** The anterior view of the eyeball.

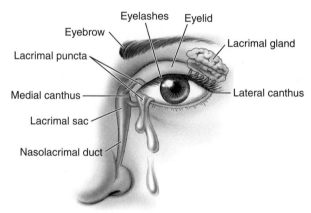

Figure 1-40 Ocular adnexa.

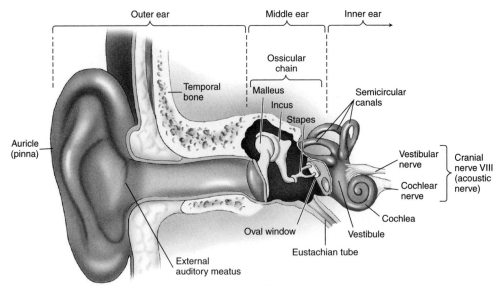

Figure 1-41 The ear.

Appendix 2
Professional Associations

Alliance of Claims Assistance Professionals (ACAP)
25500 Hawthorne Blvd., Suite 1158
Torrance, CA 90505
(888) 394-5163
Website: www.claims.org
E-mail address: askacap@charter.net

American Academy of Professional Coders (AAPC)
2480 South 3850 West, Suite B
Salt Lake City, UT 84120
(800) 626-CODE
Website: www.aapc.com
E-mail address: info@aapc.com

**American Association of Healthcare Administrative
Management (AAHAM)**
National Certification Examination Program
11240 Waples Mill Road, Suite 200
Fairfax, VA 22030
(703) 281-4043
Website: www.aaham.org
E-mail address: moayad@aaham.org

American Association of Medical Assistants (AAMA)
20 North Wacker Drive
Chicago, IL 60606
(800) 228-2262
Website: www.aama-ntl.org
E-mail address: visit website

**American College of Medical Coding Specialists
(ACMCS)**
1540 South Coast Highway, Suite 203
Laguna Beach, CA 92651
(800) 946-9402
Website: www.acmcs.org
E-mail address: info@acmcs.org

**American Health Information Management
Association (AHIMA)**
233 N. Michigan Ave., Suite 2150
Chicago, IL 60601-5800
(800) 335-5535
Website: www.ahima.org
E-mail address: info@ahima.org

American Hospital Association (AHA)
One North Franklin
Chicago, IL 60606-3421
(312) 422-3000
Website: www.aha.org
E-mail address: visit website

**American Institute of Professional Bookkeepers
(AIPB)**
6001 Montrose Road, Suite 500
Rockville, MD 20852
(800) 622-0121
Website: www.aipb.org
E-mail address: info@aipb.org

American Medical Association (AMA)
515 North State Street
Chicago, IL 60610
(800) 621-8335
Website: www.ama-assn.org
E-mail address: msc-AmerMedAssn@ama-assn.org

**American Medical Billing Association
(AMBA)**
4297 Forest Drive
Sulphur, OK 73086
(580) 622-2624
Website: www.ambanet.net/cmrs.htm
E-mail address: larry@brightok.net

American Medical Technologists (AMT)
10700 West Higgins Road, Suite 150
Rosemont, IL 60018
(800) 275-1268
Website: www.amt1.com
E-mail address: amtmail@aol.com

**Association for Healthcare Documentation Integrity
(AHDI)**
4230 Kiernan Avenue, Suite 130
Modesto, CA 95356
(800) 982-2182
Website: www.ahdionline.org
E-mail address: ahdi@ahdionline.org

Association of Registered Healthcare Professionals (ARHP)
11405 Old Roswell Road
Alpharetta, GA 30004
(888) 664-7364
Website: www.arhcp.org
E-mail address: contactus@arhc.org

Board of Medical Specialty Coding (BMSC)
P.O. Box 9402
Gaithersburg, MD 20898-9402
(800) 897-4509
Website: www.advancedmedicalcoding.com
E-mail address: info@medicalspecialtycoding.com

Health Care Compliance Association (HCCA)
6500 Barrie Road, Suite 250
Minneapolis, MN 55435
(888) 580-8373
Website: www.hcca-info.org
E-mail address: info@hcca-info.org

Healthcare Billing and Management Association (HBMA)
1540 South Coast Highway, Suite 203
Laguna Beach, CA 92651
(877) 640-4262
Website: www.hbma.com
E-mail address: info@hbma.com

Healthcare Financial Management Association (HFMA)
2 Westbrook Corporate Center, Suite 700
Westchester, IL 60154-5700
(800) 252-4362
Website: www.hfma.org
E-mail address: webmaster@hfma.com

International Association of Administrative Professionals (IAAP)
10502 NW Ambassador Drive
P. O. Box 20404
Kansas City, MO 64195-0404
(816) 891-6600
Website: www.iaap-hq.org
E-mail address: service@iaap-hq.org

International Information Systems Security Certifications Consortium, Inc. ([ISC]²)
2494 Bayshore Blvd., Suite 201
Dunedin, FL 34698
(888) 333-4458
Website: www.isc2.org
E-mail address: Isc2@asestores.com

Medical Association of Billers (MAB)
2441 Tech Center Court, Suite 111
Las Vegas, NV 89128
(702) 240-8519
Website: www.physicianswebsites.com
E-mail address: mabhelp@aol.com

Medical Group Management Association (MGMA)
American College of Medical Practice Executives (affiliate)
104 Inverness Terrace East
Englewood, CO 80112-5306
(877) 275-6462
Website: www.mgma.com
E-mail address: acmpe@mgma.com

Medical Management Institute (MMI) (a Contexo Media company)
P.O. Box 25128
Salt Lake City, UT 84125-0128
(800) 334-5724
Website: www.codingbooks.com
E-mail address: dan.mistretta@archp.org

National Center for Competency Testing (NCCT)
7007 College Blvd., Suite 705
Overland Park, KS 66211
(800) 875-4404
Website: www.ncctinc.com
E-mail address: staff@ncctinc.com

National Electronic Biller's Alliance (NEBA)
2226-A Westborough Blvd. #504, South
San Francisco, CA 94080
(650) 359-4419
Website: www.nebazone.com
E-mail address: mmedical@aol.com

National Healthcare Association (NHA)
7 Ridgedale Ave., Suite 203
Cedar Knolls, NJ 07927
(800) 499-9092
Website: www.nhanow.com
E-mail address: info@nhanow.com

Practice Management Institute (PMI)
9501 Console Drive, Suite 100
San Antonio, TX 78229
(800) 259-5562
Website: www.pmiMD.com
E-mail address: info@pmimd.com

Professional Association of Health Care Office Management (PAHCOM)
4700 Lake Avenue
Greenview, IL 60025
(800) 451-9311
Website: www.pahcom.com
E-mail address: pahcom@pahcom.com

Professional Association of Healthcare Coding Specialists (PAHCS)
218 E. Bearss Ave., #354
Tampa, FL 34613
(888) 708-4707
Website: www.pahcs.org
E-mail address: info@pahcs.org

Utilization Review Accreditation Commission (URAC)
1220 L Street, NW, Suite 400
Washington, DC 20005
(202) 216-9010
Website: www.urac.org
E-mail address: ita@urac.org

Credits

Figure A-1 Modified from the American Physical Therapy Association: *Medicare administrative contractor (MAC) jurisdictions fact sheet: June 2007*. Available at: http://www.apta.org/AM/Template.cfm?Section=Content_Folders&TEMPLATE=/CM/ContentDisplay.cfm&CONTENTID=41603. Accessed February 9, 2009.

Box A-1 From Fordney MT: *Insurance handbook for the medical office*, ed 10, St Louis, 2008, Saunders.

Box A-2 From Fordney MT: *Insurance handbook for the medical office*, ed 10, St Louis, 2008, Saunders.

Figure C-1 From Fordney MT: *Insurance handbook for the medical office*, ed 10, St Louis, 2008, Saunders.

Figure C-2 From the Iowa Medical Society, IMS Services, West Des Moines, Iowa, 1998.

Box C-1 From Fordney MT: *Insurance handbook for the medical office*, ed 10, St Louis, 2008, Saunders.

Table D-1 From Fordney MT: *Insurance handbook for the medical office*, ed 10, St Louis, 2008, Saunders.

Table E-1 From Fordney MT: *Insurance handbook for the medical office*, ed 10, St Louis, 2008, Saunders.

Figure H-1 From Fordney MT: *Insurance handbook for the medical office*, ed 10, St Louis, 2008, Saunders.

Box H-1 From Fordney MT: *Insurance handbook for the medical office*, ed 10, St Louis, 2008, Saunders.

Box H-2 From Fordney MT: *Insurance handbook for the medical office*, ed 10, St Louis, 2008, Saunders.

Box H-3 From Fordney MT: *Insurance handbook for the medical office*, ed 10, St Louis, 2008, Saunders.

Figure I-1 From Fordney MT: *Insurance handbook for the medical office*, ed 10, St Louis, 2008, Saunders.

Figure M-1 From Fordney MT: *Insurance handbook for the medical office*, ed 10, St Louis, 2008, Saunders.

Figure M-2 From Fordney MT: *Insurance handbook for the medical office*, ed 10, St Louis, 2008, Saunders.

Box M-1 From Fordney MT: *Insurance handbook for the medical office*, ed 10, St Louis, 2008, Saunders.

Figure N-1 From Fordney MT: *Insurance handbook for the medical office*, ed 10, St Louis, 2008, Saunders.

Box P-1 From Fordney MT: *Insurance handbook for the medical office*, ed 10, St Louis, 2008, Saunders.

Figure R-1 From Fordney MT: *Insurance handbook for the medical office*, ed 10, St Louis, 2008, Saunders.

Figure R-2 From Fordney MT: *Insurance handbook for the medical office*, ed 10, St Louis, 2008, Saunders.

Figure S-1 From Fordney MT: *Insurance handbook for the medical office*, ed 10, St Louis, 2008, Saunders.

Figure T-1 From Fordney MT: *Insurance handbook for the medical office*, ed 10, St Louis, 2008, Saunders.

Table T-1 From Fordney MT: *Insurance handbook for the medical office*, ed 10, St Louis, 2008, Saunders.

Figure U-1 From Fordney MT: *Insurance handbook for the medical office*, ed 10, St Louis, 2008, Saunders.

Figure 1-1 From Shiland B: *Mastering healthcare terminology*, ed 2, St Louis, 2006, Mosby.

Figure 1-2 From Shiland B: *Mastering healthcare terminology*, ed 2, St Louis, 2006, Mosby.

Figure 1-3 From Shiland B: *Mastering healthcare terminology*, ed 2, St Louis, 2006, Mosby.

Figure 1-4 From Fordney MT: Insurance handbook for the medical office, ed 10, St Louis, 2008, Saunders.

Figure 1-5 Herlihy B: *The human body in health and illness*, ed 3, St Louis, 2007, Saunders.

Figure 1-6 Herlihy B: *The human body in health and illness*, ed 3, St Louis, 2007, Saunders.

Figure 1-7 Sloane S, Fordney MT: *Saunders manual of medical transcription*, Philadelphia, 1994, Saunders.

Figure 1-8 From Shiland B: *Mastering healthcare terminology*, ed 2, St Louis, 2006, Mosby.

Figure 1-9 From Fordney MT: *Insurance handbook for the medical office*, ed 10, St Louis, 2008, Saunders.

Figure 1-10 From Fordney MT: *Insurance handbook for the medical office*, ed 10, St Louis, 2008, Saunders.

Figure 1-11 Redrawn from Marble HC: *The hand: a manual and atlas for the general surgeon*, Philadelphia, 1960, Saunders.

Figure 1-12 From Shiland B: *Mastering healthcare terminology*, ed 2, St Louis, 2006, Mosby.

Figure 1-13 Redrawn from Chabner D-E: *The language of medicine*, ed 8, St Louis, 2007, Saunders.

Figure 1-14 From Shiland B: *Mastering healthcare terminology*, ed 2, St Louis, 2006, Mosby.

Figure 1-15 From Chester GA: *Modern medical assisting*, Philadelphia, 1998, Saunders.

Figure 1-16 From Shiland B: *Mastering healthcare terminology*, ed 2, St Louis, 2006, Mosby.

Figure 1-17 From Shiland B: *Mastering healthcare terminology*, ed 2, St Louis, 2006, Mosby.

Figure 1-18 From Shiland B: *Mastering healthcare terminology*, ed 2, St Louis, 2006, Mosby.

Figure 1-19 From Shiland B: *Mastering healthcare terminology*, ed 2, St Louis, 2006, Mosby.

Figure 1-20 From Shiland B: *Mastering healthcare terminology*, ed 2, St Louis, 2006, Mosby.

Figure 1-21 From Shiland B: *Mastering healthcare terminology*, ed 2, St Louis, 2006, Mosby.

Figure 1-22 From Shiland B: *Mastering healthcare terminology*, ed 2, St Louis, 2006, Mosby.

Figure 1-23 From Shiland B: *Mastering healthcare terminology*, ed 2, St Louis, 2006, Mosby.

Figure 1-24 From Shiland B: *Mastering healthcare terminology*, ed 2, St Louis, 2006, Mosby.

Figure 1-25 From Shiland B: *Mastering healthcare terminology*, ed 2, St Louis, 2006, Mosby.

Figure 1-26 From Shiland B: *Mastering healthcare terminology*, ed 2, St Louis, 2006, Mosby.

Figure 1-27 From Shiland B: *Mastering healthcare terminology*, ed 2, St Louis, 2006, Mosby.

Figure 1-28 From Shiland B: *Mastering healthcare terminology*, ed 2, St Louis, 2006, Mosby.

Figure 1-29 From Shiland B: *Mastering healthcare terminology*, ed 2, St Louis, 2006, Mosby.

Figure 1-30 From Shiland B: *Mastering healthcare terminology*, ed 2, St Louis, 2006, Mosby.

Figure 1-31 From Shiland B: *Mastering healthcare terminology*, ed 2, St Louis, 2006, Mosby.

Figure 1-32 From Shiland B: *Mastering healthcare terminology*, ed 2, St Louis, 2006, Mosby.

Figure 1-33 From Shiland B: *Mastering healthcare terminology*, ed 2, St Louis, 2006, Mosby.

Figure 1-34 From Shiland B: *Mastering healthcare terminology*, ed 2, St Louis, 2006, Mosby.

Figure 1-35 From Shiland B: *Mastering healthcare terminology*, ed 2, St Louis, 2006, Mosby.

Figure 1-36 From Shiland B: *Mastering healthcare erminology*, ed 2, St Louis, 2006, Mosby.

Figure 1-37 From Shiland B: *Mastering healthcare terminology*, ed 2, St Louis, 2006, Mosby.

Figure 1-38 From Shiland B: *Mastering healthcare terminology*, ed 2, St Louis, 2006, Mosby.

Figure 1-39 From Shiland B: *Mastering healthcare terminology*, ed 2, St Louis, 2006, Mosby.

Figure 1-40 From Shiland B: *Mastering healthcare terminology*, ed 2, St Louis, 2006, Mosby.

Figure 1-41 From Shiland B: *Mastering healthcare terminology*, ed 2, St Louis, 2006, Mosby.